Catheter-Related Infections

Second Edition,
Revised and Expanded

INFECTIOUS DISEASE AND THERAPY

Series Editor

Burke A. Cunha

*Winthrop-University Hospital
Mineola, and
State University of New York School of Medicine
Stony Brook, New York*

1. Parasitic Infections in the Compromised Host,
   edited by Peter D. Walzer and Robert M. Genta
2. Nucleic Acid and Monoclonal Antibody Probes:
   Applications in Diagnostic Methodology,
   edited by Bala Swaminathan and Gyan Prakash
3. Opportunistic Infections in Patients with the Acquired
   Immunodeficiency Syndrome,
   edited by Gifford Leoung and John Mills
4. Acyclovir Therapy for Herpesvirus Infections,
   edited by David A. Baker
5. The New Generation of Quinolones, *edited by
   Clifford Siporin, Carl L. Heifetz, and John M. Domagala*
6. Methicillin-Resistant *Staphylococcus aureus*: Clinical
   Management and Laboratory Aspects,
   edited by Mary T. Cafferkey
7. Hepatitis B Vaccines in Clinical Practice,
   edited by Ronald W. Ellis
8. The New Macrolides, Azalides, and Streptogramins:
   Pharmacology and Clinical Applications, *edited by
   Harold C. Neu, Lowell S. Young, and Stephen H. Zinner*
9. Antimicrobial Therapy in the Elderly Patient,
   edited by Thomas T. Yoshikawa and Dean C. Norman
10. Viral Infections of the Gastrointestinal Tract:
    Second Edition, Revised and Expanded,
    edited by Albert Z. Kapikian
11. Development and Clinical Uses of *Haemophilus b*
    Conjugate Vaccines, *edited by Ronald W. Ellis
    and Dan M. Granoff*
12. *Pseudomonas aeruginosa* Infections and Treatment,
    edited by Aldona L. Baltch and Raymond P. Smith

Catheter-Related Infections

Infections

Second Edition, Revised and Expanded

edited by

Harald Seifert
Bernd Jansen
Barry M. Farr

MARCEL DEKKER   NEW YORK

Library of Congress Cataloging-in-Publication Data
A catalog record for this book is available from the Library of Congress.

ISBN: 0-8247-5854-4

This book is printed on acid-free paper.

Headquarters
Marcel Dekker, 270 Madison Avenue, New York, NY 10016, U.S.A.
tel: 212-696-9000; fax: 212-685-4540

Distribution and Customer Service
Marcel Dekker, Cimarron Road, Monticello, New York 12701, U.S.A.
tel: 800-228-1160; fax: 845-796-1772

World Wide Web
http://www.dekker.com

Preface

Published in 1997, the first edition of *Catheter-Related Infections* was well received by those with a special interest in this topic because of their work in hospital epidemiology and infection control and/or infectious diseases. Others finding the first edition useful were intensive care specialists whose patients frequently require central venous or pulmonary artery catheters and others who care for patients requiring chronic central venous catheterization. These included hematologists, oncologists, nephrologists, gastroenterologists, cardiologists and physicians in training. The first edition covered topics ranging from the basic science of catheter-related infections, such as factors like fibronectin that mediate the adherence of certain microbes to catheters (more to some catheter materials than to others) to data from epidemiologic studies and recommendations regarding the diagnosis, prevention and management of these infections.

The second edition addresses these same topics as well as some new ones, providing five chapters covering basic principles, five chapters focusing on different groups of pathogens implicated in catheter-related infections, and nine chapters discussing infections associated with different types of catheters including peritoneal dialysis catheters and central nervous system shunts as well as different types of vascular catheters. The second edition adds three new chapters - one on the epidemiology and impact of catheter-related infections by Philippe Eggimann and Didier Pittet, a second on the management of vascular catheter-related infections by Leonard Mermel and Barry Farr, and a third focusing on catheter-related urinary tract infections by Carol Chenoweth and Sanjay Saint.

Newer methods of diagnosis such as differential time-to-positivity are described in detail. Situations in which removal of the indwelling catheter is essential for cure are also contrasted with those in which the catheter may be salvaged using other types of therapy such as parenteral plus antibiotic lock therapy.

Chapter authors include some of the world's most renowned authorities in the area of catheter-related infections with representation from several continents. Many studies on catheter infections have been published in the seven years that have elapsed since publication of the first edition, so the authors of chapters from the first addition have updated their chapters with additional important references. We hope that this second edition will appeal to the same types of clinicians that found the first edition useful.

Harald Seifert
Bernd Jansen
Barry M. Farr

Contents

Contributors

Roger Bayston, M.Med.Sci., F.R.C.Path. Senior Lecturer, School of Medical and Surgical Sciences, University of Nottingham, United Kingdom

François Blot, M.D. Service de Réanimation Polyvalente, Institut Gustave Roussy, Villejuif, France

Carol E. Chenoweth, M.D. Clinical Associate Professor, Division of Infectious Diseases, Department of Internal Medicine, University of Michigan, Ann Arbor, Michigan, U.S.A.

Arnaldo L. Colombo Associate Professor, Division of Infectious Diseases, São Paulo Federal Medical School, São Paulo, Brazil

Philippe Eggimann, M.D. Medical ICU and Infection Control Program, University of Geneva Hospitals, Geneva, Switzerland

Barry M. Farr, M.D., M.Sc. Hospital Epidemiologist, The William S. Jordan, Jr. Professor of Medicine and Epidemiology, The University of Virginia Health System, Charlottesville, Virginia, U.S.A.

André Fleer, M.D., Ph.D. Medical Microbiologist, Wilhelmina Children's Hospital and Eijkman-Winkler Center for Medical Microbiology, Infectious Diseases and Inflammation, University Medical Center Utrecht, Utrecht, The Netherlands

Leo J. Gerards, M.D., Ph.D. Neonatologist, Department of Neonatology, Wilhelmina Children's Hospital, University Medical Center Utrecht, Utrecht, The Netherlands

Hend A. Hanna, M.D., M.P.H. Assistant Professor, Department of Infectious Diseases, Infection Control and Employee Health, The University of Texas M. D. Anderson Cancer Center, Houston, Texas, U.S.A.

Mathias Herrmann, M.D. Professor of Medical Microbiology and Hygiene, and Director, Institute of Medical Microbiology and Hygiene, Institutes of Infectious Disease Medicine, University of Saarland Hospital, Homburg/ Saar, University of Muenster, Muenster, Germany

Bernd Jansen Professor and Head, Department of Hygiene and Environmental Medicine, Head of Department of Hospital Hygiene and Infection Control, Johannes Gutenberg University, Mainz, Germany

R. Monina Klevens, D.D.S., M.P.H. Medical Epidemiologist, Centers for Disease Control and Prevention, National Center for Infectious Diseases, Division of Healthcare Quality Promotion, Atlanta, Georgia, U.S.A.

Wolfgang Kohnen, Ph.D. Departments of Hygiene and Environmental Medicine, and Hospital Hygiene and Infection Control, Johannes Gutenberg University, Mainz, Germany

Tannette G. Krediet Head of the Clinical Department of Neonatology, Department of Neonatology, Wilhelmina Children's Hospital, University Medical Center Utrecht, Utrecht, The Netherlands

Dennis G. Maki, M.D. Ovid O. Meyer Professor of Medicine and Head, University of Wisconsin Hospital and Clinics, Madison, Wisconsin, U.S.A.

C. Glen Mayhall, M.D. Professor, Department of Internal Medicine, Division of Infectious Diseases and Hospital Epidemiologist, Department of Healthcare Epidemiology, UTMB Hospitals and Clinics, The University of Texas Medical Branch at Galveston, Galveston, Texas, U.S.A.

Leonard A. Mermel, D.O., Sc.M., A.M. (Hon.), F.A.C.P., F.I.D.S.A. Medical Director, Department of Infection Control, Rhode Island Hospital Attending Physician, Division of Infectious Disease, Rhode Island Hospital, and Associate Professor of Medicine, Brown Medical School, Providence, Rhode Island, U.S.A.

Georg Peters, M.D. Professor of Medical Microbiology and Chairman, Institute of Medical Microbiology, University of Muenster, Muenster, Germany

Didier Pittet, M.D., M.S. Professor of Medicine, and Director, Infection Control Program, University of Geneva Hospitals, Geneva, Switzerland and Honorary Professor, Division of Investigative Science and School of Medicine, The Hammersmith Hospitals, Imperial College of Science, Technology and Medicine, London, United Kingdom

Issam Raad, M.D., F.A.C.P. Professor and Chairman (ad interim), Department of Infectious Diseases, Infection Control and Employee Health, The University of Texas M. D. Anderson Cancer Center, Houston, Texas, U.S.A.

John J. Roord, M.D., Ph.D. Pediatrician, Professor and Head, Department of Pediatrics, Free University Medical Center, Amsterdam, The Netherlands

Sanjay Saint, M.D., M.P.H. Research Investigator and Hospitalist, Ann Arbor VA Medical Center, Associate Professor of Medicine, University of Michigan School Director, VA/UM Patient Safety Enhancement Program, Ann Arbor, Michigan, U.S.A.

Tanja Schülin, M.D. Medical Microbiologist, University of Medical Centre St. Radboud, Radboud University, Nijmegen, The Netherlands

Harald Seifert, M.D. Professor of Medical Microbiology and Hygiene, Institute for Medical Microbiology, Immunology and Hygiene, University of Cologne, Cologne, Germany

Robert J. Sherertz, M.D. Chief, Infectious Diseases, Wake Forest University School of Medicine, Winston-Salem, North Carolina, U.S.A.

Jerome I. Tokars, M.D., M.P.H. Medical Epidemiologist, Centers for Disease Control and Prevention, National Center for Infectious Diseases, Division of Healthcare Quality Promotion, Atlanta, Georgia, U.S.A.

Henri A. Verbrugh, M.D., Ph.D. Professor of Medical Microbiology, and Head, Department of Medical Microbiology and Infectious Diseases, Erasmus University Medical Center, Rotterdam, The Netherlands

Andreas Voss, M.D., Ph.D. Professor and Chair Infection Control, University of Medical Centre St. Radboud, Department of Medical Microbiology and Nijmegen University Centre of Infectious Diseases, Nijmegen, The Netherlands

Sergio B. Wey   Associate Professor, Division of Infectious Diseases, São Paulo Federal Medical School, São Paulo, Brazil

Andreas F. Widmer, M.D., M.S.   Head, Infection Control, Division of Infectious Diseases and Infection Control, University of Basel Hospitals and Clinics, Basel, Switzerland

Tom F.W. Wolfs, M.D.   Pediatrician, Wilhelmina Children's Hospital Utrecht, Utrecht, The Netherlands

1

Epidemiology and Impact of Infections Associated with the Use of Intravascular Devices

Philippe Eggimann

Medical Intensive Care Unit
Department of Internal Medicine
University of Geneva Hospitals
Geneva, Switzerland

Didier Pittet

Infection Control Program
Department of Internal Medicine
University of Geneva Hospitals
Geneva, Switzerland

INTRODUCTION

Nosocomial infections are a leading cause of morbidity and mortality among hospitalized patients. They should not, however, be considered as an inevitable tribute to pay to the continuous progress in medicine, considering in particular the sophisticated diagnostic and management strategies applied to the care of complex diseases. The extent of the problem was recently highlighted in the general medical literature in the late 1990s, following a publication by the Institute of Medicine in Washington, DC. In brief, this report estimated that preventable adverse events in the United States, including nosocomial infections, were responsible for 44,000 to 98,000 deaths annually and represent a cost of $17 to $29 billion (1). Mostly based on

1

extrapolation from two studies only, this report has generated a considerable debate in the scientific community (2–9). Comparable data were published in the United Kingdom by the House of Commons in November 2000 (10). This official government report estimated that at least 100,000 infections are acquired in hospitals in England each year. These infections may be responsible for at least 5,000 deaths annually, with cost estimates as high as $1.8 billion (11).

Nosocomial infections now concern 5% to 15% of hospitalized patients and can lead to complications in 25% to 50% of those admitted to intensive care units (ICUs) (12,13). Globally, urinary tract and surgical site infections are the most frequent infections, followed by respiratory and bloodstream infections (14) (Fig. 1). Most data concerning the epidemiology of these infections concern particular types of infections in specialized wards, and general information is sparse. However, it has been repeatedly shown that intravascular devices are among the most significant risk factors for the development of nosocomial infections (15–18).

More precise epidemiological data are available for critically ill patients and those admitted to ICUs, in particular. Among these patients, pneumonia related to mechanical ventilation, intra-abdominal infections following trauma or surgery, and bacteremia or sepsis associated with the use of intravascular devices account for more than 80% of ICU-acquired infections (19,20) (Table 1).

Bloodstream infections represented 12% of all nosocomial infections reported in 10,038 patients from 1417 ICUs in the European Prevalence of Infection in Intensive Care (EPIC) study (15). The National Nosocomial Infection Surveillance (NNIS) system, which took into account only data from ICUs, reported that most nosocomial bloodstream infections are associated with the use of intravascular access, with rates substantially higher

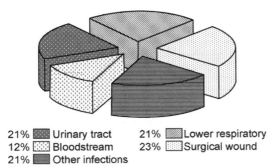

21% ▨ Urinary tract   21% ▨ Lower respiratory
12% ▨ Bloodstream   23% ▨ Surgical wound
21% ▨ Other infections

Figure 1 Proportion of nosocomial infections (*n* = 472) occurring among 4252 patients from 18 large Swiss general hospitals in 1999. Data adapted from the 2nd Swiss National Prevalence Study (14).

Table 1 Epidemiology of Leading Nosocomial Infections in Various Types of ICUs in the 1990s

	Type of ward	No. of units	No. of patients	No. of infections	Incidence-densities of nosocomial infections per 1000 patient-days					
					Overall	Bloodstream	Respiratory tract	Urinary tract	Wound/soft tissue	Other
Richards (30)[a]	Medical	112	181,993	14,177	19.8	3.3	5.3	6.1	—	4.6
Eggimann (32)[b]	Medical	1	1,050	145	34.0	3.8	12.7	5.2	7.0	2.1
Brooks (91)	Medical	1	180	12	12.3	3.0	5.1	4.1	1.0	0.0
Dettenkofer (68)	Neurology	1	505	122	25.0	5.4	7.3	7.0	—	2.4
Richards (29)[a]	Pediatric	61	110,709	6,290	14.1	4.0	4.8	2.1	1.4	1.8
Raymond (92)	Pediatric	5	710	168	16.6	3.4	8.8	2.5	1.2	0.7
Gastmeier (62)	Pediatric	72	515	78	15.3	2.1	8.9	2.3	—	2.0
Simon (75)	Pediatric	1	201	15	15.7	4.8	6.8	1.9	0.8	0.0
Gilio (53)	Pediatric	1	500	65	31.7	1.5	12.7	4.4	4.4	8.7
Legras (63)[c]	Mixed	5	1,589	344	20.3	4.1	5.7	5.2	—	5.2
Kollef (18)[d]	Mixed	2	2,000	286	32.3	—	—	—	—	—
Bradley (94)	Mixed	3	2,734	354	44.3	2.5	22.7	6.9	4.5	7.1
Brasic (61)[e]	Mixed	1	660	688	57.1	22.8	21.8	12.5	—	—
Groot (95)	Mixed	16	2,795	1,177	42.0	—	—	—	—	—
Price (96)[f]	Surgical	1	139	49	11.5	0.0	9.2	2.3	1.5	0.0
Kollef (97)	Surgical	1	327	54	47.2	9.6	15.8	—	—	18.3
Velasco (98)	Oncology	1	623	370	91.7	22.1	26.5	23.5	—	19.6
Richards (28)[a]	Coronary	93	227,451	6,698	10.6	1.8	2.6	3.7	—	2.5
Wurtz (99)	Burn	1	57	36	32.3	1.8	19.7	9.0	0.9	0.9

[a] Data adapted from reports of the NNIS database.
[b] After implementation of a global program targeted at the reduction of vascular access-related infections. Bloodstream infections include episodes of primary bacteremia (1.2/1000 patient-days) and of clinical sepsis (2.6/1000 patients-days).
[c] Bloodstream infections include episodes of primary bacteremia (1.9/1000 patient-days).
[d] Bloodstream infections include episodes of primary bacteremia (3.0/1000 patient-days).
[e] Patients hospitalized for severe infections over a 6-year period.
[f] Data reported are insufficient to extract details on incidence-densities for each type of infection.
— Data could not be extracted from the original publication.

Table 2   Definitions of Infections Associated with the Use of Intravascular Devices[a]

Criteria required for diagnosis of different types of catheter-associated infections for epidemiological surveillance

Primary bloodstream infection	Bacteremia (or fungemia) without documented distal source of infection
Clinical sepsis	Requires one of the following signs or symptoms with no other recognized cause: - fever (>38°C) - hypotension (systolic blood pressure ≤90 mmHg) - oliguria (<20 ml/hr) and the presence of all of the following conditions: - blood culture not performed or no organism detected in blood - no apparent infection at another site - physician institutes therapy for sepsis
Catheter-associated bloodstream infection	Primary bloodstream infection and presence of an intravascular access device

Criteria required for diagnosis of different types of catheter-related infections in clinical studies

Catheter colonization	Significant growth of microorganisms according to precise criteria from quantitative [Brun-Buisson technique (22); sonication, vortexing technique (24)] or semiquantitative cultures [roll-plate technique (23)] of the vascular device
Exit-site infection	Microbiologically documented: isolation of a common pathogen from the exit site (e.g., from purulent discharge) or a positive (semi)quantitative catheter culture in the presence of clinical signs of infection at the insertion site of any vascular access Clinically documented: a clinical infection (erythema, tenderness, induration, or purulence) at the insertion site
Catheter-related bloodstream infection	Primary bloodstream infection in a patient with an intravascular catheter, clinical manifestation of infection (fever, chills, and/or hypotension, and no apparent source for the bloodstream infection. One of the following should be present: - a quantitative or semiquantitative catheter culture with isolation of the same organism (i.e., identical species, antibiogram) as from the bloodstream

Table 2 Continued

Criteria required for diagnosis of different types of catheter-related infections in clinical studies

	- simultaneous quantitative blood cultures drawn percutaneously and from the catheter with a $\geq$5:1 ratio CVC versus peripheral - a differential time to positivity of $\geq$2 hr between a blood culture drawn percutaneously and a blood culture drawn from the suspected vascular catheter (27) In the absence of a positive catheter culture, defervescence after removal of an implicated catheter, without concomitant antimicrobial therapy, from a patient with primary bloodstream infection is considered as indirect evidence of catheter-related bloodstream infection

[a] *Source*: Refs. 21, 25, 100.

among patients with central venous catheters (CVCs) than among those with peripheral lines (19,20).

DEFINITIONS

One should recognize the difference between definitions used for surveillance purposes and clinical definitions. The surveillance definitions for catheter-associated bloodstream infections include all primary bloodstream infections in patients with an intravascular catheter when other sites of infection have been excluded. The clinical definitions for catheter-related infections include colonization of the device, skin exit-site infection, and microbiologically proven intravascular device-related bloodstream infection (21–27) (Table 2). Microbiological criteria remain a matter of debate among experts, and this issue will be discussed in detail in Chapter 3 of this book. However, the absence of a gold-standard reference technique may provide an explanation for the large difference in the published rates of infections. Accordingly, the clinical definition of catheter-related infections may underestimate the true rate of infections related to intravascular devices.

Important issues must be taken into consideration prior to any discussion of the epidemiology and impact of infections associated with the use of intravascular devices. According to the data regularly reported by the NNIS system, more than 85% of primary bacteremia are considered catheter-associated (28–31). The concept of bloodstream infection used includes not only primary bacteremia, but also clinical sepsis (21,32). This may overestimate the rate of infections related to intravascular devices, but it is probably more representative of the clinical reality and allows comparison of rates in surveillance studies. Although included in some reports, secondary bacteremia—by definition—should not be considered as catheter-related; it is related to another documented focus of infection.

Last but not least, infection rates usually vary according to the type of surveillance performed. In trials or studies designed to study complications associated with the use of intravascular devices, infection rates are frequently higher than in those reporting results for the surveillance of all nosocomial infections. In studies dedicated to catheter surveillance, systematic microbiological investigation might allow expression of infection rates or sites rarely investigated in overall surveys.

Finally, other caveats for surveillance and rate-reporting that may affect infection rates will not be considered in this chapter.

EPIDEMIOLOGY

Infections associated with the use of intravascular devices represent 10% to 20% of all nosocomial infections. Accordingly, they may complicate the hospital stay of 0.5% to 3% of patients admitted in ICUs, and of 3.5% to 10% of those hospitalized in general wards. In the United States, it is estimated that up to 150 million intravascular devices are inserted annually in hospitalized patients, and that 200,000 to 400,000 nosocomial bloodstream infections may occur each year (19,33).

According to the variety of definitions used in the literature, infection rates may be difficult to compare. These rates are also largely influenced by patient case-mix and the purpose of the use of vascular access (34). In this chapter, we focus on the epidemiology and impact of infections associated with the use of intravascular devices in acutely ill patients requiring short-term catheterization. The epidemiology of particular types of devices, such as long-term catheterization for hemodialysis or parenteral nutrition, and surgically implanted devices in immunocompromised patients, will be discussed elsewhere in the book.

The prevalence of bloodstream infections associated with the use of intravascular devices in selected studies performed in critically ill patients varies according to the type of disinfection used for the preparation of the skin before the insertion of a central venous catheter. Studies have repeatedly shown that chlorhexidine-based solutions, although not widely used since the early 1990s, may be more potent than those using povidone-iodine (35–42) (Table 3).

The proportion of catheter-related bloodstream infection may also be extracted from studies exploring the potential effect of antimicrobial-coated intravascular devices, mostly conducted during the second part of the 1990s. In these studies, the prevalence of catheter colonization and of catheter-

Table 3 Rates of Colonization and Catheter-Related Bloodstream Infection According to Type of Disinfectant Used for Cleansing Skin Insertion Site in Selected Series of Critically Ill Patients

Type of antisepsis; author	Year of publication	Number studied	Catheter colonization	Catheter-related bloodstream infection
Povidone-Iodine				
Maki (35)[a]	1991	227	21 (9.2%)	6 (2.6%)
Sehean (36)[b]	1993	177	12 (6.8%)	1 (0.6%)
Mimoz (37)[c]	1996	145	24 (16.6%)	4 (2.8%)
Legras (38)[d]	1997	249	31 (12.4%)	4 (1.6%)
LeBlanc (39)[e]	1999	161	23 (16.1%)	—
Humar (40)[f]	2000	116	27 (23.3%)	5/181 (2.8%)
Knasinski (41)[g]	2000	500	127 (25.4%)	20 (4.0%)
Garland (42)[h]	2001	370	76/321 (23.7%)	10/323 (3.1%)
Chlorhexidine				
Maki (35)[a]	1991	214	5 (2.3%)	1 (0.4%)
Sehean (36)[b]	1993	169	3 (1.8%)	1 (0.6%)
Mimoz (37)[c]	1996	170	12 (7.1%)	3 (1.8%)
Legras (38)[d]	1997	208	19 (9.1%)	0 (0.0%)
LeBlanc (39)[e]	1999	83	6 (7.2%)	—
Humar (40)[f]	2000	116	36 (31.0%)	4/193 (2.1%)
Knasinski (41)[g]	2000	349	33 (9.5%)	5 (1.4%)
Garland (42)[h]	2001	335	42/299 (14.1%)	11/297 (3.7%)

[a] Odds ratio for colonization: 0.25 [CI 0.10–0.66] for chlorhexidine-based skin disinfection as compared to povidone-iodine, respectively, $P < 0.01$. No significant differences for catheter-related bloodstream infections.

[b] Odds ratio for colonization: 0.22 [CI 0.06–0.75] for chlorhexidine-based skin disinfection as compared to povidone-iodine, respectively, $P < 0.01$. No significant differences for catheter-related bloodstream infections.

[c] Odds ratio for colonization: 0.43 [CI 0.22–0.82] for chlorhexidine-based skin disinfection as compared to povidone-iodine, respectively, $P < 0.01$. No significant differences for catheter-related bloodstream infections.

[d] No significant differences for catheter colonization and catheter-related bloodstream infections.

[e] Odds ratio for colonization: 0.49 [CI 0.31–0.77] for chlorhexidine-based skin disinfection as compared to povidone-iodine, respectively, $P < 0.01$.

[f] No significant differences for catheter colonization and catheter-related bloodstream infections.

[g] Odds ratio for colonization: 0.37 [CI 0.26–0.53] for chlorhexidine-based skin disinfection as compared to povidone-iodine, respectively, $P < 0.01$. Odds ratio for catheter-related bloodstream infection: 0.36 [CI 0.14–0.95] for chlorhexidine-based skin disinfection as compared to povidone-iodine, respectively, $P < 0.01$.

[h] Odds ratio for colonization: 0.6 [CI 0.4–0.8] for chlorhexidine-based skin disinfection as compared to povidone-iodine, respectively, $P < 0.01$. No significant differences for catheter-related bloodstream infections.

— Data could not be extracted from the original publication.

Table 4 Rates of Colonization and Catheter-Related Bloodstream Infection Associated with Antiseptic/Antibiotic-Impregnated and Nonimpregnated Central Venous Lines in Selected Series of Critically Ill Patients

Type of catheter; author	Year of publication	Number studied	Catheter colonization	Catheter-related bloodstream infection
Nonimpregnated				
Ramsay (43)[a]	1994	189	62 (32.8%)	4 (2.1%)
Trazzera (44)[b]	1995	99	24 (24.2%)	1 (2.3%)
Pemberton (45)[c]	1996	40	—	3 (7.5%)
Ciresi (46)[d]	1996	127	21 (16.5%)	14 (11.0%)
Bach (47)[e]	1996	117	36 (30.8%)	3 (2.5%)
Hannan (48)[f]	1996	177	71 (40.2%)	8 (4.7%)
George (49)[g]	1997	35	25 (71.4%)	3 (8.6%)
Loo (50)[h]	1997	81	25 (30.9%)	3 (3.9%)
Logghe (51)[i]	1997	342	56 (16.5%)	15 (4.4%)
Maki (52)[j]	1997	195	47 (24.1%)	9 (4.6%)
Heard (53)[k]	1998	157	82 (52.2%)	6 (3.8%)
Marik (54)[l]	1999	39	11 (28.2%)	2 (5.1%)
Raad (55)[m]	1997	136	32 (23.6%)	7 (5.0%)
Tennenberg (56)[n]	1997	145	32 (22.4%)	9 (6.4%)
van Heerden (57)[o]	1996	26	10 (38.5%)	0 —
Collin (58)[p]	1999	139	25 (18.0%)	4 (2.9%)
Sheng (59)[q]	2000	122	25 (20.5%)	2 (1.6%)
Silver-sulfadiazine/chlorhexidine-impregnated				
Ramsay (43)[a]	1994	199	46 (23.1%)	1 (0.5%)
Trazzera (44)[b]	1995	123	16 (13.0%)	4 (3.3%)
Pemberton (45)[c]	1996	32	—	2 (6.3%)
Ciresi (46)[d]	1996	124	15 (12.1%)	13 (10.5%)
Bach (47)[e]	1996	116	21 (18.1%)	0 —
Hannan (48)[f]	1996	174	47 (27.7%)	3 (1.7%)
George (49)[g]	1997	44	10 (22.7%)	1 (2.3%)
Loo (50)[h]	1997	77	12 (15.6%)	3 (3.3%)
Logghe (51)[i]	1997	338	49 (14.5%)	17 (5.0%)
Maki (52)[j]	1997	208	28 (13.5%)	2 (1.0%)
Heard (53)[k]	1998	151	60 (39.7%)	5 (3.3%)
Marik (54)[l]	1999	36	7 (19.4%)	1 (2.8%)
Tennenberg (56)[n]	1997	137	8 (5.8%)	5 (3.8%)
van Heerden (57)[o]	1996	28	4 (14.3%)	0 —
Darouiche (60)[r]	1999	382	87 (22.8%)	13 (3.4%)
Collin (58)[p]	1999	98	2 (2.0%)	1 (1.0%)
Sheng (59)[q]	2000	113	9 (7.1%)	1 (0.9%)
Minocycline/rifampin-impregnated				
Marik (54)[l]	1999	38	4 (10.5%)	0 —
Raad (55)[m]	1997	130	11 (8.0%)	0 —
Darouiche (60)[r]	1999	356	28 (7.5%)	1 (0.3%)

Notes to Table 4.

[a] Odds ratio for colonization: 0.58 [CI 0.37–0.92] for silver-sulfadiazine/chlorhexidine-impregnated as compared to nonimpregnated catheters, respectively, $P < 0.005$. No significant differences for catheter-related bloodstream infections.

[b] Odds ratio for colonization: 0.47 [CI 0.23–0.94] for silver-sulfadiazine/chlorhexidine-impregnated as compared to nonimpregnated catheters, respectively, $P < 0.005$. No significant differences for catheter-related bloodstream infections.

[c] No significant differences for catheter-related bloodstream infections.

[d] No significant differences for colonization and for catheter-related bloodstream infections.

[e] Quantitative level of bacterial colonization 52 ± 17 versus 256 ± 86 colony-forming units (CFUs) for silver-sulfadiazine/chlorhexidine-impregnated as compared to nonimpregnated catheters, respectively, $P < 0.05$. No significant differences for catheter-related bloodstream infections.

[f] Semiquantitative analysis of bacterial counts for colonization for silver-sulfadiazine/chlorhexidine-impregnated as compared to nonimpregnated catheters, $P < 0.01$. No significant differences for catheter-related bloodstream infections.

[g] Odds ratio for colonization: 0.12 [CI 0.04 0.33] for silver-sulfadiazine/chlorhexidine-impregnated as compared to nonimpregnated catheters, respectively, $P < 0.005$. No significant differences for catheter-related bloodstream infections.

[h] Catheter-tip positive cultures: for silver-sulfadiazine/chlorhexidine-impregnated as compared to nonimpregnated catheters, $P < 0.05$. No significant differences for catheter-related bloodstream infections.

[i] No significant differences for catheter-related bloodstream infections. Neutropenic cancer patients with median catheterization time of 20 days.

[j] Odds ratio for colonization: 0.56 [CI 0.36–0.89] for silver-sulfadiazine/chlorhexidine-impregnated as compared to nonimpregnated catheters, respectively, $P < 0.005$. Odds ratio for catheter-related bloodstream infections: 0.21 [CI 0.03–0.95] for silver-sulfadiazine/chlorhexidine-impregnated catheters as compared to nonimpregnated catheters, respectively, $P = 0.03$.

[k] Odds ratio for colonization only: 0.59 [CI 0.34–0.97] for silver-sulfadiazine/chlorhexidine-impregnated as compared to nonimpregnated catheters, respectively, $P = 0.04$.

[l] Semiquantitative cultures of distal segment: for minocycline/rifampin-coated as compared to nonimpregnated catheters, $P = 0.5$. No significant differences for catheter-related bloodstream infections.

[m] Odds ratio for colonization: 0.25 [CI 0.12–0.53] for minocycline/rifampin-coated as compared to nonimpregnated catheters, respectively, $P < 0.001$. The rates of catheter-related bloodstream infection per 1000 catheter-days were 7.34 for nonimpregnated and 0 for impregnated catheters ($P < 0.01$, binomial exact test).

[n] Risk reduction for colonization only: 43% for silver-sulfadiazine/chlorhexidine-impregnated as compared to nonimpregnated catheters, respectively, $P < 0.001$.

[o] Semiquantitative cultures of distal segment: for silver-sulfadiazine/chlorhexidine-impregnated as compared to nonimpregnated catheters, $P < 0.05$. No significant differences for catheter-related bloodstream infections.

[p] Kaplan-Meier estimates of the cumulative risk of colonization in the silver-sulfadiazine/chlorhexidine-impregnated catheters was significantly lower than in the noncoated catheters, $P = 0.006$. No significant differences for catheter-related bloodstream infections.

[q] Odds ratio for colonization: 0.34 [CI 0.15–0.74] silver-sulfadiazine/chlorhexidine-impregnated as compared to nonimpregnated catheters, $P = 0.006$. No significant differences for catheter-related bloodstream infections.

[r] Odds ratio for colonization: 0.35 [CI 0.23–0.52] for minocycline/rifampin as compared to silver-sulfadiazine/chlorhexidine-impregnated catheters, respectively, $P < 0.001$. Odds ratio for catheter-related bloodstream infection: 0.08 [CI 0.01–0.63] for minocycline/rifampin as compared to silver-sulfadiazine/chlorhexidine-impregnated catheters, respectively, $P < 0.0001$.

— Data could not be extracted from the original publication.

related bloodstream infections ranged from 5.8% to 71.4% and from 0.3% to 11.0%, respectively (43–60) (Table 4).

Comparisons between infection rates in different types of ICUs are more accurate when infections are reported as incidence-densities related to central venous catheterization days. According to this method, widely diffused by the NNIS system, they range between 2.3 and 16.8 episodes per 1000 catheter-days. Table 5 presents comparisons of selected reports from various types of ICUs (20,28–32,40,58,61–76).

The epidemiology of clinical sepsis is not well established. It accounts for fewer than 3% of all episodes of catheter-related infections reported to the NNIS system (28). The term *clinical sepsis* is included in the surveillance definitions for primary bloodstream infections published by the CDC to accommodate sepsis episodes where there is no pathogen cultured from blood, and as a complement to the definition of laboratory-confirmed primary bloodstream infection. This entity, which should be used for epidemiological purposes, is, however, relatively close to the definition of the syndromes of systematic inflammatory response, severe sepsis, and septic shock in response to an inflammatory or infectious process (77). At present, only few epidemiological data are available, and the impact of clinical sepsis remains to be determined (42,66,67,78–81) (Table 6).

IMPACT

Several studies have determined the impact of infections associated with the use of intravascular devices on patient morbidity and hospital costs in ICUs. A significant correlation was found between the prevalence rate of ICU-acquired infection and the mortality rate. In the EPIC study, laboratory-proven bloodstream infection, pneumonia, and clinical sepsis were independently associated with increased mortality (15).

The impact of infection is determined by the attributable part of the parameters that are considered. Accordingly, the attributable mortality of nosocomial infections is defined as the difference in the death rate of infected patients and noninfected patients in a series adjusted for the presence of other confounding factors. Several epidemiological methods may be used to determine the attributable mortality, or any other parameter associated with the acquisition of nosocomial infection. Direct estimation is a simple method in which an experienced clinician subjectively estimates if the death of a patient is related to the infection or not. This technique systematically underestimates the attributable part of the mortality. Appropriateness of evaluation protocol is another direct method that is used to estimate the prolongation of the length of stay possibly associated with the infection. Based on standardized criteria, the patient is evaluated daily to determine whether the stay in hospital is related to the underlying disease, a complication resulting from comorbidity or medical care, and/or to the presence of a nosocomial infection.

Table 5 Catheter-Associated Bloodstream Infection Rates in Selected Series of Critically Ill Patients

Author	Type of ICU	Period	Number of units	Bloodstream infections per 1000 CVC-days
NNIS[a] (30)	Medical	1997–1999	135	5.3 (3.6–7.1)[b]
NNIS[a] (28)	Coronary	1997–1999	112	4.0 (1.7–6.3)[b]
NNIS[a] (20)	Surgical	1997–1999	157	5.1 (2.6–7.0)[b]
NNIS[a] (31)[c]	Mixed	1992–1998	135	5.9 (4.0–7.8)[b]
NNIS[a] (31)[d]	Mixed	1992–1998	69	5.1 (2.6–7.0)[b]
NNIS[a] (29)	Pediatric	1997–1999	73	6.9 (4.1–9.3)[b]
Brasic (61)	Mixed	1990–1997	1	11.3
Gastmeier (62)	Mixed	1994	89	4.9
Legras (63)	Mixed	1995	5	4.8
Collin (58)[e]	Mixed	1995–1996	2	4.0
Collin (58)[f]	Mixed	1995–1996	2	1.1
Sherertz (64)[g]	Mixed	1997	6	3.3
Sherertz (64)[h]	Mixed	1997	6	2.4
Finkelstein (65)	Mixed	1997–1999	1	12.0
Luna (66)	Mixed	1998–1999	2	5.1
Humar (40)	Mixed	1998–1999	4	4.6
Eggimann (32)[i]	Medical	1995–1996	1	6.6
Eggimann (32)[j]	Medical	1997	1	2.3
Timsit (67)[k]	Medical	1995–1998	3	2.3
Timsit (67)[l]	Medical	1995–1998	3	0.7
Dettenkofer (68)	Neurological	1997–1999	1	1.9
Petrosillo (69)	HIV patients	1998–1999	17	9.6
Dimick (70)	Surgical	1998–1999	1	3.6 (2.1–5.8)[b]
Wallace (71)	Surgical	1997–1999	1	8.0
Wallace (71)	Trauma	1995–1997	1	9.1
Weber (72)	Burn	1990–1991	1	4.9
Sing-Naz (73)	Pediatric	1993	1	8.9
Sing-Naz (73)	Pediatric	1995	1	16.8
Gastmeier (74)	Pediatric	1994–1995	73	12.5 (5.7–24.7)[b]
Simon (75)	Pediatric	1998	1	10.7
Mahieu (76)	Neonatal	1998–1999	1	4.4

[a] National Nosocomial Infection Surveillance (NNIS) system.
[b] 50th percentile (25th–75th).
[c] Not major teaching hospitals.
[d] Major teaching hospitals.
[e] Patients with nonantiseptic-coated catheters.
[f] Patients with antiseptic-coated catheters.
[g] Before initiation of an educational program targeted at the reduction of catheter-related infections.
[h] After starting an educational program targeted at the reduction of catheter-related infections.
[i] Before implementation of a global strategy targeted at the reduction of catheter-related infections.
[j] After implementation of a global strategy targeted at the reduction of catheter-related infections.
[k] Including two medical ICUs and one mixed ICU. Femoral nontunneled central venous catheters.
[l] Including two medical ICUs and one mixed ICU. Femoral tunneled central venous catheters.

Table 6 Epidemiology of Different Types of Infections Associated with the Use of Intravascular Devices: Selected Series, Critically Ill Patients

Author	Characteristics of the catheter	Number studied	Catheter colonization	Clinical sepsis	Catheter-related bloodstream infections
Von Meyenfeldt (78)	Subclavian	76	4 (5.3%)	3 (3.9%)	2 (2.6%)
Von Meyenfeldt (78)	Subclavian, tunneled	63	4 (6.3%)	2 (3.2%)	2 (3.2%)
Garden (79)	Subclavian	24	—	8 (33.3%)	7 (29.2%)
Garden (79)	Subclavian, tunneled	20	—	9 (45.0%)	3 (15.0%)
Tismsit (80)[a]	Jugular	114	29 (25.4%)	18 (15.8%)	13 (11.4%)
Tismsit (80)[a]	Jugular, tunneled	117	20 (17.1%)	7 (6.0%)	4 (3.4%)
Merrer (81)[b]	Femoral	134	19 (2.4%)	6 (4.5%)	2 (0.2%)
Merrer (81)[b]	Subclavian	136	3 (0.2%)	2 (0.2%)	1 (0.1%)
Luna (66)	Subclavian (86%); femoral (9%)	130	38 (29.8%)	26 (20.0%)	9 (6.9%)
Garland (42)[c]	Povidone-iodine dressing	370	76/321 (23.7%)	44/346 (12.7%)	10/323 (3.1%)
Garland (42)[c]	Chlorhexidine dressing	335	42/299 (14.1%)	46/316 (14.6%)	11/297 (3.7%)
Timsit (67)[d]	Femoral	168	21 (12.5%)	15 (8.9%)	4 (2.4%)
Timsit (67)[d]	Femoral, tunneled	168	15 (8.9%)	5 (3.0%)	1 (0.6%)

[a] Odds ratio for colonization: 0.3 [CI 0.1–0.9] for tunneled catheters as compared to nontunneled, respectively, $P < 0.01$. No significant differences for clinical sepsis and for catheter-related bloodstream infections.

[b] Odds ratio for any catheter-related infection: 0.21 [CI 0.08–0.51] for catheters inserted at the subclavian site as compared to the femoral site, respectively, $P < 0.01$.

[c] Odds ratio for colonization: 0.6 [CI 0.4–0.8] for chlorhexidine-based skin disinfection of the insertion site as compared to povidone-iodine, respectively, $P < 0.01$. No significant differences for clinical sepsis and for catheter-related bloodstream infections.

[d] Odds ratio for colonization 0.48 [CI 0.23–0.99] for tunneled catheters as compared to nontunneled, respectively, $P = 0.045$. Odds ratio for clinical sepsis 0.25 [0.09–0.72] for tunneled catheters as compared to nontunneled, respectively, $P = 0.055$. No significant differences for catheter-related bloodstream infections.

— Not available.

Another method compares two groups of patients: those with and those without a specified nosocomial infection. Differences are expected to be attributable to the nosocomial infection. However, this technique does not take into consideration potential confounding parameters that may exist between the two groups of patients. This effect can be attenuated by including factors potentially related to death or other outcome measures in multivariate analysis. Nevertheless, these adjustments are generally insufficient and the attributable part is often overestimated. The so-called case-controlled studies (i.e., more appropriately, historical cohort studies with matching on potential confounders) are considered to be the best method to determine the impact of nosocomial infection. Infected and noninfected patients are carefully matched for several confounding factors related to the investigated parameter. Among matching variables, the ones most usually considered are age, severity of underlying disease, associated comorbidities, and number of discharge diagnoses, as well as time of exposure to risk factors. Biased evaluations of the impact are minimal with this methodological approach, apart from when case and control patients are matched too closely using variables that predict or confound the outcome of interest (82).

An analysis of the impact of nosocomial infections showed that they are responsible for a significant increase in mortality, morbidity, length of hospital stay, and resources utilization in almost all groups of patients studied (57, 69, 70, 82–90) (Table 7).

Crude mortality rates are particularly high in critically ill patients, but the attributable mortality varies according to the type of infection. The differences reported between studies may be related to some confusion between the associated and the attributable parts. In addition, some methodological bias may also play a role. Insufficient matching criteria (low case/control ratio; few and irrelevant matching parameters) may overestimate the impact, but overmatching abolishes differences between cases and controls. Cost-effectiveness analyses are based on these data and imply that the controversies in the recent literature regarding the attributable mortality of nosocomial infections concern not only epidemiologists, but also physicians-in-charge who have to select and implement preventive strategies.

FUTURE RESEARCH

More studies are required to better define the epidemiology of infections associated with the use of intravascular devices, in particular among selected and distinct populations. Methods for an appropriate comparison of rates, as well as adjustment for population case-mix, are needed. As already mentioned, the NNIS system recommends expressing catheter-associated infections as the number of infectious episodes per 1000 catheter-days to facilitate and foster benchmarking between units and hospitals. However, true risk determination requires computing infections on the days at risk only, defined

Table 7 Impact of Nosocomial Bloodstream Infection in Critically Ill Patients

Author	Type of bloodstream infection	Year of publication	Study period	Number of cases	Mortality		Attributable	
					Crude	Attributable	LOS[a](days)	Costs (US$)
Smith (83)	Nosocomial[b]	1991	1986–89	34	82%	30%	—	—
Wey (84)	Nosocomial[c]	1988	1977–84	88	57%	38%	30.0	—
Rello (85)	Nosocomial[b]	1994	1990–92	111	65%	35%[d]	—	—
Pittet (86)	Nosocomial[b]	1994	1988–90	86	50%	35%	8.0	40,000
Pittet (87)	Catheter-related	1994	1988–90	20	45%	25%	6.5	29,000
Wisplinghoff (57)	Nosocomial[e]	1998	1990–92	29	31%	16%	20.0	—
Soufir (82)	Catheter-related	1999	1990–95	38	50%	29%	—	—
DiGiovine (88)	Nosocomial[f]	1999	1994–96	68	35%	4%[g]	10.0	35,000
Rello (89)	Catheter-related	2000	1992–99	49	22%	13%[g]	20.0	4,000
Brun-Buisson (90)	Any bacteremia	2001	1998	96	52%	35%	5.5	—
Brun-Buisson (90)	Nosocomial[f]	2001	1998	28	50%	29%	8.0	—
Brun-Buisson (90)	Catheter-related	2001	1998	26	39%	12%[g]	14.0[g]	—
Dimick (70)	Catheter-related	2001	1998–99	17	56%	35%[d]	20.0	71,443[h]
Petrosillo (69)	Nosocomial[f]	2002	1998–99	65	25%	17%[d]	16.0	—

[a] LOS: Length of stay.
[b] Includes both primary and secondary bloodstream infections.
[c] Candidemia only.
[d] Attributable mortality was determined by simple comparison with the crude mortality of all patients who did not develop a bloodstream infection.
[e] *Acinetobacter baumannii* nosocomial bloodstream infections only.
[f] Includes primary bloodstream infections only.
[g] Differences are nonsignificant.
[h] Based on billing database.
— Not available.

as those on which patients are free of infection. If infection rates are expressed per patient-days, a prolonged stay will underestimate the rate of infection, whereas a ward with a high proportion of patients with a short length of stay will report a higher rate. A similar bias will occur when rates are expressed per catheter-days: the longer the duration of catheterization, the lower the rate. Considering only catheter-days at risk, and therefore excluding catheter-days after the onset of infection, will yield a more appropriate risk estimate and make benchmarking more accurate after case-mix adjustment.

This precise determination of risk estimates requires individualized surveillance data over a long period of time, which is not routinely the case in most institutions.

Better studies are needed to evaluate the impact of infection. In particular, there is a need to determine the attributable length of stay, which is a recognized surrogate marker of patient morbidity. It may provide a good estimate of the burden of infection on hospital resources that is not dependent on the accounting system or differences between countries, and may consequently be widely used for benchmarking.

Precise estimates of the financial burden of nosocomial infections is a pivotal issue for infection control practitioners competing for resources. However, cost estimation is not a straightforward exercise, and some caveats may be difficult to avoid. In particular, charges do not equal costs, charges being usually larger. Accordingly, costs may represent a more reliable estimate of the financial burden and should be preferred to charges. Such information is usually more difficult to obtain. Theoretically, the availability of a complete list of all care items and services used for each patient should be extracted from computerized systems and will allow precise determination of true resource consumption. At the present time, no such study has yet appeared in the literature, and this may be a stimulating avenue for future clinical research.

REFERENCES

1. Kohn L, Corrigan J, Donaldson M, eds. To Err is Human: Building a Safer Health System. Washington DC: Institute of Medicine, 1999.
2. Brennan TA, Leape LL, Laird NM, Hebert L, Localio AR, Lawthers AG, Newhouse JP, Weiler PC, Hiatt HH. Incidence of adverse events and negligence in hospitalized patients. Results of the Harvard Medical Practice Study I. NEJM 1991; 324:370–376.
3. Leape LL, Brennan TA, Laird N, Lawthers AG, Localio AR, Barnes BA, Hebert L, Newhouse JP, Weiler PC, Hiatt H. The nature of adverse events in hospitalized patients. Results of the Harvard Medical Practice Study II. NEJM 1991; 324:377–384.
4. Localio AR, Lawthers AG, Brennan TA, Laird NM, Hebert LE, Peterson LM, Newhouse JP, Weiler PC, Hiatt HH. Relation between malpractice claims and adverse events due to negligence. Results of the Harvard Medical Practice Study III. NEJM 1991; 325:245–251.

5. Thomas EJ, Studdert DM, Burstin HR, Orav EJ, Zeena T, Williams EJ, Howard KM, Weiler PC, Brennan TA. Incidence and types of adverse events and negligent care in Utah and Colorado. Med Care 2000; 38:261–271.
6. Leape LL. Institute of Medicine medical error figures are not exaggerated. JAMA 2000; 284:95–97.
7. Leape LL, Berwick DM. Safe health care: are we up to it? BMJ 2000; 320:725–726.
8. McDonald CJ, Weiner M, Hui SL. Deaths due to medical errors are exaggerated in Institute of Medicine report. JAMA 2000; 284:93–95.
9. Brennan TA. The Institute of Medicine report on medical errors—could it do harm? NEJM 2000; 342:1123–1125.
10. Mayor S. Hospital acquired infections kill 5000 patients a year in England. BMJ 2000; 321:1370.
11. The Committee of Public Account of the United Kingdom Parliament. The management and control of hospital acquired infection in acute NHS trusts in England. http://www.publications.parliament.uk/pa/cm199900/cmselect/cmpubacc/306/30603.htm. Accessed 1st August 2002.
12. Bates DW, Miller EB, Cullen DJ, Burdick L, Williams L, Laird N, Petersen LA, Small SD, Sweitzer BJ, Vander Vliet M, Leape LL. Patient risk factors for adverse drug events in hospitalized patients. ADE Prevention Study Group. Arch Intern Med 1999; 159:2553–2560.
13. Eggimann P, Pittet D. Infection control in the ICU. Chest 2001; 120:2059–2093.
14. Sax H, Pittet D and the Swiss-NOSO network. Interhospital differences in nosocomial infection rates–importance of case-mix adjustment. Arch Intern Med 2002; 108:180–190.
15. Vincent JL, Bihari DJ, Suter PM, Bruining HA, White J, Nicolas-Chanoin M-H, Wolff M, Spencer RC, Hemmer M. The prevalence of nosocomial infection in intensive care units in Europe. Results of the European Prevalence of Infection in Intensive Care (EPIC) study. JAMA 1995; 274:639–644.
16. Pittet D, Harbarth S, Ruef C, Francioli P, Sudre P, Pétignat C, Trampuz A, Wiedmer A. Prevalence and risk factors for nosocomial infections in four university hospitals in Switzerland. Infect Control Hosp Epidemiol 1999; 20:37–42.
17. Harbarth S, Ruef C, Francioli P, Widmer A, Pittet D. Nosocomial infections in Swiss university hospitals: a multi-centre survey and review of the published experience. *Swiss-NOSO Network*. Schweiz Med Wochenschr 1999; 129:1521–1528.
18. Kollef MH, Sherman G, Ward S, Fraser VJ. Inadequate antimicrobial treatment of infections: a risk factor for hospital mortality among critically ill patients. Chest 1999; 115:462–474.
19. Maki DG, Mermel LA, Bennett JV, Brachman PS, eds. Hospital Infections. Infections due to infusion therapy. Vol. 44. 4th ed. Philadelphia: Lippincott-Raven, 1998:689–724.
20. Monitoring hospital-acquired infections to promote patient safety—United States, 1990–1999. Morb Mortal Wkly Rep 2000; 49:149–153.
21. Garner JS, Jarvis WR, Emori TG, Toran TC, Hughes JM. CDC definitions for nosocomial infections. Am J Infect Control 1988; 16:128–140.

22. Brun-Buisson C, Abrouk F, Legrand P, Huet Y, Larabi S, Rapin M. Diagnosis of central venous catheter-related sepsis. Arch Intern Med 1987; 147:873–877.

23. Maki DG, Weise CE, Sarafin HW. A semiquantitative culture method for identifying intravenous- catheter-related infection. NEJM 1977; 296:1305–1309.

24. Sherertz RJ, Raad II, Belani A, Koo LC, Rand KH, Pickett DL, Straub SA, Fauerbach LL. Three-year experience with sonicated vascular catheter cultures in a clinical microbiology laboratory. J Clin Microbiol 1990; 28:76–82.

25. Siegman-Igra Y, Anglim AM, Shapiro DE, Adal KA, Strain BA, Farr BM. Diagnosis of vascular catheter-related bloodstream infection: a meta-analysis. J Clin Microbiol 1997; 35:928–936.

26. Kite P, Dobbins BM, Wilcox MH, McMahon MJ. Rapid diagnosis of central-venous-catheter-related bloodstream infection without catheter removal. Lancet 1999; 354:1504–1507.

27. Blot F, Nitenberg G, Chachaty E, Raynard B, Germann N, Antoun S, Laplanche A, Brun-Buisson C, Tancrè C. Diagnosis of catheter-related bacteremia: a prospective comparison of the time to positivity of hub-blood versus peripheral-blood cultures. Lancet 1999; 354:1071–1077.

28. Richards MJ, Edwards JR, Culver DH, Gaynes RP. Nosocomial infections in coronary care units in the United States. National Nosocomial Infections Surveillance System. Am J Cardiol 1998; 82:789–793.

29. Richards MJ, Edwards JR, Culver DH, Gaynes RP. Nosocomial infections in pediatric intensive care units in the United States. National Nosocomial Infections Surveillance System. Pediatrics 1999; 103:39–45.

30. Richards MJ, Edwards JR, Culver DH, Gaynes RP. Nosocomial infections in medical intensive care units in the United States. National Nosocomial Infections Surveillance System. Crit Care Med 1999; 27:887–8892.

31. Richards MJ, Edwards JR, Culver DH, Gaynes RP. Nosocomial infections in combined medical–surgical intensive care units in the United States. Infect Control Hosp Epidemiol 2000; 21:510–515.

32. Eggimann P, Harbarth S, Constantin MN, Touveneau S, Chevrolet JC, Pittet D. Impact of a prevention strategy targeted at vascular-access care on incidence of infections acquired in intensive care. Lancet 2000; 355:1864–1868.

33. Mermel LA. Prevention of intravascular catheter-related infections. Ann Intern Med 2000; 132:391–402.

34. Mermel LA, Farr BM, Sherertz RJ, Raad II, O'Grady N, Harris JS, Craven DE. Guidelines for the management of intravascular catheter-related infections. Clin Infect Dis 2001; 32:1249–1272.

35. Maki DG, Ringer M, Alvarado CJ. Prospective randomised trial of povidone-iodine, alcohol, and chlorhexidine for prevention of infection associated with central venous and arterial catheters. Lancet 1991; 338:339–343.

36. Sheehan G, Leicht K, O'Brien M, Taylor G, Rennie R. Chlorhexidine versus povidone-iodine as cutaneous antisepsis for prevention of vascular-catheter infection [abstr]. Interscience Conference on Antimicrobial Agents and Chemotherapy. Washington, DC: American Society for Microbiology, 1993:414(a1616).

37. Mimoz O, Pieroni L, Lawrence C, Edouard A, Costa Y, Samii K, Brun-Buisson C. Prospective, randomized trial of two antiseptic solutions for

prevention of central venous or arterial catheter colonization and infection in intensive care unit patients. Crit Care Med 1996; 24:1818–1823.

38. Legras A, Cattier B, Dequin PF, Boulain T, Errotin D. Etude prospective randomisée pour la prévention des infections liées aux cathéters; chlorhexidine alcoolique contre polyvidone iodée. Réanimation et Urgences 1997; 6:5–11.

39. LeBlanc A, Cobett S. IV site infection: a prospective, randomized clinical trial comparing the efficacy of three methods of skin antisepsis. Canadian Intravenous Nurses Association Journal, 1999; 15:48–50.

40. Humar A, Ostromecki A, Direnfeld J, Marshall JC, Lazar N, Houston PC, Boiteau P, Conly JM. Prospective randomized trial of 10% povidone-iodine versus 0.5% tincture of chlorhexidine as cutaneous antisepsis for prevention of central venous catheter infection. Clin Infect Dis 2000; 31:1001–1007.

41. Knasinski V, Maki DG. A prospective, randomized, controlled trial of 1% chlorhexidine 75% alcohol vs. 10% povidone iodine for cutaneous disinfection and follow-up site care with central venous and arterial catheters. (Oral presentation). National Association of Vascular Access Network Conference, 2000, San Diego, 2000.

42. Garland JS, Alex CP, Mueller CD, Otten D, Shivpuri C, Harris MC, Naples M, Pellegrini J, Buck RK, McAuliffe TL, Goldmann DA, Maki DG. A randomized trial comparing povidone-iodine to a chlorhexidine gluconate-impregnated dressing for prevention of central venous catheter infections in neonates. Pediatrics 2001; 107:1431–1436.

43. Ramsay J, Nolte F, Schwarzmann S. Incidence of Crit Care Med 1994; 22:A115.

44. Trazzera S, Stern G, Bhardway R, Sinha S, Reiser P. Examination of antimicrobial-coated central venous catheter in patients at risk for catheter-related infections in a medical intensive care unit and leukemia/bone marrow transplant unit [abstr]. Crit Care Med 1995; 23:A153.

45. Pemberton LB, Ross V, Cuddy P, Kremer H, Fessler T, McGurk E. No difference in catheter sepsis between standard and antiseptic central venous catheters. A prospective randomized trial. Arch Surg 1996; 131:986–989.

46. Ciresi DL, Albrecht RM, Volkers PA, Scholten DJ. Failure of antiseptic bonding to prevent central venous catheter-related infection and sepsis. Am Surg 1996; 62:641–646.

47. Bach A, Schmidt H, Bottiger B, Schreiber B, Bohrer H, Motsch J, Martin E, Sonntag HG. Retention of antibacterial activity and bacterial colonization of antiseptic-bonded central venous catheters. J Antimicrob Chemother 1996; 37:315–322.

48. Hannan M, Juste RN, Umasanker S, Glendenning A, Nightingale C, Azadian B, Soni N. Antiseptic-bonded central venous catheters and bacterial colonisation. Anaesthesia 1999; 54:868–872.

49. George SJ, Vuddamalay P, Boscoe MJ. Antiseptic-impregnated central venous catheters reduce the incidence of bacterial colonization and associated infection in immunocompromised transplant patients. Eur J Anaesthesiol 1997; 14:428–431.

50. Loo S, van Heerden PV, Gollege CL, Roberts BL, Power BM. Infection in central lines: antiseptic-impregnated vs standard non-impregnated catheters. Anaesth Intensive Care 1997; 25:637–639.

51. Logghe C, Van Ossel C, D'Hoore W, Ezzedine H, Wauters G, Haxhe JJ.

Evaluation of chlorhexidine and silver-sulfadiazine impregnated central venous catheters for the prevention of bloodstream infection in leukaemic patients: a randomized controlled trial. J Hosp Infect 1997; 37:145–156.

52. Maki DG, Stolz SM, Wheeler S, Mermel LA. Prevention of central venous catheter-related bloodstream infection by use of an antiseptic-impregnated catheter. A randomized, controlled trial. Ann Intern Med 1997; 127:257–266.

53. Heard SO, Wagle M, Vijayakumar E, McLean S, Brueggemann A, Napolitano LM, Edwards LP, O'Connell FM, Puyana JC, Doern GV. Influence of triple-lumen central venous catheters coated with chlorhexidine and silver sulfadiazine on the incidence of catheter-related bacteremia. Arch Intern Med 1998; 158:81–87.

54. Marik PE, Abraham G, Careau P, Varon J, Fromm RE Jr. The ex vivo antimicrobial activity and colonization rate of two antimicrobial-bonded central venous catheters. Crit Care Med 1999; 27:1128–1131.

55. Raad I, Darouiche RO, Dupuis J, Abi-Said D, Gabrielli A, Hachem R, Wall M, Harris RL, Jones J, Buzaid A, Robertson C, Shenaq S, Curling P, Burke T, Ericsson C, and the Texas Medical Center Catheter Study Group. Central venous catheter coated with minocycline and rifampine for the prevention of catheter-related colonization and bloodstream infections. A randomized, double-blind trial. Ann Intern Med 1997; 127:267 274.

56. Tennenberg S, Lieser M, McCurdy B, Boomer G, Howington E, Newman C, Wolf I. A prospective randomized trial of an antibiotic- and antiseptic- coated central venous catheter in the prevention of catheter-related infections. Arch Surg 1997; 132:1348–1351.

57. Wisplinghoff H, Perbix W, Seifert H. Risk factors for nosocomial bloodstream infections due to *Acinetobacter baumannii*: a case-control study of adult burn patients. Clin Infect Dis 1999; 28:59–66.

58. Collin GR. Decreasing catheter colonization through the use of an antiseptic-impregnated catheter: a continuous quality improvement project. Chest 1999; 115:1632–1640.

59. Sheng WH, Ko WJ, Wang JT, Chang SC, Hsueh PR, Luh KT. Evaluation of antiseptic-impregnated central venous catheters for prevention of catheter-related infection in intensive care unit patients. Diagn Microbiol Infect Dis 2000; 38:1–5.

60. Darouiche RO, Raad II, Heard SO, Thornby JI, Wenker OC, Gabrielli A, Berg J, Khardori N, Hanna H, Hachem R, Harris RL, Mayhall G, for the catheter study group. A comparison of two antimicrobial-impregnated central venous catheters. NEJM 1999; 340:1–8.

61. Barsic B, Beus I, Marton E, Himbele J, Klinar I. Nosocomial infections in critically ill infectious disease patients: results of a 7-year focal surveillance. Infection 1999; 27:16–22.

62. Gastmeier P, Schumacher M, Daschner F, Ruden H. An analysis of two prevalence surveys of nosocomial infection in German intensive care units. J Hosp Infect 1997; 35:97–105.

63. Legras A, Malvy D, Quinioux AI, Villers D, Bouachour G, Robert R, Thomas R. Nosocomial infections: prospective survey of incidence in five French intensive care units. Intensive Care Med 1998; 24:1040–1046.

64. Sherertz RJ, Ely EW, Westbrook DM, Gledhill KS, Streed SA, Kiger B, Flynn L, Hayes S, Strong S, Cruz J, Bowton DL, Hulgan T, Haponik EF. Education of physicians-in-training can decrease the risk for vascular catheter infection. Ann Intern Med 2000; 132:641–648.

65. Finkelstein R, Rabino G, Kassis I, Mahamid I. Device-associated, device-day infection rates in an Israeli adult general intensive care unit. J Hosp Infect 2000; 44:200–205.

66. Luna J, Masdeu G, Perez M, Claramonte R, Forcadell I, Barrachina F, Panisello M. Clinical trial evaluating a new hub device designed to prevent catheter-related sepsis. Eur J Clin Microbiol Infect Dis 2000; 19:655–662.

67. Timsit JF, Bruneel F, Cheval C, Mamzer MF, Garrouste-Orgeas M, Wolff M, Misset B, Chevret S, Regnier B, Carlet J. Use of tunneled femoral catheters to prevent catheter-related infection. A randomized, controlled trial. Ann Intern Med 1999; 130:729–735.

68. Dettenkofer M, Ebner W, Els T, Babikir R, Lucking C, Pelz K, Ruden H, Daschner F. Surveillance of nosocomial infections in a neurology intensive care unit. J Neurol 2001; 248:959–964.

69. Petrosillo N, Viale P, Nicastri E, Arici C, Bombana E, Casella A, Cristini F, De Gennaro M, Dodi F, Gabbuti A, Gattuso G, Irato L, Maggi P, Pallavicini F, Pan A, Pantaleoni M, Ippolito G. Nosocomial bloodstream infections among human immunodeficiency virus-infected patients: incidence and risk factors. Clin Infect Dis 2002; 34:677–685.

70. Dimick JB, Pelz RK, Consunji R, Swoboda SM, Hendrix CW, Lipsett PA. Increased resource use associated with catheter-related bloodstream infection in the surgical intensive care unit. Arch Surg 2001; 136:229–234.

71. Wallace WC, Cinat M, Gornick WB, Lekawa ME, Wilson SE. Nosocomial infections in the surgical intensive care unit: a difference between trauma and surgical patients. Am Surg 1999; 65:987–990.

72. Weber JM, Sheridan RL, Pasternack MS, Tompkins RG. Nosocomial infections in pediatric patients with burns. Am J Infect Control 1997; 25:195–201.

73. Singh-Naz N, Sprague BM, Patel KM, Pollack MM. Risk assessment and standardized nosocomial infection rate in critically ill children. Crit Care Med 2000; 28:2069–2075.

74. Gastmeier P, Hentschel J, de Veer I, Obladen M, Ruden H. Device-associated nosocomial infection surveillance in neonatal intensive care using specified criteria for neonates. J Hosp Infect 1998; 38:51–60.

75. Simon A, Bindl L, Kramer MH. [Surveillance of nosocomial infections: prospective study in a pediatric intensive care unit. Background, patients and methods]. Klin Pädiatr 2000; 212:2–9.

76. Mahieu LM, De Muynck AO, Ieven MM, De Dooy JJ, Goossens HJ, Van Reempts PJ. Risk factors for central vascular catheter-associated bloodstream infections among patients in a neonatal intensive care unit. J Hosp Infect 2001; 48:108–116.

77. Bone RC, Balk RA, Cerra FB, Dellinger RP, Fein AM, Knaus WA, Schein RM, Sibbald WJ. Definitions for sepsis and organ failure and guidelines for the use of innovative therapies in sepsis. The ACCP/SCCM consensus

conference committee. American College of Chest Physicians/Society of Critical Care Medicine. Chest 1992; 101:1644–1655.

78. von Meyenfeldt MM, Stapert J, de Jong PC, Soeters PB, Wesdorp RI, Greep JM. TPN catheter sepsis: lack of effect of subcutaneous tunnelling of PVC catheters on sepsis rate. J Parenter Enteral Nutr 1980; 4:514–517.

79. Garden OJ, Sim AJW. A comparison of tunneled and non-tunneled subclavian vein catheters: a prospective study of complications during parenteral feeding. Clin Nutr 1983; 2:51–54.

80. Timsit JF, Sebille V, Farkas JC, Misset B, Martin JB, Chevret S, Carlet J. Effect of subcutaneous tunneling on internal jugular catheter-related sepsis in critically ill patients: a prospective randomized multicenter study. JAMA 1996; 276:1416–1420.

81. Merrer J, De Jonghe B, Golliot F, Lefrant JY, Raffy B, Barre E, Rigaud JP, Casciani D, Misset B, Bosquet C, Outin H, Brun-Buisson C, Nitenberg G. Complications of femoral and subclavian venous catheterization in critically ill patients: a randomized controlled trial. JAMA 2001; 286:700–707.

82. Soufir L, Timsit JF, Mahe C, Carlet J, Regnier B, Chevret S. Attributable morbidity and mortality of catheter-related septicemia in critically ill patients: a matched, risk-adjusted, cohort study. Infect Control Hosp Epidemiol 1999; 20:396–401.

83. Smith RL, Meixler SM, Simberkoff MS. Excess mortality in critically ill patients with nosocomial bloodstream infections. Chest 1991; 100:164–167.

84. Wey SB, Motomi M, Pfaller MA, Woolson RF, Wenzel RP. Hospital-acquired candidemia. The attributable mortality and excess length of stay. Arch Intern Med 1988; 148:2642–2645.

85. Rello J, Ricart M, Mirelis B, Quintana E, Gurgui M, Net A, Prats G. Nosocomial bacteremia in a medical-surgical intensive care unit: epidemiologic characteristics and factors influencing mortality in 111 episodes. Intensive Care Med 1994; 20:94–98.

86. Pittet D, Tarara D, Wenzel RP. Nosocomial bloodstream infection in critically ill patients. Excess length of stay, extra costs, and attributable mortality. JAMA 1994; 271:1598–1601.

87. Pittet D, Wenzel RP. Nosocomial bloodstream infection in the critically ill. JAMA 1994; 272:1819–1820.

88. Di Giovine B, Chenoweth C, Watts C, Higgins M. The attributable mortality and costs of primary nosocomial bloodstream infection in the intensive care unit. Am J Respir Crit Care Med 1999; 160:976–981.

89. Rello J, Ochagavia A, Sabanes E, Roque M, Mariscal D, Reynaga E, Valles J. Evaluation of outcome of intravenous catheter-related infections in critically ill patients. Am J Respir Crit Care Med 2000; 162:1027–1030.

90. Renaud B, Brun-Buisson C. Outcomes of Primary and Catheter-related Bacteremia. A cohort and case-control study in critically ill patients. Am J Respir Crit Care Med 2001; 163:1584–1590.

91. Brooks A, Ekleberry A, McMahon J, Begle R, Johnson M, Rizzo J, Zervos MJ. Evaluation of clinical practice guidelines on outcome of infection in medical intensive care unit patients. Infect Dis Clin Pract 1999; 8:97–106.

92. Raymond J, Aujard Y. Nosocomial infections in pediatric patients: a Euro-

pean, multicenter prospective study. European Study Group. Infect Control Hosp Epidemiol 2000; 21:260–263.

93. Gilio AE, Stape A, Pereira CR, Cardoso MF, Silva CV, Troster EJ. Risk factors for nosocomial infections in a critically ill pediatric population: a 25-month prospective cohort study. Infect Control Hosp Epidemiol 2000; 21:340–342.

94. Doebbeling BN, Stanley GL, Sheetz CT, Pfaller MA, Houston AK, Annis L, Li N, Wenzel RP. Comparative efficacy of alternative hand-washing agents in reducing nosocomial infections in intensive care units. NEJM 1992; 327:88–93.

95. Groot AJ, Geubbels EL, Beaumont MT, Wille JC, de Boer AS. [Hospital infections and risk factors in the intensive care units of 16 Dutch hospitals, results of surveillance of quality assurance indicators]. Ned Tijdschr Geneeskd 2001; 145:1249–1254.

96. Price J, Ekleberry A, Grover A, Melendy S, Baddam K, McMahon J, Villalba M, Johnson M, Zervos MJ. Evaluation of clinical practice guidelines on outcome of infection in patients in the surgical intensive care unit. Crit Care Med 1999; 27:2118–2124.

97. Kollef MH, Vlasnik J, Sharpless L, Pasque C, Murphy D, Fraser V. Scheduled change of antibiotic classes: a strategy to decrease the incidence of ventilator-associated pneumonia. Am J Respir Crit Care Med 1997; 156:1040–1048.

98. Velasco E, Thuler LC, Martins CA, Dias LM, Goncalves VM. Nosocomial infections in an oncology intensive care unit. Am J Infect Control 1997; 25:458–462.

99. Wurtz R, Karajovic M, Dacumos E, Jovanovic B, Hanumadass M. Nosocomial infections in a burn intensive care unit. Burns 1995; 21:181–184.

100. O'Grady NP, Alexander M, Dellinger EP, Gerberding JL, Heard SO, Maki DG, Masur H, McCormick RD, Mermel LA, Pearson ML, Raad II, Randolph A, Weinstein RA. Guidelines for the prevention of intravascular catheter-related infections. Centers for Disease Control and Prevention. Morb Mortal Wkly Rep 2002; 51(RR-10):1–29.

2

Pathogenesis of Vascular Catheter Infections

Robert J. Sherertz

Wake Forest University School of Medicine
Winston-Salem, North Carolina, U.S.A.

Several detailed summaries of the pathogenesis of vascular catheter infections have been written in recent years (1–3). Each summary contains unique information that is worth reviewing. Information presented previously is summarized subsequently, and new understandings provided by more recent studies are discussed.

A QUANTITATIVE RELATIONSHIP EXISTS BETWEEN CATHETER COLONIZATION AND INFECTION

Like many infectious diseases, vascular catheter infection is at one end of a spectrum with colonization at the other. Clinical findings clearly correlate with quantitative catheter cultures (2,3,5–15). Studies in patients have nicely shown that the more microorganisms are removed from the surface of the catheter, the greater the likelihood of pericatheter erythema and catheter-related bloodstream infection (6–12). In an animal model, it has been further shown that the amount of inflammation around a colonized catheter (determined using a histologic index) and the likelihood of developing purulence around a catheter also correlate with the number of removeable organisms (Fig. 1) (13- 15).

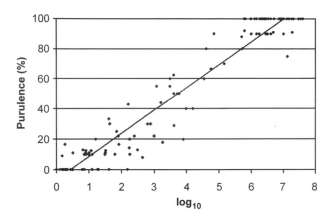

Figure 1 Association between the number of *Staphylococcus aureus* removed from the catheter and the percentage of catheters with purulence at the insertion site in a rabbit model of subcutaneous catheter infection. (From Ref. 15.)

MICROBIOLOGY OF VASCULAR CATHETER INFECTIONS

The microbiology of vascular catheter infections has changed very little over many years. The three most common organisms causing such infections are *Staphylococcus epidermidis* (and other coagulase negative staphylococci), *Staphylococcus aureus*, and *Candida* (Table 1) (1–3,6–11,16,17). *S. epidermidis* predominates in both long- and short-term catheters (17). *S. aureus* and *Candida* catheter-related infections are much more likely to be associated with positive blood cultures for unclear reasons (11). Virtually all other aerobic

Table 1 Organisms Reported in Prospective Studies in the Medical Literature to Cause Catheter-Related Bloodstream Infection

Organism	N
Coagulase negative staphylococci	27
Staphylococcus aureus	26
Yeast	17
Enterobacter	7
Serratia	5
Enterococcus	5
Klebsiella	4
Streptococcus viridans	3
Pseudomonas	3
Proteus	2
Other	1

Source: Ref. 16.

organisms known to cause nosocomial infections have been reported to cause vascular catheter infections. Anaerobic organisms and mycobacteria are extremely uncommon.

FACTORS INCREASING THE RISK OF DEVELOPING CATHETER-RELATED INFECTION: SKIN

Inserting a catheter through abnormal skin has clearly been shown to increase the risk of catheter-related infections. The prototype example of this situation is the burn patient (18). A more subtle manifestation of this same phenomenon exists in endstage HIV patients who have very high rates of *S. aureus* infection when long-term central catheters are placed (19). Although the explanation for this finding is not precisely clear, this patient group is known to have frequent dermatitis, particularly seborrheic dermatitis, and increased skin colonization +/− nasal colonization with *S. aureus* (20,21). Patients with dermatitis are known to have increased skin colonization rates with *S. aureus*, which is probably mediated by fibrinogen and fibronectin (22).

Quantitative Skin Microbiology

Data from quantitative skin microbiology have shown variations in the number of colony-forming units (cfu)/cm^2 that correlate strongly with risk of catheter-related infection (1,23,24). The findings in these studies demonstrate that peripheral catheters are exposed to lower numbers of cfu/cm^2 of skin than central venous catheters, and suggest that this may partially explain the greater risk of infection associated with central venous catheters.

Moisture at Catheter Site, Under Dressing

A pool of sweat under a plastic dressing has been shown to increase the risk of infection, but overall the risk of infection associated with plastic dressings is similar to that of gauze dressings (25).

OTHER

A number of other risk factors have been identified by multivariate analysis to increase the risk of catheter-related infection (26–38). Intrinsic risk factors include obesity, gestational age ≤32 weeks, exposure to unrelated bacteremia, second catheterization, disease of the gastrointestinal tract, chronic renal failure, and granulocytopenia (27 32). Extrinsic risk factors can be grouped by (a) catheter insertion: difficulty with insertion, inadequate aseptic technique, placing a catheter in a jugular vein or a femoral vein, type of vascular access device and how it is used; (b) catheter maintenance: increased duration of catheterization, inappropriate catheter care, contamination of the catheter hub, and increased numbers of line breaks per day; (c) hospital residence: residence within a coronary care unit or on a surgical service, transfer to another service, and (d) contamination of infusate: this can occur during manufacturing, during preparation of nutrient solutions (hyperalimentation—yeasts, 5% dextrose—Gram negative rods, lipid emulsions—Malassezia), when using multidose vials, and using warming baths for blood bank products (1–3,25,27–37). The risk of catheter-related bloodstream infection has been reported to vary as much as 50-fold, based on the type of vascular access employed, with peripheral venous catheters at one end of the spectrum and hemodialysis catheters at the other (3).

FACTORS DECREASING THE RISK OF CATHETER-RELATED INFECTION: ANTIBIOTICS

The use of systemic antibiotics during catheterization—but not at the time of insertion—decreased the risk in several studies (25,29,32,39,40). Using antibiotics as a lock solution after infusion has decreased the risk of catheter-related bloodstream infection (41–43). Although this has clearly been shown to be effective, there remain great concerns about whether this will accelerate the appearance of organisms resistant to vancomycin. The use of catheters coated with chlorhexidine and silver sulfadiazine or minocycline and rifampin have both been shown to reduce the risk of infection in comparison with uncoated catheters; and minocycline/rifampin-coated catheters were shown to be superior to chlorhexidine/silver sulfadiazine-coated catheters in randomized trials (44–46).

Improved Antisepsis

The use of chlorhexidine as a skin preparation agent has been shown to be more effective than povidone iodine (47). Maximum sterile barriers have also been shown to reduce the risk of infection in comparison with a small drape, no sterile gown, etc. (48). Educational interventions aimed at improving the technique of the physicians inserting the catheters have also been associated with lower rates of catheter-related bloodstream infection (49–51).

SOURCE OF MICROORGANISMS

Initial catheter colonization may originate from one of five major locations: skin, catheter hub, hematogenous seeding, infusion fluid, or contiguous infection (Fig. 2). Subsequent to initial colonization, a biofilm develops at a variable rate, but can be present uniformly in central venous catheters by three days after insertion (4). A striking and still unexplained finding is that approximately half of the catheters with biofilms identifiable by electron microscopy have visible bacteria that do not grow (4). The majority of the organisms that do not grow in routine cultures are coagulase negative staphylococci when studied using molecular probes (Guy Cook, Bacterin, Inc., Boseman, MT; personal communication). For catheters with microorganisms

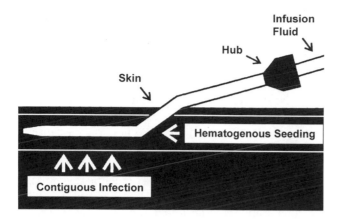

Figure 2 Sources of vascular catheter infection. Vascular catheter infection develops most commonly from organisms originating at the skin surface, followed by the catheter hub, and then much less frequently from infusion fluid, hematogenous seeding, or contiguous infection.

that can be grown by culture, the time course of their appearance is variable. In intensive care unit (ICU) patients, the sequence of initial colonization is first from the skin (average 5.1 days from insertion), then from hematogenous seeding (average 8.6 days), and finally from the catheter hub (average 13.1 days) in about equal proportions, with other sources being much less common (<5%). In long-term catheters, the majority of colonization originates from the hub (5). These findings suggest that early colonization relates to the insertion process and later colonization to line breaks, with hematogenous seeding being a risk in patients who develop bloodstream infection from a source elsewhere in the body. The risk of hematogenous seeding associated with long-term catheters has not been clearly defined.

A recent study by Atela et al. utilized molecular typing techniques and surveillance cultures of the vascular catheter skin exit site and catheter hub in an ICU patient population to evaluate the source of microorganisms (52). Approximately half of the organisms colonizing catheter tips were found to match up with either skin strains (early) or hub strains (later, >8 days after insertion); the source of the other half was not identified. The finding of organisms originating from the skin early and from the hub later is consistent with other studies (1–3). The high frequency of isolates for sources other than skin or hub is likely to be explained by the finding that in ICU patients, up to 50% of organisms colonizing the catheter tip may have arrived hemagenously (5,28). Another possibility is suggested by a study by Frebourg et al. (53). Twenty of 54 patients with coagulase-negative staphylococci (CNS) on their vascular catheter had a matching strain (using molecular typing) in their nose. This raised the possibility that, like *S. aureus*, the nose may be a source for CNS infecting vascular catheters. An additional new finding from the study by Atela et al. was that CNS strains were found to change dynamically on the skin, whereas other organisms were more likely to maintain persistent colonization (52). The dynamic nature of skin colonization by CNS is not yet understood, but may be quite important in understanding the pathogenesis of catheter-related infections.

Two clinical studies raise the possibility that certain strains of CNS are more transmissible or better able to cause catheter-related infection. Nouwen et al. found that two genotypes of CNS predominated (74%) as a cause of catheter-related infections in a group of hematology oncology patients (54). In a more mixed group of patients with CNS catheter-related infections, Worthington et al. found that 25% of the isolates have identical genotypes (55). The competitive advantage of the clonal isolates has not yet been identified and deserves further study to better understand the mechanism.

Biofilm

The importance of biofilm formation in vascular catheter infections is becoming increasingly apparent. The greatest progress in understanding the importance of biofilms in the pathogenesis of catheter-related infection has occurred with *S. epidermidis*. Initial attachment appears to be mediated by a protein autolysin (AtlE) (56,57). Subsequent adherence and biofilm formation are mediated by polysaccharide intercellular adhesin (PIA) (58–60). In a rat model, *S. epidermidis* isolates lacking AtlE or PIA are significantly less likely ($P < 0.05$) to cause catheter infection, peripheral bacteremia, and metastatic infection (61,62). Even more interesting in this regard is that the *ica* operon that encodes for PIA in *S. epidermidis* can also be found in *S. aureus* isolates from patients with catheter-related infection or prosthetic joint infection, suggesting that the ability to form biofilm may be more conserved in staphylococci than previously appreciated (63,64). The *ica* locus appears to be regulated by the *agr* quorum-sensing system (65). *S. aureus* strains that are *agr*-positive are unlikely to form biofilms (6%), whereas *agr*-negative strains form biofilms 78% of the time. Importantly, blockers that can inhibit *S. aureus* quorum sensing increase biofilm formation. Since quorum-sensing blockers are being considered as adjuncts to antibiotic therapy, this could actually negatively affect *S. aureus* by augmenting biofilm formation. This could paradoxically decrease the efficacy of antibiotics by increasing the amount of drug necessary to kill the organism 100- to 1000-fold.

THE INTERACTION BETWEEN CATHETER-RELATED THROMBOSIS AND INFECTION

There are a number of recent studies examining the relationship between thrombosis and indwelling vascular catheters. Ultrasound studies have shown that early (≤24 h) catheter-related thrombosis occurs near the site of insertion and later (>24 h) thrombosis occurs near the catheter tip (66). Catheters left in place for more than a few days will be encased by a fibrin sleeve, which will be transformed into a collagen tunnel covered by endothelial cells within a few months (67). A number of factors further affect the natural history of clot formation. Peripherally inserted central venous catheters (PICC) appear to have a higher risk of thrombosis than centrally inserted catheters (68). Some studies suggest that there is even a hierarchy of thrombosis risk for central catheters: femoral catheters > subclavian catheters > internal jugular catheters (34,69). Tip position can even further modify the risk of thrombosis for central venous catheters; peripheral location (axillosubclavian-innominate) or right atrium > superior vena cava (70–73). Catheter material may affect the risk with silicone having up to a threefold greater risk than other materials (74). Some recent data suggest that antibodies to certain blood coagulation factors, such as inhibitors to factors V and VIII, may increase the risk of catheter-related thrombosis through as yet unclear mechanisms (75,76). Bone marrow harvesting appears to induce a short-term hypercoaguable state (77). There are some data in pediatric oncology patients that suggest that genetic risk factors for intravascular thrombosis such as factor V Leiden, etc. may increase the risk of catheter-related thrombosis (78,79), but this seems less clear with adults (80,81).

An ongoing speculation is whether there is a link between catheter-related infection and catheter-related thrombosis; in particular, which comes first (82–85). Such speculations have been amplified by a number of studies with heparin-coated central venous catheters, which have shown a reduction in both catheter-related thrombosis and catheter-related infection (86,87). In these studies, heparin is attached to the catheter via benzalkonium chloride, which has substantial antibacterial properties and may be the source of the reduction in risk of infection. Whether the risk of thrombosis was reduced in these studies by the bound heparin, the benzalkonium chloride, or both has not been determined. This association has assumed even greater importance since the realization that there is a statistically significant increase in the risk of deep venous thrombosis associated with femoral venous catheterization (34,88), which can be prevented by using heparin-bonded catheters (86,87). Recent in vitro studies have shown that surface manipulations of polyurethane can lead to differences in protein and platelet deposition with associated differences in bacterial adherence (89). No in vivo data exist to show whether such observations will have clinical significance.

FUTURE RESEARCH

Recent work clearly suggests that we need to understand why certain strains of *S. aureus* and *S. epidermidis* are much more likely to cause catheter-related infections. In particular, can a better understanding of biofilm formation lead to interventions that reduce the risk of infection without having to resort to antibiotic coatings that may engender resistance to antibiotics used therapeutically? Another area deserving attention is to develop a better understanding of the relationship between catheter colonization and clot formation, especially since there are hints suggesting that catheter colonization may come first.

REFERENCES

1. Maki DG. Infections caused by intravascular devices used for infusion therapy: pathogenesis, prevention, and management. In: Bisno AL, Waldvogel FA, eds. Infections Associated with Indwelling Medical Devices. Washington, D.C.: ASM Press, 1994:155–212.
2. Sherertz RJ. Pathogenesis of vascular catheter-related infections. In: Seifert H, Jansen B, Farr BM, eds. Catheter-Related Infections. New York: Marcel Dekker, Inc., 1997:1–30.
3. Sherertz RJ. Pathogenesis of vascular catheter infections. In: Waldvogel FA, Bisno AL, eds. Infections Associated with Indwelling Medical Devices. ASM Press, 2000:111–125.
4. Raad I, Costerton W, Sabharwal U, Sacilowski M, Anaissie E, Bodey GP. Ultrastructural analysis of indwelling vascular catheters: a quantitative relationship between luminal colonization and curation of placement. J Infect Dis 1993; 168:400–407.
5. Sherertz RJ, Heard SO, Raad II. Diagnosis of triple-lumen catheter infection: comparison of roll plate, sonication, and flushing methodologies. J Clin Microbiol 1997; 35:641–646.
6. Maki DG, Weise CE, Sarafin HW. A semi-quantitative culture method for identifying intravenous-catheter-related infection. N Engl J Med 1977; 296:1305–1309.
7. Cleri DJ, Corrado ML, Seligman SJ. Quantitative culture of intravenous catheters and other intravascular inserts. J Infect Dis 1980; 141:781–786.
8. Bjornson HS, Colley R, Bower RH, Duty VP, Schwartz-Fulton JT, Fischer JE. Association between microorganism growth at the catheter insertion site and colonization of the catheter in patients receiving total parenteral nutrition. Surgery 1982; 92:721–727.
9. Brun-Buisson C, Abrouk F, Legrand P, Huet Y, Larabi S, Rapin M. Diagnosis of central venous catheter-related sepsis. Critical level of quantitative tip cultures. Arch Intern Med 1987; 147:873–877.
10. Heard SO, Davis RF, Sherertz RJ, Mikhail MS, Gallagher RC, Layon AJ, Gallagher TJ. Influence of sterile protective sleeves on the sterility of pulmonary artery catheters. Crit Care Med 1987; 15:499–502.
11. Sherertz RJ, Raad II, Belani A, Koo LC, Rand KH, Pickett DL, Straub SA, Fauerbach LL. Three-year exerience with sonicated vascular catheter cultures in a clinical microbiology laboratory. J Clin Microbiol 1990; 28:76–82.
12. Siegman-Igra Y, Anglim AM, Shapiro DE, Adal KA, Strain BA, Farr BM. Diagnosis of vascular catheter-related bloodstream infection: a meta-analysis. J Clin Microbiol 1997; 35:928–936.

13. Carruth WA, Byron MP, Solomon DD, White WL, Stoddard GJ, Marosok RD, Sherertz RJ. Subcutaneous, catheter-related inflammation in a rabbit model correlates with peripheral vein phlebitis in human volunteers. J Biomed Mater Res 1994; 28:259–267.

14. Sherertz RJ, Carruth WA, Marosok RD, Espeland MA, Johnson RA, Solomon DD. Contribution of vascular catheter material to the pathogenesis of infection: the enhanced risk of silicone in vivo. J Biomed Mat Res 1995; 29:635–645.

15. Bassetti S, Hu J, D'Agostino RB, Sherertz RJ. In vitro zones of inhibition of coated vascular catheters predict efficacy in prevention catheter infection with *Staphylococcus aureus* in vivo. Eur J Clin Microbiol Infect Dis 2000; 19:612–617.

16. Hampton AA, Sherertz RJ. Vascular-access infections in hospitalized patients. Surg Clin N Amer 1988; 68:57–71.

17. Widmer AF. Intravenous-related infections. In: Wenzel RP, ed. Prevention and Control of Nosocomial Infections. Baltimore: Williams & Wilkins, 1997:771–805.

18. Franceschi D, Gerding RL, Phillips G, Fratianne RB. Risk factors associated with intravascular catheter infections in burned patients: a prospective, randomized study. Journal of Trauma Injury Infection & Critical Care 1989; 29:811–816.

19. Raviglione MC, Battan R, Pablos-Mendez A, Aceves-Casillas P, Mullen MP, Taranta A. Infections associated with Hickman catheters in patients with acquired immunodeficiency syndrome. Am J Med 1989; 86:780–786.

20. Shapiro M, Smith KJ, James WD, Giblin WJ, Margolis DJ, Foglia AN, McGinley K, Leyden JJ. Cutaneous microenvironment of human immunodeficiency virus (HIV)-seropositive and HIV-seronegative individuals, with special reference to *Staphylococcus aureus* colonization. J Clin Microbiol 2000; 38:3174–3178.

21. Nguyen MH, Kauffman CA, Goodman RP, Squier C, Arbeit RD, Singh N, Wagener MM, Yu VL. Nasal carriage of and infection with *Staphylococcus aureus* in HIV-infected patients. Ann Intern Med 1999; 130:221–225.

22. Cho SH, Strickland I, Tomkinson A, Fehringer AP, Gelfand EW, Leung DY. Preferential binding of *Staphylococcus aureus* to skin sites of Th2-mediated inflammation in a murine model. J Invest Derm 2001; 116:658–663.

23. Maki DG. Marked differences in insertion sites for central venous, arterial and peripheral IV catheters: the major reason for differing risks of catheter-related infection? Program and abstracts of the thirtieth Interscience Conference on Antimicrobial Agents and Chemotherapy, Atlanta, GA, October 1990. Abstract #712.

24. Bertone SA, Fisher MC, Mortensen JE. Quantitative skin cultures at potential catheter sites in neonates. Infect Control Hosp Epidemiol 1994; 15:315–318.

25. Maki DG, Ringer M. Evaluation of dressing regimens for prevention of infection with peripheral intravenous catheters. JAMA 1987; 258:2396–2403.

26. Maki DG, Mermel LA. Infections due to infusion therapy. In: Bennett JV, Brachman PS, eds. Hospital Infections. Philadelphia: Lippincott-Raven, 1998:725–740.

27. Newman KA, Reed WP, Schimpff SC, Bustamante CI, Wade JC. Hickman

catheters in association with intensive cancer chemotherapy. Support Care Cancer 1993; 1:92–97.

28. Maki DG, Will L. Risk factors for central venous catheter-related infection with the ICU: a prospective study of 345 catheters. Programs and abstracts of the thirtiety Interscience Conference on Antimicrobial Agents and Chemotherapy, Atlanta, GA, October 1990. Abstract #205.

29. Pittet D. Intravenous catheter-related infections: current understanding. Programs and abstracts of the thirty-second Interscience Conference on Antimicrobial Agents and Chemotherapy, Anaheim, CA, 1992. Abstract #411.

30. Ena J, Cercenado E, Martinez D, Bouza E. Cross-sectional epidemiology of phlebitis and catheter-related infections. Infect Control Hosp Epidemiol 1992; 13:15–20.

31. Almirall J, Gonzalez J, Rello J, Campistol JM, Montoliu J, Puig de la Bellacasa J, Revert L, Gatell JM. Infection of hemodialysis catheters: incidence and mechanisms. Am J Nephrol 1989; 9:454–459.

32. Garland JS, Buck RK, Maloney P, Durkin DM, Toth-Lloyd S, Duffy M, Szocik P. McAuliffe TL, Goldmann D. Comparison of 10% povidone-iodine and 0.5% chlorhexidine gluconate for the prevention of peripheral intravenous catheter colonization in neonates: a prospective trial. Ped Infect Dis J 1995; 14:510–516.

33. Conly JM, Grieves K, Peters BA. A prospective, randomized study comparing transparent and dry gauze dressings for central venous catheters. J Infect Dis 1989; 159:310–319.

34. Merrer J, De Jonghe B, Golliot F, Lefrant JY, Raffy B, Barre E, Rigaud JP, Casciani D, Misset B, Bosquet C, Outin H, Brun-Buisson C, Nitenberg G; French Catheter Study Group in Intensive Care. Complications of femoral and subclavian venous catheterization in critically ill patients: a randomized controlled trial. JAMA 2001; 286:700–707.

35. Duthoit D, Devleeshouwer C, Paesmans M, et al. Infection of totally implantable chamber catheters in cancer patients: multivariate analysis of risk factors. Programs and abstracts of the thirty-third Interscience Conference on Antimicrobial Agents and Chemotherapy, New Orleans, LA, October 1993. Abstract #416.

36. Sherertz RJ, Gledhill KS, Hampton KD, Pfaller MA, Givner LB, Abramson JS, Dillard RG. Outbreak of *Candida* bloodstream infections associated with retrograde medication administration in a neonatal intensive care unit. J Ped 1992; 120:455–461.

37. Mermel LA, McCormick RD, Springman SR, Maki DG. The pathogenesis and epidemiology of catheter-related infection with pulmonary artery Swan-Ganz catheters: a prospective study utilizing molecular subtyping. Am J Med 1991; 91(suppl 3B):197S–205S.

38. Moro ML, Vigano EF, Cozzi Lepri A. Risk factors for central venous catheter-related infections in surgical and intensive care units. Infect Control Hosp Epidemiol 1994; 15:253–264.

39. Rello J, Coll P, Net A, Prats G. Infection of pulmonary artery catheters: epidemiologic characteristics and multivariate analysis of risk factors. Chest 1993; 103:132–136.

40. Sherertz RJ, Falk RJ, Huffman KA, Thomann CA, Mattern WD. Infections associated with subclavian Uldall catheters. Arch Intern Med 1983; 143:52–56.

41. Barriga FJ, Varas M, Potin M, Sapunar F, Rojo H, Martinez A, Capdeville V, Becker A, Vial PA. Efficacy of a vancomycin solution to prevent bacteremia associated with indwelling central venous catheter in neutropenic and non-neutropenic cancer patients. Med Ped Oncol 1997; 28:196–200.

42. Carratala J, Niubo J, Fernandez-Sevilla A, Juve E, Castellsague X, Berlanga J, Linares J, Gudiol F. Randomized, double-blind trial of an antibiotic-lock technique for prevention of gram-positive central venous catheter-related infection in neutropenic patients with cancer. Antimicrob Ag Chemother 1999; 43:2200–2204.

43. Henrickson KJ, Axtell RA, Hoover SM, Kuhn SM, Pritchett J, Kehl SC, Klein JP. Prevention of central venous catheter-related infections and thrombotic events in immunocompromised children by the use of vancomycin/ciprofloxacin/heparin flush solution: a randomized, multicenter, double-blind trial. J Clin Oncol 2000; 18:1269–1278.

44. Raad I, Darouiche R, Dupuis J, Abi-Said D, Gabrielli A, Hachem R, Wall M, Harris R, Jones J, Buzaid A, Robertson C, Shenaq S, Curling P, Burke T, Ericsson C. Texas Medical Center Catheter Study Group. Ann Intern Med 1997; 127:267–275.

45. Maki DG, Stolz SM, Wheeler S, Mermel LA. Prevention of central venous catheter-related bloodstream infection by use of an antiseptic-impregnated catheter. A randomized, controlled trial. Ann Intern Med 1997; 127:257–265.

46. Darouiche RO, Raad II, Heard SO, Thornby JI, Wenker OC, Gabrielli A, Berg J, Khardori N, Hanna H, Hachem R, Harris RL, Mayhall G. Catheter Study Group. A comparison of two antimicrobial-impregnated central venous catheters. N Engl J Med 1999; 340:1–8.

47. Maki DG, Alvarado CJ, Ringer MA. A prospective, randomized trial of povidone-iodine, alcohol and chlorhexidine for prevention of infection with central venous and arterial catheters. Lancet 1991; 338:339–343.

48. Raad II, Hohn DC, Gilbreath BJ, Suleiman N, Hill LA, Bruso PA, Marts K, Mansfield PF, Bodey GP. Prevention of central venous catheter-related infections by using maximal sterile barrier precautions during insertion. Infect Control Hosp Epidemiol 1994; 15:231–238.

49. Sherertz RJ, Ely EW, Westbrook DM, Gledhill KS, Streed SA, Kiger B, Flynn L, Hayes S, Strong S, Cruz J, Bowton DL, Hulgan T, Haponik EF. Education of training physicians can decrease the risk of vascular catheter infections. Ann Intern Med 2000; 132(18):641–648.

50. Eggimann P, Harbarth S, Constantin MN, Touveneau S, Chevrolet JC, Pittet D. Impact of a prevention strategy targeted at vascular-access care on incidence of infections acquired in intensive care. Lancet 2000; 355:1864–1868.

51. Coopersmith CM, Rebmann TL, Zack JE, Ward MR, Corcoran RM, Schallom ME, Sona CS, Buchman TG, Boyle WA, Polish LB, Fraser VJ. Effect of an education program on decreasing catheter-related bloodstream infections in the surgical intensive care unit. Crit Care Med 2002; 30:59–64.

52. Atela I, Coll P, Rello J, Quintana E, Barrio J, March F, Sanchez F, Barraquer P, Ballus J, Cotura A, Prats G. Serial surveillance cultures on skin and catheter

hub specimens from critically ill patients with central venous catheters: molecular epidemiology of infection and implications for clinical management and research. J Clin Microbiol 1997; 35:1784–1790.

53. Frebourg NB, Cauliez B, Lemeland J-F. Evidence for nasal carriage of methicillin-resistant staphylococci colonizing intravascular devices. J Clin Microbiol 1999; 37:1182–1185.

54. Nouwen JL, van Belkum A, de Marie S, Sluijs J, Wielenga JJ, Kluytmans JA, Verbrugh HA. Clonal expansion of *Staphylococcus epidermidis* strains causing Hickman catheter-related infections in a hemato-oncologic department. J Clin Microbiol 1998; 36: 2696–2702.

55. Worthington T, Lambert PA, Elliott TSJ. Is hospital-acquired intravascular catheter-related sepsis associated with outbreak strains of coagulase-negative staphylococci? J Hosp Infect 2000; 46:130–134.

56. Heilmann C, Gerke C, Perdreau-Remington F, Gotz F. Characterization of Tn917 insertion mutuants of *Staphylococcus epidermidis* affected in biofilm formation. Infect Immun 1996; 64:227–232.

57. Heilmann C, Hussain M, Peters G, Gotz F. Evidence for autolysin-mediated primary attachment of *Staphylococcus epidermidis* to a polystyrene surface. Mol Microbiol 1997; 24:1013–1024.

58. Mack D, Fischer W, Krokotsch A, Leopold K, Hartmann R, Egge H, Laufs R. The intercellular adhesion involved in biofilm accumulation of *Staphylococcus epidermidis* is a linear β-1, 6-linked glucosaminoglycan: purification and structural analysis. J Bacteriol 1996; 178:175–183.

59. Mack D, Nedelmann M, Krokotsch A, Schwarzkopf A, Heesemann J, Laufs R. Characterization of transposon mutants of biofilm-producing *Staphylcoccus epidermidis* impaired in the accumulative phase of biofilm production: genetic identification of a hexosamine-containing polysaccharide intercellular adhesion. Infect Immun 1994; 62:3244–3253.

60. Mack D, Siemssen N, Laufs R. Parallel induction by glucose of adherence and a polysaccharide antigen specific for plastic-adherent *Staphylococcus epidermidis*: evidence for functional relation to intercellular adhesion. Infect Immun 1992; 60:2048–2057.

61. Rupp ME, Ulphani JS, Fey PD, Mack D. Characterization of *Staphylococcus epidermidis* polysaccharide intercellular adhesion/hemagglutinin in the pathogenesis of intravascular catheter-associated infection in a rat model. Infect Immun 1999; 67:2656–2659.

62. Rupp ME, Fey PD, Heilmann C, Gotz F. Characterization of the importance of *Staphylococcus epidermidis* autolysin and polysaccharide intercellular adhesion in the pathogenesis of intravascular catheter-associated infection in a rat model. J Infect Dis 2001; 183:1038–1042.

63. Arciola CR, Baldassarri L, Montanaro L. Presence of *ica*A and *ica*D genes and slime production in a collection of staphylococcal strains from catheter-associated infections. J Clin Microbiol 2001; 39:2151–2156.

64. Fowler VG, Fey PD, Reller LB, Chamis AL, Corey GR, Rupp ME. The intercellular adhesion locus *ica* is present in clinical isolates of *Staphylococcus aureus* from bacteremic patients with infected and uninfected joints. Med Microbiol Immunol 2001; 189:127–131.

65. Vuong C, Saenz HL, Gotz F, Otto M. Impact of the *agr* quorum-sensing system on adherence to polystyrene in *Staphylococcus aureus*. J Infect Dis 2000; 182:1688–1693.
66. Everitt NJ, Krupowicz DW, Evans JA, McMahon MJ. Ultrasonographic investigation of the pathogenesis of infusion thrombophlebitis. Br J Surg 1997; 84:642–645.
67. Xiang DZ, Verbeken EK, van Lommel AT, Stas M, de Wever I. Composition and formation of the sleeve enveloping a central venous catheter. J Vasc Surg 1998; 28:260–271.
68. Kuriakose P, Colon-Otero G, Paz-Fumagalli R. Risk of deep venous thrombosis associated with chest versus arm central venous subcutaneous port catheters: a 5-year single-institution retrospective study. J Vasc Interv Radiol 2002; 13:179–184.
69. Trerotola SO, Kuhn-Fulton J, Johnson MS, Shah H, Ambrosius WT, Kneebone PH. Tunneled infusion catheters: increased incidence of symptomatic venous thrombosis after subclavian versus internal jugular access. Radiol 2000; 217:89–93.
70. Kearns PJ, Coleman S, Wehner JH. Complications of long arm-catheters: a randomized trial of central vs peripheral tip location. JPEN 1996; 20, 20–24.
71. Cohn DE, Mutch DG, Rader JS, Farrell M, Awantang R, Herzog TJ. Factors predicting subcutaneous implanted central venous port function: the relationship between catheter tip location and port failure in patients with gynecologic malignancies. Gyn Oncol 2001; 83:533–536.
72. Luciani A, Clement O, Halimi P, Goudot D, Portier F, Bassot V, Luciani JA, Avan P, Frija G, Bonfils P. Catheter-related upper extremity deep venous thrombosis in cancer patients: a prospective study based on Doppler US. Radiol 2001; 220:655–660.
73. Gilon D, Schechter D, Rein AJ, Gimmon Z, Or R, Rozenman Y, Slavin S, Gotsman MS, Nagler A. Right atrial thrombi are related to indwelling central venous catheter position: insights into time course and possible mechanism of formation. Am Heart J 1998; 135:457–462.
74. Mhic Iomhair M, Lavelle SM. The antithrombotic effect of some EURO-BIOMAT project test polymers in vivo. Technol & Health Care 1996; 4:385–388.
75. Sands JJ, Nudo SA, Moore KD, Ortel TL. Antibodies to prothrombin, factor V, and B$_2$-glycoprotein I and vascular access thrombosis. ASAIO J 2001 Sept–Oct; 47(5):507–510.
76. Collins PW, Khair KS, Liesner R, Hann IM. Complications experienced with central venous catheters in children with congenital bleeding disorders. Br J Haematol 1997; 99:206–208.
77. Sletnes KE, Holte H, Halvorsen S, Jakobsen E, Wisloff F, Kvaloy S. Activation of coagulation and deep vein thrombosis after bone marrow harvesting and insertion of a Hickman-catheter in ABMT patients with malignant lymphoma. Bone Marrow Transplantation 1996; 17:577–581.
78. Wermes C, Prondzinski M von D, Lichtinghagen R, Barthels M, Welte K, Sykora K-W. Clinical relevance of genetic risk factors for thrombosis in paediatric oncology patients with central venous catheters. Eur J Pediatr 1999; 158:S143.

79. Knofler R, Siegert E, Lauterbach I, Taut-Sack H, Siegert G, Gehrisch S, Muller D, Rupprecht E, Kabus M. Clinical importance of prothrombotic risk factors in pediatric patients with malignancy-impact of central venous lines. Eur J Pediatr 1999; 158, S147–S150.

80. Riordan M, Weiden PL. Factor V Leiden mutation does not account for central venous catheter-related thrombosis. Am J Hematol 1998; 58:150–152.

81. Leebeek FWG, Stadhouders NAM, van Stein D, Gomez-Garcia EB, Kappers-Klunne MC. Hypercoagulability states in upper-extremity deep venous thrombosis. Am J Hematol 2001; 67:15–19.

82. Press OW, Ramsey PG, Larson EB, Fefer A, Hickman RO. Hickman catheter infections in patients with malignancies. Med 1984; 63:189–200.

83. Raad II, Luna M, Khalil S-AM, Costerton JW, Lam C, Bodey GP. The relationship between the thrombotic and infectious complications of central venous catheters. JAMA 1994; 271:1014–1016.

84. Timsit JF, Farkas JC, Boyer JM, Martin JB, Misset B, Renaud B, Carlet J. Central vein catheter-related thrombosis in intensive care patients: incidence, risk factors, and relationship with catheter-related sepsis. Chest 1998; 114:207–213.

85. Eastman ME, Khorsand M, Maki DG, Williams EC, Kim K, Sondel PM, Schiller JH, Albertini MR. Central venous device-related infection and thrombosis in patients treated with moderate dose continuous-infusion interleukin-2. Cancer 2001; 91:806–814.

86. Krafte-Jacobs B, Sivit CJ, Meijia R, Pollack MM. Catheter-related thrombosis in critically ill children: comparison of catheters with and without heparin-bonding. J Pediatr 1995; 126:50–54.

87. Pierce CM, Wade A, Mok Q. Heparin-bonded central venous lines reduce thrombotic and infective complications in critically ill children. Intensive Care Med 2000; 26:967–972.

88. Mian NZ, Bayly R, Schreck DM, Besserman EB, Richmand D. Incidence of deep venous thrombosis associated with femoral venous catheterization. Acad Emerg Med 1997; 4:1118–1121.

89. Baumgartner JN, Cooper SL. Bacterial adhesion on polyurethane surfaces conditioned with thrombus components. ASAIO J 1996; 42:M476–M479.

3

Diagnosis of Catheter-Related Infections

François Blot

Service de Réanimation Polyvalente
Institut Gustave Roussy
Villejuif, France

INTRODUCTION

Intravascular devices are used increasingly in new areas of medical care, including antineoplastic therapy in oncology/hematology, treatment of chronic infectious diseases, total parenteral nutrition, and management of critically ill patients. Central venous catheters (CVCs) are a leading source of nosocomial infections, and catheter-related infection (CRI) poses a number of problems in terms of risk factors, diagnosis, treatment, and prevention. Intravascular CRIs result in increased hospital costs, duration of hospitalization, and patient morbidity (1).

Clinical findings are not sufficient to establish the diagnosis of infections related to a CVC (2–4); the present chapter will only superficially deal with the description of clinical diagnosis. A definite diagnosis of CRI usually requires the removal of the catheter for catheter-tip culture, and catheter-tip culture methods will be described later. However, over 75% of CVCs that are removed because of suspicion of CRI are removed unnecessarily, since the septic focus may be found in another anatomic site (2). Diagnostic techniques have been proposed to establish the diagnosis of CRI and to avoid unjustified removal of the catheter. This chapter will focus mainly on the microbiological diagnosis of CRI, with and without catheter removal.

PATHOGENESIS

Pathogenesis of vascular CRI is detailed in another chapter. However, it is important to address briefly the main routes of colonization of catheters, which may influence the diagnostic approach to CRIs.

Colonization of the catheter may occur by means of two major pathways that have been traditionally opposed: the extraluminal or the intraluminal route. In fact, these two pathways to CRI occur at different times in the course of catheterization (5). The extraluminal route (from the cutaneous entry site) predominates for short-term catheters (i.e., < 30 days), such as those inserted in the intensive care unit. Conversely, endoluminal contamination is the most frequent route of microbial seeding in prolonged indwelling vascular catheters, thus predominating in patients with total parenteral nutrition or in cancer patients with long-term catheters for chemotherapy (6). Linares et al., investigating 135 subclavian catheters in patients on total parenteral nutrition, concluded that the catheter hub was the source of infection in 14 (70%) of 20 episodes of catheter-related bloodstream infections (CR-BSIs) (7). Logically, the authors concluded that the most common site of origin of organisms causing CRI was the catheter hub, in this setting.

Other routes for CRIs include hematogenous seeding of the catheter during an episode of secondary bacteremia, or contamination of the infusate. Overall, in clinical practice, about 65% of the CRIs originate from the skin, 30% from the contaminated hub, and 5% from other pathways (5). In a study by Cercenado et al., among 125 patients hospitalized in intensive care units and medical and surgical wards, 56.5% of CRIs had an external origin, 22.5% had an internal origin, and 15% had both origins (8).

The accuracy of each diagnostic approach is dependent on the main pathway of colonization involved. Diagnostic techniques which explore the external surface of the catheter are mainly designed for short-term catheters contaminated by the extraluminal route. Methods exploring both external and internal surfaces of the catheter tip are obviously appropriate for diagnosing either short-term or long-term intravascular CRIs. This point will be detailed later in this chapter.

In summary, short-term catheter-related infections will be better diagnosed by techniques exploring the extraluminal pathway of colonization, from the cutaneous entry site of the catheter. Conversely, long-term catheter-related infections are better diagnosed by techniques exploring the endoluminal pathway of colonization, from the hub of the catheter.

DEFINITIONS AND CLINICAL DIAGNOSIS

CRIs may be separated into localized and systemic infections. Localized infections, such as exit-site infections, pocket infections, or tunnel infections, are confined to the catheter and surrounding tissues. Systemic infections are catheter-related bloodstream infections (CR-BSIs), i.e., bacteremia or septicemia. Infusate-related bloodstream infections are included in the category of systemic infections, as well as infectious complications such as septic thrombophlebitis, endocarditis, or metastatic infection (9).

Clinical findings are not sufficient to establish the diagnosis of infections related to a CVC. Except in some very typical cases, local or systemic signs of infection lack sensitivity or specificity. In a clinical study on 101 intravenous catheters from 82 patients, local inflammation was not significantly associated with CRI, with the exception of gross pus on the catheter exit site (4). In a more recent study, the rate of colonized CVCs was similar whatever the indication for catheter removal was: systemic sepsis (36.7%), local sepsis (36.4%), CVC no longer needed (31.3%), or death (30%) (10). This finding underlines the lack of specificity of clinical suspicion of CRI based on local or systemic signs of infection.

Local Infections

Superficial signs of infection are often, but not always, present in cases of colonization of the catheter surface; inflammation at the catheter exit site may be lacking in as many as 70% of CR-BSIs. Conversely, inflammation is not always due to infection, whereas purulence around the CVC and bacteremia have great specificity but are poorly sensitive (1). The presence of components of inflammation may be helpful for the diagnosis of peripheral CRI, but is rare in CVC-related infections. In the classical study by Maki et al. (11), local inflammation was present in only 64% of catheters that were positive on semiquantitative culture, and in as many as 18% of culture-negative ones. Among 142 catheters used for total parenteral nutrition, CRI was associated with the presence of erythema larger than 4 mm in diameter at the insertion site (12). In this study, however, there was no significant association between CRI and either swelling, tenderness, or extravasation of fluid at the insertion site (12).

Definitions of exit-site, pocket, and tunnel infections and of superficial suppurative thrombophlebitis are given in Table 1 (1). Exit-site infections are characterized by inflammation localized in the immediate area of the catheter exit site. Exit-site infections can often be cured by means of antibiotics and local care (13), except if *Staphylococcus aureus* or *Pseudomonas aeruginosa* are cultured from the exit site. Conversely, catheter removal is required to achieve cure in most tunnel (13) and pocket infections.

Superficial suppurative thrombophlebitis is frequently associated with thrombosis and bacteremia. Burn patients particularly are exposed to this complication. Signs of local inflammation are commonly present in the upper extremities. Conversely, thrombophlebitis is often difficult to identify when catheters are inserted in the lower extremities, since local signs of inflammation may be absent in as many as two-thirds of patients. Therefore, suppu-

Table 1 Commonly Used Definitions of Catheter-Related Infections

Local infections
  Exit-site infections: erythema, increased warmth, tenderness, induration,
    or purulence within 2 cm of the skin at the exit site of the catheter.
  Pocket infections of totally implanted devices: erythema and necrosis of the skin
    over the reservoir, or purulent exudate in the subcutaneous pocket containing
    the reservoir.
  Tunnel infections: erythema, tenderness, and induration in the tissues overlying the
    catheter and >2 cm from the exit site.
  Superficial suppurative thrombophlebitis: inflammation of the vein wall due to the
    presence of microorganisms.
Systemic infections
  Catheter-related bloodstream infections: isolation of the same organism (identical
    species, antibiogram) from a catheter segment culture and from the blood of a
    patient with accompanying clinical symptoms of bloodstream infections, in the
    absence of another apparent source of infection.
  Infusate-related bloodstream infections: isolation of the same microorganism from
    infusate and from separate percutaneous blood cultures, without another
    identifiable source of infection.

Source: Ref. 1.

rative thrombophlebitis may be revealed tardily by a picture of septic shock, or by pulmonary abscesses. A duration of intravenous catheterization greater than four days is an important risk factor for suppurative thrombophlebitis.

Systemic Infections

Catheter-related bloodstream infections are defined in Table 1 (1). Fever, with or without chills, is the most sensitive finding, but it has poor specificity for the diagnosis of CR-BSI (1), especially in critically ill or cancer patients. In the absence of laboratory confirmation, the cure of the sepsis syndrome or return to a normal temperature after removal of an implicated catheter from a patient with BSI may be considered indirect evidence of CR-BSI (1,14). Fever, chills, or hypotension at the time of catheter connection should also increase the suspicion of CRI. Finally, a CR-BSI is likely when the bacteremia or fungemia is due to a common skin organism (such as coagulase-negative staphylococci, propionibacterium, micrococcus, *Bacillus* sp.), *S. aureus*, or *Candida* spp., and no apparent source of sepsis is identified except the catheter (14). In contrast, patients with catheter-tip cultures positive for *S. aureus* have a high risk to develop bacteremia from this microorganism, whereas the risk is lower for coagulase-negative staphylococci (15).

Thoracic central vein suppurative thrombophlebitis occurs in patients with CVCs. The systemic findings of sepsis overshadow any local finding of venous occlusion; a superior vena cava syndrome is rare in this setting. When a CR-BSI fails to be resolved after catheter removal and despite appropriate antimicrobial therapy, a suppurative thrombophlebitis should be suspected.

In summary, local or systemic signs of infection lack sensitivity or specificity, and are not sufficient to establish the diagnosis of CRI. Inflammation at the exit site is not always due to infection, and may be lacking in 70% of CR-BSI. Purulence around the catheter has great specificity, but is poorly sensitive. Fever is the most sensitive finding, but it has poor specificity for the diagnosis of CR-BSI. The cure of the sepsis syndrome after removal of an implicated catheter from a patient with BSI is indirect evidence of CR-BSI. Fever, chills, or hypotension at the time of catheter connection should also increase the suspicion of CRI. Finally, a CR-BSI is likely when the BSI is due to a common skin organism such as coagulase-negative staphylococci, *S. aureus*, or *Candida* spp., without apparent source of sepsis except the catheter.

CATHETER-TIP CULTURE TECHNIQUES

Qualitative Broth Culture

Traditionally, a definite diagnosis of CRI requires removal of the catheter, or a guidewire exchange, for culture of the catheter tip (16,17). Qualitative broth culture of the catheter tip was the only method available until 1977: The catheter segment was immersed in broth and incubated. The main concern was that broth cultures could not distinguish between colonization and infection (5). In studies employing the culture technique by immersion in liquid medium, the actual rate of CRI was overestimated (11).

Broth cultures are highly sensitive. When broth cultures are negative, the probability of CRI is low. Conversely, considering that removing a catheter may provide opportunity for contaminating it, and that microorganisms from distant sites of infection can "seed" the catheter, the clinical relevance of a positive catheter culture in broth is poor. Interestingly, the effect of the skin exit site and the subcutaneous tunnel on the accuracy of CVC-tip cultures has been studied in an in vitro model (18). The authors showed that pulling a catheter through a contaminated area resulted in clinical contamination. When such a phenomenon occurs, quantitation of microorganisms may help to differentiate between contamination and significant colonization. In addition, using this model, Harris et al. showed that organisms growing on the distal segment of the catheter can be dislodged from the surface of the catheter when it is pulled through an agar tunnel (18).

Semiquantitative Catheter-Tip Culture

Since 1977, semiquantitative catheter-tip culture techniques have been proposed to replace qualitative broth cultures. The roll plate method has been proposed by Maki et al. (11), in which the external surface of the distal segment of the catheter is rolled on a blood agar plate, which is subsequently incubated at 37°C for 48 h (Table 2). Two-hundred and fifty catheters were studied, from 198 patients; most of them were inserted in a peripheral vein (Table 3). A threshold of 15 colony-forming units (cfu) was correlated with local signs of inflammation. The roll plate method is historically the first technique that distinguishes infection from contamination, and it is much more specific in diagnosing CRI than catheter culture in broth.

However, this technique, which explores only the external surface of the catheter, has some important limitations. First, the threshold of 15 or more colonies on the plate was designated as positive semiquantitative culture because local inflammation was more frequent (16/25 versus 30/225) with catheters yielding 15 or more colonies (11). However, correlation with clinical criteria of infection is not precise in the study. Only four cases of bacteremia have been reported. In each case, a confluent growth (colony count $\geq 10^3$) of the infecting pathogen was observed, so that the accuracy of the 15 cfu threshold is debatable. Second, most of the devices analyzed were peripheral short-term catheters, so that extrapolation to CVCs may be hazardous. In particular, the accuracy of the roll plate method with long-term intravascular devices, for which the intraluminal route of colonization predominates, remains to be determined. Third, although it has optimal sensitivity, the technique lacks specificity (20–50%) (5). In 1983, Moyer et al. showed that positive and negative predictive values were 25 and 100%, respectively, using this threshold (4).

Other thresholds for significant colonization of the catheter have been evaluated in several studies. Collignon et al. studied 780 tips from central CVCs inserted in 440 critically ill patients (19). The results were correlated with clinical data for 30 bacteremic episodes, 14 of which were CR-BSIs. When five or more colonies per plate were taken as a positive result, instead of 15 cfu, the sensitivity and specificity of the method were 92% and 83%, respectively, with a negative predictive value of 99.8%. However, given the low incidence of CR-BSIs [2%], the positive predictive value was only 8.8% in the population studied. The positive predictive value was only slightly improved (9.8%) when the threshold for significant colonization of the catheter was increased to 100 cfu (19). This value is notably insufficient for a reference technique.

Three years later, Kristinsson et al. studied prospectively 236 CVCs using roll plate culture, combined with tip-flush and ultrasonication techniques (20). The results of culture showed a bimodal distribution: All the patients with CRI had more than 50 cfu by the semiquantitative culture, and all but one had more than 100 colonies. Although the negative predictive values were high (99% and 93% for thresholds of 15 and 100 colonies, respectively), the positive predictive values remained limited (46% and 56%, respectively). Finally, similar findings were reported by Rello et al. in critically ill patients, using thresholds of 15 and 50 colonies (21). Although sensitivity, negative predictive value, and even (to a lesser degree) specificity proved to be

Table 2 Methods of Catheter-Tip Culture

Semiquantitative catheter-tip culture method[a]

At the time of catheter removal, any antimicrobial ointment or blood present on the skin around the catheter should be removed. The catheter is withdrawn with sterile forceps, the externalized portion being kept directed upward and away from the skin surface. For short peripheral catheters, the entire length is aseptically amputated and cultured. For longer catheters, the distal 5- to 7-cm catheter segment is sectioned and cultured. Catheter segments are transported to the laboratory in a sterile tube. In the laboratory, the catheter-tip segment is transferred to the surface of a 10-cm, 5% sheep-blood agar plate for semi-quantitative culturing. While downward pressure is exerted with a flamed forceps, the catheter is rolled back and forth across the surface at least four times. Plates are subsequently incubated at 37°C. All colony types appearing on the plate are enumerated, and all organisms recovered are fully identified.

Quantitative tip-flush culture technique[b]

The intradermal segment is separated from the intravascular catheter segment. A needle is inserted into the proximal end of the intravascular segment, which is immersed in 2 ml or 10 ml of trypticase soy broth, depending on the size of the insert, and flushed three times. The broth is serially diluted 100-fold, and 0.1 ml of the dilution is streaked onto blood agar. After incubation, the number of cfu is calculated by multiplying the number of colonies by 10 times the dilution factor, and dividing by the volume of broth in which the insert has been immersed.

Quantitative culture technique after catheter vortexing[c]

After removal, the distal 5- to 6-cm catheter segment is sectioned in a sterile tube. One milliliter of sterile water is dripped onto the catheter and the tube is vortexed for 1 min, then 0.1 ml of the suspension is sampled and plated over a 5% horse-blood agar plate. The plate is incubated at 37°C and examined daily for 5 days. All colony types are identified by colony morphology, Gram stain, and standard microbiologic techniques. The colonies are enumerated, and the counts are corrected for the initial 1/10 dilution.

Quantitative culture technique after catheter ultrasonication[d]

After removal, the catheter tip is placed in 10 ml of tryptic soy broth, sonicated for 1 min (55 000 Hz, 125 W), and then vortexed for 15 s. A 0.1-ml sample of the broth is added to either 0.9 ml (1:10 dilution) or 9.9 ml (1:100 dilution) of saline and vortexed. Then, 0.1 ml of these dilutions and 0.1 ml of the sonicated broth are surface-plated, using a wire loop on blood agar.

---

[a] From Ref. 11.
[b] From Ref. 24.
[c] From Ref. 17.
[d] From Ref. 25.

Table 3   Catheter-Tip Culture Methods

	No.	Setting	Method	CVC/periph	CRIs (%)	Mean duration of placement	Threshold (cfu/ml)
Maki (11)	250	All hosp.	Roll plate	CVC 33 periph 217	10	3 days	15
Brun-Buisson (17)	331	ICU	Vortexing	CVC only	11	5 days	1,000
Sherertz (25)	1,681	All hosp.	Sonication	CVC + periph	12	ND	100

No.: number of catheters studied.
ICU: intensive care unit.
CVC: central venous catheter.
periph: peripheral catheter.
CRI: catheter-related infection.
cfu/ml: colony-forming units per milliliter.

satisfactory, the positive predictive values were less than 50%, whatever the threshold chosen.

Interestingly, the results of 197 CVC semiquantitative tip cultures plated at the bedside were compared with those cultured in the laboratory, to determine if bedside plating provides a better yield (22). The last 6 cm of each catheter was divided into two 3-cm subsegments—a distal segment (including the tip), and one just proximal to that. Each segment was plated either at the bedside or in the laboratory during the first period, and alternately during the second half of the study. Among 31 positive tip cultures, only 10 were simultaneously positive at the bedside and in the laboratory. Cultures were exclusively positive in 18 cases at the bedside, whereas laboratory plating resulted in only three positive cases. This finding suggests that cultures plated at bedside could be more sensitive than roll plate cultures performed in the laboratory. This result supports the premise that the delay associated with routine laboratory culture of the catheter tips may result in loss of viable organisms. As suggested by Cooper and Hopkins (23) and Collignon et al. (19), it is conceivable that organisms, such as *Candida* sp., that thrive in moist environments may not survive for a prolonged period on dry plastic surfaces.

Despite these concerns, the semiquantitative culture technique is considered to be easy and fast, and it remains the most common method used world-wide in microbiology laboratories. However, physicians should be aware of the limitations of this catheter-tip culture technique.

Quantitative Catheter-Tip Culture Techniques

Conversely to the roll plate method, the first quantitative culture technique proposed by Cleri et al. explored only the internal part of the CVC (24). Using a tip-flush technique with a threshold of positivity of 10^3 cfu/ml, a good correlation with catheter-related bacteremia was shown. In the aforementioned study by Kristinsson et al. (20), a positive culture from the inside of the catheter, using the tip-flush technique, was one of the best predictors of infection, although a false negative was recorded in a patient with CR-BSI.

However, flushing the inside of the catheter segment may be difficult sometimes. The method is cumbersome and is therefore not routinely performed in microbiological laboratories. Therefore, the quantitative culture technique has been simplified for routine clinical practice, using catheter vortexing in sterile water (17). This catheter-tip culture technique by Brun-Buisson et al. is described in Table 2. A threshold of 10^3 cfu/ml correlated with signs of systemic infection (fever, chills, hypotension or septic shock), with or without catheter-associated bacteremia, and exhibited high specificity (88%) and sensitivity (97.5%) in critically ill patients with CVC in place for several days (Table 3). Both the external and the internal surface of the catheter are explored by this technique.

Another technique for quantitative catheter-tip culture, using ultrasonication to dislodge bacteria adherent to the catheter, gave similar results (25) (Table 2). The sonication method allows quantitation of the number of cfu removed from a catheter for levels between 10^2 and 10^7 cfu. For catheter cultures in which $\geq 10^2$ cfu grew, the risk of positive blood cultures for the same organism was correlated to the number of organisms recovered from the catheter (Table 3). Similar to the method described by Brun-Buisson et al. (17), both the external surface and the internal lumen of the catheter were explored. Disadvantages of the method include the need for additional equipment and the difficulty of standardizing the ultrasound. In addition, a high energy level of ultrasound waves may kill gram-negative bacteria and decrease the sensitivity of the test.

Culture of the Subcutaneous Catheter Segment

The culture of the subcutaneous catheter segment, in addition to the catheter-tip culture, was first studied by Maki et al. (11). When CVCs were removed, a 5- to 7-cm proximal segment, beginning several centimeters inside the skin–catheter interface, was cultured. In all cases with positive semiquantitative culture, the segment that had traversed the intracutaneous wound showed notably heavier growth than the tip. However, the relevance of this additional culture remained unclear.

Among 101 catheters in place for an average of ten days in medical–surgical patients (including patients with burns), no significant difference was noted between the cultures of transcutaneous catheter segments and those of the tip segments by either broth or roll plate techniques, although subcutaneous segments were colonized slightly more often (4).

In a more recent clinical trial, several culture techniques (sonication and roll plate methods for tip and subcutaneous segments, and flush cultures of all lumens of triple-lumen catheters) were compared (26). To define significant catheter colonization, a composite index (any of the seven types of cultures meeting quantitative criteria)* was used. Sonication of the subcutaneous segment was the most sensitive method of detecting colonization (58%), followed by sonication of the catheter tip (53%).

However, in an analysis using data derived from two prospective, randomized studies, the quantitative culture of the subcutaneous catheter segment did not add to the diagnostic yield of catheter-tip cultures, nor aid in identifying CR-BSIs (27). Therefore, it can be concluded that culturing the subcutaneous segment of the catheter is not indicated in clinical practice.

In situ semiquantitative cultures of the subcutaneous segment (without catheter removal) have also been proposed (28) (see section on "Culture of the Exit Site and Hub of the Catheter").

Distinctive Features for Diagnosis in Ports and Pulmonary Artery Catheters

The diagnosis of CRI may be slightly more complex with some types of intravascular devices, such as totally implanted access ports or pulmonary artery catheters. The issue will be addressed in detail in Chapters 14 and 15, respectively.

Briefly, besides the intravascular portion of the catheter, the reservoir of totally implanted access ports constitutes an additional source of infection (29). The accumulation of infected clots under the silicone septum of the reservoir of venous access ports could be the source of bloodstream infections, even without catheter-tip colonization. Douard et al. investigated prospectively all the ports removed over a 16-month period, assessing the accuracy of quantitative cultures of the tip and septum (i.e., the internal part of the venous access port). In this setting, the tip culture was only 46% sensitive, whereas septum culture was 93% sensitive for confirming CRI (29). Thus, when a venous access port is removed because of suspected CRI, the catheter tip and the port itself should both be cultured. The presence of deposits of fibrin containing clusters of bacteria inside the reservoir of the port may explain the limited efficacy of antibiotic-lock techniques in the treatment of venous access port-related bacteremia (30).

Diagnostic criteria for pulmonary artery CRIs are somewhat complex as well. The need to culture the distal segments of both the pulmonary artery catheter and the indwelling introducer in order to diagnose pulmonary artery CRIs has been underlined. Valles et al. showed that the yield of catheter-tip

---

*Composite index for diagnosis of catheter colonization: ≥ 15 colony-forming units (cfu) by the roll-plate method (either for tip segment [method 1] or subcutaneous segment [2]); ≥ 100 cfu by sonication (either for tip segment [3] or subcutaneous segment [4]); or ≥ 100 cfu by flush culture or a ratio of catheter lumen blood cfu to peripheral lumen blood cfu of ≥ 5 (for either the proximal [5], middle [6], or distal [7] lumen of the catheter).

cultures increased from 68%, when only the Swan-Ganz catheter was cultured, to 91% when both the Swan-Ganz catheter and the introducer tips were cultured (31). Recently, we reported that introducer and Swan-Ganz catheter colonizations were dissociated (only one of the devices was colonized) in six of seven episodes of CRI (32). Introducers were mainly colonized within the first five days, whereas Swan-Ganz catheter colonization occurred later (usually after the fifth day), suggesting that contamination of introducers and pulmonary artery catheters could be caused either by early extraluminal colonization originating from the skin or by the introduction of bacteria via the endoluminal route, due to repeated manipulations.

Comparison of Catheter Culture Techniques.
Methodological Comment

Quantitative or semiquantitative cultures of catheters are recommended by the Guidelines for the Management of Intravascular CRI (1), whereas qualitative broth cultures, which have high sensitivity but very poor specificity, are not recommended.

The different mechanisms of colonization of the intravascular part of the catheter may explain the discrepancy between the catheter-tip culture techniques. As previously mentioned, the extraluminal route predominates for short-term catheters, whereas endoluminal contamination is most frequent in cases of prolonged catheterization (6). The optimal technique for determining that the catheter is the source of BSI should be independent of the duration of placement and the route (extra- or intraluminal) of colonization.

Furthermore, the selection and the interpretation of diagnostic tests affect the information they provide. The values of sensitivity and specificity are dependent on the definition used for the diagnosis of CR-BSI, which may result in potential incorporation bias (33). Receiver operating characteristic (ROC) analysis* has been used for selecting among several alternative diagnostic tests and for selecting optimal cutoff values for a positive result. ROC analysis provides an effective way to determine which of many different tests proposed for the diagnosis of CR-BSI offers the best overall performance (33). In a meta-analysis focusing on the diagnostic tools for CRI (34), ROC analysis showed that the diagnostic accuracy of various culture techniques

---

*Receiver operating characteristic (ROC) analysis is performed to distinguish variation in the decision threshold from actual differences in accuracy. The results of studies evaluating a specific test method are plotted as true positive rates (sensitivity) against false positive rates (1 − specificity) in an ROC space. In these plots, a single point represents the two estimated parameters (sensitivity and specificity) from each study. Sensitivity and specificity are calculated according to variations of cutoff values. (Sensitivity and specificity depend on the cutoff value used to define a positive test; e.g., a stricter cutoff will increase specificity but decrease sensitivity.) The overall accuracy of a test is conveyed by the areas under the ROC curve, and the areas under the ROC curves generated for each method may be compared (33,35).

increased with better quantitation (i.e., quantitative > semiquantitative > qualitative methods). Quantitative CVC-tip cultures had the highest pooled sensitivity and specificity (>90%) when compared with semiquantitative or qualitative (broth) cultures (34).

In a recent study, Kite et al. reported that the specificity of the tip roll method (55%) was lower than the specificity of tip flush (76%) and endoluminal brush (98%) techniques, whereas the sensitivity of all methods was greater than 90% (35). When several culture techniques were compared for the diagnosis of triple-lumen CRI, sonication of the catheter tip (a quantitative culture technique) was 20% more sensitive than the roll plate method (26). The greater sensitivity of the sonication method was attributed to its greater ability to detect catheter lumen colonization, compared to the roll plate method (82% versus 57%, respectively). Therefore, the vortexing or ultrasonication methods proposed for quantitative catheter-tip culture (17,25), which take into account the external and internal surfaces of the device, appear to be the most appropriate for the diagnosis of CRI, whatever the route of colonization and the duration of placement.

Finally, in the light of quantitative catheter-tip culture results, the following definitions may be proposed for contamination, colonization, and infection of a CVC. Contamination corresponds to a catheter-tip culture under the threshold of the method used (e.g., $< 10^3$ cfu/ml using the vortexing technique), without any clinical sign of infection. Colonization of the catheter may be defined by a positive catheter-tip culture (e.g., $\geq 10^3$ cfu/ml using the vortexing technique), without any clinical sign of infection. Local and systemic infections are defined by a positive catheter-tip culture in a patient with clinical local or systemic signs of infection. In fact, there is probably a continuum between contamination, colonization, and eventual infection (17): Contaminated catheters with intermediate (i.e., 10^2 to 10^3 cfu/ml) bacterial concentrations growing from them may cause silent infection and eventually lead to overt clinical sepsis if they remain intravascular for longer periods (17).

In summary, qualitative broth cultures, which have high sensitivity but very poor specificity, are not recommended. Semiquantitative roll plate cultures, which explore only the external surface of the catheter, are highly sensitive but lack specificity. Quantitative catheter-tip cultures using vortexing or sonication, which explore either internal and external surfaces of the catheter, have the highest pooled sensitivity and specificity (>90%) when compared with semiquantitative or broth cultures. Quantitative cultures are equally effective in short- and long-term catheterizations.

GUIDEWIRE EXCHANGE

Guidewire exchange of CVCs suspected of CRI has been proposed as a compromise solution between diagnostic techniques with and without removal of the catheter. If the first catheter is found to be significantly colonized, the second catheter is removed and a new line inserted on a new site (9). Considering that in about 80% of suspected CRI, the catheter is not the source of infection, guidewire exchange could prevent many of the noninfectious complications associated with puncture of a new site.

Guidewire exchange has been proposed as a reasonable step in the early management of patients on total parenteral nutrition (36). In such a setting, Bonadimani et al. reported that guidewire replacement was successful in treating 91.6% of patients with suspected CRI (37). The design of the study did not allow definite conclusions.

In fact, the value and safety of guidewire exchange in cases where CRI is suspected remain highly controversial. Several complications or contraindications are attributed to guidewire exchanges. Although this technique is associated with fewer mechanical complications and less discomfort than new-site replacement, the guidewire exchange could be linked to a greater (although nonsignificant) risk of CRI (38,39). If guidewire exchange is used, meticulous aseptic technique is necessary (39), and the method may be proposed only in the absence of clinical signs of local inflammation. Obviously, a purulent discharge at the insertion site precludes guidewire exchange of the catheter. Recently, the CDC Guidelines for the Prevention of Intravascular Catheter-Related Infections took a more stringent position on guidewire exchanges (40): "Replacement of temporary catheters over a guidewire in the presence of bacteremia is not an acceptable replacement strategy, because the source of infection is usually colonization of the skin tract from the insertion site to the vein."

Other experts consider this position somewhat excessive. In particular, the recent revision of the XIIth Consensus Conference on Intravascular Catheter-Related Infections of the French Society of Critical Care (41) considered guidewire exchange to be acceptable in case of low suspicion of CRI, in patients with strictly stable conditions without clinical signs of local inflammation. Only in this setting can such a standpoint be considered reasonable, considering that more than 75% of CVCs that are removed because of suspicion of CRI are removed unnecessarily (2).

In summary, guidewire exchange of catheters suspected of CRI may prevent many of the noninfectious complications associated with puncture of a new site, but at the expense of a possibly greater risk of CRI. Guidewire exchange should not be performed in patients with bacteremia and high risk of CRI. In special situations, guidewire exchange could be proposed in stable patients with low suspicion of CRI and without skin inflammation or purulence.

DIAGNOSIS OF CRI WITHOUT CATHETER REMOVAL

Whatever the type of catheter-tip culture technique, the limitation of all these techniques is that the diagnosis is always retrospective. Only about 15 to 25%

of CVCs removed because of suspicion of infection actually prove to be infected after quantitative catheter-tip cultures (2,14). In an observational study, the rate of colonized CVCs was similar whatever the indication for catheter removal (sepsis, CVC no longer needed, or death) (10). This finding underlines the lack of specificity of clinical suspicion of CRI.

In addition, Widmer et al. showed that the clinical impact of culturing CVCs on the treatment of critically ill patients was limited (16). In 96% of the episodes leading to removal of the catheter, no clinical impact was observed, whereas in the remaining 4%, clinical decisions were guided mainly by the concurrent positive blood cultures. In this striking and slightly provocative study, the authors stated that newer laboratory techniques that do not require removal of the catheter were needed to guide therapeutic decisions.

For all these reasons, diagnostic techniques have been proposed to establish the diagnosis of CRI in situ, avoiding unjustified removal of the catheter and the potential risks associated with placement of a new catheter at a new site.

If a short peripheral catheter is suspected to be infected, it should be immediately removed and cultured, considering that peripheral catheters are intended to be used for only a few days (1). On the other hand, it may be desirable to establish the diagnosis and eventually treat the infection without removing the CVC, assuming that the clinical situation is not life-threatening and the catheter is still needed. This is especially the case in infections with less-virulent organisms such as coagulase-negative staphylococci. Indeed, severe sepsis or deep local infections (tunnel or pocket infection, thrombophlebitis) are indications for immediate removal of the suspected CVCs. In other settings, several diagnostic tests without removal of the intravascular device have been proposed.

Culture of the Exit Site and Hub of the Catheter

Culture of skin and the exit site of the catheter, or cultures of the hub, have high sensitivity and a high negative predictive value; they are, therefore, mainly destined to rule out the diagnosis of CRI (8).

Cultures of the catheter entry site reflect mainly the extraluminal contamination way, which predominates for short-term catheters. The basic method and some variants are described in Table 4. This diagnostic technique was first proposed by Bjornson et al. in 1982 in patients receiving total parenteral nutrition (42) (Table 5). In this study, the growth of more than 1000 organisms at the catheter site was significantly associated with CRI.

Guidet et al. studied the value of quantitative skin culture using a threshold of 15 cfu (43). The method was considered to be useful for assessing catheter colonization in critically ill patients, whatever the reason for CVC removal (suspicion of CRI or not). The skin culture was always positive in case

Table 4 Methods of Skin and Hub Cultures

Culture of the skin at the catheter insertion site[a]

Cutaneous specimens may be obtained with a dry or a moistened swab, after removal of the dressing. No antiseptic agent is needed. The cotton swab may be moistened with 0.01 M phosphate-buffered saline (PBS), using the blister of the device. The swab may then be rubbed on the skin in two perpendicular directions on a predefined area surrounding the insertion point of the catheter (e.g, 2 × 2 cm, or 6 × 4 cm; a template may be used). Other authors propose to swab the sterile cotton applicator from top to bottom in 10 back-and-forth strokes, in the predefined area, followed by a second set of 10 back-and-forth strokes at right angles to the first. The cotton swab is then pulled back into the protective tube, which contains 1.0 ml of PBS, and vortexed for 90 seconds. In the Culturette® system, 0.5 ml of a Stuart medium are used. Finally, a 0.1-ml sample of this solution (and eventually a 1:100 dilution of this solution) is plated on blood agar, and colonies are counted after incubation for 24 and 48 hours at 35°C.

Culture of the catheter hub[b]

The catheter is clamped in order to avoid any blood contamination, and the luer lock is removed aseptically. After cleaning the outside of the hub with a disinfectant, the inner hub sample is taken using a swab that is introduced into the hub and rubbed repeatedly against its interior surface. The swab is then streaked onto an agar plate for semiquantitative culture.

[a] From Refs. 8, 43, 44, 47.
[b] From Refs. 7, 8, 43, 48.

of catheter colonization and always negative in the absence of catheter colonization. In patients with total parenteral nutrition, Armstrong et al. showed that CRI was associated with site colonization by 50 or more cfu of an organism other than coagulase-negative staphylococci (12). In addition, CRI was present if signs of inflammation were present in combination with site colonization by 50 or more cfu of coagulase-negative staphylococci. Finally, Mahé et al. found that sensitivity, specificity, and positive and negative predictive values of skin culture for detection of CVC colonization in ICU patients were 92.3%, 52.7%, 32%, and 96.7%, respectively (44). In this study, the relative risk of CVC colonization when skin culture was positive was 9.44 ($p < 0.0001$). Conversely, in patients on total parenteral nutrition, Sitges-Serra et al. showed, as expected, that skin cultures were not sensitive in diagnosing CRI during an outbreak due to coagulase-negative staphylococci (45).

The value of surveillance skin cultures, without suspicion of CRI, has been assessed by Snydman et al. in patients with tunneled catheters (46). The sensitivity for diagnosing a catheter-tip colonization was 95%, the specificity was 76%, the positive predictive value was 61%, and the negative predictive value was 98%. All these values increased to 100%, 84%, 67%, and 100%, respectively, when only the skin cultures obtained during the week before

Table 5 Hub and Skin Exit-Site Culture Methods

	Skin/Hub	No.	Setting	Suspicion of CRI/No suspicion	CVC/peri.	CRIs (%)
Snydman (56)	Skin	59	TPN	No	CVC	24
Bjornson (42)	Skin	74	TPN		CVC	26
Cercenado (8)	Skin + Hub	139	All hosp.	Yes 79/No 60	CVC 95 Peri 44	38
Armstrong (12)	Skin	152	TPN		CVC	13
Guidet (43)	Skin	50	ICU	Yes 20/No 30	CVC	20
Guidet (43)	Hub	50	ICU	Yes 20/No 30	CVC	20
Raad (47)	Skin	132	Cancer	Yes 15/No 132	CVC	20
Mahé (44)	Skin	134	ICU	Yes 60/No 74	CVC	
Segura (50)	Skin + Hub	41	TPN	Yes	CVC	32

No.: number of catheters studied.
ICU: intensive care unit.
TPN: total parenteral nutrition.
CVC: central venous catheter.
peri: peripheral catheter.
CRI: catheter-related infection.
cfu: colony forming units.
T = targeted, S = surveillance cultures.
* criterion: catheter-related bacteremia.
Se: sensitivity.
Sp: specificity.
NPV: negative predictive value.
PPV: positive predictive value.

removal of the catheter were considered. These encouraging results may be explained in part by the short duration of catheterization in the study (<30 days). Raad et al. compared the values of targeted (usually when CRI is suspected) and surveillance skin cultures (done routinely 1 and 3 months after insertion of the CVC) in 132 cancer patients with long-term CVCs (47). Targeted skin cultures were associated with a sensitivity of 75%, specificity of 100%, positive predictive value of 100%, and negative predictive value of 92%. Conversely, surveillance skin cultures had sensitivity and positive predictive values of only 18% and 25%, respectively. The results of only two of the 87 initial surveillance skin cultures were positively concordant with results of subsequent quantitative catheter cultures or skin cultures at 3 months after CVC insertion. Similarly, Fan et al. reported in 1988 that the sensitivity of twice-weekly surveillance skin culture was only 38% in patients with CVCs used for total parenteral nutrition (48). Therefore, unlike targeted quantitative skin cultures (when CRI is suspected), surveillance skin cultures have low sensitivity and positive predictive values (49).

Diagnostic criterion	Mean duration of placement	Threshold (cfu)	Se (%)	Sp (%)	NPV (%)	PPV (%)
Roll plate	20 days	$>0/?$ cm^2	95	76	98	61
Roll plate		$10^3/25$ cm^2	68	91	91	68
Vortexing	15 (1–21) d	15/10 cm^2	T:97	T:68	T:99	T:34
	5 (1–15) d				All:96	All:66
Roll plate		50/5 cm^2	45	94	92	53
Vortexing	7 days	15/9 cm^2	100		100	
Vortexing	7 days	>0	45			
Roll plate + Sonication	>3 months	$10^3/24$ cm^2	T:75 S:18	T:100 S:92	T:92 S:93	T:100 S:25
Vortexing	10 days	15/25 cm^2	92	52	96	32
Roll plate	22 days	>0			96*	100*

In these studies, the choice of the diagnostic criterion of CRI may have influenced the accuracy of the diagnostic method evaluated. In particular, using the semiquantitative roll plate culture, which explores only the external surface of the catheter, may induce a bias in favor of skin cultures, which also explore the extraluminal pathway of colonization (12). The population studied (ICU patients with short-term catheters, or cancer patients with long-term CVCs) is an important factor influencing the results of these studies. In addition, conflicting results may be in part explained by differences in the methods. Bjornson et al., Raad et al., and Mahé et al., cultured a 24- to 25-cm^2 area around the insertion site (42,44,47), whereas Cercenado et al. and Guidet et al. cultured a 9- to 10-cm^2 area (8,43). In the study by Armstrong et al., a small area of skin approximately 2.5 cm in diameter was cultured (12). Skin samples have been obtained by rubbing dry (8,12) or premoistened (42,44,47) swabs over the area surrounding the point of insertion of the catheter. Premoistened skin swabs, using the Culturette® system, have also been performed. Finally, thresholds of positivity ranging from 15 (43) to 1000 cfu (42,47) have been used in these different studies.

Cultures of the hub of the catheter (Table 4) reflect mainly the endoluminal contamination route, which predominates for long-term catheters such as those used in cancer patients and could be more useful than skin cultures in this subset of patients (7). In an aforementioned study (43), Guidet et al. assessed the diagnostic value of 50 CVC hub cultures in critically ill patients, with a median duration of catheterization of 7 days (Table 5). The contribution of the catheter hub culture alone was minimal, since there was no case of catheter colonization with negative skin cultures and positive hub cultures, suggesting that the main route of catheter colonization was via the skin in this subset of patients. Similar findings were reported by Fortun et al. in 124 patients with nontunneled short-term CVCs (28): The sensitivity of hub and skin cultures analyzed individually was less than 62%. Conversely, when Raad et al. studied the value of skin cultures in cancer patients with long-term CVCs, the only false-negative result of the quantitative skin culture had been diagnosed by hub culture (47). Similarly, in patients on total parenteral nutrition, Sitges-Serra et al. showed that an infected hub was associated with an infected tip in 15 of 17 episodes of CRI due to coagulase-negative staphylococci (45).

Interestingly, in rare cases, authentic hub-related bacteremias (with negative catheter-tip cultures) may be observed. Douard et al. reported that 16 of 58 episodes of bacteremia were diagnosed by positive hub culture, whereas the tip cultures remained negative (49). The authors concluded that CVC-tip culture should be associated with hub cultures.

As reported for surveillance skin cultures, Fan et al. reported that the sensitivity of daily surveillance catheter hub culture was only 34.5% in 142 patients with parenteral nutrition (48). When either the hub or the skin culture result was considered as an indication of CRI, the sensitivity increased to 79.3%. The positive and the negative predictive values of the combined result were 44.2% and 93.3%, respectively.

Segura et al. investigated the predictive value for CR-BSI of hub and skin cultures in patients on total parenteral nutrition managed without removal of the central line (50) (Table 5). A conservative strategy, based on the results of superficial cultures, was compared with immediate removal of the catheter in patients with suspected CRI. The negative predictive value of combined skin and hub cultures was 96%. A positive hub culture had a 100% positive predictive value for CR-BSI. Only 1 out of 41 catheters was removed unnecessarily using the conservative strategy, compared with 7 out 18 catheters in the group with immediate withdrawal (51). Similarly, Cercenado et al. studied the value of combined skin and hub ("superficial") cultures in 139 intravascular (long central and short peripheral) catheters, in a mixed population of inpatients located in different hospital wards (8). The predictive value of positive superficial cultures in the diagnosis of CRI was 66.2%, and that of negative cultures was 96.7%. In the aforementioned study by Fortun et al. (28), the sensitivity of the combined skin and hub cultures increased to 86.2%. Therefore, in patients with suspected CRI but with negative superficial cultures, the possibility of CRI may reasonably be ruled out (8,28,48).

In addition, in this latter study, the value of in situ semiquantitative culture of the subcutaneous segment (after removing the catheter only 2 cm) was studied (28). Although the sensitivity was similar, the specificity and the positive predictive value of subcutaneous segment cultures were significantly higher (94% and 88.5%, respectively) than skin and hub cultures. Sensitivity of the combined subcutaneous segment and hub cultures and of the combined skin and hub cultures were similar (84.3% and 86.2%, respectively); the specificity of the latter combination was higher than the former (82% versus 59.7%). However, despite these encouraging results, the actual value of the in situ semiquantitative culture of the subcutaneous segment is not clearly defined.

Finally, the limitation of skin and hub cultures is that both of these techniques generally exhibit a poor specificity (8,42). In addition, by definition, skin and hub cultures cannot be proposed for patients with totally implanted ports. Gram staining of skin and hub swabs could be helpful for early diagnosis of CRI (51) (see section on "Gram Staining of Pericatheter Skin and Hub").

In summary, targeted skin cultures are very useful in ruling out the diagnosis when the culture is negative (high negative predictive value), mainly in patients with short-term catheters, such as critically ill patients. The optimal threshold of positivity of quantitative skin cultures remains to be determined (between 15 and 1000 cfu). Conversely, unlike targeted quantitative skin cultures (when CRI is suspected), surveillance skin cultures have a low sensitivity. In patients with long-term CVC, such as patients with cancer or total parenteral nutrition, hub cultures exhibit a high sensitivity (but poor specificity), and could be more useful in ruling out the diagnosis in this setting. Although surveillance hub culture is poorly sensitive, combined skin and hub cultures could be more useful. However, the actual place of hub cultures in the routine, and their safety, remain to be determined.

Central Quantitative Blood Cultures

Quantitative blood cultures drawn from the CVC (hub–blood cultures) involve measuring the number of microorganisms present in blood drawn through the hub of the CVC while the catheter is in position. When a bacteremia is linked to a CRI, the number of microorganisms retrieved by the hub–blood culture is high, due to a purging effect of the infected lumen of the catheter. Several methods are available for quantitative blood cultures: pour plate cultures, lysis-centrifugation technique, and direct inoculation onto agar media (Table 6). The lysis-centrifugation technique has proven to be effective in the rapid isolation of organisms from mixed cultures and is more sensitive than standard broth culture in detecting low levels of bacte-

Table 6   Methods of Paired and Unpaired Quantitative Blood Cultures

Pour plate cultures[a]
  The connection of the CVC and the venous line are externally disinfected. A
  sample of 5 ml of blood is drawn into a heparinized disposable syringe through the
  hub of the catheter. The syringe is immediately brought to the microbiology
  laboratory. One milliliter of blood is mixed with 10 to 20 ml of molten liquid
  tryptic soy/Mueller-Hinton agar at 45/46°C, poured into a sterile petri dish,
  allowed to solidify, and incubated for 48 h at 37°C, and the colonies are counted.
  When paired quantitative blood cultures are performed, the same volume of blood
  is obtained from a peripheral vein, immediately after (or before) the hub–blood
  culture, by standard venipuncture and placed in a heparinized tube.
Lysis-centrifugation technique (Isolator, DuPont Co)[b]
  Blood is inoculated into tubes with saponin, a cell-lysing agent. The content of the
  tube is mixed with a Vortex, and the tube is centrifuged. The supernatant (lysate) is
  removed with a syringe, and the concentrate is then inoculated onto agar plates.
  Plates are examined after overnight incubation, and the number of cfu is
  determined.
Direct inoculation of blood on agar media[c]
  Blood is inoculated directly onto agar plates. The blood is dispersed over the agar
  by gentle rotation. Plates are incubated for 48 h at 37°C, and colonies are counted.
  Mixing the blood with molten agar is not necessary with this method.

[a] From Refs. 46, 55.
[b] From Ref. 62.
[c] From Ref 60.

remias caused by species of Enterobacteriaceae and yeasts, although contaminants are more frequent than in broth cultures (52,53). In addition,
Isolator® 1.5-ml microbial tubes are useful in the neonatal intensive care unit
because they are designed for small volumes of blood (0.5 to 1.5 ml) (54).
Finally, the technique eliminates the need to perform bedside inoculations
and obviates the need for immediate transfer of the blood to the laboratory.
However, the lysis-centrifugation technique is more expensive than the simple
pour plate technique.
    Quantitative blood cultures, drawn solely from the catheter, have been
tested in several studies (4,55,56) (Table 7a). Among 100 courses of total

Table 7a   Quantitative Central Blood Culture Methods

	No.	Setting	CRIs (%)	Culture method	Mean duration of placement	Threshold (cfu)	Se (%)	Sp (%)
Moyer (4)	67	All hosp	27	Pour plate	10 days	>25	80	100
Snydman (46)	100	TPN	12	Pour plate	14 days	>15	42	92
Capdevila (57)	107	All hosp	20	Pour plate	19 days	>100	82	100
Andremont (55)	205	Cancer	29	Pour plate		>1000	20	99

parenteral nutrition in 69 patients, the results of pour plate cultures of blood obtained from central lines and cultures of intravascular segments did not correlate. Nevertheless, the pathogen was isolated from the pour plate prior to the positive blood culture results and the removal of the line segment in three courses with CRI (56). Among 67 catheters in place for an average of 10 days, Moyer et al. showed that quantitative blood cultures drawn through the catheter, using the pour plate technique with a threshold of 25 colonies, had a high positive predictive value for the diagnosis of CRI. (4). Using a cutoff value of >100 cfu/ml with the pour plate technique, the sensitivity and specificity of an isolated quantitative catheter blood culture were 82% and 100%, respectively, in 64 patients with catheters remaining in situ for a mean of 19 (3 to 65) days (57).

In 179 cancer patients, the microbial concentrations in samples of blood collected via the hubs of 205 CVCs were determined using a pour plate technique (55). The semiquantitative measurement of the number of micro-organisms present in blood drawn through the catheter (using a threshold of 10^3 cfu/ml) had a specificity of 99%, but a sensitivity of only 20% for catheter-tip colonization. The decrease of the threshold to 10^2 or 10 cfu/ml reduced the specificity of the method significantly. Quantitative central blood cultures are characterized by a high specificity and a high positive predictive value, allowing affirmation of the diagnosis of CRI in case of positivity.

As reported in several studies, antibiotic treatment did not affect the results of quantitative blood cultures for assessing CRI (4,55,57).

Paired Central and Peripheral Quantitative Blood Cultures

The sensitivity of hub–blood culture is increased when a simultaneous blood culture is drawn from a peripheral vein. The comparison of the microbial count between hub and peripheral blood cultures shows an overload of bacteria in the central blood culture, compared to the peripheral blood culture, when a CRI is present. Conversely, when the bloodstream infection is not related to a CRI, the microbial counts are similar. In 1979, Wing et al. first used differential quantitative blood cultures in a patient who had a permanent indwelling hyperalimentation catheter, with suspected bacteremic CRI (58). Blood drawn from the peripheral vein had 25 colonies per ml, whereas blood drawn through the hub had more than 10,000 colonies per ml. When the CVC was removed, the catheter tip was found to be infected with the same organisms that were present in the blood.

The value of differential quantitative blood cultures has been assessed in several studies (Table 7b). When quantitative blood cultures are drawn simultaneously from the catheter and a peripheral vein, a significant differential colony count of 4:1 to 10:1 for the CVC versus the peripheral vein culture is indicative of CRI (49,57,59,60), although some discrepancies between differential quantitative blood cultures and semiquantitative catheter cultures have been reported (61).

Table 7b   Paired Quantitative Central Blood Culture Methods

	No.	Setting	CRIs (%)	Culture method	Threshold (ratio)	Se (%)	Sp (%)
Raucher (60)	28	Children	25	Direct inoculation	10:1	100	100
Capdevila (57)	107	All hosp.	20	Pour plate	4:1	94	100
Paya (61)	44	All hosp.		Isolator	+ 30 cfu	47	73
Flynn (53)	13	Cancer + TPN	61	Isolator 1.5	5:1		100
Fan (63)	24	TPN	37	Pour plate	7:1	78	100
Douard (62)	58	Bacteremic adults	(all)	Isolator 1.5	3:1	83	100
Quilici (64)	283	ICU	19	Pour plate	8:1	93	99

No.: number of catheters studied.
ICU: intensive care unit.
TPN: total parenteral nutrition.
CRI: catheter-related infection.
cfu: colony-forming units.
Se: sensitivity.
Sp: specificity.

In an animal experiment, Flynn et al. showed that the difference in bacterial concentration in non-CR-BSI did not exceed fivefold (59). The authors used a similar threshold in a study of 13 pediatric patients with suspected CRI (53). In another pediatric study, a colony count more than 50% greater in the catheter than in peripheral specimens was considered as indicative of CRI (54), but the major methodological biases contained in the study did not allow to consider this threshold as accurate.

Raucher et al. showed that a tenfold or greater difference in bacterial concentrations between the two specimens was indicative of CR-BSI in children with Broviac catheters (60). Using as the cutoff value a significant differential colony count of 4:1, a sensitivity of 94% and a specificity and a positive predictive value of 100% were obtained in patients hospitalized in internal medicine and surgery wards, and intensive care units (57). Using pediatric Isolator® (DuPont) tubes in 58 bacteremic adult patients, a specificity and a positive predictive value of 100%, with slightly lower sensitivity (83%) and negative predictive value (78%), have been reported using a cutoff value of 3:1 (49). In fact, the differential colony count most often exceeds 50 or 100 in cases of proven CRI. In pediatric oncology and hematology patients, the colony counts from catheter blood samples were 30-fold higher than the colony counts from peripheral samples in patients with CRI (62). Fan et al. considered the test to be indicative of CR-BSI if bacterial colonies in the catheter blood specimen were sevenfold more frequent than identical colonies in the peripheral blood specimen, in 24 patients on TPN with suspected CRI (63). Sensitivity of the test was 77.8%, specificity was 100%, and overall accuracy was 91.7%. The two infected catheters that gave false-negative results with quantitative blood cultures were mainly colonized on the outer surface.

Paired quantitative blood cultures have been validated mainly for long-term catheters such as those used for parenteral nutrition or cancer therapy, and more recently for short-term catheters in the intensive care unit (64). Quilici et al. studied the value of pour plate cultures of blood drawn simultaneously from 283 catheters and from the peripheral vein in 190 critically ill adult patients. Receiver operating characteristic curve analysis was carried out by varying the catheter/peripheral cfu ratio. The combined sensitivity and specificity were most satisfactory at a ratio of 8:1. With use of this threshold, differential blood cultures had a sensitivity of 92.8% and a specificity of 98.8%. The specificity was 100% when the catheters were removed because of suspected CRI (64).

The usefulness of comparative quantitative cultures of central venous and peripheral blood specimens has been studied in patients with CRI treated without catheter removal. In these cases, the serial quantitation of bacteremia may demonstrate rapidly decreasing blood concentrations of viable organisms following initiation of therapy with appropriate antibiotics (59). However, the main argument for successful in situ therapy remains the rapid resolution of clinical signs of sepsis and of peripheral blood cultures.

In the aforementioned meta-analysis by Siegman-Igra et al., the paired quantitative method appeared to be the most accurate of the blood culture methods evaluated by means of the Youden index (sensitivity + specificity − 1), although this trend remained statistically insignificant (34).

In summary, using thresholds between 15 and 1000 cfu/ml, hub–blood cultures are highly specific but poorly sensitive for the diagnosis of CRI. When quantitative blood cultures are drawn simultaneously from the catheter and a peripheral vein, a significant differential colony count of 4 to 10:1 for the CVC versus the peripheral vein culture is indicative of CRI, with a specificity of 90 to 100% and a sensitivity of about 80%. However, the technique is rarely used in clinical practice, mainly because of relative complexity and cost.

Paired Central and Peripheral Nonquantitative Blood Cultures

The measurement of the differential time to positivity between hub–blood and peripheral blood cultures has been proposed as a further promising method for the diagnosis of CRI in situ (65). In clinical microbiology practice, the time to blood culture positivity may be measured using automatic devices (e.g., radiometric methods). A given cutoff value, linked to the metabolism and to the number of microorganisms initially present in the bottle, indicates that bacterial or fungal multiplication has occurred in the bottle. The higher the initial bacterial inoculum, the quicker this cutoff value is reached. In an in vitro study (66), a linear relationship between the initial concentration of various microorganisms and the time to positivity of culture has been shown for all species tested. Similar results have been reported using continuous-monitoring blood culture systems for the diagnosis of CRI due to coagulase-negative staphylococci, with an average decrease of 1.5 h to positivity for each tenfold increase in concentration (67). Consequently, for central and peripheral blood cultures, comparing the times elapsing between bottle inoculation and the detection of positivity could constitute an alternative method to quantitative blood cultures.

In a retrospective study of 64 cancer patients with long-term catheters (66), earlier positivity of central versus peripheral vein blood cultures was shown to be highly predictive of CRI. The differential time to positivity was significantly greater in patients with CRI than in the patients for whom CRI was ruled out or thought unlikely. A cutoff limit of 2 h had sensitivity and specificity above 95% for the diagnosis of CRI (66). These results have been confirmed by a prospective study (65) in which a definite diagnosis of CRI could be made in 16 of the 17 patients who had a positive result of a blood sample from the CVC at least 2 h earlier, in comparison to a peripheral blood culture. The overall sensitivity was 91%, and specificity was 94%. In another study of 107 cancer patients, a receiver-operating characteristic curve was constructed to determine the optimum threshold of the test; a cutoff point of 3 h was associated with 100% specificity and 81% sensitivity (68).

For an accurate interpretation of the differential time to positivity, a rigorous method is mandatory. The first milliliters of blood drawn via the catheter should be used for culture and not discarded, and only aerobic bottles are needed. Using both aerobic and anaerobic bottles could alter the inoculum present in each bottle and add to the difficulty in interpreting the time to positivity. For multiple-lumen catheters, blood should be drawn from the distal port, which corresponds to the portion of the device cultured (65). However, in pediatric oncology patients with multilumen, long-term CVCs, the estimated sensitivity of a culture drawn from a single lumen was only 84%, suggesting that drawing blood cultures from all lumens could be useful in this setting (69).

The value of this technique, based on the results of blood cultures, may be higher in patients with long-term catheters—which are predominantly colonized by an endoluminal route—than in patients with short-term CVCs, such as critically ill patients. Two studies suggest that sensitivity and specificity of the method could be lower in intensive care unit patients (70,71). However, because of methological biases, these studies allow no definitive conclusion for critically ill patients at the moment (72). Conversely, Raad et al. have compared the diagnostic value of the differential time to positivity in 90 cancer patients with short-term (<30 days of placement) and long-term (>30 days) catheters (73). By multiple logistic regression analysis, a differential time to positivity greater than 2 h was highly predictive of bacteremic CRI. Sensitivity, specificity, and negative and positive predictive values were 94%, 91%, 95%, and 88%, respectively, for short-term CVCs, and 94%, 89%, 89% and 85%, respectively, for long-term devices. Finally, Seifert et al. showed recently that differential time to positivity compared favorably with paired quantitative blood cultures for the diagnosis of CR-BSIs in neutropenic patients with short-term nontunneled catheters (median, 10 days; range 1–38 days). The sensitivity of the method was 82% and the specificity was 88% (74). More studies should be helpful in reaching a better understanding of the accuracy of the technique in critically ill patients with short-term catheters.

The value of the absolute time to positivity of blood cultures could have some additional significance. When the absolute time to positivity was studied a posteriori in cancer patients, the median time to positivity of the hub–blood culture was significantly lower in patients with CRI than in other cases, and a time to positivity greater than 24 h excluded a CRI (65). However, in patients with coagulase-negative staphylococci bacteremia, other authors found no difference between contaminated samples and true bacteremia in the time to detection of positive blood cultures (75,76).

Dissociated results of paired blood cultures (i.e., when one of the paired blood cultures is positive) are more difficult to interpret. The reliability of blood cultures obtained through intravascular catheters remains controversial. Wormser et al. showed that catheter blood cultures were 96% sensitive and 98% specific for the detection of septicemia (77). Conversely, DesJardin et al. reported that culture of blood drawn through the CVC had low positive predictive value, apparently less than from a peripheral venipuncture, in cancer patients (78). Similarly, in critically ill surgical patients, the specificity and positive predictive value of blood cultures drawn through a catheter were lower than those obtained from a peripheral venipuncture, whereas both types of cultures had an excellent negative predictive value (79). Therefore, a positivity of the hub–blood culture only, which may reflect either a contamination of the sample or a definite CRI, needs clinical interpretation and requires confirmation. Such situations should be analyzed as a dynamic process: When the first dissociated pair (catheter positive/venipuncture negative) is recorded, an additional pair (catheter positive/venipuncture negative or catheter positive/venipuncture positive) usually indicates a CRI (65). Conversely, if no other positive blood culture is recorded (i.e., only one catheter positive/venipuncture negative pair), this pattern reflects a contamination during sampling (65). This is in agreement with the interpretation of multiple positive blood cultures for distinguishing true bacteremia and pseudobacteremia due to coagulase-negative staphylococci (80). When only the peripheral blood culture is positive (catheter negative/venipuncture positive), we are likely to be facing a true bacteremia related to another focus of infection, except when skin microorganisms such as coagulase-negative staphylococci are involved (65,78).

Critically ill patients often present problems with peripheral venous access for obtaining blood samples. Some of these problems can be overcome with indwelling arterial catheters. For the vast majority of blood tests, if sufficient dead space is removed from the catheter tubing, the source of the blood does not influence the result of the test. Levin et al. showed that the results of blood cultures taken from the arterial line were frequently equivalent (83% equivalent results among 90 parallel blood culture sets) to those taken from venipuncture (81). When discordant, the growth of gram-positive bacteria almost certainly reflects contamination or arterial line colonization, whereas the growth of gram-negative bacteria may have to be considered as reflecting bacteremia (81). Therefore, arterial blood cultures are a satisfactory alternative when peripheral venipuncture is not possible for paired blood cultures.

In summary, the measurement of the differential time to positivity between hub–blood and peripheral blood cultures constitutes an alternative method to quantitative blood cultures. In cancer patients, a cutoff limit of 2 h in favor of the blood culture drawn on the catheter has sensitivity and specificity above 90% for the diagnosis of CRI. The value of this technique, based on the results of blood cultures, could be higher in patients with long-term catheters than in patients with short-term CVCs, such as critically ill patients. The practicability of the method may have some limitations in clinical practice. First, although many clinical microbiology laboratories use continually monitored blood-culture systems, that may be not the case all over the world, mainly in developing countries. Second, a 24-h capability in the microbiology laboratory (including on weekends) or the ability to process blood cultures on the ward are rather uncommon. Therefore, whatever the accuracy of the method, the technique may be somewhat difficult to perform routinely around the clock.

RAPID DIAGNOSIS OF CRI BY USING DIRECT EXAMINATION

An overnight incubation is usually necessary for microbiological cultures of a catheter segment, exit site, or blood samplings. Therefore, whatever the diagnostic strategy chosen (removal of the catheter or not), an early diagnosis and a microbiological orientation would be very useful for the clinician.

Direct Examination of the Catheter Tip

The direct examination of the catheter tip has been proposed by Cooper and Hopkins (23). Gram stain of the catheter tip was 100% sensitive and 97% specific for the diagnosis of catheter-tip colonization based on semiquantitative cultures, with negative and positive predictive values of 100 and 84%, respectively. Using a gram-stained impression smear of the external surface of the CVC fixed on a glass slide, Collignon et al. reported 83% sensitivity and 81% specificity, whereas the positive predictive value was only 44%, due to the low prevalence of bacteremic CRI in the study group (82). Acridine-orange staining of the CVC has also been proposed, but compared with the culture method, direct examination lacked sensitivity (83). Acridine-orange staining seems to be less accurate than Gram staining. Other authors reported that Gram staining of catheter segments failed to diagnose CRI, and above all showed that the technique was time-consuming and impractical in clinical practice (84). More recently, the utility of a centrifuged-prepared Gram stain of sonication broth as a rapid test for the diagnosis of CRI was assessed (85). Similarly, no correlation was found between this test and the diagnosis of CRI established by the sonication technique. In fact, the clinical utility of these techniques is limited in routine, except in cases when a rapid diagnosis is needed in a patient with severe sepsis.

The rapid diagnosis of fungal infection of intravascular catheters in newborns, by scanning electron microscopy examination of removed central or umbilical catheters, has been proposed (86). Scanning electron microscopy identified fungi in the biomaterials covering the catheter surface in a few hours. However, the actual significance of this complex technique is not defined in other settings and in clinical practice. The tests described in the following section may be more promising for the clinical practice than direct examination of the catheter tip.

Gram Staining of Pericatheter Skin and Hub

The value of Gram staining the pericatheter skin and the connection in detecting CRI was the focus of a Spanish study (51). A CRI was considered to be present if the same microorganism was isolated from the catheter tip, skin and/or hub, and blood cultures. Taken together, the sensitivity, specificity, and positive and negative predictive values for Gram staining of the skin and hub were 80%, 82%, 35%, and 97%, respectively. Therefore, as previously shown for the skin cultures, the negative results of Gram staining skin and hub swabs could be useful to quickly rule out the presence of CRI.

Acridine-Orange Leucocyte Cytospin Test

Direct examination of blood drawn from the catheter using the acridine-orange leucocyte cytospin (AOLC) test is a rapid method for the diagnosis of CRI. The AOLC test allows detection of bacteria from a small sample (50 µl) of blood aspirated from the catheter (87). The cytospin allows the production of a monolayer from the sample onto a slide. Acridine-orange is an intercalating agent used to stain DNA on the slide, which may then be examined using ultraviolet microscopy with oil immersion. The AOLC test was first tested in a population of infants with suspected catheter sepsis, defined by quantitative blood cultures (88). The AOLC test was 87% sensitive and 94% specific in the diagnosis of CRI. The results were available in an hour.

The same group showed that the AOLC test was not as reliable for the detection of CRI in adults. This could be due to a lower quantitative level of bacteremia in adults than in neonates (87), leading to a lower sensitivity of the test. Therefore, Tighe et al. reported a modification of the test, using an endoluminal brush to release a larger number of organisms colonizing the catheter. After the brush is used, a shower of fibrin and organisms released from the wall of colonized catheters is subsequently aspirated and identified using the AOLC test (87). Two groups of 50 adult patients with suspected sepsis and a CVC, in whom the decision to remove the catheter had been made, were compared. In the first group, a blood sample was withdrawn from the catheter for the AOLC test; in the second group, an endoluminal brush was used to "sweep" the catheter before collection of the blood sample. Results of the AOLC test were compared with culture of the catheter tip. The test was positive in only 12% of the infected catheters in group 1 (no brush), compared to 83% of the infected catheters in cases with endoluminal brushing. The AOLC test produced no false positives in either group. Despite these encouraging data with the endoluminal brush, the theoretical risk of embolization or subsequent bacteremia should be considered. Previously, the same group had proposed an endoluminal brush technique, with a threshold of 10^2 cfu/ml, for in situ diagnosis of CRI (89).

More recently, Kite et al. conducted a similar study in 124 adult surgical patients, using the AOLC test and Gram stain for rapid diagnosis of CRI without catheter removal (35). The Gram stain and AOLC test is simple, rapid (30 min), inexpensive, and requires two 50 μl-samples of catheter blood treated with EDTA, and the use of light and ultraviolet microscopy (Table 8). No endoluminal brushing was used. CRIs were defined using a composite criterion based on the results of three methods, which allow the differential

Table 8   Rapid Diagnosis of CR-BSI Without Catheter Removal

Gram stain and acridine-orange leucocyte cytospin (AOLC) test[a]

A 1-ml sample of blood (treated with edetic acid) is aspirated from the catheter lumen for the Gram stain and AOLC test, which require two 50-μl samples of catheter blood. Each sample is placed into 12-mm by 75-mm polystyrene tubes to which is added 1.2 ml formalin (10% by volume) saline (0.025 mol/l) solution, and the mixture left for 2 min. 2.8 ml 0.19 mol/l saline is then added to each tube, followed by centrifugation at 352 g for 5 min. The supernatant is decanted and the cellular deposit is homogenized by vortexing for 5 s and then transferred to a cytospin cupule that contains a microscope slide. The cellular suspension is centrifuged at 153 g for 5 min in a cytocentrifuge. A monolayer of leucocytes and microorganisms is placed on each of two microscope slides, which are heat-dried on a 60°C hotplate for 3 min and then stained with either 1 in 10,000 (weight/volume) acridine-orange or Gram stain and viewed by ultraviolet and light microscopy. A minimum of 100 high-power fields are examined, and the presence of any microorganisms within the cellular monolayer (on either slide) is considered a positive result.

---

[a] From Ref. 88.

assessment of both endoluminal and extraluminal portions of the CVC. A sensitivity of 96%, a specificity of 91%, a negative predictive value of 97%, and a positive predictive value of 91% were reported for the diagnosis of bacteremic CRI with both tests taken together (35). The Gram stain and AOLC test have a threshold of 1000 microorganisms per milliliter of blood; considering that peripheral blood contained less than 250 cfu/ml, the technique was unlikely to detect bacteremia unrelated to the catheter. The operational values reported are similar to those obtained using the measurement of the differential time to positivity (65).

Interestingly, although the specificity of the method was high in both studies, the AOLC test had a very much higher sensitivity (96%) in the recent study by Kite et al. (35) than in the first group (no brush; sensitivity 12%) of the former study by Tighe et al. (87). The reasons for this finding are unclear. Microbiological techniques are similar in both studies. The use of Gram stain in the latter study cannot account for this discrepancy, considering that the concordance between Gram stain and AOLC test was excellent (35). Finally, the theoretical risk of toxicity of acridine-orange, an intercalating agent, may justify some precautions in the microbiology laboratories. Despite these concerns, this promising technique allows a rapid diagnosis (< 1 h), and could be used in the near future to establish the diagnosis of CRI without catheter removal and to guide an early targeted antimicrobial therapy, or conversely, to avoid unnecessary use of antibiotics, particularly glycopeptides.

Gram Staining of Blood Drawn From the Catheter

Gram staining of blood drawn from the catheter is a simple method for the diagnosis of CRI, enabling a preliminary identification of the pathogen. Kite et al. suggested that the AOLC test could be more accurate in cases of gram-negative bacteremia if bacterial counts are low, and if red blood cells are poorly lysed (35). Nevertheless, the authors showed a high concordance between the results of the Gram stain and the AOLC test (only one discrepant result with positive Gram stain and negative AOLC test). Using the Gram staining alone, for direct examination of blood drawn from the catheter during 23 episodes of CRI, Moonens et al. reported a 100% specificity but a lower sensitivity (78% for definite CRI, 61% for suspected and definite CRI taken together) (90).

OTHER TECHNIQUES

Recently, Elliott et al. proposed a serological test for the diagnosis of CRI due to coagulase-negative staphylococci (CNS) (91). To our knowledge, this innovative approach is the only one of this type described to date. The authors compared 67 patients suspected of having CRI due to CNS and 67 control patients with a CVC, but without CRI. Ten milliliters of blood were obtained in both groups, and serum antibody levels of both IgG and IgM against a short-chain lipoteichoic acid antigen isolated from CNS were determined, using an ELISA technique. Significant differences between the mean IgG and IgM titers of the test group and the control group were observed. Using an IgG titer of 20,000, the test had a sensitivity of 75% and a specificity of 90%.

This method has several limitations, however, which precluded its use in clinical practice at that time.

1. The criteria used in the study for the diagnosis of CRI are debatable. None of the microbiological techniques usually considered as reference were used, including quantitative catheter-tip cultures or paired blood cultures. Only a clinical criterion was used, which commonly lacks specificity. In addition, only one positive blood culture with isolation of CNS was required, probably leading to the inclusion of "false bacteremias."

2. Despite significant differences between IgG levels, there was an overlap between the control group and the group with suspected CRI, leading to a 75% sensitivity. Although the authors state that the test compares favorably with other diagnostic methods, it is clearly lower than the sensitivity and specificity of quantitative (Sp and Se > 92%) (64) or qualitative (Sp and Se > 90%) (65,73) paired blood cultures.

3. Only staphylococci are detected. However, as many as 30 to 40% (92), or even more than 55% (93) of the CRIs are due to Enterobacteriaceae, *Pseudomonas* sp., *S. aureus*, or yeasts, the severity of which may be far greater than that of CNS bacteremia. In addition, the antigen used is common to *S. epidermidis* and *S. aureus* strains. A diagnostic method allowing identification of the microorganism responsible for sepsis (and especially to distinguish between CNS and *S. aureus* strains, and to identify Gram-negative rods and yeasts) is mandatory when a CRI is suspected.

4. Finally, the usefulness of the method in terms of rapidity of diagnosis can be a matter of controversy. Although the authors consider that the diagnosis can be made without having to wait for blood culture results, the algorithm proposed suggests that the value of the ELISA result alone is limited when the results of blood cultures are not available. Similar results have been reported in a study recently published by the same group (94). Serological tests have also been proposed by this group for rapid diagnosis of endocarditis caused by gram-positive cocci (95).

Further studies are needed before serological tests can be proposed in routine. However, the concept of this method is innovative in the field of catheter infections. Indirect diagnostic methods, such as those developed for community-acquired pneumonia (e.g., legionella urinary antigen) could offer new perspectives in this setting. The usefulness of serological methods for the diagnosis of CRI remains to be confirmed.

Other tests that have been proposed, such as C-reactive protein and nitro-blue tetrazolium tests, have not proved to be useful in the diagnosis of CRI.

COST-EFFECTIVENESS OF DIAGNOSTIC TESTS

Nosocomial catheter-related bloodstream infections account for estimated excess hospital costs ranging from $34,000 to $56,000 per infection (40,96). As shown for attributable morbidity and mortality (97), these added costs are probably overestimated because of imperfect adjustment. True additional costs could be lower after adjustment for severity factors during the ICU stay and before the event. Pittet et al. estimated that additional costs were $29,000 per survivor in critically ill patients (98). In a Spanish study, each episode of CR-BSI represented an additional cost of about $3,100 (99). Attributable mortality, excess length of stay, and costs are lower for CR-BSI than for bacteremia of other origin (100).

Few studies have focused on the cost-effectiveness of diagnostic strategies. In 1997, Siegman-Igra et al. estimated the total hospital laboratory cost for each test, including costs for personnel, minutes of test time, supplies, reagents, equipment maintenance, and laboratory overhead (34) (Table 9). Finally, the overall cost of each accurate test result was calculated by using the cost of the test and the pooled sensitivity and specificity for the test. The costs of antibiotic therapy in cases of true-positive and false-positive results,

Table 9   Estimated Cost for Each Microbiologic Method

Test method	Estimated cost ($)	
	per test	per accurate result
Diagnostic methods after catheter removal		
Qualitative catheter segment culture	57	467
Semiquantitative catheter segment culture	39	401
Quantitative catheter segment culture	89	415
Direct examination	22–47	ND
Diagnostic methods without catheter removal		
Unpaired qualitative catheter blood culture	38	271
Unpaired quantitative catheter blood culture	60	198
Paired quantitative catheter blood culture	120	282
Differential time to positivity of blood cultures[a]	38–57	ND
Gram stain and AOLC test	60–90	ND

AOLC: acridine-orange leucocyte cytospin.
[a] Considering that aerobic (± anaerobic) bottles are used for peripheral blood cultures, and only an aerobic bottle for the hub–blood culture.
Source: Ref. 34.

and the costs of catheters and catheter replacement, were included in the calculation.

Among the catheter-tip culture techniques, the estimated cost per test was about 2.5-fold greater for quantitative ($88) than for semiquantitative culture ($38), but was similar ($415 versus $401) when calculated per accurate result. In the same analysis, the unpaired quantitative catheter blood cultures offered the lowest cost per accurate test result ($198 versus $282 for paired quantitative blood cultures) (34).

Since this meta-analysis, new diagnostic tools have been described. The Gram stain and AOLC test are considered to be inexpensive (35). Considering the total time for doing both a Gram stain and an AOLC test as 20–30 min, as reported by Kite et al., a cost of about $60 to $90 per test may be estimated (101). Differential time to positivity of blood cultures may also be used for diagnosing CRI. Although paired blood cultures are taken, only aerobic bottles are needed, and the total laboratory cost of qualitative blood cultures has been shown to be about one-third lower than that of quantitative blood cultures ($38 versus $60) (34). In addition, this procedure may avoid both unjustified removal of the CVC when the differential time to positivity between central and peripheral blood cultures is short, and unjustified prolonged antibiotic treatment when the differential time to positivity is long.

The cost-effectiveness of these new techniques is likely, but subsequent prospective studies are required to assess whether these tests actually change clinicians' decisions about catheter replacement, which has been estimated to cost $582 per replacement for nontunneled catheters (101).

CONCLUSIONS

New techniques have been recently proposed for diagnosing CRI. The most promising techniques seem to be the direct examination of blood drawn from the catheter, using the acridine-orange leucocyte cytospin test and Gram stain, and the differential time to positivity of paired blood cultures. However, the value of these recently described diagnostic tools requires confirmation by other investigators, in other settings, before either method can be recommended for routine use (101). Both techniques could be more accurate for long-dwelling catheters, such as those used in cancer patients, than for short-term catheters. This is consistent with identification of the CVC lumen as the predominant source of infection in patients with long-term catheterization (35). The easier method to set up immediately would be the differential time to positivity test, given that many clinical microbiology laboratories use continuous-monitoring blood culture systems, and provided that many physicians investigate a newly occurring fever by drawing simultaneous catheter and venipuncture blood cultures (100).

These latter methods are mainly destined to establish the diagnosis of CRI without removal of the catheter. However, paired blood cultures with measurement of the differential time to positivity can be performed exclusively in clinically stable patients, without local (purulence or cellulitis) or systemic (severe sepsis or septic shock) signs of severity. The Gram stain and AOLC test are destined to establish or to rule out the diagnosis of CRI within 30 min. In unstable septic patients, however, the technique should be used exclusively to guide an early targeted antibiotic therapy, rather than to attempt to save a potentially seriously colonized catheter.

In case of septic shock of undetermined origin in a patient with a CVC, or when local signs of infection are present, the catheter needs to be removed immediately and a semiquantitative—or, if possible, a quantitative—culture of the catheter tip (and eventually of the port) needs to be performed (5). Empirical antibiotics should be started immediately, eventually guided by the results of the Gram stain and AOLC test. In stable patients, techniques with high sensitivity and negative predictive value (such as skin cultures) and methods with high specificity and positive predictive value of bacteremic CRI (such as paired blood cultures or the Gram stain and AOLC test) could be proposed to avoid the removal of the CVC, which is unjustified in most cases. The recent recommendations for the Management of Intravascular CRI will be helpful for clinicians in the decision-making process (1).

A decisional tree for the diagnosis of CRI is proposed in Fig. 1.

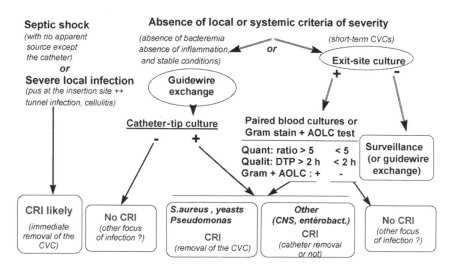

AOLC: acridine-orange leucocyte cytospin
AB: antibiotic treatment
Quant: quantitative blood cultures
Qualit: nonquantitative blood cultures
CNS: coagulase-negative staphylococci

(From Ref 5.)

Figure 1 Proposed decisional tree for the diagnosis of catheter-related infections.

REFERENCES

1. Mermel LA, Farr BM, Sherertz RJ, Raad II, O'Grady N, Harris JS, Craven DE. Guidelines for the management of intravascular catheter-related infections. Infect Control Hosp Epidemiol 2001; 22:222–242.
2. Ryan JA, Abel RM, Abbott WM, Hopkins CC, Chesney TMC, Colley R, Phillips K, Fisher JE. Catheter complications in total parenteral nutrition. A prospective study of 200 consecutive patients. N Engl J Med 1974; 290: 757–761.
3. Raad II, Sabbagh MF, Rand KH, Sherertz RJ. Quantitative tip culture methods and the diagnosis of central venous catheter-related infections. Diagn Microbiol Infect Dis 1992; 15:13–20.
4. Moyer MA, Edwards LD, Farley L. Comparative culture methods on 101 intravenous catheters. Routine, semiquantitative, and blood culture. Arch Intern Med 1983; 143:66–69.
5. Blot F, Brun-Buisson C. Current approaches to the diagnosis and prevention of catheter-related infections. Curr Opinion Crit Care 1999; 5:341–349.
6. Raad I, Costerton W, Sabharwal U, Sacilowski M, Anaissie F, Bodey GP. Ultrastructural analysis of indwelling vascular catheters: a quantitative relationship between luminal colonization and duration of placement. J Infect Dis 1993; 168:400–407.
7. Linares J, Sitges-Serra A, Garau J, Perez JL, Martin R. Pathogenesis of catheter sepsis: a prospective study with quantitative and semiquantitative cultures of catheter hub and segments. J Clin Microbiol 1985; 21:357–360.
8. Cercenado E, Ena J, Rodriguez-Creixems M, Romero I, Bouza E. A conservative procedure for the diagnosis of catheter-related infections. Arch Intern Med 1990; 150:1417–1420.
9. Pearson ML and the Hospital Infection Control Practices Advisory Committee. Guideline for prevention of intravascular device-related infections. Infect Control Hosp Epidemiol 1996; 17:438–473.
10. Juste RN, Hannan M, Glendenning A, Azadian B, Soni N. Central venous blood culture: a useful test for catheter colonisation? Intensive Care Med 2000; 26:1373–1375.
11. Maki DG, Weise CE, Sarafin HW. A semiquantitative culture method for identifying intravenous-catheter-related infection. N Engl J Med 1977; 296:1305–1309.
12. Armstrong CW, Mayhall CG, Miller KB, Newsome HH, Sugerman HJ, Dalton HP, Hall GO, Hunsberger S. Clinical predictors of infection of central venous catheters used for total parenteral nutrition. Infect Control Hosp Epidemiol 1990; 11:71–78.
13. Benezra D, Kiehn TE, Gold JWM, Brown AE, Turnbull ADM, Armstrong D. Prospective study of infections in indwelling central venous catheters using quantitative blood cultures. Am J Med 1988; 85:495–498.
14. Raad II, Bodey GP. Infectious complications of indwelling vascular catheters. Clin Infect Dis 1992; 15:197–210.
15. Peacock SJ, Eddelston M, Emptage A, King A, Crook DWM. Positive intravenous line tip cultures as predictors of bacteraemia. J Hosp Infection 1998; 40:35–38.

16. Widmer AF, Nettleman M, Flint K, Wenzel RP. The clinical impact of culturing central venous catheters. A prospective study. Arch Intern Med 1992; 152:1299–1302.

17. Brun-Buisson C, Abrouk F, Legrand P, Huet Y, Larabi S, Rapin M. Diagnosis of central venous catheter-related sepsis. Critical level of quantitative tip cultures. Arch Intern Med 1987; 147:873–877.

18. Harris GJ, Rosenquist MD, Kealey GP. An in vitro model for studying the effect of the subcutaneous tunnel and the skin exit site on the accuracy of central venous catheter tip cultures. J Burn Care Rehabil 1992; 13:628–631.

19. Collignon PJ, Soni N, Pearson IY, Woods WP, Munro R, Sorrell TC. Is semiquantitative culture of central vein catheter tips useful in the diagnosis of Cathéter-associated bacteremia? J Clin Microbiol 1986; 24:532–535.

20. Kristinsson KG, Burnett IA, Spencer RC. Evaluation of three methods for culturing long intravascular catheters. J Hosp Infect 1989; 14:183–191.

21. Rello J, Coll P, Prats G. Evaluation of culture techniques for diagnosis of catheter-related sepsis in critically ill patients. Eur J Clin Microbiol Infect Dis 1992; 11:1192–1193.

22. Hnatiuk OW, Pike J, Stoltzfus D, Lane W. Value of bedside plating of semiquantitative cultures for diagnosis of central venous catheter-related infections in ICU patients. Chest 1993, 103:896–899.

23. Cooper GL, Hopkins CC. Rapid diagnosis of intravascular catheter-associated infection by direct Gram staining of catheter segments. N Engl J Med 1985; 312:1142–1147.

24. Cleri DJ, Corrado ML, Seligman SJ. Quantitative culture of intravenous catheters and other intravascular inserts. J Infect Dis 1980; 141:781–786.

25. Sherertz RJ, Raad II, Belani A, Koo LC, Rand KH, Pickett DL, Straub SA, Fauerbach LL. Three-year experience with sonicated vascular catheter cultures in a clinical microbiology laboratory. J Clin Microbiol 1990; 28:76–82.

26. Sherertz RJ, Heard SO, Raad II. Diagnosis of triple-lumen catheter infection: comparison of roll plate, sonication and flushing methodologies. J Clin Microbiol 1997; 35:641–646.

27. Raad II, Hanna HA, Darouiche RO. Diagnosis of catheter-related bloodstream infections: is it necessary to culture the subcutaneous catheter segment? Eur J Clin Microbiol Infect Dis 2001; 20:566–568.

28. Fortun J, Perez-Molina JA, Asensio A, Calderon C, Casado JL, Mir N, Moreno A, Guerrero A. Semiquantitative culture of subcutaneous segment for conservative diagnosis of intravascular catheter-related infection. J Parenter Enteral Nutr 2000; 24:210–214.

29. Douard MC, Arlet G, Longuet P, Troje C, Rouveau M, Ponscarme D, Eurin B. Diagnosis of venous access port-related infections. Clin Infect Dis 1999; 29:1197–1202.

30. Longuet P, Douard MC, Arlet G, Molina JM, Benoit C, Leport C. Venous access port-related bacteremia in patients with acquired immunodeficiency syndrome or cancer: the reservoir as a diagnostic and therapeutic tool. Clin Infect Dis 2001; 32:1776–1783.

31. Valles J, Rello J, Matas L, Fontanals D, Baigorri F, Saura P, Artigas A. Impact of using an indwelling introducer on diagnosis of Swan-Ganz pul-

monary artery catheter colonization. Eur J Clin Microbiol Infect Dis 1996; 15:71–75.

32. Blot F, Chachaty E, Raynard B, Antoun S, Bourgain JL, Nitenberg G. Mechanisms and risk factors of infection of pulmonary artery catheters and introducer sheaths in cancer patients admitted to an intensive care unit. J Hosp Infection 2001; 48:289–297.

33. Farr BM, Shapiro D. Diagnostic tests: distinguishing good tests from bad and even ugly ones. Infect Control Hosp Epidemiol 2000; 21:278–284.

34. Siegman-Igra Y, Anglim AM, Shapiro DE, Adal KA, Strain BA, Farr BM. Diagnosis of vascular catheter-related bloodstream infection: a meta-analysis. J Clin Microbiol 1997; 35:928–936.

35. Kite P, Dobbins BM, Wilcox MH, McMahon MJ. Rapid diagnosis of central-venous-catheter-related bloodstream infection without catheter removal. Lancet 1999; 354:1504–1507.

36. Bozzetti F, Terno G, Bonfanti G, Scarpa D, Scotti A, Ammatuna M, Bonalumi MG. Prevention and treatment of central venous catheter by exchange via a guidewire. Ann Surg 1983; 198:48–52.

37. Bonadimani B, Sperti C, Stevanin A, Cappellazzo F, Militello C, Petrin P, Pedrazzoli S. Central venous catheter guidewire replacement according to the Seldinger technique: usefulness in the management of patients on total parenteral nutrition. J Parenter Enteral Nutr 1987; 11:267–270.

38. Cobb DK, High KP, Sawyer RG, Sable CA, Adams RB, Lindley DA, Pruett TL, Schwenzer KJ, Farr BM. A controlled trial of scheduled replacement of central venous and pulmonary-artery catheters. N Engl J Med 1992; 327:1062–1068.

39. Cook D, Randolph A, Kernerman P, Cupido C, King D, Soukup C, Brun-Buisson C. Central venous catheter replacement strategies: a systematic review of the literature. Crit Care Med 1997; 25:1417–1424.

40. Centers for Disease Control and Prevention. Guidelines for the prevention of intravascular catheter-related infections. MMWR 2002; 51:1–29.

41. Commission des Référentiels de la Société de Réanimation de Langue Française. Réactualisation de la XIIe Conférence de Consensus sur les Infections liées aux cathéters veineux centraux en réanimation. Réanimation 2003. In press.

42. Bjornson HS, Colley R, Bower RH, Duty VP, Schwartz-Fulton JT, Fisher JE. Association between microorganism growth at the catheter insertion site and colonization of the catheter in patients receiving total parenteral nutrition. Surgery 1982; 92:720–725.

43. Guidet B, Nicola I, Barakett V, Gabillet JM, Snoey E, Petit JC, Offenstadt G. Skin versus hub cultures to predict colonization and infection of central venous catheter in intensive care patients. Infection 1994; 22:43–52.

44. Mahé I, Fourrier F, Roussel-Delvallez M, Martin G, Chopin C. Predictive value of skin culture in central venous catheter colonization. Réan Urg 1998; 7:17–24.

45. Sitges-Serra A, Puig P, Linares J, Perez JL, Farrero N, Jaurrieta E, Garau J. Hub colonization as the initial step in an outbreak of catheter-related sepsis due to coagulase negative staphylococci during parenteral nutrition. J Parenter Enteral Nutr 1984; 8:668–672.

46. Snydman DR, Pober BR, Murray SA, Gorbea HF, Majka JA, Perry LK. Predictive value of surveillance skin cultures in total-parenteral-nutrition-related infection. Lancet 1982; 2(8312):1385–1388.

47. Raad II, Baba M, Bodey GP. Diagnosis of catheter-related infections: the role of surveillance and targeted quantitative skin cultures. Clin Infect Dis 1995; 20:593–597.

48. Fan ST, Teoh-Tchan CH, Lau KF, Chu KW, Kwan AKW, Wong KK. Predictive value of surveillance skin and hub cultures in central venous catheter sepsis. J Hosp Infect 1988; 12:191–198.

49. Douard MC, Clementi E, Arlet G, Marie O, Jacob L, Schremmer B, Rouveau M, Garrouste MT, Eurin B. Negative catheter tip culture and diagnosis of catheter-related bacteremia. Nutrition 1994; 10:397–404.

50. Segura M, Llado L, Guirao X, Piracés M, Herms R, Alia C, Sitges-Serra A. A prospective study of a new protocol for in situ diagnosis of central venous catheter related bacteraemia. Clin Nutr 1993; 12:103–107.

51. Leon M, Garcia M, Herranz MA, Gonzalez V, Martinez A, Castillo F, Andres E, Leon C, Huet J. Diagnostic value of Gram staining of peri-catheter skin and the connection in the prediction of intravascular-catheter-related bacteremia. Enferm Infecc Microbiol Clin 1998; 16:214–218.

52. Kiehn TE, Wong B, Edwards FF, Armstrong D. Comparative recovery of bacteria and yeasts from lysis–centrifugation and a conventional blood culture system. J Clin Microbiol 1983; 18:300–304.

53. Flynn PM, Shenep JL, Strokes D, Barrett FF. Differential quantitation with a commercial blood culture tube for diagnosis of catheter-related infection. J Clin Microbiol 1988; 26:1045–1046.

54. Ruderman JW, Morgan MA, Klein AH. Quantitative blood cultures in the diagnosis of sepsis in infants with umbilical and Broviac catheters. J Pediatr 1988; 112:748–751.

55. Andremont A, Paulet R, Nitenberg G, Hill C. Value of semiquantitative cultures of blood drawn through catheter hubs for estimating the risk of catheter tip colonization in cancer patients. J Clin Microbiol 1988; 26:2297–2299.

56. Snydman DR, Murray SA, Kornfeld SJ, Majka JA, Ellis CA. Total parenteral nutrition-related infections. Prospective epidemiologic study using semi-quantitative methods. Am J Med 1982; 73:695–699.

57. Capdevila JA, Planes AM, Palomar M, Gasser I, Almirante B, Pahissa A, Crespo E, Martinez-Vazquez JM. Value of differential quantitative blood cultures in the diagnosis of catheter-related sepsis. Eur J Clin Microbiol Infect Dis 1992; 11:403–407.

58. Wing EJ, Norden CW, Shadduck RK, Winkelstein A. Use of quantitative bacteriologic techniques to diagnose catheter-related sepsis. Arch Intern Med 1979; 139:482–483.

59. Flynn PM, Shenep JL, Strokes DC, Barrett FF. "In situ" management of confirmed central venous catheter-related bacteremia. Pediatr Infect Dis 1987; 6:729–734.

60. Raucher HS, Hyatt AC, Barzilai A, Harris MB, Weiner MA, LeLeiko NS, Hodes DS. Quantitative blood cultures in the evaluation of septicemia in children with Broviac catheters. J Pediatr 1984; 104:29–33.

61. Paya CV, Guerra L, Marsh HM, Farnell MB, Washington J, Thompson RL.

Limited usefulness of quantitative culture of blood drawn through the device for diagnosis of intravascular-device-related bacteremia. J Clin Microbiol 1989; 27:1431–1433.

62. Douard MC, Arlet G, Leverger G, Paulien R, Waintrop C, Clementi E, Eurin B, Schaison G. Quantitative blood cultures for diagnosis and management of catheter-related sepsis in pediatric hematology and oncology patients. Intensive Care Med 1991; 17:30–35.

63. Fan ST, Teoh-Chan CH, Lau KF. Evaluation of central venous catheter sepsis by differential quantitative blood culture. Eur J Clin Microbiol Infect Dis 1989; 8:142–144.

64. Quilici N, Audibert G, Conroy MC, Bollaert PE, Guillemin F, Welfringer P, Garric J, Weber M, Laxenaire MC. Differential quantitative blood cultures in the diagnosis of catheter-related sepsis in intensive care units. Clin Infect Dis 1997; 25:1066–1070.

65. Blot F, Nitenberg G, Chachaty E, Raynard B, Germann N, Antoun S, Laplanche A, Brun-Buisson C, Tancrede C. Diagnosis of catheter-related bacteraemia: a prospective comparison of the time to positivity of central vs. peripheral blood cultures. Lancet 1999; 354:1071–1077.

66. Blot F, Schmidt E, Nitenberg G, Tancrede C, Leclercq B, Laplanche A, Andremont A. Earlier positivity of central-venous versus peripheral-blood cultures is highly predictive of catheter-related sepsis. J Clin Microbiol 1998; 36:105–109.

67. Rogers MS, Oppenheim BA. The use of continuous monitoring blood culture systems in the diagnosis of catheter related sepsis. J Clin Pathol 1998; 51:635–637.

68. Malgrange VB, Escande MC, Theobald S. Validity of earlier positivity of central venous blood cultures in comparison with peripheral blood cultures for diagnosing catheter-related bacteremia in cancer patients. J Clin Microbiol 2001; 39:274–278.

69. Robinson JL. Sensitivity of a blood culture drawn through a single lumen of a multilumen, long term, indwelling, central venous catheter in pediatric oncology patients. J Pediatr Hematol Oncol 2002; 24:72–74.

70. Mermel LA, Josephson S, Binns L. Diagnosis of catheter-related bloodstream infection by differential growth rates of catheter-drawn and percutaneously drawn blood cultures [abstr]. 38th Interscience Conference on Antimicrobial Agents and Chemotherapy, San Diego, 1998:K5.

71. Rijnders BJA, Verwaest C, Peetermans WE, Wilmer A, Vandecasteele S, Van Eldere J, Van Wijngaerden E. Difference in time to positivity of hub–blood versus nonhub–blood cultures is not helpful for the diagnosis of catheter-related bloodstream infection in critically ill patients. Crit Care Med 2001; 29:1399–1403.

72. Blot F. Why should paired blood cultures not be useful for diagnosing catheter-related bacteremia in critically ill patients? Crit Care Med 2002; 30:1402–1403.

73. Raad II, Hanna HA, Alakech B, Chatzinikolaou I, Johnson MM, Tarrand J. Differential time to positivity: a useful method for diagnosing catheter-related bloodstream infections. Ann Intern Med 2004; 140:18–25.

74. Seifert H, Cornely O, Seggewiss K, Decker M, Stefanik D, Wisplinghoff H,

Fatkenheuer G. Bloodstream infection in neutropenic cancer patients related to short-term nontunnelled catheters determined by quantitative blood cultures, differential time to positivity, and molecular epidemiological typing with pulsed-field gel electrophoresis. J Clin Microbiol 2003; 41:118–123.

75. Khatib R, Riederer KM, Clark JA, Khatib S, Briski LE, Wilson FM. Coagulase-negative staphylococci in multiple blood cultures: Strain relatedness and determinants of same-strain bacteremia. J Clin Microbiol 1995; 33:816–820.

76. Souvenir D, Anderson DE Jr, Palpant S, Mroch H, Askin S, Anderson J, Claridge J, Eiland J, Malone C, Garrison MW, Watson P, Campbell DM. Blood cultures positive for coagulase-negative staphylococci: antisepsis, pseudobacteremia, and therapy of patients. J Clin Microbiol 1998; 36:1923–1926.

77. Wormser GP, Onorato IM, Preminger TJ, Culver D, Martone WJ. Sensitivity and specificity of blood cultures obtained through intravascular catheters. Crit Care Med 1990; 18:152–156.

78. DesJardin JA, Falagas ME, Ruthazer R, Griffith J, Wawrose D, Schenkein D, Miller K, Snydman DR. Clinical utility of blood cultures drawn from indwelling central venous catheters in hospitalized patients with cancer. Ann Intern Med 1999; 131:641–647.

79. Martinez JA, DesJardin JA, Aronoff M, Supran S, Nasraway SA, Snydman DR. Clinical utility of blood cultures drawn from central venous or arterial catheters in critically ill surgical patients. Crit Care Med 2002; 30:7–13.

80. Archer GL. Coagulase-negative *Staphylococci* in blood cultures: the clinician's dilemma. Infect Control 1985; 6:12–13.

81. Levin PD, Hershch M, Rudensky B, Yinnon AM. The use of arterial line as a source for blood cultures. Intensive Care Med 2000; 26:1350–1354.

82. Collignon P, Chan R, Munro R. Rapid diagnosis of intravascular catheter-related sepsis. Arch Intern Med 1987; 147:1609–1612.

83. Coutlee F, Lemieux C, Paradis JF. Value of direct catheter staining in the diagnosis of intravascular catheter-related infection. J Clin Microbiol 1988; 26:1088–1090.

84. Spencer RC, Kristinsson KG. Failure to diagnose intravascular-associated infection by direct Gram staining of catheter segments. J Hosp Infection 1986; 7:305–306.

85. Kelly M, Wciorka LR, McConico S, Peterson LR. Sonicated vascular catheter-tip cultures. Quantitative association with catheter-related sepsis and the non-utility of an adjuvant cytocentrifuge Gram stain. Am J Clin Pathol 1996; 105:210–215.

86. Sbarbati A, Fanos V, Bernardi P, Tato L. Rapid diagnosis of fungal infection of intravascular catheters in newborns by scanning electron microscopy. Scanning 2001; 23:376–378.

87. Tighe MJ, Kite P, Thomas D, Fawley WN, McMahon MJ. Rapid diagnosis of catheter related sepsis using the acridine-orange leukocyte cytospin test and an endoluminal brush. JPEN 1996; 20:215–218.

88. Rushforth JA, Hoy CM, Kite P, Puntis JW. Rapid diagnosis of central venous catheter sepsis. Lancet 1993; 342:402–403.

89. Kite P, Dobbins BM, Wilcox MH, Fawley WN, Kindon AJ, Thomas D, Tighe MJ, McMahon MJ. Evaluation of a novel endoluminal brush method for in situ diagnosis of catheter related sepsis. J Clin Pathol 1997; 50:278–282.

90. Moonens F, El Alami S, van Gossum A, Struelens MJ, Serruys E. Usefulness of Gram staining of blood collected from total parenteral nutrition catheter for rapid diagnosis of catheter-related sepsis. J Clin Microbiol 1994; 32:1578–1579.

91. Elliott TSJ, Tebbs SE, Moss HA, Worthington T, Spare MK, Faroqui MH, Lambert PA. A novel serological test for the diagnosis of central venous catheter-associated sepsis. J Hosp Infection 2000; 40:262–266.

92. Richards MJ, Edwards JR, Culver DH, Gaynes RP, and the National Nosocomial Infections Surveillance System. Nosocomial infections in medical intensive care units in the United States. Crit Care Med 1999; 27:887–892.

93. Groeger JS, Lucas AB, Thaler HT, Friedlander-Klar H, Brown AE, Kiehn TE, Armstrong D. Infectious morbidity associated with long-term use of venous access devices in patients with cancer. Ann Intern Med 1993; 119:1168–1174.

94. Worthington T, Lambert PA, Traube A, Elliott TS. A rapid ELISA for the diagnosis of intravascular catheter related sepsis caused by coagulase negative staphylococci. J Clin Pathol 2002; 55:41–43.

95. Connaughton M, Lang S, Tebbs SE, Littler WA, Lambert PA, Elliott TS. Rapid serodiagnosis of gram-positive bacterial endocarditis. J Infect 2001; 42:140–144.

96. Dimick JB, Pelz RK, Consunji R, Swoboda SM, Hendrix CW, Lipsett PA. Increased resource use associated with catheter-related bloodstream infection in the surgical intensive care unit. Arch Surg 2001; 136:229–234.

97. Soufir L, Timsit JF, Mahe C, Carlet J, Régnier B, Chevret S. Attributable morbidity and mortality of catheter-related septicemia in critically ill patients: a matched, risk-adjusted, cohort study. Infect Control Hosp Epidemiol 1999; 20:396–401.

98. Pittet D, Hulliger S, Auckenthaler R. Intravascular device-related infections in critically ill patients. J Chemother 1995; 7:55–66.

99. Rello J, Ochagavia A, Sabanes E, Roque M, Mariscal D, Reynaga E, Valles J. Evaluation of outcome of intravenous catheter-related infections in critically ill patients. Am J Respir Crit Care Med 2000; 162:1027–1030.

100. Renaud B, Brun-Buisson C. Outcomes of primary and catheter-related bacteremia. A cohort and case-control study in critically ill patients. Am J Respir Crit Care Med 2001; 163:1584–1590.

101. Farr BM. Accuracy and cost-effectiveness of new tests for diagnosis of catheter-related bloodstream infections. Lancet 1999; 354:1487–1488.

Management of Intravascular Catheter-Related Infections

Leonard A. Mermel

*Division of Infectious Disease, Rhode Island Hospital
and Brown Medical School
Providence, Rhode Island*

Barry M. Farr

*The University of Virginia Health System and
The University of Virginia School of Medicine
Charlottesville, VA*

INTRODUCTION

Some 80,000 patients in U.S. intensive care units (ICUs) develop central venous catheter-related infections each year (1,2), and even more do so throughout the rest of the health system (3). The variable outcome of catheter-related infections reflects the fact that a myriad of microbes may cause such infections. *Staphylococcus aureus* and *Candida* species are associated with the greatest morbidity and mortality (4,5). Despite the potential seriousness of such infections, scant data exist in the literature regarding evidence-based management. Guidelines have been recently published to assist clinicians caring for patients with catheter-related infections (3,6), and many of the chapters in this book include sections on the management of infections related to particular devices and pathogens. The purpose of this chapter is to summarize some of the salient features of the published guidelines regarding management and to discuss some of the controversial management issues.

DIAGNOSIS OF CRBSI

Appropriate management of catheter-related bloodstream infection (CRBSI) depends first upon accurate diagnosis. A large majority of ICU patients with an indwelling CVC and a new fever, but with no local signs of inflammation at the catheter site, have the CVC removed and cultures performed and are shown to have no catheter-related infection (7). False-positive blood cultures among such patients have been associated with overdiagnosis and excessive therapy, resulting in prolonged hospital stays and extra costs ranging from $4100 to $4385 (8,9). Unnecessary antibiotic therapy also helps to add selective pressure favoring the survival and proliferation of antibiotic-resistant pathogens in healthcare facilities, where they result in more costly infections and a higher risk of mortality with serious infections. Because many patients with CRBSI have infection from normal skin flora, which are also frequent causes of false-positive blood cultures due to contamination during specimen collection, there must be a way of distinguishing true-positive from false-positive blood cultures.

One study found that 154 (90%) of 171 cultures growing coagulase-negative staphylococci (CNS) were likely to be false-positives (10). Of these 171 patients, 130 (76%) had only one positive set of blood cultures, and 40 (24%) had two or more positive sets. Of the 40 with two or more positive sets, 23 (62%) had symptoms compatible with bloodstream infection, but for three of the patients each set contained a different species of CNS. Another three patients had two or more sets growing the same species, but pulsed-field gel electrophoresis showed that each set contained a different strain. This left only 17% of the patients with CNS-positive blood cultures that appeared to be true causes of bloodstream infection.

Most hospital laboratories do not have access to molecular typing or, if they do, usually not in a timely manner that could help interpret clinical isolates for an individual patient. For this reason, national guidelines have recommended that at least two sets of blood cultures collected from different sites should show what appears to be the same strain of the same species (i.e., with the same antibiogram plus any other readily identifiable features such as colonial color, morphology, etc., that might be used to recognize a particular strain) before considering a bloodstream infection due to skin flora like CNS (11). Percutaneously drawn samples are less likely to be contaminated than those drawn from an indwelling catheter (8), but up to half of the positive percutaneously drawn cultures may still represent false-positive cultures (12–14).

A problem of underdiagnosis could be equally important, however, since 70% of patients with CRBSI due to CVCs had no inflammation at the site of the CVC (15,16). For this reason, patients with an indwelling catheter and onset of a new fever without another obvious source must be evaluated for possible CRBSI.

Evaluation of a new fever should involve collection of two sets of blood cultures (3). For ICU patients with continuing fever and negative routine blood cultures, specialized blood culture collection bottles may improve the yield of diagnosing occult candidemia and should be considered (17). For patients who have an indwelling CVC, the diagnosis of CRBSI should be suspected even in the absence of local inflammatory signs, because for such patients a new fever and/or rigors without localizing symptoms are often related to CRBSI (18). For adult patients, blood cultures should use a sample of at least 10 ml (and preferably 20 ml) of blood per set of blood cultures (19). For most patients with short-term catheters, both sets of cultures should be obtained percutaneously, because false-positive cultures have been shown to be significantly more likely when drawn from the hub of an indwelling catheter (8,20). To minimize the false-positive rate of percutaneously drawn cultures, an alcohol-based antiseptic should be used for skin preparation before phlebotomy. One recent study showed that 70% isopropyl alcohol appeared to be as effective for this purpose as two other alcohol-containing preps, tincture of iodine, and a commercial product that contains povidone iodine and 70% isopropyl alcohol (21). Isopropyl alcohol has the advantage of being less costly and is associated with a lower rate of skin reactions than is tincture of iodine.

For patients with long-term catheters (i.e., those in place for weeks to months), one of the two sets of blood cultures should be from the indwelling catheter. This has been shown to yield important diagnostic information when using either quantitative blood cultures or qualitative blood cultures that are continuously monitored for positivity. Blood drawn from the catheter that turns culture-positive more than two hours earlier than blood drawn from a peripheral vein has been shown to suggest that the catheter is the source of infection (22,23). With quantitative blood cultures, a concentration of bacteria 5- to 10-fold higher in blood from the catheter has been shown to indicate catheter-related infection as the source of the bacteremia (24). The way in which differential time to positivity works with qualitative cultures is related to the principle upon which the paired quantitative cultures work. A sample with a higher inoculum will be detected as positive earlier than one with a lower inoculum, so the continuously monitored qualitative blood cultures are in effect providing an inexpensive form of quantitative culture by measuring and comparing time to positivity for the two samples.

When a catheter is removed because of suspected catheter infection and infection is not already confirmed (e.g., through paired blood cultures using differential time to positivity), then catheter segments should be submitted for culture to confirm the diagnosis. This is usually done by removing the catheter with aseptic technique, following careful antiseptic preparation surrounding the catheter exit site, and then truncating the distal 5-cm segment into a sterile container for transport to the laboratory. The catheter tip should undergo culture using a semiquantitative method (the most widely used approach in hospital laboratories) or a quantitative method, which costs somewhat more but is also somewhat more accurate (24). The costs per accurate result are similar for the two methods (24). Routine culture of the 5-cm segment just beneath the catheter–skin interface may not be necessary (25).

REMOVAL OF THE INFECTED CATHETER

A common clinical question is whether to leave an intravascular catheter in place in a patient who has CRBSI. The usual answer in the past has been to remove the infected device, thereby removing a foreign body at the site of an infection. This is because foreign bodies have been shown to promote continuing infection despite antibiotic therapy, and removal allows the immune response to handle any remaining infection better. The catheter should always be removed for severe infections and for proven infections involving short-term catheters. In the case of long-term catheters, for which there may be a greater incentive to try treating through the infection, tunnel infection is usually associated with failure of therapy and the necessity to remove the catheter.

Different pathogens have been associated with different outcomes when the catheter has been left in place while attempting antibiotic therapy of catheter infection. According to the results of a multivariate analysis in one study (26), for example, for CRBSI due to CNS there was a threefold higher risk of recurrent CRBSI if the catheter was not removed. In the only published study of this question, there did not appear to be an increased risk of death from CRBSI due to CNS when the catheter was not removed, but the study was retrospective and had relatively low statistical power to address this question (26).

The outcome has appeared to be different in cases of CRBSI due to *S. aureus* or *Candida*. For *S. aureus*, one observational study found a four-fold higher risk of death if the catheter was left in situ for greater than 48 h after the onset of bacteremia (27). Another group of investigators found a 6.5-fold higher independent risk of relapse or death if the catheter was left in place; 13 (56%) of 23 patients from whom the catheter was not removed died (28). In the latter study, 80% of the patients were hemodialysis patients, for whom removal of a dialysis catheter may be problematic because of limited veins available for dialysis access. A more recent study among hemodialysis patients, however, found that none of 50 cases of CRBSI due to *S. aureus* resulted in death, suggesting the need for additional carefully controlled studies of this question (29). For *Candida* CRBSI, there was a two- to tenfold higher independent risk of death in two studies when the catheter was left in situ after the first positive blood culture (30,31). Other studies in children and adults have reached similar conclusions, but only by univariate analysis (32–34). Of note, approximately 70% of patients with significant growth of *S. aureus* or *Candida* from a catheter tip have been found to have concomitant CRBSI, and the likelihood of CRBSI in the presence of significant growth from a catheter tip is two to three times greater with *S. aureus* or *Candida* as compared with CNS (35,36).

Based on the findings noted above, patients with significant growth of *S. aureus* or *Candida* from a catheter tip should certainly have blood cultures drawn (if not already ordered) so as not to miss an associated bloodstream infection. If CRBSI is documented, infection due to either of these two pathogens usually warrants removal of the catheter. The exception might be a patient with a long-dwelling tunneled catheter and *S. aureus* CRBSI of lumenal origin with rapidly clearing bacteremia. In this circumstance, parenteral and antibiotic lock therapy may be associated with a clinical cure and catheter salvage (37,38). Antibiotic lock therapy has usually failed in published reports of attempts with fungal infections (39,40–42), so it seems necessary to remove the catheter when any fungal infection is present (3). Many patients with CNS CRBSIs, especially those involving implanted or tunneled devices, can be managed by initiating appropriate antimicrobial therapy and closely following such patients clinically, taking repeated blood cultures. Patients with unremitting bacteremia (e.g., $\geq$2–3 days) or those without clinical improvement, despite use of appropriate antibiotics, should have their catheters removed. Also, patients with CRBSI due to almost any pathogen and who have prosthetic intravascular devices in place (e.g., prosthetic valve, pacemaker, defibrillator, etc.) should be managed with expedient catheter removal in addition to appropriate antimicrobial therapy.

ANTIBIOTIC LOCK THERAPY

Eradicating microbial pathogens from the surface of intravascular catheters is difficult. Bacteria and fungi on the catheter surface are less susceptible to the host immune response (43,44) and to the antimicrobial activity of various classes of antibiotics (44,45). Despite exposure to the supratherapeutic concentrations used in an antibiotic lock, the microbe usually survives unless therapy is repeated for hours at a time, over a period of a couple of weeks. Even then, attempts to eradicate bacteria associated with a thrombus can be unsuccessful (46).

Antibiotic lock therapy provides a new approach to treatment, without removing the catheter, by infusing parenteral antibiotics through the catheter and then locking an even higher concentration into the catheter during periods in which the catheter will not normally be used (e.g., over an 8- to 12-h period each night) (37–42). This is usually accomplished by preparing an antibiotic solution that has appropriate activity against the etiologic agent in a concentration of 1–5 mg/ml mixed with 50–100 U of heparin or saline, in sufficient volume to fill the lumen of the catheter (usually from 2 to 5 ml). Such therapy, usually given over a two-week period, has been successful in salvaging the infected catheter in a large majority of patients who require long-term vascular access and who have infections due to a variety of pathogens (37–41,47–52). Compared to a couple of weeks of parenteral therapy alone, the addition of ALT has increased the probability of salvage by about 25%, according to one recent review of the published data (3). All 40 hemodialysis patients in one study were cured and their catheters salvaged, including all 12 cases with *S. aureus* infection (37,38). The mean duration of follow-up without relapse in that study was 20.5 months.

These data suggest that uncomplicated, mild-to-moderate infection of long-dwelling tunneled or hemodialysis catheters (including some cases due to *S. aureus*) may be treated without catheter removal if infection is confined to the lumen of the catheter (i.e., in the absence of tunnel or exit-site infection) (3). In one study, the success rate was only 43% when ALT was used for infected subcutaneous ports (46). Vancomycin has been shown to be stable in both total parenteral nutrition solutions and heparin solutions at room temperature for a 24-h period, allowing for concurrent therapy during TPN infusion and/or for antibiotic lock with heparin overnight, if indicated (53). Another study showed that heparin could be kept for 72 h at body temperature with seven different antibiotics, without losing a favorable ratio of antibiotic concentration to mean inhibitory concentration (54). Two studies have suggested that two weeks of ALT alone may be as effective as several days of systemic therapy followed by two weeks of ALT (48,51). However, most clinicians would not feel comfortable treating patients infected with high-risk microbes (e.g., *S. aureus* or *Candida*) or those in high-risk situations, without full-course parenteral therapy (47).

DURATION OF SYSTEMIC THERAPY

For CNS CRBSI, 5 to 7 days of parenteral therapy are usually sufficient if the catheter is removed. If a long-dwelling catheter is left in place, then 10 to 14 days of therapy, along with ALT, should be given (3). For most other bacterial pathogens, the recommended duration of therapy has been 10 to 14 days with catheter removal, or the same duration plus antibiotic lock if a long-dwelling catheter is to be salvaged (3).

An area of ongoing debate concerns the optimal duration of treatment of *S. aureus* CRBSI. In a study of 103 consecutive adult patients with *S. aureus* bacteremia, 67% were due to intravascular catheter infections. One in four patients had endocarditis, and only one in five patients with *S. aureus* endocarditis had physical findings of a new murmur or embolic skin lesions (55). In addition, transthoracic and transesophageal echocardiography revealed evidence of endocarditis in 27% and 100% of cases, respectively ($p = 0.0005$). Because of the propensity toward endocarditis and potentially elusive physical findings, transesophageal echocardiography has been recommended to determine the treatment duration for clinically uncomplicated *S. aureus* CRBSI (56), and recent guidelines have reached similar conclusions (3). However, short-course therapy (e.g., 2 weeks) for *S. aureus* bacteremia is not without hazard (57). Interestingly, relapse despite a negative transesophageal echocardiogram is not usually due to endocarditis missed by this form of echocardiography, but instead results from initially unrecognized metastatic infections (55). Recent evidence also suggests that patients should not be given short-course therapy if their *S. aureus* bacteremia does not clear within 72 h of initiating of appropriate antimicrobial therapy and catheter removal (58–60). In sum, patients with *S. aureus* CRBSI, who have a negative transesophageal echocardiogram, are without prosthetic heart valves, and whose symptoms and bacteremia resolve quickly with appropriate management may be candidates for an antibiotic course of less than four weeks. All others should be managed with four weeks of antimicrobial therapy.

Beta-lactam antibiotics should be used for treating *S. aureus* bacteremia when the isolate is susceptible, unless the patient has a serious allergy. For patients with penicillin allergy without anaphylaxis or angioedema, a first-generation cephalosporin can be used without eliciting an allergic response in 90% of patients. Those with serious allergic manifestations can be treated with vancomycin. Vancomycin should not be used for therapy of *S. aureus* susceptible to beta-lactam therapy (61–64). Patients with *S. aureus* endocarditis treated with vancomycin have had higher failure rates and slower clearance of bacteremia than usually observed with beta-lactam therapy. Patients with candidemia should be treated with amphotericin B or caspofungin (65), or with fluconazole (for susceptible species such as *Candida albicans*) for two weeks following conversion of blood cultures to negative. A randomized trial of patients with candidemia without neutropenia (72% due to candidal CRBSI) has shown that fluconazole (400 mg/day for adult patients) was as effective and less toxic than amphotericin B (0.5 mg/kg/day) given for the same length of time (66). However, this trial was conducted at a time when *Candida* species were more likely to be susceptible to fluconazole. Therefore, fluconazole should be used with caution for candidemic patients infected with species other than *C. albicans*, unless susceptibility data are available.

REFERENCES

1. Mermel LA. Prevention of intravascular catheter-related infections. Ann Intern Med 2000; 132:391–402.
2. Mermel LA. Correction: catheter-related bloodstream infections. Ann Intern Med 2000; 133:395.
3. Mermel LA, Farr BM, Sherertz RJ, Raad II, O'Grady N, Harris JS, Craven DE.

Guidelines for the management of intravascular catheter-related infection. Clin Infect Dis 2001; 32:1249–1272.

4. Arnow PM, Quimosing EM, Beach M. Consequences of intravascular catheter sepsis. Clinical Infectious Diseases 1993; 16:778–784.

5. Byers KE, Adal KA, Anglim AM, Farr BM. Case fatality rate for catheter-related bloodstream infections CRBSI: a meta-analysis. Infect Control Hosp Epidemiol 1995; 16(part 2 suppl):23.

6. Mermel LA, Farr BM, Sherertz RJ. Reply. Clin Infect Dis 2001; 33:1949–1951.

7. Rello J, Coll P, Prats G. Evaluation of culture techniques for diagnosis of catheter-related sepsis in critically ill patients letter. Eur J Clin Micro Infect Dis 1992; 11:1192–1193.

8. Bates DW, Goldman L, Lee TH. Contaminant blood cultures and resource utilization. The true consequences of false-positive results. JAMA 1991; 265:365–369.

9. Little JR, Murray PR, Traynor PS, Spitznagel E. A randomized trial of povidone-iodine compared with iodine tincture for venipuncture site disinfection: effects on rates of blood culture contamination. Am J Med 1999; 107:119–125.

10. Kim SD, McDonald LC, Jarvis WR, McAllister SK, Jerris R, Carson LA, Miller JN. Determining the significance of coagulase-negative staphylococci isolated from blood cultures at a community hospital: a role for species and strain identification. Infect Control Hosp Epidemiol 2000; 21:213–217.

11. Centers for Disease Control and Prevention. Recommendations for preventing the spread of vancomycin resistance: Recommendations of the Hospital Infection Control Practices Advisory Committee (HICPAC). MMWR 1995; 44(RR-12):1–13.

12. Weinstein MP, Towns ML, Quartey SM, Mirrett S, Reimer LG, Parmigiani G, Reller B. The clinical significance of positive blood cultures in the 1990's: a prospective comprehensive evaluation of the microbiology, epidemiology, and outcome of bacteremia and fungemia in adults. Clin Infect Dis 1997; 24:584–602.

13. MacGregor RR, Beaty HN. Evaluation of positive blood cultures. Arch Intern Med 1972; 130:84–87.

14. Aronson MD, Bor DH. Blood cultures. Ann Intern Med 1987; 106:246–253.

15. Pittet D, Chuard C, Rae AC, Auckenthaler R. Clinical diagnosis of central venous catheter line infections: a difficult job [abstract 453]. Abstracts and Programs of the 31st Interscience Conference of Antimicrobial Agents and Chemotherapy, (Chicago) Washington, DC: American Society for Microbiology, 1991.

16. Safdar N, Maki DG. Inflammation at the insertion site is not predictive of catheter-related bloodstream infection with short-term, noncuffed central venous catheters. Crit Care Med 2002; (30):2632–2635.

17. Meyer MH, Letscher-Bru V, Jaulhac B, Waller J, Candolfi E. Comparison of Mycosis IC/F and plus Aerobic/F media for diagnosis of fungemia by the bactec 9240 system. J Clin Microbiol 2004; 42:773–777.

18. Velez LA, Mermel LA, Zilz MA, Maki DG. Epidemiologic and microbiologic features of nosocomial bloodstream infection NBSI implicating a vascular

catheter source: a case–case control study of 85 vascular catheter-related and 101 secondary NBSIs. Programs and Abstracts of the 2nd Annual Meeting of the Society for Hospital Epidemiology of America. Baltimore, April 1992, Infection Control and Hospital Epidemiology [13], 562, 1992.

19. Mermel LA, Maki DG, Detection of bacteremia in adults: consequences of culturing and inadequate volume of blood. Ann Intern Med 1993; 119: 270–272.

20. Martinez JA, DesJardin JA, Aronoff M, Supran S, Nasraway SA, Snydman DR. Clinical utility of blood cultures drawn from central venous or arterial catheters in critically ill surgical patients. Crit Care Med 2002; 30:7–13.

21. Calfee DP, Farr BM. Comparison of four antiseptic preparations for skin in the prevention of contamination of percutaneously-drawn blood cultures: a randomized trial. J Clin Micro 2002; 40:1660–1665.

22. Blot F, Schmidt E, Nitenberg G. Earlier positivity of central venous versus peripheral blood cultures is highly predictive of catheter related sepsis. J Clin Micro 1998; 36:105–109.

23. Raad I, Hanna HA, Alakech B, Chatzinikolaou I, Johnson MM, Tarrand J. Differential time to positivity. a useful method for diagnosing catheter-related bloodstream infections. Ann Intern Med 2004; 140:18–25.

24. Siegman-Igra Y, Anglim AM, Shapiro DE, Adal KA, Strain BA, Farr BM. Diagnosis of vascular catheter-related bloodstream infection: a meta-analysis. J Clin Micro 1997; 35:928–936.

25. Raad II, Hanna IIA, Darouiche R. Diagnosis of catheter-related bloodstream infections: is it necessary to culture the subcutaneous catheter segment? Eur J Clin Micro Infect Dis 2001; 20:566–568.

26. Raad I, Davis S, Khan A, Tarrand J, Elting L, Bodey GP. Impact of central venous catheter removal on the recurrence of catheter-related coagulase-negative staphylococcal bacteremia. Infect Control Hosp Epidemiol 1992; 13:215–221.

27. Malanoski GJ, Samore MM, Pefanis A, Karchmer AW. *Staphylococcus aureus* bacteremia: minimal effective therapy and unusal infectious complications associated with arterial sheath catheters. Arch Intern Med 1995; 155:1161–1166.

28. Fowler VG, Sanders LL, Sexton DJ. Outcome of *Staphylococcus aureus* bacteremia according to compliance with recommendations of infectious diseases specialist: experience with 244 patients. Clin Infect Dis 1998; 27:478–486.

29. Peacock SJ, Curtis N, Berendt AR, Bowler IC, Winearls CG, Maxwell P. Outcome following haemodialysis catheter-related *Staphylococcus aureus* bacteremia. J Hosp Infect 1999; 41:223–228.

30. Nguyen MH, Peacock JE, Tanner DC, Therapeutic approaches in patients with candidemia. Evaluation in a multicenter, prospective, observational study. Arch Intern Med 1995; 155:2429–2435.

31. Nucci M, Colombo AL, Silveira F, Risk factors for death in patients with candidemia. Infect Control Hosp Epidemiol 1998; 9:846–850.

32. Eppes SC, Troutman JL, Gutman LT. Outcome of treatment of candidemia in children whose central catheters were removed or retained. Pediatric Infect Dis J 1989; 8:99–104.

33. Dato VM, Dajani AS. Candidemia in children with central venous catheters: role of catheter removal and amphotericin B therapy. Pediatric Infect Dis J 1990; 9:309–341.

34. Lecciones JA, Lee JW, Navarro E. Vascular catheter-associated fungemia in patients with cancer: analysis of 155 episodes. Clin Infect Dis 1992; 14:875–883.

35. Peacock SJ, Eddleston M, Emptage A, King A, Crook DW. Positive intravenous line tip cultures as predictors of bacteremia. J Hosp Infect 1998; 40:35–38.

36. Sherertz RJ, Raad I, Belani A. Three year experience with sonicated vascular catheter cultures in a clinical microbiology laboratory. J Clin Micro 1990; 28:76–82.

37. Capdevila JA, Segarra A, Planes AM, Gasser I, Gavalda J, Pahissa A. Long term follow-up of patients with catheter related sepsis (CRS) treated without catheter removal [Abstract J3]. Programs and Abstracts of the 35th Interscience Conference of Antimicrobial Agents and Chemotherapy, (San Francisco) Washington, DC: American Society for Microbiology, 1995.

38. Capdevila JA, Segarra A, Planes AM. Successful treatment of haemodialysis catheter-related sepsis without catheter removal. Nephrol Dial Transplant 1993; 8:231–234.

39. Krzywda EA, Andris DA, Edmiston CE. Treatment of Hickman catheter sepsis using antibiotic lock technique. Infect Control Hosp Epidemiol 1995; 16:596–598.

40. Benoit JL, Carandang G, Sitrin M. Intraluminal antibiotic treatment of central venous catheter infections in patients receiving parenteral nutrition at home. Clin Infect Dis 1995; 21:1286–1288.

41. Johnson DC, Johnson FL, Goldman S. Preliminary results treating persistent central venous catheter infections with the antibiotic lock technique in pediatric patients. Pediatric Infect Dis J 1994; 13:930–931.

42. Arnow PM, Kushner R. Malassezia furfur catheter infection cured with antibiotic lock therapy. Am J Med 1982; 90:128–130.

43. Zimmerli W, Lew PD, Waldvogel FA. Pathogenesis of foreign body infection evidence for a local granulocyte defect. J Clin Invest 1984; 73:1191–1200.

44. Costerton JW, Stewart PS, Greenberg EP. Bacterial biofilms: a common cause of persistent infections. Science 1999; 284:1318–1322.

45. Zimmerli W, Frei R, Widmer AF, Rajacic Z. Microbiological tests to predict treatment outcome in experimental device-related infections due to *Staphylococcus aureus*. J Antimicrob Chemo 1994; 33:959–967.

46. Longuet P, Douard MC, Arlet G. Venous access port-related bacteremia in patients with acquired immunodeficiency syndrome or cancer: the reservoir as a diagnostic and therapeutic tool. Clin Infect Dis 2001; 32:1776–1783.

47. Rao JS, O'Meara A, Harvey T. A new approach to the management of Broviac catheter infection. J Hosp Infect 1992; 22:109–116.

48. Messing B, Man F, Colimon R. Antibiotic lock technique is an effective treatment of bacterial catheter-related sepsis during parenteral nutrition. Clin Nutr 1990; 9:220–227.

49. Capdevila JA, Barbera J, Gavalda J. Diagnosis and conservative management CM of infection related to long term venous catheterization CI in AIDS patients [Abstract J55]. Programs and Abstracts of the 34th Interscience

Conference of Antimicrobial Agents and Chemotherapy, (Orlando, FL) Washington, DC: American Society for Microbiology, 1994.

50. Williams N, Carlson GL, Scott NA. Incidence and management of catheter-related sepsis in patients receiving home parenteral nutrition. Br J Surg 1994; 81:392–394

51. Messing B, Peitra-Cohen S, Debure A, Beliah M, Bernier JJ. Antibiotic-lock technique: a new approach to optimal therapy for catheter-related sepsis in home-parenteral nutrition patients. JPEN 1988; 12:185–189.

52. Douard MC, Arlet G, Leverger G, Paulien R, Waintrop C, Clementi E, Eurin B, Schaison G. Quantitative blood cultures for diagnosis and management of catheter-related sepsis in pediatric hematology and oncology patients. Intens Care Med 1991; 17:30–35.

53. Yao JD, Arkin CF, Karchmer AW. Vancomycin stability in heparin and total parenteral nutrition solutions: novel approach to therapy of central venous catheter-related infections. JPEN 1992; 16:268–274.

54. Saxinger LM, Williams KE, Lyon M. Stability of antibiotics in heparin at 37C toward antibiotic locks for central venous catheter related infections [abstract 626]. Programs and Abstracts of the 39th Interscience Conference on Antimicrobial Agents and Chemotherapy, (San Francisco). Washington, DC: American Society for Microbiology, 1999.

55. Fowler VG, LI J, Corey GR, Boley J, Marr KA, Gopal AK, Kong LK, Gottlieb G, Donovan CL, Sexton DJ, Ryan T. Role of echocardiography in evaluation of patients with *Staphylococcus aureus* bacteremia: experience in 103 patients. J Amer Coll Cardiol 1997; 30:1072–1078.

56. Rosen AB, Fowler VG, Corey GR. Cost-effectiveness of transesophageal echocardiography to determine the duration of therapy for intravascular catheter-associated *Staphylococcus aureus* bacteremia. Ann Intern Med 1999; 20:810–820.

57. Jernigan JA, Farr BM. Short-course Therapy of Catheter-related *Staphylococcus aureus* Bacteremia: A Meta-analysis. Annals of Internal Medicine 1993; 1194:304–311.

58. Raad I, Sabbagh MF. Optimal duration of therapy for catheter-related *Staphylococcus aureus* Bacteremia: a study of 55 cases and review. Clin Infect Dis 1992; 14:75–82.

59. Fowler VG Jr, Olsen MK, Corey GR, Woods CW, Cabell CH, Reller LB, Cheng AC, Dudley T, Oddone EZ. Clinical identifiers of complicated *Staphylococcus aureus* bacteremia. Arch Intern Med 2003; 163:2066–2072.

60. Chang FY, MacDonald BB, Peacock JE Jr, Muscher DM, Triplett P, Mylotte JM, O'Donnel A, Wagener MM, Yu VL. A prospective multicenter study of *Staphylococcus aureus* bacteremia: incidence of endocarditis, risk factors for mortality, and clinical impact of methicillin resistance. Medicine (Baltimore) 2003; 82:322–332.

61. Hartstein AI, Mulligan ME, Morthland VH, Kwok RY. Recurrent *Staphylococcus aureus* bacteria. J Clin Micro 1992; 30:670–674.

62. HICPAC. Recommendations for preventing the spread of vancomycin resistance. Hospital Infection Control Practices Advisory Committee (HICPAC). Infect Control Hosp Epidemiol 1995; 16:105–113.

63. Small PM, Chambers HF. Vancomycin for *Staphylococcus aureus* endocarditis

in intravenous drug abusers. Antimicrob Agents Chemother 1990; 34:1227–1231.

64. Chang FY, Peacock JE Jr, Musher DM, Triplett P, MacDonald BB, Mylotte JM, O'Donnell A, Wagener MM, Yu VL. *Staphylococcus aureus* bacteremia: recurrence and the impact of antibiotic treatment in a prospective multicenter study. Medicine (Baltimore) 2003; 82:323–339.

65. Mora-Duarte J, Betts R, Rotstein C, Colombo AL, Thompson-Moya L, Smietana J, et al. Caspofungin Invasive Candidiasis Study Group. Comparison of caspofungin and amphotericin B for invasive candidiasis. N Eng J Med 2002; 347:2020–2029.

66. Rex JH, Bennett JE, Sugar AM. A randomized trial comparing fluconazole with amphotericin B for the treatment of candidemia in patients without neutropenia. N Eng J Med 1994; 331:1325–1330.

5

Prevention and Control of Catheter-Related Infections

Bernd Jansen and Wolfgang Kohnen
Department of Hygiene and Environmental Medicine
Department of Hospital Hygiene and Infection Control
Johannes Gutenberg University
Mainz, Germany

INTRODUCTION

Since their introduction in 1945, polymeric catheters have gained widespread acceptance in all fields of medicine. Currently, they are used for various therapeutic and diagnostic purposes such as infusion therapy, administration of blood products, or hemodynamic monitoring of ICU patients. Thus, they represent major progress in modern medicine.

It is estimated that more than half of all patients admitted to a hospital, either in the United States, Europe, or elsewhere, will receive an intravascular catheter. In the United States this represents 15 to 20 million patients, some of whom will be at high risk of catheter-related infection (CRI). The annual frequency of CRI in the United States has been reported to be approximately 850,000 cases (1). Because CRIs are major causes of primary nosocomial bloodstream infection, they represent an important patient risk factor influencing morbidity and mortality, and also hospital economics. In former studies, for example, it was estimated that CRI led to a cost increase of approximately $3,000 to $6,000 per case, due to therapy and prolonged hospital stay (2,3).

Especially in intensive care units (ICU), there is a substantially higher risk for patients to acquire a catheter-related bloodstream infection. In the United States there is a total of 15 million central venous catheter (CVC)-days annually, reflecting the widespread use of such devices in critically ill patients (4). The average rate of CVC-related bloodstream infections has been reported to be 5.3 per 1000 catheter-days, but recent data from Germany show a somewhat lower rate of 2.2 per 1000 catheter-days in such settings (5). In ICU patients the attributable costs have been estimated even higher, with figures ranging from approximately $34,000 to $56,000 (6,7). The attributable mortality of CVC-related bloodstream infections remains unclear, because recent studies that controlled for the severity of illness could not demonstrate an increase (6,8). If all hospitals are considered, the attributable mortality is estimated to lie between 12% and 25%, with an underlying estimated figure of approximately 250,000 CVC-related bloodstream infections occurring each year (9).

Additional special features of CRIs contribute to their importance and enhance their impact on patient health and economics. First, despite considerable progress in evaluating new diagnostic tools for CRI there still remain difficulties in finding an accurate diagnosis. This may lead to a considerable number of unnecessarily removed catheters (with associated cost increase), whereas a failure in diagnosis may have severe consequences for the patient. Second, failure of antibiotic treatment in many cases of established CRI and the subsequent necessity for catheter removal also considerably contribute to morbidity and to cost increase.

For all these reasons, effective prevention of CRI is of paramount importance. In the last 10 to 20 years, a large number of studies on various aspects of CRI such as epidemiology, pathogenesis, therapy, and prevention have been published, and they have substantially increased our knowledge about these unique infections. Surely, this research has also inspired the development of preventive measures. The aim of this chapter is to give a comprehensive overview of current strategies in the prevention of CRIs, carefully considering their individual benefits and shortcomings.

BASIC CONSIDERATIONS

For effective prevention, a basic understanding of the underlying mechanisms leading to CRI is essential. These include the pathogenesis and epidemiology as well as patient risk factors and are intensively discussed in the respective chapters in this book. In the following, certain aspects of these issues will be addressed that are relevant with regard to prevention of CRI.

Factors Contributing to the Establishment of CRI

A variety of different factors may contribute to the development and establishment of a CRI. The nature and specific abilities of the pathogen involved are important, for example. Gram-positive organisms such as coagulase-negative staphylococci (CoNS) and *Staphylococcus aureus* are main causative organisms due to their occurence on skin and mucous membranes and their adherence capability, but in recent years CRIs involving Gram-negative microorganisms and fungi have been increasingly observed, especially in immunocompromised patients. Thus, modern preventive strategies must not only aim at Gram-positive bacteria as the most frequent isolated organisms, but must also take into account Gram-negative bacteria and fungi. Although CRIs occur in immunocompromised as well as in immunocompetent hosts, immunosuppression of a patient is an important risk factor for CRI in terms of severity and outcome. Other patient risk factors include extremes of age, burns and other major trauma, major skin lesions, and severe underlying diseases.

The catheter itself, with its specific properties, may also play a particular role in the generation of associated infection. In addition to the chemical composition, surface topography, and thrombogenicity of a specific material, the type of catheter and its particular application may display different risks for CRI.

Additional important factors that can influence the risk for CRI are insertion technique, location of catheter placement, hygienic care of catheters, frequency of manipulations at the catheter system, duration of catheterization, etc. Some of these factors may significantly contribute to CRI, as has been pointed out by a variety of clinical studies and will be addressed more intensively in the next part of the chapter. A summary of the most important risk factors discussed so far is given in Table 1.

Pathogenesis

There are three principal routes by which microorganisms may adhere to and colonize an IV catheter (1):

1. Colonization by migration along the external catheter surface to the catheter tip.
2. Colonization by contamination of the catheter hub or the infusate along the internal catheter surface.
3. Hematogenous spread of microorganisms from a distant site of infection.

Although the first pathway seems to be the most frequent one in the pathogenesis of CRI, the other two routes are important also with regard to preventive measures, and current prevention strategies must consider all the different pathways. Most of these are "hygienic" measures and will be discussed later in detail. Strategies aimed at the catheter material have been developed in recent years and require a basic understanding of the mechanisms by which microorganisms adhere to and colonize a catheter. Therefore,

Table 1 Risk Factors for Catheter-Related Infection (CRI)

Patient factors	• Extremes of age
	• Burns, trauma
	• Surgical patient, ICU patient
	• Immunocompromised patient
	• Severe skin lesion
	• Severe underlying disease
Catheter	• Chemical composition (e.g., PVC)
	• Surface topography
	• Thrombogenicity
	• Type (steel cannula, peripheral, central venous, etc.)
Catheterization	• Insertion technique
and catheter care	• Skill of medical personnel
	• Access route
	• Duration of placement
	• Catheter dressing
	• Interval of catheter and infusion system exchange
	• Frequency of manipulations
	• Kind of medicaments administered (e.g., parenteral nutrition)

some of the principal adherence and colonization mechanisms will be discussed here.

There is evidence from many investigations that adherence to medical devices (mainly synthetic polymers) is the first and most important step in the pathogenesis of foreign-body-associated infection (10–12). This holds true also for CRI. Accumulation on the polymer surface, production of extracellular substances by microorganisms (slime, glycocalix), and involvement of host factors (e.g., blood and tissue proteins, platelets) lead to the formation of a compact matrix (biofilm) on a device surface that is able to interfere with host defense mechanisms and resist antibiotic attack (12,13).

Principally, the mechanisms of microbial interaction with synthetic surfaces can be divided into unspecific and specific mechanisms (11). Unspecific interactions will dominate if microorganisms adhere to a native, uncoated catheter surface in the absence of specific host factors, e.g., the adherence of *Staphylococcus epidermidis* to a pure polymer in a protein-free medium. These unspecific mechanisms include van der Waals forces and electrostatic and hydrophobic interactions, and have been extensively studied in a large number of investigations (10,11). Unspecific adherence can be described either by using the DLVO model or by a thermodynamical approach, provided that specific physicochemical features of the microcorganisms, the properties of the solid surface (medical device), and the properties of the surrounding medium are known or can be determined experimentally. Regarding CRI, unspecific adherence of skin microorganisms (e.g., *S. epidermidis*) to a native catheter surface may only occur very early, at the time of insertion. After insertion, however, virtually all foreign-body materials soon become coated by glycoproteins derived from fluid or matrix phases containing fibrinogen, fibronectin, collagen, and other proteins (10,14). This coating process leads to a fibrin sheath or, more generally, to a biofilm around the catheter, resulting in a major change of the physicochemical properties of the surface. It is well known that *S. aureus* binds to plastic surfaces via fibronectin as a mediator of adherence (15, 16), but mediator-dependent adherence has been shown also for CoNS. Blood platelets seem to play another major role, especially in the adherence of *S. aureus* (17,18). Further, specific factors on the bacterial surface of CoNS have been elucidated as adhesins (19–22), e.g., polysaccharide intercellular adhesin (PIA) (23) and an accumulation-associated protein (AAP) (24). Discovering the genetic basis for the expression of PIA has led to more insight into the complex nature of specific adherence, especially of CoNS (25). This and other recent findings in the molecular pathogenesis especially of staphylococci are discussed in detail in Chapter 7.

Basic Approaches for the Prevention of CRI

Considering that microbial adherence is an essential step in the pathogenesis of foreign-body infection and CRI, inhibition of adherence appears to be a very attractive approach for prevention. All important steps in the pathogenesis—such as adhesion, accumulation, and biofilm formation—represent possible targets against which prevention strategies may be directed (Table 2). Although there is now a more detailed insight into the molecular pathogenesis of device-related infection, this has not yet led to strategies directed against specific adherence mechanisms, especially because it is as yet unkown whether a specific adhesin (e.g., protein, polysaccharide) is genus- or species-specific, or merely strain-specific. Therefore, most of the recently developed strategies have focused on the modification of medical devices, especially catheters.

Alteration of the material surface (e.g., of a polymeric catheter) leads to a change in specific and unspecific interactions with microorganisms. In a previous study we showed for a large series of different modified polymers—each with unique physicochemical properties—that the unspecific adherence of *S. epidermidis* KH6 could not be inhibited by surface modification, although that was thermodynamically predicted (26). We hypothesized that there is a certain "minimum of bacterial adherence" that is independent of the nature of the device surface. Nevertheless, surface modification of polymeric medical devices may lead to a reduced microbial adherence via altered interactions with proteins and platelets.

Table 2 Possible Strategies Directed Against Specific Factors in the Pathogenesis of CRI

Step in pathogenesis	Possible preventive strategy
Adhesion	Antiadhesive surfaces by polymer surface modification
	Inhibition of specific adherence mechanisms
	Antimicrobial devices
Accumulation	Inhibition of specific factors involved in accumulation, e.g., antibodies against PS/A, AAP
	Antimicrobial devices
Biofilm formation	Antimicrobial devices
	Interference with quorum sensing
	Electrical current, ultrasound + antimicrobials

The development of so-called antimicrobial polymers aims predominantly at the prevention of microbial colonization rather than microbial adherence. Catheters or parts of the catheter system containing antibiotics, disinfectants, or metals have been evaluated experimentally or in clinical trials, and are in part commercially available and already used in clinical applications. Destruction of the biofilm by enzymes or ultrasound plus subsequent antibiotic therapy, as well as the electrical enhancement of antibiotic penetration through biofilms (27–30), are therapeutic strategies rather than preventive measures and will be discussed elsewhere in this book.

PREVENTION STRATEGIES AIMED AT CATHETERIZATION AND CATHETER CARE

As was pointed out in the previous section, there is a variety of risk factors for CRI, and due to the particular pathogenesis, there exist several possible routes by which a catheter can become contaminated and thus infected. It is the goal of this chapter to review current prevention strategies that are directed against some of the most important risk factors and are mainly based on hygienic principles. Concerning infection control measures, in the last three years actual guidelines for the prevention of CRI have been published in the United Kingdom, the United States, and in Germany (9,31,32). These guidelines are evidence-based and the recommendations given are categorized, differentiating between strong and less-strong recommendations, unresolved issues, recommendations that are required by law. More or less, they comprise all of the issues important for the prevention of CRI. The key features of measures applicable to almost all kinds of intravascular catheters are presented in the following section. For a more detailed insight, the reader is referred to the respective guidelines.

Catheter Insertion

Education of Medical Personnel

Continuing education of health care workers involved in catheterization has been shown to be of benefit in preventing CRI. Sherertz et al. reported that a one-day course on infection control practices and on procedures of vascular access insertion was shown to reduce the infection rate by 73%, from 3.3 to 2.4 per 1000 CVC days (33). Eggiman et al. recently showed a 64% decrease in the incidence density of exit-site catheter infection and a 67% decrease in BSI after implementation of a global strategy targeted at the reduction of CRIs in critically ill patients. Moreover, the incidence density of all nosocomial infection was reduced by 35% (34).

Indication for Catheterization

An important measure to help avoid CRI is to question whether a patient needs an IV catheter any longer. With a catheter in place—especially a central venous catheter—the indication to continue catheterization should be made daily, because it has been shown from various studies that the cumulative risk of CRI increases with prolonged catheterization, even though the incidence per catheter day does not change (35–38). Also, there may be clinical situations in which a patient needs only short-term peripheral IV access, which carries a lower risk of infection. Thus, efforts to minimize the duration of catheterization—if possible—could be beneficial to reducing the risk of CRI.

Catheter Type and Material

It was emphasized that in an individual situation, the choice of the catheter type (e.g., peripheral instead of central) may be of benefit in order to avoid CRI. When using steel cannulae rather than polymeric catheters for short-term access, due to their low adherence properties, the possible advantage must be weighed against the risk of infiltration of intravenous (IV) fluids into the subcutaneous tissue (39,40). On the basis of several studies, some recommendations for the choice of the appropriate catheter type can be given. Concerning the basic polymer material, it has been shown that polyvinylchloride (PVC), and even polyethylene are unsuitable, due to their higher thrombogenicity and vulnerability for infection (41–45). Catheters made from silicone, polyurethane, or fluoropolymers are thus preferable (39). A study by Sherertz et al., however, demonstrated an increased risk for infection also with silicone catheters (46).

The all-purpose, multilumen catheter is frequently used in many ICU units, although in a number of cases single-lumen catheters could also be used. It is yet unclear if there is a greater risk associated with multilumen catheters (47–49), but single-lumen catheters should be applied for longer periods whenever possible, as well as for cost reasons. If it is anticipated that a catheter will remain in place for more than one or two months, the implantation of a tunnelled, cuffed catheter (Hickman or Broviac) or a totally implantable catheter system (e.g., Port-a-Cath™) should be considered, because their use is associated with a significantly lower risk for CRI than with other types of CVCs.

The value of antimicrobial catheters in preventing CRI and actual recommendations on their use will be discussed later in this chapter.

Catheter Insertion Site

The location of IV access may influence the patient's risk for CRI, the density of skin flora at the catheter insertion site being the crucial parameter. Although no study has satisfactorily elucidated different infectious risks for jugular, subclavian, or femoral access, the jugular vein—especially the internal jugular vein (36)—is supposed to be associated with a lower risk of mechanical complication but a higher risk of infection. The opposite holds for the subclavian vein (50–52). Therefore, in adult patients the subclavian route should be preferred due to its lower rate of infectious complications. For patients in whom the jugular or subclavian site cannot be used, the femoral vein access site can be an alternative (53,54), but the risk for deep venous thrombosis is higher with femoral vein insertion (55). In pediatric patients, the femoral route has been associated with fewer mechanical complications and an infection rate equivalent to that of nonfemoral access (56,57).

Aseptic Measures and Barrier Precautions

With each IV catheterization, the intact skin's barrier against microorganisms is locally penetrated, and the catheter itself acts as a port of entry for microbes into the bloodstream. Thus, it is mandatory that strict antiseptic and aseptic conditions are followed during insertion of a catheter. This is valid for all types of catheters, but especially for central venous catheters. Handwashing with an antiseptic solution (preferably alcohol) should precede each catheterization and is also of great importance for each later manipulation of the catheter or tubing system. Use of sterile gloves is strictly recommended with central venous catheters and should even be taken into consideration during insertion of peripheral IV catheters in highly immunocompromised patients.

The benefit of using maximal sterile barrier precautions to reduce the risk of CRI has been elucidated in two studies. In one study it was shown that the use of masks, caps, sterile gloves, gowns, and a large drape during insertion of nontunnelled, noncuffed central venous catheters leads to a more than sixfold reduction in catheter-related septicemia, compared to a control group in which only sterile gloves and small sterile drapes were used (58). In the other study, on Swan-Ganz pulmonary artery catheters, the application of such barrier precautions was associated with a twofold lower risk of infection (59). It is concluded that these measures are cost-effective, beneficial to the patient, and thus strongly recommended, at least for the insertion of central venous catheters.

IV Teams

The skill of the person or the team performing catheterization is an important factor contributing to minimize the risk of CRI. A number of studies have shown that catheter insertion and catheter maintenance by a team of specially trained physicians, technicians, and nurses is associated with a lower risk of CRI and proves to be highly cost-effective (60–65). Thus, a considerable number of hospitals in the United States have established such teams, whereas in most European countries IV teams are rarely instituted. The implementation of specially trained personnel is undoubtedly of benefit, but understaffing, on the other hand, might be an additional risk factor for CRI, as was demonstrated in a study by Fridkin et al. (66). The impact of a sufficient staffing level of educated medical personnel on the quality of care, and thus on infection rates, has been confirmed in a more recent study by Needleman et al. (67).

Cutaneous Antisepsis

Because of the particular pathogenesis of CRI, skin disinfection at the insertion site is mandatory, since contamination of the catheter by the patient's own microflora during insertion is supposed to be one of the major causes of infection. However, even strict cutaneous antisepsis is not able to reduce all the resident flora, especially in deeper skin areas. Current protocols in the United States and in the United Kingdom emphasize the use of 2% chlorhexidine-based preparations, as a result of comparative investigations of chlorhexidine with, e.g., PVP-iodine (32,68–72). Although chlorhexidine seems to be superior for cutaneous antisepsis in catheterization (73), alcoholic antiseptics are frequently used for this purpose in Germany and other European countries. As with every antiseptic or disinfectant, the recommended concentrations and duration of the application have to be carefully followed to obtain maximum success.

Antimicrobial Prophylaxis

Systemic antimicrobial prophylaxis during catheter insertion is still a controversial issue. In two trials, one-randomized and one nonrandomized (74,75), a reduction of CRI was demonstrated, whereas other controlled studies showed no benefit (76–79). Recently, a systematic review of the prophylactic use of antibiotics prior to the insertion of tunnelled long-term CVCs revealed that the prophylactic use of vancomycin/teicoplanin decreased the number of Gram-positive infections (80). Nevertheless, at present routine systemic administration of antibiotics prior to or during catheter insertion is not recommended.

Catheter Care

A general principle in catheter care is to restrict manipulations at the catheter or the infusion system to a necessary minimum (1,81). Each health care worker managing patients with IV catheters (especially those in ICU) should always be aware that the catheter is a conduit of the bloodstream to the environment, with numerous risks of microbial contamination. Handwashing and wearing sterile gloves before each manipulation are essential, particularly in the case of central venous lines in high-risk patients.

Catheter Site Dressings

To protect the insertion site of a catheter properly and to have an opportunity to inspect the site daily for suspicion of infection, transparent dressings have been introduced. There has been some controversy in the literature regarding the benefits and shortcomings of such dressings compared with sterile gauze (82–86). In a former meta-analysis it was concluded that the risk of catheter tip infection is significantly increased by use of transparent rather than gauze dressings for both peripheral and central venous catheters (87). Accumulation of moisture under the polymeric dressing was associated with increased microbial contamination at the insertion site. Other studies, however, found no significant differences (85,86,88). The development of new dressings with high permeability and increased water vapor transmission rates, thus allowing no penetration of moisture and microbes from the outside but permitting the evaporation of water vapor, has further minimized the risk of moisture build-up under the dressings (89). Thus, in the current U.S., U.K., and German guidelines the use of either transparent or gauze dressings is recommendend.

Replacement of the dressing is necessary if it has become damp, loosened, or soiled (9). Especially for short-term central venous catheters (including hemodialysis and pulmonary artery catheters), gauze dressings should be replaced every two days and transparent dressings at least every seven days, whereas dressings used on implanted or tunneled CVC sites should be replaced no more than once a week.

Topical Antimicrobials

To minimize the risk of microbial ascension from the insertion site along the catheter surface, topical antimicrobials have been applied. Results with a polyantibiotic ointment consisting of polymyxin, neomycin, and bacitracin were indeterminate (90), whereas on the other hand its use was associated with an increased frequency of *Candida* catheter colonizations.

The use of topical polyvinylpyrrolidone-iodine (povidone-iodine) on the catheter site seems to be of benefit in patients with hemodialysis catheters (91,92). However, the most beneficial effects were observed among the group of nasal carriers of *S. aureus*. Mupirocin, which is mainly applied for the eradication of methicillin-resistant *S. aureus* in nasal carriers, has also shown some success in the reduction of CRI, used either as local treatment or to decontaminate nasal staphylococcal carriage in hemodialysis patients (93–95). However, prolonged use of mupirocin ointment may lead to the development of mupirocin resistance in both coagulase-negative staphylococci (CoNS) and *S. aureus* (96,97). Furthermore, mupirocin may exhibit a negative effect, at least on polyurethane catheters (98,99).

Studies with other antibiotic iontments have also led to conflicting results (90,100,101). Thus, except for hemodialysis patients (9,32), the routine application of topical antimicrobials on the catheter site is not recommended.

Replacement of Catheters and Administration Sets

A frequently arising question in catheter care and still a matter of debate is how long a particular catheter can be left in place if no infection is suspected. It must be emphasized again that the responsible physician should assess daily whether a catheter is further needed. If a catheter is no longer necessary, it should be removed to avoid possible complications such as infection. Furthermore, most guidelines recommend that catheters inserted in emergency situations should be replaced as soon as possible, e.g., within 24–48 hours.

In case of peripheral IV catheters, the U.S. guidelines still emphasize a routine replacement every 72–96 hours to reduce the risk of phlebitis (9). However, in recent studies it was shown that the risk of phlebitis and infection is not increased if the catheters are not exchanged routinely (102–104). Thus, in the recently published German guideline a routine replacement of peripheral IV catheters is no longer recommended (32).

Concerning central venous catheters, two clinical trials could not demonstrate a benefit in regard to infection rates if central venous catheters were replaced at scheduled time intervals, compared to changing a catheter only if necessary (105,106). Bonawitz et al. found no significant differences in catheter colonization between CVCs that were replaced on day 3 or on day 7 (107).

In a literature review, scheduled guidewire exchanges as a tool to prevent CRI did not result in lower infection rates (108). It is now common practice to change a malfunctioning central venous catheter over a guidewire by the Seldinger technique. The main purpose is to avoid complications associated with the new venous puncture (e.g., pneumothorax and other mechanical complications) and to have a new catheter in place quickly, especially in high-risk patients with limited IV access. There have been a number of studies on the benefits and shortcomings of the Seldinger technique versus new venous puncture (105,109–111), but up to now it has not been conclusively demonstrated whether or not a guidewire exchange leads to increased infection rates. Nevertheless, replacement of a central venous catheter by the guidewire technique in the presence of known infection is not regarded as an acceptable strategy. In the actual U.S. guideline, use of the Seldinger technique is recommended for the exchange of a malfunctioning catheter in the absence of infection, or in selected patient situations. Concerning replacement recommendations for the other types of intravascular catheters, or in pediatric patients, the reader is referred to the respective chapters in this book that discuss specific catheters.

The exchange interval for administration sets is in most U.S. hospitals every 72 hours, based on controlled trials (112–114). Exceptions are the administration of blood products, lipid emulsions, and total parenteral nutrition (115–120). In those cases the administration systems should be replaced more frequently, e.g., within 24 hours. Infusions of lipid emulsions alone should be completed within 12 hours of hang time, and those of blood and blood products even in 4 hours (9) (German guideline: 6 hours).

In-Line Filters

To minimize the risk of CRI due to extrinsic contamination by the infusate, in-line filters with a pore size of 0.22–0.45µm have been proposed as a means of retaining bacteria and endotoxins, (121,122). In-line filters are able to reduce the incidence of infusion-related phlebitis (123,124). However, most of them are not able to prevent the passage of endotoxins; they frequently have to be exchanged and may become blocked, with an even higher risk of contamination. Because of the relatively high costs associated with their use, along with doubtful benefit for minimizing CRI, they cannot be recommended for routine use to prevent CRI at present (9,32,81).

Other Measures

Because thrombosis and fibrin deposits on the catheter surface might enhance microbial adherence and thus promote infection, anticoagulant flush solutions are frequently used to prevent catheter thrombosis. In a meta-analysis, Randolph et al. (125) evaluated the effect of heparin prophylaxis (3 U/ml in TPN, 5000 U every 6 or 12 h flush, or 2500 U low-molecular-weight heparin subcutaneously) in patients with short-term CVCs, showing that the risk of catheter-related central venous thrombosis can be reduced. However, no relevant difference in the rate for CR-BSI was observed. Because heparin solutions usually contain antimicrobial preservatives, a certain effect on the rate of CRI can also be expected.

The addition of nontoxic, biodegradable antiseptics to IV fluids as a measure to avoid fluid contamination and thereby to minimize the risk of hub contamination was proposed in another study (126). Replacement of heparin in flush solutions by substances with intrinsic antimicrobial activity, such as EDTA, might be of further benefit in reducing the risk of catheter-related bacteremia (127). Raad et al. (128) have proposed the use of minocycline plus EDTA as a lock solution because of the antibiofilm properties of this combination. However, no randomized trials with this approach have been conducted so far. Three further studies in neutropenic patients with long-term catheters have shown the usefulness of flushing and filling the catheter lumen with antibiotic solution and allowing it to dwell in for a certain time (antibiotic lock) (129–131). In a recent article, Allon (132) reported the efficacy of an antibiotic lock solution, comprising taurolidine and citrate, in increasing the bacteremia-free survival of catheters at 90 days in patients undergoing hemodialysis (94% versus 47% in the control group, p < 0.001). In the current guidelines, routine use of antibiotic lock solutions for the prevention of CRI is not recommended.

The risk of phlebitis due to the administration of certain drugs (e.g., potassium chloride, lidocaine, antimicrobials) may be reduced by using intravenous additives such as hydrocortisone (133,134). The topical application of glyceril trinitrate or antiinflammatory agents such as cortisone near the catheter site has effectively reduced the incidence of infusion-related thrombophlebitis, and thus has increased the life span of the catheters (135–137). However, the mechanism by which transdermal glyceryl trinitrate acts in preventing infusion phlebitis is still unclear, and further studies on the mechanism, efficacy, and cost-effectiveness of glyceryl trinitrate and other substances are needed before a general recommendation for such measures can be given.

Surveillance

In daily routine, the catheter site has to be inspected visually or by palpation for signs of infection. All data concerning insertion and maintenance of a catheter should be documented in a standardized form. Catheter tips should be microbiologically cultured only if CRI is suspected.

Because skin colonization is thought to be an important risk factor for CRI, a few studies have dealt with surveillance cultures of skin and hub to find correlations between the extent of contamination and the development of CRI (138–140). However, despite a sensitivity of approximately 80%, the positive predictive value was only 44% in one study (139), and further studies are needed to evaluate the significance of surveillance cultures in the diagnosis and prevention of CRI.

Maki suggested surveillance of intravascular device-related bacteremias as a valuable tool in infection control, provided all blood isolates—especially CoNS—are identified to species level, the antibiotic phenotype is determined by standardized methods, and bloodstream isolates are saved for two years to be available for future epidemiological studies (141).

Documentation of catheter-related bloodstream infection rates according to defined criteria, and comparison of the data with the infection rates of other comparable hospitals and wards, are also essential in order to recognize any trends regarding increase or decrease of CRI and CRI–BSI in a given unit. Data from the National Nosocomial Infections Surveillance (NNIS) system revealed that between 1990 and 1999 bloodstream infection rates decreased in medical (nonsurgical) ICUs by 44%, in pediatric ICUs by 32%, and in surgical ICUs by 31% (142). If one assumes that 80–90% of bloodstream infections are line-associated, this decrease can be traced to a substantial decrease in CRI. More recently, a German report by Zuschneid et al. (143) on infection rates in ICUs that participate in the German system for surveillance of nosocomial infections (KISS) showed a decrease in primary BSIs from 2.1 to 1.5 per 1000 CVC days, corresponding to an overall relative reduction of 28.6% during a two-year observational period in a total of 84 ICUs. Although reasons for this reduction are difficult to determine, in addition to new research findings, improved guidelines, intensified education of medical personnel, and introduction of specific prevention measures it is assumed that a modification of behaviour under surveillance is at least partially resonsible for the decrease in infection rates. Therefore, the authors concluded that surveillance is an important factor in infection control and should be recommended for ICUs everywhere. That conclusion is also supported by other studies on the influence of surveillance on infection rates (144,145).

Comparison of Current Guidelines

In 2002, the revised U.S. guideline for the prevention and control of intravascular catheter-related infections was published (9), and replacing the former guideline from 1996 (146). As was the case with its predecessor, this guideline is intended to provide evidence-based recommendations for the prevention of CRI and to address medical personnel involved in catheter insertion and catheter care, as well as persons responsible for surveillance and control of infections in hospitals, outpatient facilities, and home health-care settings. This guideline was prepared by a group of expert professionals from various fields, e.g., critical care medicine, infectious diseases, health-care infection control, surgery, anaesthesiology, interventional radiology, pulmonary medicine, pediatrics, and nursing. The recommendations are divided into categories I A–C, II, and "unresolved issue" (Table 3) to inform the user on the strength of the respective recommendations.

The recently published German recommendations provided by the Commission for Hospital Hygiene and Infection control at the Robert Koch-Institut (RKI) (32) are similar to the U.S. guideline. They are evidence-based and also use categorized recommendations (Table 3). A separate chapter is provided for each different catheter type (peripheral catheters, CVCs, arterial and pulmonary artery catheters, hemodialysis catheters, umbilical catheters, partially and totally implanted catheters) and for infusion therapy in general.

The U.K. guideline, "Preventing Infections Associated with Central Venous Catheters," dates from the year 2001 and is part of the general guidelines for preventing hospital-acquired infections that are part of the

Table 3 Categories for the Grade of Recommendations Used in Different National Guidelines for Prevention of Catheter-Related Infections

Guideline	Grade of recommendations
U.S.A.	Category IA: Strongly recommended for implementation and strongly supported by well-designed experimental, clinical, and epidemiological studies
	Category IB: Strongly recommended for implementation and strongly supported by some experimental, clinical, and epidemiological studies, and a strong theoretical rationale
	Category IC: Required by state or federal regulations, rules, or standards
	Category II: Suggested for implementation and supported by suggestive clinical or epidemiological studies or a theoretical rationale
	Unresolved issue: Represents an unresolved issue for which evidence is insufficient or no consensus regarding efficacy exists
U.K.	Category 1: Generally consistent findings in a range of evidence derived from a majority of acceptable studies
	Category 2: Evidence based on a single acceptable study, or a weak or inconsistent finding in multiple acceptable studies
	Category 3: Limited scientific evidence that does not meet all the criteria of "acceptable studies," or an absence of directly applicable studies of good quality. This includes published expert opinion derived from systematically retrieved and appraised professional, national, and international guidelines
	Note: All recommendations are endorsed equally and none is regarded as optional, independent from the category
Germany	Category IA: Strongly recommended for implementation in all hospitals, supported by well-designed experimental or epidemiological studies
	Category IB: Strongly recommended for implementation in all hospitals, supported by expert opinions and consensus opinion of the Commission of Hospital Hygiene at the Robert Koch-Institute (RKI)
	Category II: Recommended for implementation in most hospitals, based on clinical and epidemiological studies, or on a theoretical rationale
	Category III: No recommendation or unresolved issue; measures with unproven efficacy or with no consensus opinion
	Category IV: Measures required by law, rules, or standards

Table 4 Selected Recommendations for the Prevention of Catheter-Related Infections: Comparison of Three National Guidelines

Preventive measure	U.S.A.	U.K.	Germany
Catheter insertion			
Education of medical personnel	Yes	—	Yes
Catheter type and material			
Preferential use of single-lumen catheters	Yes	Yes	Yes
Preference of PUR and Teflon catheters	—	—	Yes
Use of antimicrobial catheters in high-risk adult population when other preventive measures have not decreased infection rates	Yes	Yes	Unresolved issue
Catheter insertion site			
Choice of subclavian rather than jugular or femoral vein for CVCs	Yes	Yes	Yes
Preparation of insertion site with chlorhexidine-containing antiseptics	Yes	Yes	No preference of CHX
Use of maximum sterile barriers during insertion of CVCs	Yes	Yes	Yes
Use of specially educated personnel(IV teams)	Yes	—	—
Antimicrobial prophylaxis	No	No	No
Catheter care			
Catheter site dressings			
Use of either gauze or transparent dressings	Yes	Yes	Yes
Exchange of damp, dirty, or loosened dressings	Yes	Yes	Yes
Use of topical antimicrobials	No	No	No
Replacement of catheters and administration sets			
Exchange of peripheral IV catheters every 72–96 h	Yes	—	No routine exchange
No routine exchange of nontunneled CVCs	Yes	Yes	Yes
Removal of a catheter no longer needed	Yes	Yes	Yes
Exchange of administration sets every 72 h	Yes	Yes	Yes
Exchange of administration sets within 24 h if lipids or blood (products) are administered	Yes	Yes	Infusion time for lipids 12 h, blood 6 h
Use of in-line filters	No	—	No
Surveillance			
Daily inspection of catheter site	Yes	—	Yes
Recording of operator, date, and time of catheter insertion, dressing changes and removal	Yes	—	—
Documentation of infection rates of CR-BSI according to a standardized protocol with accepted definitions for CRI allowing interhospital comparison.	Yes	—	—

Source: Refs. 9,31,32.

"Epic Project: Developing National Evidence-Based Guidelines for Preventing Healthcare-Associated Infections" (31). The evidence of the recommendations is graded in categories 1–3 (Table 3), but all recommendations are endorsed equally and none is regarded as optional. They are divided into seven distinct interventions, namely, selection of catheter type and insertion site; aseptic technique during catheter insertion; cutaneous antisepsis; catheter and catheter site care; catheter replacement strategies; and antibiotic prophylaxis.

Since most of the recommendations in all three of the aforementioned guidelines are based on the same evidence from the literature or on expert opinions, they do not differ very much one from the other. The most relevant differences among these actual national guidelines are summarized in Table 4.

PREVENTION STRATEGIES AIMED AT THE MODIFICATION OF CATHETERS AND RELATED DEVICES

In Section II of this chapter, the basic considerations regarding prevention of CRI by developing innovative catheter systems have been discussed. It seems obvious that due to the particular pathogenesis of CRI, approaches directed against the bacterial colonization of a device are very promising. Catheters made out of a material that is antiadhesive, or at least colonization-resistant in vivo, would be the most suitable candidates to avoid colonization and subsequent infection. In the last 15–20 years there have been a large number of studies dealing with this problem, in part using different strategies. A general overview is given in Table 5. Most of the studies have been performed with intravascular catheters. A few studies have dealt with the development of infection-resistant CAPD, ventricular, or urinary catheters and will be discussed at the end of this section, together with modified devices that are used along with catheterization such as cuffs or hubs—but are not actually catheters themselves.

Experimental Approaches

Antiadhesive Polymer Materials

The most attractive approach to obviating foreign body-associated infections, and in particular CRI, would be to develop a medical material that proves to be resistant to microbial adherence, even after insertion into the bloodstream and despite the ever-occurring interactions of the device surface with host factors such as proteins and cells. There is evidence that the intrinsic properties of a material might be of advantage regarding resistance to infection. Thus, improvement of the surface texture, tailoring the protein adsorption characteristics, and improving the antithrombogenicity of a given

Table 5 Prevention Strategies Aimed at Modification of Catheters and Devices

---

A. Catheters and devices used in modification processes
Intravascular catheters
Urinary catheters
Ventricular catheters
CAPD catheters
Catheter hub
Cuffs
Dressings
Tubing systems

B. Process of modification
Modification of basic polymers (antiadhesive polymers)
Incorporation or superficial bonding of antimicrobial substances
    (antimicrobial polymers)
  • antibiotics
  • antiseptics
  • metals with antimicrobial activity

---

material would be key features in the development of innovative, infection-resistant materials. However, this goal has not yet been reached satisfactorily.

Several research groups have tried to develop polymers with new surface properties leading to a reduction of bacterial adhesion. Bridgett et al. studied the adherence of three isolates of *S. epidermidis* to polystyrene surfaces that were modified with a copolymer of polyethylene oxide and polypropylene oxide (147). A substantial reduction in bacterial adhesion was achieved in vitro with all surfactants tested. Similar results were found by Desai et al., who investigated the adhesion of *S. epidermidis*, *S. aureus*, and *Pseudomonas aeruginosa* to polymers that were surface-modified with poly(ethylene oxide) (148). They observed reductions in adherent bacteria between 70 and 95%, compared to the untreated polymer. A photochemical coating of polymers was used by Dunkirk et al., demonstrating that the coating reduced adhesion of a variety of bacterial strains (149). Tebbs et al. compared the adherence of five *S. epidermidis* strains to a polyurethane catheter and to a commercial hydrophilic, coated polyurethane catheter (Hydrocath™) (150). Adhesion of three strains to the coated catheters was considerably reduced. Bacterial coloniziation was further reduced by the addition of benzalkonium chloride to a hydrophilic polyurethane (Hydrocath™) catheter (151). Our own approaches to develop anti-infective materials involved the modification of polymer surfaces by radiation or glow discharge techniques. For example, 2-hydroxymethylmethacrylate (HEMA) was covalently bonded to a polyurethane surface by means of radiation grafting, leading to a reduced in vitro adhesion of *S. epidermidis* (152,153).

More recent work on surface modification of polymer materials to prevent bacterial adhesion involved the use of sulfonated polyethylene oxide as a surfactant in a polyurethane (154), or the introduction of glycerophosphorylcholine as a chain extender in polyurethane (155). Both approaches lead to increased water uptake and to lower bacterial adhesion. An overview mainly of experimental research on the surface modification of polymers, and on binding macromolecules such as albumin to surfaces in order to prevent bacterial adherence, is given in Refs. (156,157).

So far none of such modified polymers has been used in clinical applications, with the exception of the hydrophilic, polyvinylpyrrolidone-coated Hydrocath™ catheter based on polyurethane. Its relatively low thrombogenicity and low in vitro bacterial adherence should be of benefit also in regard to infection resistance, but this has not yet been demonstrated in a clinical trial.

A major disadvantage of all the previously described approaches, which aim primarily at the modification of the surface properties of basic materials for catheters or related devices, is the fact that—for thermodynamical reasons—the creation of surfaces that show a "zero" adhesion is probably not feasible. We have demonstrated in an experimental study, which investigated the relationship between bacterial adhesion and the free surface enthalpy of adhesion of a large number of differently modified polymers, that it obviously seems to be impossible to develop a polymer surface that shows an absolute bacterial "zero" adherence in vitro (26). Hence, in our opinion it seems impossible to design an absolute antiadhesive material that retains its properties even in the more complex in vivo situation, in which the native surface properties are masked by adsorption of bacterial and host components.

Incorporation of Antimicrobial Agents

The loading of medical polymers with antimicrobial substances, either for therapeutic or for preventive purposes, has a long tradition. The best known anti-infective, polymeric drug delivery systems are the polymethylmethacrylate (PMMA)-gentamicin bone cement and the PMMA-gentamicin beads (Septopal™) used for treatment of bone and soft tissue infections (158,159). Vascular prostheses made of Dacron™ have been treated with various antibiotic substances to create infection-resistant grafts, but they have had no routine clinical application up to now (160–162).

In recent years, catheters or parts of the catheter system have been coated with antimicrobial drugs, and some of these antimicrobial devices are already commercially available. The main principle of such devices is that an antimicrobial substance (e.g., an antibiotic, disinfectant, or metal ion) is bound superficially to a catheter—either directly or by means of a carrier—or incorporated into the interior of the polymer. If such a device comes into contact with an aqueous environment the drug is released into the near vicinity. The amount of the antimicrobial substance released is influenced by the processing parameters, loading dose, applied technique, molecular size of the drug, and the physicochemical properties of the polymeric device. A high antimicrobial concentration is reached (at least initially) in the very near vicinity of the device surface, mostly exceeding the MIC and MBC of susceptible organisms. Most such materials exhibit a release pattern according to first-order kinetics, with an initally high drug release and afterwards an exponential decrease of the released drug. However, more sophisticated drug-release systems with defined release kinetics have also been developed.

It is not yet clear whether such a device is capable of inhibition of microbial adherence per se, but at least an elimination of already adherent microorganims should be achieved for the entire time the antimicrobial compound is being released in the necessary concentrations. Thus, such materials are especially suitable to prevent CRI in short-term catheters which originates from contamination during the insertion or from hub contamination.

Antibiotics: There is a large number of studies on the bonding of antibiotics to biomaterials. Solovskiij et al. prepared polymers to which ampicillin and 6-aminopenicillanic acid were covalently bonded and which inhibited the in vitro growth of *S. aureus* (163). However, most studies have focused on the incorporation or superficial coating of antimicrobials rather than on covalent bonding by chemical reaction. For example, Sherertz et al. used a rabbit model to investigate intravascular catheters coated with several antimicrobial compounds (dicloxacillin, clindamycin, fusidic acid, and chlorhexidine) (164). The frequency of catheter infections was significantly reduced, compared with the control group, when the dicloxacillin-coated catheter was used. We have investigated the incorporation of flucloxacillin, clindamycin, and ciprofloxacin into polyurethane polymers and have demonstrated a considerable reduction in the in vitro adherence of *S. epidermidis* (152,165). As a further approach, a commercially available central venous, hydrophilic-coated polyurethane catheter (Hydrocath™) was loaded with the glycopeptide teicoplanin (166,167). In in vitro studies, as well as in a mouse model, the capability of this catheter to prevent colonization with *S. epidermidis* and *S. aureus*, respectively, for a period of at least 48 hours was proven, rendering the catheter suitable to prevent early-onset infection (166,168). To extend the antimicrobial spectrum of such a catheter to include Gram-negative bacteria and fungi, a combination of teicoplanin with silver was incorporated into Hydrocath™-catheters, which exhibited considerable activity against *S. epidermidis*, *Escherichia coli*, and *Candida albicans* (169).

Kamal et al. have evaluated the efficacy of a cefazolin-containing catheter in a prospective, randomized trial (170). Raad and Darouiche et al. reported on the efficacy of a central venous catheter coated with minocycline and rifampicin to prevent catheter-related bacteremia (171). This commercially available catheter is already in clinical use and will be discussed later in further detail. More recent work on antibiotic-containing catheters has included the adsorption of cefamandole nafate on functionalized urethane catheters, which were then used to coat a commercial central venous catheter (172), or the use of an antibacterial substance (rifampin) in combination with an antifungal substance (miconazole) in a polyurethane catheter (173).

A disadvantage of all those approaches might result from the risk of developing resistance against the antimicrobial agents, especially if antibiotics considered to be first-line drugs in the therapy of infections are used as an active part of the modified catheters.

Antiseptics: Antimicrobial substances that are different from antibiotics, such as antiseptics, have been used to develop new catheter materials. The disinfectant Irgasan™, for example, was incorporated into several polymer catheters and showed a reduction of infections in rabbits (174). We used the hydrophilic Hydrocath™ catheter to incorporate iodine, leading to a polyvinylpyrrolidone iodine-complex on the inner and outer catheter surfaces (175). In vitro adherence of various microorganisms (*Staphylococcus* spp., *Escherichia coli*, *Candida* sp., *Pseudomonas* sp.) was completely inhibited during the time of iodine release. After iodine exhaustion, reloading of the catheter was possible. Tebbs and Elliot incorporated benzalkonium chloride into triple-lumen Hydrocath™ catheters and demonstrated the long-lasting antimicrobial activity of the catheters against staphylococci, and a somewhat lesser activity against Gram-negative bacteria and *C. albicans* (151).

The most promising development in this field in recent years was a catheter using a combination of an antiseptic (chlorhexidine) and silver-sulfadiazine. This catheter will be discussed in detail later.

Metals: Among metals with antimicrobial activity, silver has raised the interest of many investigators because of its good antimicrobial action and low toxicity. Silver has also been used extensively for the development of infection-resistant urinary catheters as discussed later.

Sioshansi et al. used ion implantation to deposit silver-based coatings on a silicone rubber surface, which thereafter demonstrated antimicrobial activity (176). Also, silver-copper surface films, sputter-coated onto catheter materials, showed antibacterial activity against *P. aeruginosa* biofilm formation (177). In more recent research, an ion beam technique applying low-implantation energy has been used for the formation of silver nanoparticles on the surface of polymers which exhibited an improved effect on bacterial adhesion (178). We developed an antimicrobial polymer by binding silver ions to an acid-modified, negatively charged polyurethane surface (26). Another approach involved loading a hydrophilic polyurethane catheter with silver nitrate (179). Also, surface-coated polyurethane catheters with a silver surface thickness of 15–20 Å were investigated regarding their biocompatibility and antimicrobial efficacy, showing markedly decreased adherence of Gram-positive and Gram-negative microorganisms in vitro (180).

Further interest has been raised in devices in which silver is distributed in the form of nanoparticles, or in combination with other elements such as carbon and platinum. The Erlanger silver catheter, for example, uses a microdispersed silver technology to increase the quantity of available ionized silver (181). The Oligon catheters are composed of polyurethane in which carbon, silver, and platinum particles are incorporated, which leads to an electrochemically driven release of silver ions in the outer and inner vicinity of the catheter surface. However, a peripherally implanted central catheter based on this technology (Olimpicc™, Vygon, UK, Ltd.,) has been withdrawn from the market, at least in Germany, due to mechanical problems associated with this type of catheter. A more recent development is the Oligon Vantex catheter (182), and other approaches include catheters with active iontophoresis technology, in which microorganisms are repelled by electrical current generated from a carbon-impregnated catheter (183), or where low-amperage current is produced by two electrically charged parallel silver wires helically wrapped around the proximal segment of a silicone catheter (184).

Clinical Studies with Antimicrobial Catheters

Only few of the aforementioned approaches have led to the development of commercially available catheters (Table 6). The two currently best-known catheters that are also in clinical use – (preferably in the United States) – are the catheter containing chlorhexidine and silversulfadiazine (Arrowgard blue, Arrow International, USA) and the catheter containing minocycline and rifampin (Cook Spectrum, Cook Critical Care, USA). There is now a considerable number of clinical studies and meta-analysis reports that have been published concerning these catheters which will be discussed in the next section.

Chlorhexidine-Silversulfadiazine (CHSS) Catheters

This catheter, which became available approximately 10 years ago, is polyurethane-based and impregnated with minute amounts of chlorhexidine and silversulfadiazine (ArrowGard, Arrow International, USA). A synergistic effect of chlorhexidine and sulfadiazine has been shown in vitro (185). This first-generation CHSS catheter is coated only on the exterior surface and exhibits antimicrobial properties for approximately 15 days. Since its introduction, more than 8 million of these catheters have been sold worldwide. Up to now there has been a considerable number of randomized clinical trials performed with this type of catheter. If one excludes studies published only as abstracts and those studies investigating only catheter colonization, and not

Table 6 Examples of Commercially Available Antimicrobial Intravascular Catheters

Catheter trade name	Manufacturer	Principle
ArrowGard[a]	Arrow International,	Chlorhexidine +
ArrowGard Plus	USA	Silversulfadiazine
Cook Spectrum	Cook Critical Care, USA	Minocycline + Rifampin
AMC Thromboshield	Baxter, USA	Benzalkoniumchloride-Heparin
Vantex Oligon	Edwards Life Sciences, USA	Silver, Carbon, Platinum

[a] Only externally coated.

CR-BSI, there remain at least 11 controlled trials, which is by far the greatest number of such studies available for an antimicrobial catheter (186–196). In the study with the greatest patient numbers, which also used molecular methods for the confirmation of CR-BSI, the CHSS catheter was associated with a two-fold reduction in the incidence of catheter colonization and a fivefold reduction of CR-BSI (RR: 0.21, p = 0.03) (192). As of 2002, 6 meta-analyses or systematic reviews have been published (4,197–201). Veenstra et al. (198) investigated randomized clinical trials with CHSS versus control catheters up to 1998 and found summary odds ratios for catheter colonization of 0.44 (95% confidence interval: 0.36–0.54, p < 0.001) and of 0.56 for CR-BSI (95% confidence interval: 0.37–0.84, p = 0.005). Also Mermel (4) concluded from an analysis of six prospective studies that short-term use of CHSS catheters reduces the risk for CR-BSI. In one study (191) with longer catheter dwelling times (mean duration 20 days), no such difference in the incidence of CR-BSI was observed, probably reflecting less antimicrobial efficacy over time due to a loss of activity to 25% of the baseline value after 10 days in situ. Because the first-generation CHSS catheters are coated only externally, with longer duration of placement also, colonization of the inner lumen due to hub contamination might be of greater relevance. For these reasons, a new second-generation CHSS catheter which is coated both internally and externally and which exhibits enhanced chlorhexidine activity has recently been developed. Clinical trials with this new type of catheter are currently being performed.

Development of resistance to chlorhexidine has been demonstrated in vitro (202). However, in vivo resistance to either chlorhexidine or silver-sulfadiazine associated with the use of the antimicrobial catheter has not yet been observed, although an outbreak of urinary tract infections with a multiple antibiotic-resistant and also chlorhexidine-resistant *Proteus mirabilis* strain has been described, in which a broad use of chlorhexidine in the institution was assumed to be responsible for the chlorhexidine resistance (203).

Anaphylactoid reactions, probably due to chlorhexidine have been reported, from Japan and from the United Kingdom (204).

Minocycline-Rifampin (MR) Catheters

Raad et al. (171,205) reported about the broad-spectrum activity against Gram-negative and Gram-positive organisms and *C. albicans* of a minocy-cline–rifampin (MR) catheter based on in vitro and animal data. This catheter has been marketed as the Cook Spectrum™ catheter (Cook Critical Care, USA) and is coated on the inner and outer surfaces with minocycline and rifampin, which act either synergistically or additively in combination. In a prospective randomized clinical trial (206), the MR catheter was compared with an uncoated control catheter and demonstrated a statistically significant decrease in catheter colonization (8 versus 26% for the control catheter, $p <$ 0.001) and in CR-BSI (0 versus 5%, $p <$ 0.01). In a large multicenter trial, the MR catheter was compared with the CHSS catheter (207). It was found that the antibiotic-coated catheter was three times less likely to be colonized (7.8 versus 22.6% for the CHSS catheter, $p <$ 0.001) and 12-fold less likely to lead to CR-BSI (0.3% versus 3.4%, $p <$ 0.002). This difference has been explained by the fact that MR catheters are coated internally and externally, in contrast to the first generation CHSS catheter, that the combination of minocycline and rifampin shows better surface activity than chlorhexidine, and finally that the MR catheters retain surface antimicrobial activity longer in situ (201).

Although resistance against minocycline and rifampin could not be detected in clinical trials, this remains of concern because in vitro development of resistance has been demonstrated (208).

Other Intravascular Antimicrobial Catheters

Only a few clinical trials have been performed with antimicrobial catheters other than the CHSS or the MR catheter. Kamal et al. have evaluated the efficacy of a cefazolin-containing catheter (in which cefazolin was bound to benzalkonium chloride) in a prospective, randomized trial (170). There was a significant sevenfold decrease in catheter colonization as determined by the semiquantitative tip culture method (209); no CR-BSI was observed in this study. In a more recent comparative study before and after the routine use of cefazolin catheters in the ICU, the authors reported a marked reduction in the rate of CR-BSI, from 11.5 to 5.1 infections per 1000 catheter days (210).

Another interesting phenomenon was detected in a meta-analysis of prospective studies of Swan-Ganz pulmonary artery catheters (211). Heparin is now commonly bonded to the external surface of Swan-Ganz catheters to enhance their antithrombogenicity (212), and heparin-bonded catheters obviously showed a lower frequency of CRI. In in vitro studies it has already been demonstrated that coating with heparin reduces bacterial adherence, but it was assumed that the surfactant benzalkonium chloride, to which heparin is bonded, was mainly responsible for the anti-infective properties of these Swan-Ganz catheters. Thus, catheters coated internally and externally with benzalkoniumchloride (Becton Dickinson, UK) have been developed and were tested in two randomized trials (213,214). In the study by Moss et al. (213), a reduction in catheter colonization of both internal and external surfaces was observed (21 coated catheters colonized versus 38 uncoated control catheters, $p = 0.0016$), but a benefit for reducing CR-BSI could not be shown. In the study by Jaeger et al. (214), no differences in catheter colonization and incidence of CR-BSI between the coated and the uncoated catheters were seen.

A few more clinical studies have been performed with silver-containing intravascular catheters. In a randomized prospective study among hemato-oncological patients, a silversulfate-polyurethane catheter (Fresenius AG, Germany) was associated with a significantly lower rate of CR-BSI compared to the control group (10.2% versus 22.5%, $p = 0.01$) (215). In three trials the Erlanger silver catheter, in which the silver is microdispersed, was evaluated (181,216,217). In the adult population, a reduction in catheter colonization and in "catheter-associated sepsis" was observed, but the authors used criteria for determining CR-BSI that differed from most other studies. A more recent clinical investigation failed to show a statistically significant difference in the colonization rate of the silver catheter compared to a control catheter (217). Ranucci et al. (182) compared the Vantex Oligon catheter, composed of silver, carbon, and platinum (Edwards Life Sciences, Irvine, CA), with a benzalkonium chloride-treated catheter (Edwards Life Sciences, Irvine, CA) in a prospective randomized trial. Use of the Vantex Oligon catheter decreased the rate for catheter colonization by 11%, while the rate for CR-BSI did not differ significantly between the Oligon and the control group.

Critical Evaluation of Antimicrobial Catheters

The majority of clinically important (e.g., randomized and prospective) studies have been performed with the chlorhexidine-silversulfadiazine (CHSS) catheters and, to a lesser extent, with the minocycline-rifampin (MR) catheter. Most of the studies with the CHSS catheter have revealed a trend toward lowering the incidence of CR-BSI. In the meta-analysis of Veenstra et al. (198), for example, it was shown that use of the CHSS-catheter in short-term catheterization reduced the risk for CR-BSI approximately by half. Only in one study (191) was no effect shown, probably due to the prolonged mean duration of catheterization in this study. With the MR catheters, two important studies so far (206,207) have shown a benefit in reducing the incidence of CR-BSI, one directly comparing the MR catheter with the CHSS catheter. Reasons for a better performance of the MR catheter have already been discussed (e.g., coating of the MR catheter on both surfaces and longer-lasting surface activity of the antibiotic combination in comparison to chlorhexidine). However, in our opinion it is clear that more controlled trials of good quality—especially from independent investigator groups—are needed for the MR catheter, in order to finally judge on the superiority of one of these catheters.

The cost-effectiveness of such impregnated catheters has recently been evaluated. Maki deduced from his trial (192) that in settings where the incidence of CR-BSI is greater than 3.3 per 1000 catheter days, the use of CHSS catheter would be cost-effective. Veenstra et al. (218) estimated a cost saving of from $68 to $391 on the basis of a multivariate sensitivity analysis. A recent analysis from the same group (219) came to the conclusion that MR catheters are cost-effective for patients catheterized for at least one week and lead to overall cost savings when patients are catheterized for two weeks or longer.

These analyses, together with the promising clinical results—at least for the CHSS and MR catheters—concerning the reduction of the incidence of CR-BSI, have led to the adoption of recommendations for the use of antimicrobial catheters in the form of current guidelines. In the U.S. guideline, for example, the use of antimicrobial or antiseptic-impregnated catheters in adults with an expected catheter duration time of greater than 5 days is emphasized (Category IB; see also Table 3) if, after implementing a comprehensive strategy to reduce rates of CR-BSI, the CR-BSI rate remains above the goal set by the individual institution, based on benchmark rates (9). The UK guideline (31) recommends considering the use of an antimicrobial-impregnated central venous catheter for adult patients who require short-term (<10 days) central venous catheterization and who are at high risk for CR-BSI. No recommendations are given for the use of such catheters in pediatric patients. In the actual German guideline (32), the use of antimicrobial catheters is still a matter of debate and regarded as a controversial issue (Category III; see also Table 3), reflecting in part the very limited clinical experiences with such catheters in Germany so far.

Although antimicrobial catheters obviously have the potential to decrease line-associated bloodstream infections and thus contribute to less patient morbidity and mortality, and even to considerable cost savings, there remain open questions that may jeopardize the application of such catheters. The two major points of criticism are the possible side effects: anaphylactoid reactions associated with the CHSS catheter (such as the cases reported from Japan and the United Kingdom), and the concern about development of microbial resistance against the agents used, e.g., either chlorhexidine, or silversulfadiazine and minocycline, or rifampin. Although resistance has not been demonstrated in the clinical trials with antimicrobial catheters, this is still a matter of concern that should be carefully monitored when using such catheters and should be an important issue in forthcoming clinical studies. As microorganisms embedded in biofilms are inactivated or killed only at far higher antimicrobial concentrations than are necessary for sessile bacteria, the decrease in concentration due to the drug release from the antimicrobial devices may lead to subinhibitory or sublethal activity, thus promoting the development of resistance. In *Pseudomonas stutzeri*, for example, a resistance against chlorhexidine could be achieved through repeated passages of the organisms in the presence of subinhibitory concentrations of chlorhexidine (202,220). Also, for the combination of minocycline and rifampin a 10- to 16-fold increase for *S. epidermidis* after exposure to concentrations below the minimum inhibitory concentration (MIC) was observed (208). Because all catheters come into contact with the normal skin flora, resistance could be induced and thus limit the use of rifampin as a valuable agent in severe staphylococcal infections (221).

Other open questions refer to the design of the studies performed so far with antimicrobial catheters. For example, all published studies with CHSS catheters have been conducted with the externally coated catheter (Arrow-Gard), especially the comparative trial MR versus CHSS catheters. Clinical studies with the new internally and externally coated CHSS catheter (ArrowGard Plus) (222) are required for a better comparison of the antibiotic-impregnated and the antiseptic-impregnated catheters, especially in view of longer catheter dwelling times. Concerning the MR catheter, its efficacy in preventing CR-BSI caused by organisms such as *Candida*, *Pseudomonas*, or *Enterococci* is doubtful due to the antimicrobial spectrum of minocycline and rifampin. More clinical investigations that also address this issue, especially from independent authors, are needed for this catheter in the future. In studies where the proof of catheter colonization is essential to establish the diagnosis of CR-BSI, methods for culturing bacteria or yeasts from the catheter should be employed which are influenced little or none by the antimicrobial substances used for coating or impregnation. Furthermore, almost none of the studies published so far have looked at the influence of the use of antimicrobial catheters on patient mortality. Secondary endpoints such as length of stay and the amount of antibiotic use should also be included in future studies.

In conclusion, it can be stated that especially the CHSS and the MR catheter show a significant trend toward a benefit in decreasing the incidence of CR-BSI, and they also seem to be cost-effective. However, in a recently published critical article on the value of antimicrobial catheters, 11 randomized studies were analyzed and yielded several methodological flaws. Moreover, in this review, no significant clinical benefit associated with the use of such catheters for the purpose of reducing CR-BSI or improving patient outcomes could be delineated (223). The actual U.S. guideline (9) uses the following formulation: "The decision to use chlorhexidine/silversulfadiazine- or minocycline/rifampin-impregnated catheters should be based on the need to enhance prevention of CR-BSI after standard procedures have been implemented (e.g., educating personnel, using maximal sterile barrier precautions, ...) and then balanced against the concern for emergence of resistant pathogens and the cost of implementing this strategy."

Modified Devices Used in Catheterization

As an alternative approach, protective cuffs have been developed for central venous catheters. These cuffs were coated with silver compounds to increase the anti-infective effect and attached to the catheter prior to insertion, to act as a tissue-interface barrier and thus to inhibit bacterial migration from the skin along the catheter. The VitaCuff™ (Vitaphore Corporation, USA), for example, consists of a detachable cuff made of biodegrable collagen to which silver ions are chelated. Several studies have been undertaken to assess the ability of such cuffs to prevent CRI and have yielded conflicting results. In a prospective, randomized, multicenter trial it was found that catheters, inserted with the cuff were three times less likely to be colonized on removal than were control catheters, and nearly four times less likely to produce bacteremia (224). Similar results were observed in another study (225), whereas Groeger et al. found no difference in the frequency of CR-BSI between the test and the control group (226). A reason for the controversial results might be that Groeger et al. used the cuff in patients with long-term catheterization, in whom hub colonization may be a more important factor for CRI than extraluminal contamination, against which the cuff confers protection. Also, in a study by Dahlberg et al. (227), use of the impregnated cuffs had no influence on the incidence of CR-BSI. Smith et al. found a reduction in the colonization of skin sites and hubs for the impregnated cuff patients, but no significant difference in CR-BSI between the VitaCuff™ and the control group (228). It is assumed that extrusion of the silver cuff from the catheter tunnel tract to the skin may be a reason for the limited ability of the cuff to prevent CRI in short-term CVCs.

Because hub contamination is regarded as the second most important step in catheter colonization and subsequent infection, hubs have also been modified. In one approach, a povidone-iodine-saturated sponge was developed to encase the hub and showed a significant reduction in CR-BSI compared to a control hub (229). A novel CVC hub (Segur-Lock™, Inibsa Laboratories) with a reservoir containing iodinated alcohol proved to be effective in decreasing rates of CR-BSI in a clinical trial (4 versus 16% for the control hub, $p < 0.01$) (230). However, this result could not be confirmed in a subsequent trial (231).

The Biopatch™ antimicrobial dressing (Johnson and Johnson, USA) is a hydrophilic polyurethane foam dressing impregnated with chlorhexidine gluconate, designed to release chlorhexidine and to inhibit microbial growth at the catheter entry site for at least 7 days. Two randomized clinical trials have investigated this new type of dressing. In one study, a significant reduction in catheter colonization was found (232), and the other demonstrated a significant reduction in the incidence of CR-BSI (1.2 versus 3.3% for the control group, $p < 0.01$) (233). Garland et al. conducted a randomized clinical trial to assess the efficacy of the Biopatch™ in prevention of CRI in neonates (234). Neonates randomized to the Biopatch™ group were less likely to have colonized CVC tips than control neonates, in whom skin disinfection with povidone-iodine was performed. The rate of CR-BSI did not differ between the two groups. However, the risk of local contact dermatitis under the Biopatch dressing was high, especially in low-birthweight infants. This observation, together with the fact that the Biopatch™ shall be not removed if in place, thus preventing visual daily inspection of the catheter entry site, may limit the use of this antimicrobial dressing.

A novel catheter system, equipped with a diaphragm instead of a stopcock for drawing blood specimens from arterial lines, proved to be associated with a sixfold lower rate of fluid contamination than systems using standard stopcocks (235). Another approach designed to reduce the risk of transmission of blood-borne infections to health care workers led to the design and introduction of needleless devices (236–239). At present, there are only few data available on the benefit of such systems, but it seems that technical problems arise with the use of such systems and will have to be solved before these devices should be evaluated in longer trials.

Until now, in the recently published guidelines, none of these modified devices are recommended as tools for the prevention of CRI.

Anti-Infective Catheters Other Than CVCs

A number of studies have been published on anti-infective urinary catheters. Aminoglycosides such as dibekacin sulfate or kanamycin, as well as cephalotin or cefoxitin, have been bonded to hydrophilic polymers, polyethylene, and silicone rubber catheters and evaluated experimentally or in part in clinical studies, showing some effectiveness in the prevention of urinary catheter-associated infection. Most studies, however, have dealt with the development of silver-containing urinary catheters. Liedberg et al. investigated the interaction between silver alloy-coated urinary catheters and *P. aeruginosa* and demonstrated supression of in vitro biofilm formation (240). In a randomized clinical trial, the incidence of catheter-associated urinary tract infection was reduced (241). In another prospective study involving 482 hospitalized patients, Johnson et al. observed a similar rate of catheter-associated urinary tract infections in patients with a silver-oxide urinary catheter, compared to patients with normal catheters (242). Riley et al. could not confirm such results in their study on silver-impregnated urinary catheters (243). In a meta-analysis performed by Saint et al. (244), the authors reported that silver alloy urinary catheters were more effective in reducing bacteriuria than silver-oxide catheters.

In recent years, clinical trials with silver-hydrogel urinary catheters (e.g., Bardex IC Foley catheter, Bard, USA) have been performed, all showing reduction of catheter-associated UTI (245–247). In a new approach, Gaonkar et al. (248) have evaluated the in vitro long-term efficacy of latex and silicone urinary catheters impregnated with chlorhexidine and silversulfadiazine—with and without the addition of the antiseptic triclosan—demonstrating a broad-spectrum, long-lasting effect against microbial colonization on the outer surface of the catheters. In a recent article, Stickler has referred to the fact that frequent application of chlorhexidine in patients undergoing intermittent bladder catheterization has led to the development of chlorhexidine resistance in organisms such as *Pseudomonas stuartii*, *P. aeruginosa*, and *P. mirabilis* (249). He stated that the catheterized urinary tract, with its mixed population, would be a greater challenge for a biocide-containing device than the vascular tract, thereby warning against the reintroduction of chlorhexidine for the prevention of catheter-related UTI.

Recently, Niel-Weise and colleagues (250) performed a systematic literature review of clinical trials and meta-analyses with silver urinary catheters. They concluded that there is to date insufficient evidence to recommend the use of silver urinary catheters, and that more randomized clinical trials with a good standard of internal quality are needed.

Trooskin et al. developed an infection-resistant continuous ambulatory peritoneal dialysis (CAPD) catheter by binding penicillin to the silicone elastomer via the cationic surfactant tridodecylmethylammonium chloride (TDMAC). In vivo studies with rats, the antibiotic-bonded catheters were more resistant to colonization after exit-site and intraluminal bacterial challenges (251). As already reported for urinary catheters, the technology using chlorhexidine and silversulfadiazine as impregnating agents has also been used, together with triclosan, for the development of a new type of antimicrobial CAPD catheter (252). In a rat animal model, the exit site of the implanted catheter was inoculated with *S. aureus* 7 days postimplantation, none of the modified catheters were colonized intraperitoneally (control group: 100%), and only 12.5% of the modified catheters at the exit site (control group: 100%).

Infection of central nervous systems (hydrocephalus) shunts is a major problem in patients with ventricular drainage. Therefore, efforts have also been made to develop infection-resistant hydrocephalus shunts or other neurological prostheses. Bridgett et al. reported on the reduced staphylococcal adherence to Hydromer™-coated—and thus hydrophilic—cerebrospinal fluid shunts, but there were technical difficulties in achieving a uniform Hydromer layer on the silicone rubber (253). Bayston et al. have published a considerable body of experimental work on impregnation of silicone shunt catheters with various antimicrobials (254–257). In particular, a combination of rifampin and clindamycin proved to be clearly superior to other agents tested. In a newer study, it could be shown that the rifampin and clindamycin-impregnated catheters are able to kill adhered staphylococci completely within 48 to 52 hours (258,259).

We have also developed a method for incorporating rifampin and other hydrophobic antibiotics into silicone ventricular catheters (260). A rifampin-loaded catheter is capable of inhibiting in vitro adherence of staphylococci. In an animal model using New Zealand white rabbits, catheters were implanted into the ventricular space and infection was induced by inoculation of certain dosages of *S. epidermidis* or *S. aureus* (261). None of the animals that received the rifampin-loaded catheter showed clinical signs of infection, nor could the infecting strain be recovered from the catheter, brain tissue, or cerebrospinal fluid. In contrast, all animals with the uncoated catheters showed signs of severe meningitis or ventriculitis, and the infecting strains were cultivated in each case from the catheter and from surrounding tissue. As an improvement of the catheter, especially to prevent staphylococci from developing resistance to rifampin, a combination of rifampin and trimethoprim was used for the impregnation process (262).

Recently, two cases in which the rifampin catheter was successfully used for the treatment of patients with a complicated course of shunt infection were reported (263). Further, a silicone catheter with a combination of three antimicrobials (rifampin, fusidic acid, and mupirocin) has been described, with a long-lasting drug release of up to ~100 days. However, no animal or clinical data are available so far for this type of catheter (264). Zabramski et al. (265) performed a prospective, randomized clinical trial with an external ventricular drain catheter coated with minocycline and rifampin. The antibiotic-impregnated catheters were one-half as likely to become colonized as the control catheters (17.9 versus 36.7%, $p < 0.0012$), and CSF cultures were seven times less frequently positive in patients with the modified catheters than in the control group (1.3 versus 9.4%, $p = 0.002$).

For a more detailed discussion on antimicrobial CSF shunt catheters and related devices, see Chapter 16.

OTHER APPROACHES TO THE PREVENTION OF CRI

There is only a limited number of studies on innovative approaches to the prevention of foreign-body infection and CRI which do not aim at the modification of the medical device (implant or catheter). A very interesting approach to prevent biofilm formation as a prerequisite for CRI has been suggested by Khoury et al. (28). They found that by application of an external stimulus, e.g., an electric field together with antibiotics, the killing of biofilm-embedded bacteria is dramatically enhanced (e.g., killing of *P. aeruginosa* by tobramycin). Although it is more a therapeutical strategy rather than a preventive measure, the use of electric current might be useful for the prevention of CRI, as has been pointed out before. Related approaches aiming at eradication of biofilms include the combined use of ultrasound together with antibiotics (29,30), and possibly the bactericidal effect of extracorporeal shock waves on *S. aureus* (266).

A polysaccharide was isolated from a *S. epidermidis* strain that appears to be involved in adhesion to synthetic polymers such as silicone (19,20). Active immunization of rabbits with this polysaccharide-adhesin (PS/A) factor led to reduced bacteremia caused by catheters contaminated with the specific *S. epidermidis* strain (267). In a further study, *S. epidermidis* prosthetic valve endocarditis was successfully prevented by active and passive immunization of the rabbits (268).

In a multicenter trial on the efficacy of vaccination with staphylococcal toxoid in patients with CAPD catheters, no increase of the intraperitoneal bactericidal activity and no reduction of catheter-associated peritonitis or exit-site infection was observed (269). Further, it has been proposed to develop monoclonal antibodies against fibronectin and other mediators of bacterial (staphylococcal) adherence to inhibit the specific adherence process (270). Because there is now more insight into the molecular pathogenesis of CRIs—especially those caused by staphylococci—future strategies might involve, for example, blocking of the gene operon detected in *S. epidermidis*, which is responsible for autoaggregation and biofilm formation (25). It was shown that antibodies directed against the accumulation-associated protein (AAP) are able to prevent *S. epidermidis* biofilm formation in vitro (24). A better understanding of quorum sensing—a cell-to-cell communication process also responsible for the regulation of biofilm formation—may lead to new concepts of how biofilm formation can be prevented, e.g., on the basis of chemical substances that disturb microbial communication (271,272). Danese has recently given an overview of potential future strategies with nonbactericidal antibiofilm approaches (273).

CONCLUDING REMARKS

Because of the difficulties in treatment of CRIs and because of their impact on morbidity and even mortality, as well as on cost increase, prevention of CRI remains a major goal in the medicine of today. The preceding sections of this chapter have tried to highlight actual preventive strategies, based on advances in catheterization technique and care, and on innovative technology. Since the first CDC guidelines for prevention of intravascular infection appeared in 1983 (274), we have learned much more about different aspects of CRI, and a considerable number of well-performed, controlled clinical studies have contributed to our actual practice in intravascular catheterization. This improved knowledge has now led to a variety of evidence-based recommendations for the prevention of CRI, which have been precipitated in national (e.g., U.S., U.K. or German) directions. Because it would be beyond the scope of this chapter to give detailed instructions for the daily management of catheters and prevention of CRI, the reader is referred to the recently published guidelines (9,31,32), which should be translated into institution-specific recommendations.

The development of new catheters based on modified, anti-infective materials, and other innovative approaches in this field, will surely lead to a further reduction in the incidence of CRI in the future. Some of the new developments such as antimicrobial catheters have already been adopted in current national guidelines, but still more clinical studies of good quality are needed to better define their impact on reducing CR-BSI and patient morbidity and mortality, and to recommend a broader use of these promising devices. However, it should be remembered that the best technology will fail to prevent CRI if hygienic standard procedures such as education of personnel and use of maximal barrier precautions are not, or not adequately, implemented. The main risks for CRI result from lack of aseptic technique, inappropriate insertion site care, and lack of necessary technical skills. A multiple-approach prevention strategy targeted at catheter insertion and catheter care and based on actual recommendations from the respective national guidelines, which are evidence-based, together with the use of even more sophisticated and improved innovative catheter materials, might help to combat the threat of infections associated with vascular access.

REFERENCES

1. Widmer AF. IV-related infection. In: Wenzel RP, ed. Prevention and Control of Nosocomial Infection. Williams and Wilkins, 1993:556–579.
2. Arnow PM, Quimosing EM, Beach M. Consequences of intravascular catheter sepsis. Clin Infect Dis 1993; 16(6):778–784.
3. Maki DG. Nosocomial bacteremia. An epidemiologic overview. Am J Med 1981; 70(3):719–732.
4. Mermel LA. Prevention of intravascular catheter-related infections. Ann Intern Med 2000; 132(5):391–402.
5. Gastmeier P, Weist K, Ruden H. Catheter-associated primary bloodstream infections: epidemiology and preventive methods. Infection 1999; 27(suppl 1): S1–S6.
6. Rello J, Ochagavia A, Sabanes E, Roque M, Mariscal D, Reynaga E, Valles J. Evaluation of outcome of intravenous catheter-related infections in critically ill patients. Am J Respir Crit Care Med 2000; 162(3 Pt 1):1027–1030.
7. Dimick JB, Pelz RK, Consunji R, Swoboda SM, Hendrix CW, Lipsett PA. Increased resource use associated with catheter-related bloodstream infection in the surgical intensive care unit. Arch Surg 2001; 136(2):229–234.
8. DiGiovine B, Chenoweth C, Watts C, Higgins M. The attributable mortality and costs of primary nosocomial bloodstream infections in the intensive care unit. Am J Respir Crit Care Med 1999; 160(3):976–981.
9. O'Grady NP, Alexander M, Dellinger EP, Gerberding JL, Heard SO, Maki DG, Masur H, McCormick RD, Mermel LA, Pearson ML, Raad II,

Randolph A, Weinstein RA. Guidelines for the prevention of intravascular catheter-related infections. Centers for Disease Control and Prevention. MMWR Recomm Rep 2002; 51(RR-10):1–29.

10. Dankert J, Host AH, Feijen J. Biomedical polymers: bacterial adhesion, colonization and infection. In: Williams DF, ed. Critical Reviews in Biocompatibility. Boca Raton, FL: CRC Press, 1986:219–301.

11. Jansen B, Peters G, Pulverer G. Mechanisms and clinical relevance of bacterial adhesion to polymers. J Biomater Appl 1988; 2(4):520–543.

12. Jansen B, Schumacher-Perdreau F, Peters G, Pulverer G. New aspects in the pathogenesis and prevention of polymer-associated foreign-body infections caused by coagulase-negative staphylococci. J Invest Surg 1989; 2(4): 361–380.

13. Peters G, Schumacher-Perdreau F, Jansen B, Bey M, Pulverer G. Biology of *Staphylococcus epidermidis* slime. In: Pulverer G, Quie P, Peters G, eds. Clinical Significance and Pathogenicity of Coagulase-Negative Staphylococci. Stuttgart: Gustav Fischer Verlag, 1987:15–32.

14. Gristina AG. Biomaterial-centered infection: microbial adhesion versus tissue integration. Science 1987; 237(4822):1588–1595.

15. Herrmann M, Vaudaux PE, Pittet D, Auckenthaler R, Lew PD, Schumacher-Perdreau F, Peters G, Waldvogel FA. Fibronectin, fibrinogen, and laminin act as mediators of adherence of clinical staphylococcal isolates to foreign material. J Infect Dis 1988; 158(4):693–701.

16. Vaudaux P, Suzuki R, Waldvogel FA, Morgenthaler JJ, Nydegger UE. Foreign body infection: role of fibronectin as a ligand for the adherence of *Staphylococcus aureus*. J Infect Dis 1984; 150(4):546–553.

17. Herrmann M, Lai QJ, Albrecht RM, Mosher DF, Proctor RA. Adhesion of *Staphylococcus aureus* to surface-bound platelets: role of fibrinogen/fibrin and platelet integrins. J Infect Dis 1993; 167(2):312–322.

18. Herrmann M, Suchard SJ, Boxer LA, Waldvogel FA, Lew PD. Thrombospondin binds to *Staphylococcus aureus* and promotes staphylococcal adherence to surfaces. Infect Immun 1991; 59(1):279–288.

19. Muller E, Hubner J, Gutierrez N, Takeda S, Goldmann DA, Pier GB. Isolation and characterization of transposon mutants of *Staphylococcus epidermidis* deficient in capsular polysaccharide/adhesin and slime. Infect Immun 1993; 61(2):551–558.

20. Tojo M, Yamashita N, Goldmann DA, Pier GB. Isolation and characterization of a capsular polysaccharide adhesin from *Staphylococcus epidermidis*. J Infect Dis 1988; 157(4):713–722.

21. Timmerman CP, Fleer A, Besnier JM, DeGraaf L, Cremers F, Verhoef J. Characterization of a proteinaceous adhesin of *Staphylococcus epidermidis* which mediates attachment to polystyrene. Infect Immun 1991; 59(11):4187–4192.

22. Rupp ME, Archer GL. Hemagglutination and adherence to plastic by *Staphylococcus epidermidis*. Infect Immun 1992; 60(10):4322–4327.

23. Mack D, Siemssen N, Laufs R. Parallel induction by glucose of adherence and a polysaccharide antigen specific for plastic-adherent *Staphylococcus epidermidis*: evidence for functional relation to intercellular adhesion. Infect Immun 1992; 60(5):2048–2057.

24. Hussain M, Herrmann M, von Eiff C, Perdreau-Remington F, Peters G. A 140-kilodalton extracellular protein is essential for the accumulation of *Staphylococcus epidermidis* strains on surfaces. Infect Immun 1997; 65(2):519–524.

25. Ziebuhr W, Heilmann C, Gotz F, Meyer P, Wilms K, Straube E, Hacker J. Detection of the intercellular adhesion gene cluster (ica) and phase variation in *Staphylococcus epidermidis* blood culture strains and mucosal isolates. Infect Immun 1997; 65(3):890–896.

26. Jansen B, Kohnen W. Prevention of biofilm formation by polymer modification. J Ind Microbiol 1995; 15(4):391–396.

27. Ascher DP, Shoupe BA, Maybee D, Fischer GW. Persistent catheter-related bacteremia: clearance with antibiotics and urokinase. J Pediatr Surg 1993; 28 (4):627–629.

28. Khoury AE, Lam K, Ellis B, Costerton JW. Prevention and control of bacterial infections associated with medical devices. ASAIO J 1992; 38(3): M174–M178.

29. Rediske AM, Roeder BL, Brown MK, Nelson JL, Robison RL, Draper DO, Schaalje GB, Robison RA, Pitt WG. Ultrasonic enhancement of antibiotic action on *Escherichia coli* biofilms: an in vivo model. Antimicrob Agents Chemother 1999, 43(5):1211–1214.

30. Rediske AM, Roeder BL, Nelson JL, Robison RL, Schaalje GB, Robison RA, Pitt WG. Pulsed ultrasound enhances the killing of *Escherichia coli* biofilms by aminoglycoside antibiotics in vivo. Antimicrob Agents Chemother 2000; 44(3):771–772.

31. Pratt RJ. Guidelines for preventing infections associated with the insertion and maintenance of central venous catheters. Journal of Hospital Infection 2001; 47(suppl):S47–S66.

32. Trautmann M, Jansen B, Frey P, Hummler H, Rasche M, Scheringer I, Schwalbe B. Prävention Gefäßkatheter-assoziierter Infektionen. Bundesgesundheitsbl Gesundheitsforsch Gesundheitsschutz 2002; 45:907–924.

33. Sherertz RJ, Ely EW, Westbrook DM, Gledhill KS, Streed SA, Kiger B, Flynn L, Hayes S, Strong S, Cruz J, Bowton DL, Hulgan T, Haponik EF. Education of physicians-in-training can decrease the risk for vascular catheter infection. Ann Intern Med 2000; 132(8):641–648.

34. Eggimann P, Harbarth S, Constantin MN, Touveneau S, Chevrolet JC, Pittet D. Impact of a prevention strategy targeted at vascular-access care on incidence of infections acquired in intensive care. Lancet 2000; 355(9218):1864–1868.

35. Gil RT, Kruse JA, Thill-Baharozian MC, Carlson RW. Triple- vs single-lumen central venous catheters. A prospective study in a critically ill population. Arch Intern Med 1989; 149(5):1139–1143.

36. Richet H, Hubert B, Nitemberg G, Andremont A, Buu-Hoi A, Ourbak P, Galicier C, Veron M, Boisivon A, Bouvier AM. Prospective multicenter study of vascular-catheter-related complications and risk factors for positive central-catheter cultures in intensive care unit patients. J Clin Microbiol 1990; 28(11):2520–2525.

37. Miller JJ, Venus B, Mathru M. Comparison of the sterility of long-term central venous catheterization using single lumen, triple lumen, and pulmonary artery catheters. Crit Care Med 1984; 12(8):634–637.

38. Ullman RF, Gurevich I, Schoch PE, Cunha BA. Colonization and bacteremia related to duration of triple-lumen intravascular catheter placement. Am J Infect Control 1990; 18(3):201–207.
39. Band JD, Maki DG. Steel needles used for intravenous therapy. Morbidity in patients with hematologic malignancy. Arch Intern Med 1980; 140(1):31–34.
40. Tully JL, Friedland GH, Baldini LM, Goldmann DA. Complications of intravenous therapy with steel needles and Teflon catheters. A comparative study. Am J Med 1981; 70(3):702–706.
41. Maki DG, Ringer M. Risk factors for infusion-related phlebitis with small peripheral venous catheters. A randomized controlled trial. Ann Intern Med 1991; 114(10):845–854.
42. Sheth NK, Rose HD, Franson TR, Buckmire FL, Sohnle PG. In vitro quantitative adherence of bacteria to intravascular catheters. J Surg Res 1983; 34 (3):213–218.
43. Collins RN, Braun PA, Zinner SH, Kass EH. Risk of local and systemic infection with polyethylene intravenous catheters. A prospective study of 213 catheterizations. N Engl J Med 1968; 279(7):340–343.
44. Maki DG, Goldman DA, Rhame FS. Infection control in intravenous therapy. Ann Intern Med 1973; 79(6):867–887.
45. Mitchell A, Atkins S, Royle GT, Kettlewell MG. Reduced catheter sepsis and prolonged catheter life using a tunnelled silicone rubber catheter for total parenteral nutrition. Br J Surg 1982; 69(7):420–422.
46. Sherertz RJ, Carruth WA, Marosok RD, Espeland MA, Johnson RA, Solomon DD. Contribution of vascular catheter material to the pathogenesis of infection: the enhanced risk of silicone in vivo. J Biomed Mater Res 1995; 29(5):635–645.
47. Yeung C, May J, Hughes R. Infection rate for single lumen v triple lumen subclavian catheters. Infect Control Hosp Epidemiol 1988; 9(4):154–158.
48. McCarthy MC, Shives JK, Robison RJ, Broadie TA. Prospective evaluation of single and triple lumen catheters in total parenteral nutrition. JPEN J Parenter Enteral Nutr 1987; 11(3):259–262.
49. Clark-Christoff N, Watters VA, Sparks W, Snyder P, Grant JP. Use of triple-lumen subclavian catheters for administration of total parenteral nutrition. JPEN J Parenter Enteral Nutr 1992; 16(5):403–407.
50. Collignon P, Soni N, Pearson I, Sorrell T, Woods P. Sepsis associated with central vein catheters in critically ill patients. Intensive Care Med 1988; 14(3):227–231.
51. Horowitz HW, Dworkin BM, Savino JA, Byrne DW, Pecora NA. Central catheter-related infections: comparison of pulmonary artery catheters and triple lumen catheters for the delivery of hyperalimentation in a critical care setting. JPEN J Parenter Enteral Nutr 1990; 14(6):588–592.
52. Pinilla JC, Ross DF, Martin T, Crump H. Study of the incidence of intravascular catheter infection and associated septicemia in critically ill patients. Crit Care Med 1983; 11(1):21–25.
53. Lazarus HM, Creger RJ, Bloom AD, Shenk R. Percutaneous placement of femoral central venous catheter in patients undergoing transplantation of bone marrow. Surg Gynecol Obstet 1990; 170(5):403–406.

54. Williams JF, Seneff MG, Friedman BC, McGrath BJ, Gregg R, Sunner J, Zimmerman JE. Use of femoral venous catheters in critically ill adults: prospective study. Crit Care Med 1991; 19(4):550–553.

55. Trottier SJ, Veremakis C, O'Brien J, Auer AI. Femoral deep vein thrombosis associated with central venous catheterization: results from a prospective, randomized trial. Crit Care Med 1995; 23(1):52–59.

56. Venkataraman ST, Thompson AE, Orr RA. Femoral vascular catheterization in critically ill infants and children. Clin Pediatr (Phila) 1997; 36(6):311–319.

57. Goldstein AM, Weber JM, Sheridan RL. Femoral venous access is safe in burned children: an analysis of 224 catheters. J Pediatr 1997; 130(3):442–446.

58. Raad II, Hohn DC, Gilbreath BJ, Suleiman N, Hill LA, Bruso PA, Marts K, Mansfield PF, Bodey GP. Prevention of central venous catheter-related infections by using maximal sterile barrier precautions during insertion. Infect Control Hosp Epidemiol 1994; 15(4 Pt 1):231–238.

59. Mermel LA, McCormick RD, Springman SR, Maki DG. The pathogenesis and epidemiology of catheter-related infection with pulmonary artery Swan-Ganz catheters: a prospective study utilizing molecular subtyping. Am J Med 1991; 91(3B):197S–205S.

60. Faubion WC, Wesley JR, Khalidi N, Silva J. Total parenteral nutrition catheter sepsis: impact of the team approach. JPEN J Parenter Enteral Nutr 1986; 10(6):642–645.

61. Keohane PP, Jones BJ, Attrill H, Cribb A, Northover J, Frost P, Silk DB. Effect of catheter tunnelling and a nutrition nurse on catheter sepsis during parenteral nutrition. A controlled trial. Lancet 1983; 2(8364):1388–1390.

62. Nelson DB, Kien CL, Mohr B, Frank S, Davis SD. Dressing changes by specialized personnel reduce infection rates in patients receiving central venous parenteral nutrition. JPEN J Parenter Enteral Nutr 1986; 10(2):220–222.

63. Tomford JW, Hershey CO, McLaren CE, Porter DK, Cohen DI. Intravenous therapy team and peripheral venous catheter-associated complications. A prospective controlled study. Arch Intern Med 1984; 144(6):1191–1194.

64. Tomford JW, Hershey CO. The i.v. therapy team: impact on patient care and costs of hospitalization. NITA 1985; 8(5):387–389.

65. Soifer NE, Borzak S, Edlin BR, Weinstein RA. Prevention of peripheral venous catheter complications with an intravenous therapy team: a randomized controlled trial. Arch Intern Med 1998; 158(5):473–477.

66. Fridkin SK, Pear SM, Williamson TH, Galgiani JN, Jarvis WR. The role of understaffing in central venous catheter-associated bloodstream infections. Infect Control Hosp Epidemiol 1996; 17(3):150–158.

67. Needleman J, Buerhaus P, Mattke S, Stewart M, Zelevinsky K. Nurse-staffing levels and the quality of care in hospitals. N Engl J Med 2002; 346(22):1715–1722.

68. Henderson DK. Bacteremia due to percutaneous intravascular devices. In: Mandell GL, Douglas RG, Bennet JE, eds. Principles and Practice of Infectious Diseases. New York: Churchill Livingstone, 1990:2189–2199.

69. Rutala WA. APIC guideline for selection and use of disinfectants. Am J Infect Control 1990; 18(2):99–117.

70. Mimoz O, Pieroni L, Lawrence C, Edouard A, Costa Y, Samii K, Brun-

Buisson C. Prospective, randomized trial of two antiseptic solutions for prevention of central venous or arterial catheter colonization and infection in intensive care unit patients. Crit Care Med 1996; 24(11):1818–1823.

71. Humar A, Ostromecki A, Direnfeld J, Marshall JC, Lazar N, Houston PC, Boiteau P, Conly JM. Prospective randomized trial of 10% povidone-iodine versus 0.5% tincture of chlorhexidine as cutaneous antisepsis for prevention of central venous catheter infection. Clin Infect Dis 2000; 31(4):1001–1007.

72. Garland JS, Buck RK, Maloney P, Durkin DM, Toth-Lloyd S, Duffy M, Szocik P, McAuliffe TL, Goldmann D. Comparison of 10% povidone-iodine and 0.5% chlorhexidine gluconate for the prevention of peripheral intravenous catheter colonization in neonates: a prospective trial. Pediatr Infect Dis J 1995; 14(6):510–516.

73. Maki DG, Ringer M, Alvarado CJ. Prospective randomised trial of povidone-iodine, alcohol, and chlorhexidine for prevention of infection associated with central venous and arterial catheters. Lancet 1991; 338(8763):339–343.

74. Bock SN, Lee RE, Fisher B, Rubin JT, Schwartzentruber DJ, Wei JP, Callender DP, Yang JC, Lotze MT, Pizzo PA. A prospective randomized trial evaluating prophylactic antibiotics to prevent triple-lumen catheter-related sepsis in patients treated with immunotherapy. J Clin Oncol 1990; 8(1):161–169.

75. AlSibai MB, Harder EJ, Faskin RW, Johnson GW, Padmos MA. The value of prophylactic antibiotics during the insertion of long-term indwelling silastic right atrial catheters in cancer patients. Cancer 1987; 60(8):1891–1895.

76. McKee R, Dunsmuir R, Whitby M, Garden OJ. Does antibiotic prophylaxis at the time of catheter insertion reduce the incidence of catheter-related sepsis in intravenous nutrition? J Hosp Infect 1985; 6(4):419–425.

77. Ranson MR, Oppenheim BA, Jackson A, Kamthan AG, Scarffe JH. Double-blind placebo controlled study of vancomycin prophylaxis for central venous catheter insertion in cancer patients. J Hosp Infect 1990; 15(1):95–102.

78. Rackoff WR, Weiman M, Jakobowski D, Hirschl R, Stallings V, Bilodeau J, Danz P, Bell L, Lange B. A randomized, controlled trial of the efficacy of a heparin and vancomycin solution in preventing central venous catheter infections in children. J Pediatr 1995; 127(1):147–151.

79. Ljungman P, Hagglund H, Bjorkstrand B, Lonnqvist B, Ringden O. Peroperative teicoplanin for prevention of gram-positive infections in neutropenic patients with indwelling central venous catheters: a randomized, controlled study. Support Care Cancer 1997; 5(6):485–488.

80. van de Wetering MD, van Woensel JB. Prophylactic antibiotics for preventing early central venous catheter Gram positive infections in oncology patients. Cochrane Database Syst Rev 2003; (2):CD003295.

81. Maki DG, Mermel LA. Infections due to infusion therapy. In: Bennett JV, Brachmann PS, eds. Hospital Infections. Philadelphia: Lippincott-Raven, 1998: 689–724.

82. Craven DE, Lichtenberg DA, Kunches LM, McDonough AT, Gonzalez MI, Heeren TC, McCabe WR. A randomized study comparing a transparent polyurethane dressing to a dry gauze dressing for peripheral intravenous catheter sites. Infect Control 1985; 6(9):361–366.

83. Dickerson N, Horton P, Smith S, Rose RC III. Clinically significant central venous catheter infections in a community hospital: association with type of dressing. J Infect Dis 1989; 160(4):720–722.

84. Conly JM, Grieves K, Peters B. A prospective, randomized study comparing transparent and dry gauze dressings for central venous catheters. J Infect Dis 1989; 159(2):310–319.

85. Maki DG, Ringer M. Evaluation of dressing regimens for prevention of infection with peripheral intravenous catheters. Gauze, a transparent polyurethane dressing, and an iodophor-transparent dressing. JAMA 1987; 258(17): 2396–2403.

86. Ricard P, Martin R, Marcoux JA. Protection of indwelling vascular catheters: incidence of bacterial contamination and catheter-related sepsis. Crit Care Med 1985; 13(7):541–543.

87. Hoffmann KK, Weber DJ, Samsa GP, Rutala WA. Transparent polyurethane film as an intravenous catheter dressing. A meta-analysis of the infection risks. JAMA 1992; 267(15):2072–2076.

88. Hoffmann KK, Western SA, Kaiser DL, Wenzel RP, Groschel DH. Bacterial colonization and phlebitis-associated risk with transparent polyurethane film for peripheral intravenous site dressings. Am J Infect Control 1988; 16(3):101–106.

89. Thomas S, Loveless P, Hay NP. Comparative review of the properties of six semipermeable film dressings. Pharm J 1988; 241:784.

90. Maki DG, Band JD. A comparative study of polyantibiotic and iodophor ointments in prevention of vascular catheter-related infection. Am J Med 1981; 70(3):739–744.

91. Levin A, Mason AJ, Jindal KK, Fong IW, Goldstein MB. Prevention of hemodialysis subclavian vein catheter infections by topical povidone-iodine. Kidney Int 1991; 40(5):934–938.

92. Fong IW. Prevention of haemodialysis and peritoneal dialysis catheter related infection by topical povidone-iodine. Postgrad Med J 1993; 69(suppl 3):S15–S17.

93. Hill RL, Casewell MW. Reduction in the colonization of central venous cannulae by mupirocin. J Hosp Infect 1991; 19(suppl B):47–57.

94. Boelaert JR, De Baere YA, Geernaert MA, Godard CA, Van Landuyt HW. The use of nasal mupirocin ointment to prevent *Staphylococcus aureus* bacteraemias in haemodialysis patients: an analysis of cost-effectiveness. J Hosp Infect 1991; 19(suppl B):41–46.

95. Sesso R, Barbosa D, Leme IL, Sader H, Canziani ME, Manfredi S, Draibe S, Pignatari AC. *Staphylococcus aureus* prophylaxis in hemodialysis patients using central venous catheter: effect of mupirocin ointment. J Am Soc Nephrol 1998; 9(6):1085–1092.

96. Zakrzewska-Bode A, Muytjens HL, Liem KD, Hoogkamp-Korstanje JA. Mupirocin resistance in coagulase-negative staphylococci, after topical prophylaxis for the reduction of colonization of central venous catheters. J Hosp Infect 1995; 31(3):189–193.

97. Miller MA, Dascal A, Portnoy J, Mendelson J. Development of mupirocin resistance among methicillin-resistant *Staphylococcus aureus* after widespread

use of nasal mupirocin ointment. Infect Control Hosp Epidemiol 1996; 17(12): 811–813.

98. Rao SP, Oreopoulos DG. Unusual complications of a polyurethane PD catheter. Perit Dial Int 1997; 17(4):410–412.

99. Riu S, Ruiz CG, Martinez-Vea A, Peralta C, Oliver JA. Spontaneous rupture of polyurethane peritoneal catheter. A possible deleterious effect of mupirocin ointment. Nephrol Dial Transplant 1998; 13(7):1870–1871.

100. Zinner SH, Denny-Brown BC, Braun P, Burke JP, Toala P, Kass EH. Risk of infection with intravenous indwelling catheters: effect of application of antibiotic ointment. J Infect Dis 1969; 120(5):616–619.

101. Norden CW. Application of antibiotic ointment to the site of venous catheterization-a controlled trial. J Infect Dis 1969; 120(5):611–615.

102. Bregenzer T, Conen D, Widmer AF. Routine replacement of peripheral IV-catheters is not necessary: a prospective study. Can J Infect Dis 1995; 6(C): 245C.

103. Bregenzer T, Conen D, Sakmann P, Widmer AF. Is routine replacement of peripheral intravenous catheters necessary? Arch Intern Med 1998; 158(2): 151–156.

104. Cornely OA, Bethe U, Pauls R, Waldschmidt D. Peripheral Teflon catheters: factors determining incidence of phlebitis and duration of cannulation. Infect Control Hosp Epidemiol 2002; 23(5):249–253.

105. Eyer S, Brummitt C, Crossley K, Siegel R, Cerra F. Catheter-related sepsis: prospective, randomized study of three methods of long-term catheter maintenance. Crit Care Med 1990; 18(10):1073–1079.

106. Uldall PR, Merchant N, Woods F, Yarworski U, Vas S. Changing subclavian haemodialysis cannulas to reduce infection. Lancet 1981; 1(8234):1373.

107. Bonawitz SC, Hammell EJ, Kirkpatrick JR. Prevention of central venous catheter sepsis: a prospective randomized trial. Am Surg 1991; 57(10):618–623.

108. Cook D, Randolph A, Kernerman P, Cupido C, King D, Soukup C, Brun-Buisson C. Central venous catheter replacement strategies: a systematic review of the literature. Crit Care Med 1997; 25(8):1417–1424.

109. Cobb DK, High KP, Sawyer RG, Sable CA, Adams RB, Lindley DA, Pruett TL, Schwenzer KJ, Farr BM. A controlled trial of scheduled replacement of central venous and pulmonary-artery catheters. N Engl J Med 1992; 327 (15):1062–1068.

110. Armstrong CW, Mayhall CG, Miller KB, Newsome HH Jr, Sugerman HJ, Dalton HP, Hall GO, Gennings C. Prospective study of catheter replacement and other risk factors for infection of hyperalimentation catheters. J Infect Dis 1986; 154(5):808–816.

111. Snyder RH, Archer FJ, Endy T, Allen TW, Condon B, Kaiser J, Whatmore D, Harrington G, McDermott CJ. Catheter infection. A comparison of two catheter maintenance techniques. Ann Surg 1988; 208(5):651–653.

112. Josephson A, Gombert ME, Sierra MF, Karanfil LV, Tansino GF. The relationship between intravenous fluid contamination and the frequency of tubing replacement. Infect Control 1985; 6(9):367–370.

113. Maki DG, Botticelli JT, LeRoy ML, Thielke TS. Prospective study of replacing administration sets for intravenous therapy at 48- vs 72-hour intervals. 72 hours is safe and cost-effective. JAMA 1987; 258(13):1777–1781.

114. Snydman DR, Donnelly-Reidy M, Perry LK, Martin WJ. Intravenous tubing

containing burettes can be safely changed at 72 hour intervals. Infect Control 1987; 8(3):113–116.

115. McKee KT Jr, Melly MA, Greene HL, Schaffner W. Gram-negative bacillary sepsis associated with use of lipid emulsion in parenteral nutrition. Am J Dis Child 1979; 133(6):649–650.

116. Jarvis WR, Highsmith AK, Allen JR, Haley RW. Polymicrobial bacteremia associated with lipid emulsion in a neonatal intensive care unit. Pediatr Infect Dis 1983; 2(3):203–208.

117. Crocker KS, Noga R, Filibeck DJ, Krey SII, Markovic M, Steffee WP. Microbial growth comparisons of five commercial parenteral lipid emulsions. JPEN J Parenter Enteral Nutr 1984; 8(4):391–395.

118. Hanna HA, Raad I. Blood products: a significant risk factor for long-term catheter-related bloodstream infections in cancer patients. Infect Control Hosp Epidemiol 2001; 22(3):165–166.

119. Avila-Figueroa C, Goldmann DA, Richardson DK, Gray JE, Ferrari A, Freeman J. Intravenous lipid emulsions are the major determinant of coagulase-negative staphylococcal bacteremia in very low birth weight newborns. Pediatr Infect Dis J 1998; 17(1):10–17.

120. Melly MA, Meng HC, Schaffner W. Microbial growth in lipid emulsions used in parenteral nutrition. Arch Surg 1975; 110(12):1479–1481.

121. Baumgartner TG, Schmidt GL, Thakker KM, Sitren HS, Cerda JJ, Mahaffey SM, Copeland EM III. Bacterial endotoxin retention by inline intravenous filters. Am J Hosp Pharm 1986; 43(3):681–684.

122. Freeman JB, Litton AA. Preponderance of gram-positive infections during parenteral alimentation. Surg Gynecol Obstet 1974; 139(6):905–908.

123. Falchuk KH, Peterson L, McNeil BJ. Microparticulate-induced phlebitis. Its prevention by in-line filtration. N Engl J Med 1985; 312(2):78–82.

124. Maddox RR, John JF Jr, Brown LL, Smith CE. Effect of inline filtration on postinfusion phlebitis. Clin Pharm 1983; 2(1):58–61.

125. Randolph AG, Cook DJ, Gonzales CA, Andrew M. Benefit of heparin in central venous and pulmonary artery catheters: a meta-analysis of randomized controlled trials. Chest 1998; 113(1):165–171.

126. Freeman R, Holden MP, Lyon R, Hjersing N. Addition of sodium metabisulphite to left atrial catheter infusates as a means of preventing bacterial colonisation of the catheter tip. Thorax 1982; 37(2):142–144.

127. Root JL, McIntyre OR, Jacobs NJ, Daghlian CP. Inhibitory effect of disodium EDTA upon the growth of *Staphylococcus epidermidis* in vitro: relation to infection prophylaxis of Hickman catheters. Antimicrob Agents Chemother 1988; 32(11):1627–1631.

128. Raad I, Buzaid A, Rhyne J, Hachem R, Darouiche R, Safar H, Albitar M, Sherertz RJ. Minocycline and ethylenediaminetetraacetate for the prevention of recurrent vascular catheter infections. Clin Infect Dis 1997; 25(1):149–151.

129. Henrickson KJ, Axtell RA, Hoover SM, Kuhn SM, Pritchett J, Kehl SC, Klein JP. Prevention of central venous catheter-related infections and thrombotic events in immunocompromised children by the use of vancomycin/ciprofloxacin/heparin flush solution: A randomized, multicenter, double-blind trial. J Clin Oncol 2000; 18(6):1269–1278.

130. Carratala J, Niubo J, Fernandez-Sevilla A, Juve E, Castellsague X, Berlanga

J, Linares J, Gudiol F. Randomized, double-blind trial of an antibiotic-lock technique for prevention of gram-positive central venous catheter-related infection in neutropenic patients with cancer. Antimicrob Agents Chemother 1999; 43(9):2200–2204.

131. Schwartz C, Henrickson KJ, Roghmann K, Powell K. Prevention of bacteremia attributed to luminal colonization of tunneled central venous catheters with vancomycin-susceptible organisms. J Clin Oncol 1990; 8(9):1591–1597.

132. Allon M. Prophylaxis against dialysis catheter-related bacteremia with a novel antimicrobial lock solution. Clin Infect Dis 2003; 36(12):1539–1544.

133. Sketch MH, Cale M, Mohiuddin SM, Booth RW. Use of percutaneously inserted venous catheters in coronary care units. Chest 1972; 62(6):684–689.

134. Bassan MM, Sheikh-Hamad D. Prevention of lidocaine-infusion phlebitis by heparin and hydrocortisone. Chest 1983; 84(4):439–441.

135. Wright A, Hecker JF, Lewis GB. Use of transdermal glyceryl trinitrate to reduce failure of intravenous infusion due to phlebitis and extravasation. Lancet 1985; 2(8465):1148–1150.

136. Woodhouse CR. Movelat in the prophylaxis of infusion thrombophlebitis. Br Med J 1979; 1(6161):454–455.

137. O'Brien BJ, Buxton MJ, Khawaja HT. An economic evaluation of transdermal glyceryl trinitrate in the prevention of intravenous infusion failure. J Clin Epidemiol 1990; 43(8):757–763.

138. Guidet B, Nicola I, Barakett V, Gabillet JM, Snoey E, Petit JC, Offenstadt G. Skin versus hub cultures to predict colonization and infection of central venous catheter in intensive care patients. Infection 1994; 22(1):43–48.

139. Fan ST, Teoh-Chan CH, Lau KF. Evaluation of central venous catheter sepsis by differential quantitative blood culture. Eur J Clin Microbiol Infect Dis 1989; 8(2):142–144.

140. Raad II, Baba M, Bodey GP. Diagnosis of catheter-related infections: the role of surveillance and targeted quantitative skin cultures. Clin Infect Dis 1995; 20(3):593–597.

141. Maki DG. Infections caused by intravascular devices used for infusion therapy: pathogenesis, prevention and management. In: Bisno AL, Waldvogel FA, eds. Infections associated with indwelling medical devices. Washington D.C.: ASM Press, 1994:155–212.

142. Anonymous. Monitoring Hospital-Acquired Infections to Promote Patient Safety—United States 1990–1999. MMWR 2000; 49(08):149–153.

143. Zuschneid I, Schwab F, Geffers C, Ruden H, Gastmeier P. Reducing central venous catheter-associated primary bloodstream infections in intensive care units is possible: data from the German nosocomial infection surveillance system. Infect Control Hosp Epidemiol 2003; 24(7):501–505.

144. Haley RW, Culver DH, White JW, Morgan WM, Emori TG, Munn VP, Hooton TM. The efficacy of infection surveillance and control programs in preventing nosocomial infections in US hospitals. Am J Epidemiol 1985; 121(2):182–205.

145. Yoo S, Ha M, Choi D, Pai H. Effectiveness of surveillance of central catheter-related bloodstream infection in an ICU in Korea. Infect Control Hosp Epidemiol 2001; 22(7):433–436.

146. Pearson ML. Guideline for prevention of intravascular device-related infections. I. Part, Intravascular device-related infections: an overview. The Hospital Infection Control Practices Advisory Committee. Am J Infect Control 1996; 24(4):262–277.

147. Bridgett MJ, Davies MC, Denyer SP. Control of staphylococcal adhesion to polystyrene surfaces by polymer surface modification with surfactants. Biomaterials 1992; 13(7):411–416.

148. Desai NP, Hossainy SF, Hubbell JA. Surface-immobilized polyethylene oxide for bacterial repellence. Biomaterials 1992; 13(7):417–420.

149. Dunkirk SG, Gregg SL, Duran LW, Monfils JD, Haapala JE, Marcy JA, Clapper DL, Amos RA, Guire PE. Photochemical coatings for the prevention of bacterial colonization. J Biomater Appl 1991; 6(2):131–156.

150. Tebbs SE, Sawyer A, Elliott TS. Influence of surface morphology on in vitro bacterial adherence to central venous catheters. Br J Anaesth 1994; 72(5):587–591.

151. Tebbs SE, Elliott TS. Modification of central venous catheter polymers to prevent in vitro microbial colonisation. Eur J Clin Microbiol Infect Dis 1994; 13(2):111–117.

152. Jansen B, Schareina S, Steinhauser H, Peters G, Schumacher-Perdreau F, Pulverer G. Development of polymers with antiinfective properties. Polym Mater Sci Eng 1987; 57:43–46.

153. Jansen B. New concepts in the prevention of polymer-associated foreign body infections. Zentralbl Bakteriol 1990; 272(4):401–410.

154. Han DK, Park KD, Kim YH. Sulfonated poly(ethylene oxide)-grafted polyurethane copolymer for biomedical applications. J Biomater Sci Polym Ed 1998; 9(2):163–174.

155. Baumgartner JN, Yang CZ, Cooper SL. Physical property analysis and bacterial adhesion on a series of phosphonated polyurethanes. Biomaterials 1997; 18(12):831–837.

156. Kohnen W, Jansen B. Changing Material Surface Chemistry for Preventing Bacterial Adhesion. In: An YH, Friedman RJ, eds. Handbook of Bacterial Adhesion. Totowa, NJ: Humana Press, 2000:581–589.

157. An YH, Blair BK, Martin KL, Friedman RJ. Macromolecule Surface Coating for Preventing Bacterial Adhesion. In: An YH, Friedman RJ, eds. Handbook of Bacterial Adhesion. Totowa, NJ: Humana Press, 2000:609–625.

158. Marcinko DE. Gentamicin-impregnated PMMA beads: an introduction and review. J Foot Surg 1985; 24(2):116–121.

159. Welch A. Antibiotics in acrylic bone cement. In vitro studies. J Biomed Mater Res 1978; 12(5):679–700.

160. Moore WS, Chvapil M, Seiffert G, Keown K. Development of an infection-resistant vascular prosthesis. Arch Surg 1981; 116(11):1403–1407.

161. Powell TW, Burnham SJ, Johnson G Jr, A passive system using rifampin to create an infection-resistant vascular prosthesis. Surgery 1983; 94(5):765–769.

162. McDougal EG, Burnham SJ, Johnson G Jr, Rifampin protection against experimental graft sepsis. J Vasc Surg 1986; 4(1):5–7.

163. Solovskij MV, Ulbrich K, Kopecek J. Synthesis of N-(2-hydroxypropyl)methacrylamide copolymers with antimicrobial activity. Biomaterials 1983; 4(1):44–48.

164. Sherertz RJ, Carruth WA, Hampton AA, Byron MP, Solomon DD. Efficacy of antibiotic-coated catheters in preventing subcutaneous *Staphylococcus aureus* infection in rabbits. J Infect Dis 1993; 167(1):98–106.

165. Jansen B, Peters G. Modern strategies in the prevention of polymer-associated infections. J Hosp Infect 1991; 19(2):83–88.

166. Jansen B, Jansen S, Peters G, Pulverer G. In-vitro efficacy of a central venous catheter ('Hydrocath') loaded with teicoplanin to prevent bacterial colonization. J Hosp Infect 1992; 22(2):93–107.

167. Jansen B. Beschichtung von Kathetern und Inplantaten mit Teicoplanin zur Prävention von Fremdkörperinfektionen. Chemotherapie Journal 1996; 11 (suppl):42–44.

168. Romano G, Berti M, Goldstein BP, Borghi A. Efficacy of a central venous catheter (Hydrocath) loaded with teicoplanin in preventing subcutaneous staphylococcal infection in the mouse. Zentralbl Bakteriol 1993; 279(3):426–433.

169. Jansen B, Ruiten D, Pulverer G. In-vitro activity of a catheter loaded with silver and teicoplanin to prevent bacterial and fungal colonization. J Hosp Infect 1995; 31(3):238–241.

170. Kamal GD, Pfaller MA, Rempe LE, Jebson PJ. Reduced intravascular catheter infection by antibiotic bonding. A prospective, randomized, controlled trial. JAMA 1991; 265(18):2364–2368.

171. Raad I, Darouiche R, Hachem R, Sacilowski M, Bodey GP. Antibiotics and prevention of microbial colonization of catheters. Antimicrob Agents Chemother 1995; 39(11):2397–2400.

172. Donelli G, Francolini I, Piozzi A, Di Rosa R, Marconi W. New polymer-antibiotic systems to inhibit bacterial biofilm formation: a suitable approach to prevent central venous catheter-associated infections. J Chemother 2002; 14(5):501–507.

173. Schierholz JM, Fleck C, Beuth J, Pulverer G. The antimicrobial efficacy of a new central venous catheter with long-term broad-spectrum activity. J Antimicrob Chemother 2000; 46(1):45–50.

174. Kingston D, Seal DV, Hill ID. Self-disinfecting plastics for intravenous catheters and prosthetic inserts. J Hyg (Lond) 1986; 96(2):185–198.

175. Jansen B, Kristinsson KG, Jansen S, Peters G, Pulverer G. In-vitro efficacy of a central venous catheter complexed with iodine to prevent bacterial colonization. J Antimicrob Chemother 1992; 30(2):135–139.

176. Sioshansi P. New processes for surface treatment of catheters. Artif Organs 1994; 18(4):266–271.

177. McLean RJ, Hussain AA, Sayer M, Vincent PJ, Hughes DJ, Smith TJ. Antibacterial activity of multilayer silver-copper surface films on catheter material. Can J Microbiol 1993; 39(9):895–899.

178. Davenas J, Thevenard P, Philippe F, Arnaud MN. Surface implantation treatments to prevent infection complications in short term devices. Biomol Eng 2002; 19(2–6):263–268.

179. Gatter N, Kohnen W, Jansen B. In vitro efficacy of a hydrophilic central venous catheter loaded with silver to prevent microbial colonization. Zentralbl Bakteriol 1998; 287(1–2):157–169.

180. Jansen B, Rinck M, Wolbring P, Strohmeier A, Jahns T. In vitro evaluation of the antimicrobial efficacy and biocompatibility of a silver-coated central venous catheter. J Biomater Appl 1994; 9(1):55–70.

181. Boswald M, Lugauer S, Regenfus A, Braun GG, Martus P, Geis C, Scharf J, Bechert T, Greil J, Guggenbichler JP. Reduced rates of catheter-associated infection by use of a new silver-impregnated central venous catheter. Infection 1999; 27(suppl 1):S56–S60.

182. Ranucci M, Isgro G, Giomarelli PP, Pavesi M, Luzzani A, Cattabriga I, Carli M, Giomi P, Compostella A, Digito A, Mangani V, Silvestri V, Mondelli E. Impact of oligon central venous catheters on catheter colonization and catheter-related bloodstream infection. Crit Care Med 2003; 31(1):52–59.

183. Liu WK, Tebbs SE, Byrne PO, Elliott TS. The effects of electric current on bacteria colonising intravenous catheters. J Infect 1993; 27(3):261–269.

184. Raad I, Hachem R, Zermeno A, Dumo M, Bodey GP. In vitro antimicrobial efficacy of silver iontophoretic catheter. Biomaterials 1996; 17(11):1055–1059.

185. Quesnel LB, Al Najjar AR, Buddhavudhikrai P. Synergism between chlorhexidine and sulphadiazine. J Appl Bacteriol 1978; 45(3):397–405.

186. Bach A, Schmidt H, Bottiger B, Schreiber B, Bohrer H, Motsch J, Martin E, Sonntag HG. Retention of antibacterial activity and bacterial colonization of antiseptic-bonded central venous catheters. J Antimicrob Chemother 1996; 37(2):315–322.

187. Hannan M, Juste RN, Umasanker S, Glendenning A, Nightingale C, Azadian B, Soni N. Antiseptic-bonded central venous catheters and bacterial colonisation. Anaesthesia 1999; 54(9):868–872.

188. Ciresi DL, Albrecht RM, Volkers PA, Scholten DJ. Failure of antiseptic bonding to prevent central venous catheter-related infection and sepsis. Am Surg 1996; 62(8):641–646.

189. Pemberton LB, Ross V, Cuddy P, Kremer H, Fessler T, McGurk E. No difference in catheter sepsis between standard and antiseptic central venous catheters. A prospective randomized trial. Arch Surg 1996; 131(9):986–989.

190. George SJ, Vuddamalay P, Boscoe MJ. Antiseptic-impregnated central venous catheters reduce the incidence of bacterial colonization and associated infection in immunocompromised transplant patients. Eur J Anaesthesiol 1997; 14(4):428–431.

191. Logghe C, Van Ossel C, D'Hoore W, Ezzedine H, Wauters G, Haxhe JJ. Evaluation of chlorhexidine and silver-sulfadiazine impregnated central venous catheters for the prevention of bloodstream infection in leukaemic patients: a randomized controlled trial. J Hosp Infect 1997; 37(2):145–156.

192. Maki DG, Stolz SM, Wheeler S, Mermel LA. Prevention of central venous catheter-related bloodstream infection by use of an antiseptic-impregnated catheter. A randomized, controlled trial. Ann Intern Med 1997; 127(4):257–266.

193. Tennenberg S, Lieser M, McCurdy B, Boomer G, Howington E, Newman C, Wolf I. A prospective randomized trial of an antibiotic- and antiseptic-coated central venous catheter in the prevention of catheter-related infections. Arch Surg 1997; 132(12):1348–1351.

194. Collin GR. Decreasing catheter colonization through the use of an antiseptic-impregnated catheter: a continuous quality improvement project. Chest 1999; 115(6):1632–1640.

195. Heard SO, Wagle M, Vijayakumar E, McLean S, Brueggemann A, Napolitano LM, Edwards LP, O'Connell FM, Puyana JC, Doern GV. Influence of triple-lumen central venous catheters coated with chlorhexidine and silver sulfadiazine on the incidence of catheter-related bacteremia. Arch Intern Med 1998; 158(1):81–87.

196. Sheng WH, Ko WJ, Wang JT, Chang SC, Hsueh PR, Luh KT. Evaluation of antiseptic-impregnated central venous catheters for prevention of catheter-related infection in intensive care unit patients. Diagn Microbiol Infect Dis 2000; 38(1):1–5.

197. Haxhe JJ, D'Hoore W. A meta-analysis dealing with the effectiveness of chlorhexidine and silver-sulfadiazine impregnated central venous catheters. J Hosp Infect 1998; 40(2):166–168.

198. Veenstra DL, Saint S, Saha S, Lumley T, Sullivan SD. Efficacy of antiseptic-impregnated central venous catheters in preventing catheter-related bloodstream infection: a meta-analysis. JAMA 1999; 281(3):261–267.

199. Marin MG, Lee JC, Skurnick JH. Prevention of nosocomial bloodstream infections: effectiveness of antimicrobial-impregnated and heparin-bonded central venous catheters. Crit Care Med 2000; 28(9):3332–3338.

200. Pai MP, Pendland SL, Danziger LH. Antimicrobial-coated/bonded and -impregnated intravascular catheters. Ann Pharmacother 2001; 35(10):1255–1263.

201. Crnich CJ, Maki DG. The promise of novel technology for the prevention of intravascular device-related bloodstream infection. I. Pathogenesis and short-term devices. Clin Infect Dis 2002; 34(9):1232–1242.

202. Tattawasart U, Maillard JY, Furr JR, Russell AD. Development of resistance to chlorhexidine diacetate and cetylpyridinium chloride in *Pseudomonas stutzeri* and changes in antibiotic susceptibility. J Hosp Infect 1999; 42(3):219–229.

203. Dance DA, Pearson AD, Seal DV, Lowes JA. A hospital outbreak caused by a chlorhexidine and antibiotic-resistant *Proteus mirabilis*. J Hosp Infect 1987; 10(1):10–16.

204. Oda T, Hamasaki J, Kanda N, Mikami K. Anaphylactic shock induced by an antiseptic-coated central venous [correction of nervous] catheter. Anesthesiology 1997; 87(5):1242–1244.

205. Raad I, Darouiche R, Hachem R, Mansouri M, Bodey GP. The broad-spectrum activity and efficacy of catheters coated with minocycline and rifampin. J Infect Dis 1996; 173(2):418–424.

206. Raad I, Darouiche R, Dupuis J, Abi-Said D, Gabrielli A, Hachem R, Wall M, Harris R, Jones J, Buzaid A, Robertson C, Shenaq S, Curling P, Burke T, Ericsson C. Central venous catheters coated with minocycline and rifampin for the prevention of catheter-related colonization and bloodstream infections. A randomized, double-blind trial. The Texas Medical Center Catheter Study Group. Ann Intern Med 1997; 127(4):267–274.

207. Darouiche RO, Raad II, Heard SO, Thornby JI, Wenker OC, Gabrielli A, Berg J, Khardori N, Hanna H, Hachem R, Harris RL, Mayhall G. A com-

parison of two antimicrobial-impregnated central venous catheters. Catheter Study Group. N Engl J Med 1999; 340(1):1–8.

208. Tambe SM, Sampath L, Modak SM. In vitro evaluation of the risk of developing bacterial resistance to antiseptics and antibiotics used in medical devices. J Antimicrob Chemother 2001; 47(5):589–598.

209. Maki DG, Weise CE, Sarafin HW. A semiquantitative culture method for identifying intravenous-catheter-related infection. N Engl J Med 1977; 296 (23):1305–1309.

210. Kamal GD, Divishek D, Kumar GC, Porter BR, Tatman DJ, Adams JR. Reduced intravascular catheter-related infection by routine use of antibiotic-bonded catheters in a surgical intensive care unit. Diagn Microbiol Infect Dis 1998; 30(3):145–152.

211. Mermel LA, Stolz SM, Maki DG. Surface antimicrobial activity of heparin-bonded and antiseptic-impregnated vascular catheters. J Infect Dis 1993; 167(4):920–924.

212. Hoar PF, Wilson RM, Mangano DT, Avery GJ, Szarnicki RJ, Hill JD. Heparin bonding reduces thrombogenicity of pulmonary-artery catheters. N Engl J Med 1981; 305(17):993–995.

213. Moss HA, Tebbs SE, Faroqui MH, Herbst T, Isaac JL, Brown J, Elliott TS. A central venous catheter coated with benzalkonium chloride for the prevention of catheter-related microbial colonization. Eur J Anaesthesiol 2000; 17(11): 680–687.

214. Jaeger K, Osthaus A, Heine J, Ruschulte H, Kuhlmann C, Weissbrodt H, Ganser A, Karthaus M. Efficacy of a benzalkonium chloride-impregnated central venous catheter to prevent catheter-associated infection in cancer patients. Chemotherapy 2001; 47(1):50–55.

215. Goldschmidt H, Hahn U, Salwender HJ, Haas R, Jansen B, Wolbring P, Rinck M, Hunstein W. Prevention of catheter-related infections by silver coated central venous catheters in oncological patients. Zentralbl Bakteriol 1995; 283(2):215–223.

216. Carbon RT, Lugauer S, Geitner U, Regenfus A, Boswald M, Greil J, Bechert T, Simon SI, Hummer HP, Guggenbichler JP. Reducing catheter-associated infections with silver-impregnated catheters in long-term therapy of children. Infection 1999; 27(suppl 1):S69–S73.

217. Stoiser B, Kofler J, Staudinger T, Georgopoulos A, Lugauer S, Guggenbichler JP, Burgmann H, Frass M. Contamination of central venous catheters in immunocompromised patients: a comparison between two different types of central venous catheters. J Hosp Infect 2002; 50(3):202–206.

218. Veenstra DL, Saint S, Sullivan SD. Cost-effectiveness of antiseptic-impregnated central venous catheters for the prevention of catheter-related bloodstream infection. JAMA 1999; 282(6):554–560.

219. Marciante KD, Veenstra DL, Lipsky BA, Saint S. Which antimicrobial impregnated central venous catheter should we use? Modeling the costs and outcomes of antimicrobial catheter use. Am J Infect Control 2003; 31(1):1–8.

220. Russell AD, Tattawasart U, Maillard JY, Furr JR. Possible link between bacterial resistance and use of antibiotics and biocides. Antimicrob Agents Chemother 1998; 42(8):215.

221. Farr BM. Antimicrobial catheters: value and safety. Crit Care Med 2000; 28(9):3366–3367.

222. Sampath L, Tambe S, Modak S. Comparison of the efficacy of antiseptic and antibiotic catheters impregnated on both their luminal and outer surface. Program and Abstracts of the 39th Interscience Conference on Antimicrobial Agents and Chemotherapy of the American Society for Microbiology Sept 26–29, San Francisco 1999.

223. McConnell SA, Gubbins PO, Anaissie EJ. Do antimicrobial-impregnated central venous catheters prevent catheter-related bloodstream infection? Clin Infect Dis 2003; 37(1):65–72.

224. Maki DG, Cobb L, Garman JK, Shapiro JM, Ringer M, Helgerson RB. An attachable silver-impregnated cuff for prevention of infection with central venous catheters: a prospective randomized multicenter trial. Am J Med 1988; 85(3):307–314.

225. Flowers RH III, Schwenzer KJ, Kopel RF, Fisch MJ, Tucker SI, Farr BM. Efficacy of an attachable subcutaneous cuff for the prevention of intravascular catheter-related infection. A randomized, controlled trial. JAMA 1989; 261(6): 878–883.

226. Groeger JS, Lucas AB, Coit D, LaQuaglia M, Brown AE, Turnbull A, Exelby P. A prospective, randomized evaluation of the effect of silver impregnated subcutaneous cuffs for preventing tunneled chronic venous access catheter infections in cancer patients. Ann Surg 1993; 218(2):206–210.

227. Dahlberg PJ, Agger WA, Singer JR, Yutuc WR, Newcomer KL, Schaper A, Rooney BL. Subclavian hemodialysis catheter infections: a prospective, randomized trial of an attachable silver-impregnated cuff for prevention of catheter-related infections. Infect Control Hosp Epidemiol 1995; 16(9):506–511.

228. Smith HO, DeVictoria CL, Garfinkel D, Anderson P, Goldberg GL, Soeiro R, Elia G, Runowicz CD. A prospective randomized comparison of an attached silver-impregnated cuff to prevent central venous catheter-associated infection. Gynecol Oncol 1995; 58(1):92–100.

229. Halpin DP, O'Byrne P, McEntee G, Hennessy TP, Stephens RB. Effect of a betadine connection shield on central venous catheter sepsis. Nutrition 1991; 7(1):33–34.

230. Segura M, Alvarez-Lerma F, Tellado JM, Jimenez-Ferreres J, Oms L, Rello J, Baro T, Sanchez R, Morera A, Mariscal D, Marrugat J, Sitges-Serra A. A clinical trial on the prevention of catheter-related sepsis using a new hub model. Ann Surg 1996; 223(4):363–369.

231. Luna J, Masdeu G, Perez M, Claramonte R, Forcadell I, Barrachina F, Panisello M. Clinical trial evaluating a new hub device designed to prevent catheter-related sepsis. Eur J Clin Microbiol Infect Dis 2000; 19(9):655–662.

232. Hanazaki K, Shingu K, Adachi W, Miyazaki T, Amano J. Chlorhexidine dressing for reduction in microbial colonization of the skin with central venous catheters: a prospective randomized controlled trial. J Hosp Infect 1999; 42(2):165–168.

233. Maki DG. The efficacy of a chlorhexidine-impregnated sponge (biopatch) for the prevention of intravascular catheter-related infection: a prospective, randomized, controlled, multicenter trial (abstract 1430). Program and

abstracts of the 40th Interscience Conference on Antimicrobial Agents and Chemotherapy of the American Society for Microbiology, Toronto 2000.

234. Garland JS, Alex CP, Mueller CD, Otten D, Shivpuri C, Harris MC, Naples M, Pellegrini J, Buck RK, McAuliffe TL, Goldmann DA, Maki DG. A randomized trial comparing povidone-iodine to a chlorhexidine gluconate-impregnated dressing for prevention of central venous catheter infections in neonates. Pediatrics 2001; 107(6):1431–1436.

235. Crow S, Conrad SA, Chancy-Rowell C, King JW. Microbial contamination of arterial infusions used for hemodynamic monitoring: a randomized trial of contamination with sampling through conventional stopcocks versus a novel closed system. Infect Control Hosp Epidemiol 1989; 10(12):557–561.

236. Adams KS, Zehrer CL, Thomas W. Comparison of a needleless system with conventional heparin locks. Am J Infect Control 1993; 21(5):263–269.

237. Danzig LE, Short LJ, Collins K, Mahoney M, Sepe S, Bland L, Jarvis WR. Bloodstream infections associated with a needleless intravenous infusion system in patients receiving home infusion therapy. JAMA 1995; 273(23):1862–1864.

238. Kellermann S, Shay D, Howard J, Feusner J, Goes C, Jarvis W. Bloodstream infections associated with needleless devices used for central venous catheter access in children receiving home health care. Program and Abstracts of the 35th Interscience Conference on Antimicrobial Agents and Chemotherapy of the American Society for Microbiology 1995: Abstract J11, 258.

239. Vassallo D, Blanc-Jouvan M, Bret M, Coronel B, Kasparian S, Mosnier S, Mercatella A, Moskovtechenko JF. *Staphylococcus aureus* septicemia and a needleless system of infusion. Program and Abstracts of the 35th Interscience Conference on Antimicrobial Agents and Chemotherapy of the American Society for Microbiology 1995: Abstract J12, 259.

240. Liedberg H, Ekman P, Lundeberg T. *Pseudomonas aeruginosa*: adherence to and growth on different urinary catheter coatings. Int Urol Nephrol 1990; 22(5):487–492.

241. Liedberg H, Lundeberg T. Silver alloy coated catheters reduce catheter-associated bacteriuria. Br J Urol 1990; 65(4):379–381.

242. Johnson JR, Roberts PL, Olsen RJ, Moyer KA, Stamm WE. Prevention of catheter-associated urinary tract infection with a silver oxide-coated urinary catheter: clinical and microbiologic correlates. J Infect Dis 1990; 162(5):1145–1150.

243. Riley DK, Classen DC, Stevens LE, Burke JP. A large randomized clinical trial of a silver-impregnated urinary catheter: lack of efficacy and staphylococcal superinfection. Am J Med 1995; 98(4):349–356.

244. Saint S, Elmore JG, Sullivan SD, Emerson SS, Koepsell TD. The efficacy of silver alloy-coated urinary catheters in preventing urinary tract infection: a meta-analysis. Am J Med 1998; 105(3):236–241.

245. Bologna RA, Tu LM, Polansky M, Fraimow HD, Gordon DA, Whitmore KE. Hydrogel/silver ion-coated urinary catheter reduces nosocomial urinary tract infection rates in intensive care unit patients: a multicenter study. Urology 1999; 54(6):982–987.

246. Verleyen P, De Ridder D, Van Poppel H, Baert L. Clinical application of the Bardex IC Foley catheter. Eur Urol 1999; 36(3):240–246.

247. Lai KK, Fontecchio SA. Use of silver-hydrogel urinary catheters on the incidence of catheter-associated urinary tract infections in hospitalized patients. Am J Infect Control 2002; 30(4):221–225.

248. Gaonkar TA, Sampath LA, Modak SM. Evaluation of the antimicrobial efficacy of urinary catheters impregnated with antiseptics in an in vitro urinary tract model. Infect Control Hosp Epidemiol 2003; 24(7):506–513.

249. Stickler DJ. Susceptibility of antibiotic-resistant Gram-negative bacteria to biocides: a perspective from the study of catheter biofilms. J Appl Microbiol 2002; 92(suppl):163S–170S.

250. Niel-Weise BS, Arend SM, van den Broek PJ. Is there evidence for recommending silver-coated urinary catheters in guidelines? J Hosp Infect 2002; 52 (2):81–87.

251. Trooskin SZ, Donetz AP, Baxter J, Harvey RA, Greco RS. Infection-resistant continuous peritoneal dialysis catheters. Nephron 1987; 46(3):263–267.

252. Kim CY, Kumar A, Sampath L, Sokol K, Modak S. Evaluation of an antimicrobial-impregnated continuous ambulatory peritoneal dialysis catheter for infection control in rats. Am J Kidney Dis 2002; 39(1):165–173.

253. Bridgett MJ, Davies MC, Denyer SP, Eldridge PR. In vitro assessment of bacterial adhesion to Hydromer-coated cerebrospinal fluid shunts. Biomaterials 1993; 14(3):184–188.

254. Bayston R, Milner RD. Antimicrobial activity of silicone rubber used in hydrocephalus shunts, after impregnation with antimicrobial substances. J Clin Pathol 1981; 34(9):1057–1062.

255. Bayston R, Zdroyewski V, Barsham S. Use of an in vitro model for studying the eradication of catheter colonisation by *Staphylococcus epidermidis*. J Infect 1988; 16(2):141–146.

256. Bayston R, Barsham S. Catheter colonisation: a laboratory model suitable for aetiological, therapeutic and preventive studies. Med Lab Sci 1988; 45(3):235–239.

257. Bayston R, Grove N, Siegel J, Lawellin D, Barsham S. Prevention of hydrocephalus shunt catheter colonisation in vitro by impregnation with antimicrobials. J Neurol Neurosurg Psychiatry 1989; 52(5):605–609.

258. Bayston R, Lambert E. Duration of protective activity of cerebrospinal fluid shunt catheters impregnated with antimicrobial agents to prevent bacterial catheter-related infection. J Neurosurg 1997; 87(2):247–251.

259. Bayston R, Ashraf W, Bhundia C. Mode of action of an antimicrobial shunt catheter. Eur J Pediatr Surg 2000; 12:S56.

260. Schierholz J, Jansen B, Jaenicke L, Pulverer G. In-vitro efficacy of an antibiotic releasing silicone ventricle catheter to prevent shunt infection. Biomaterials 1994; 15(12):996–1000.

261. Hampl J, Schierholz J, Jansen B, Aschoff A. In vitro and in vivo efficacy of a rifampin-loaded silicone catheter for the prevention of CSF shunt infections. Acta Neurochir (Wien) 1995; 133(3–4):147–152.

262. Kohnen W, Schaper J, Klein O, Tieke B, Jansen B. A silicone ventricular catheter coated with a combination of rifampin and trimethoprim for the prevention of catheter-related infections. Zentralbl Bakteriol 1998; 287(1–2):147–156.

263. Hampl JA, Weitzel A, Bonk C, Kohnen W, Roesner D, Jansen B. Rifampin-impregnated silicone catheters: a potential tool for prevention and treatment of CSF shunt infections. Infection 2003; 31(2):109–111.
264. Schierholz JM, Pulverer G. Investigation of a rifampin, fusidic-acid and mupirocin releasing silicone catheter. Biomaterials 1998; 19(22):2065–2074.
265. Zabramski JM, Whiting D, Darouiche RO, Horner TG, Olson J, Robertson C, Hamilton AJ. Efficacy of antimicrobial-impregnated external ventricular drain catheters: a prospective, randomized, controlled trial. J Neurosurg 2003; 98(4):725–730.
266. von Eiff C, Overbeck J, Haupt G, Herrmann M, Winckler S, Richter KD, Peters G, Spiegel HU. Bactericidal effect of extracorporeal shock waves on *Staphylococcus aureus*. J Med Microbiol 2000; 49(8):709–712.
267. Kojima Y, Tojo M, Goldmann DA, Tosteson TD, Pier GB. Antibody to the capsular polysaccharide/adhesin protects rabbits against catheter-related bacteremia due to coagulase-negative staphylococci. J Infect Dis 1990; 162(2): 435–441.
268. Takeda S, Pier GB, Kojima Y, Tojo M, Muller E, Tosteson T, Goldmann DA. Protection against endocarditis due to *Staphylococcus epidermidis* by immunization with capsular polysaccharide/adhesin. Circulation 1991; 84(6): 2539–2546.
269. Poole-Warren LA, Hallett MD, Hone PW, Burden SH, Farrell PC. Vaccination for prevention of CAPD associated staphylococcal infection: results of a prospective multicentre clinical trial. Clin Nephrol 1991; 35(5):198–206.
270. Vaudaux P, Yasuda H, Velazco MI, Huggler E, Ratti I, Waldvogel FA, Lew DP, Proctor RA. Role of host and bacterial factors in modulating staphylococcal adhesion to implanted polymer surfaces. J Biomater Appl 1990; 5(2):134–153.
271. Perez-Giraldo C, Rodriguez-Benito A, Moran FJ, Hurtado C, Blanco MT, Gomez-Garcia AC. Influence of N-acetylcysteine on the formation of biofilm by *Staphylococcus epidermidis*. J Antimicrob Chemother 1997; 39(5):643–646.
272. Balaban N, Giacometti A, Cirioni O, Gov Y, Ghiselli R, Mocchegiani F, Viticchi C, Del Prete MS, Saba V, Scalise G, Dell'Acqua G. Use of the quorum-sensing inhibitor RNAIII-inhibiting peptide to prevent biofilm formation in vivo by drug-resistant *Staphylococcus epidermidis*. J Infect Dis 2003; 187(4):625–630.
273. Danese PN. Antibiofilm approaches: prevention of catheter colonization. Chem Biol 2002; 9(8):873–880.
274. Simmons BP. CDC guidelines for the prevention and control of nosocomial infections. Guideline for prevention of intravascular infections. Am J Infect Control 1983; 11(5):183–199.

6

Catheter-Related *Staphylococcus aureus* Infection

Barry M. Farr

University of Virginia Health System
Charlottesville, Virginia, U.S.A.

INTRODUCTION

Staphylococcus aureus is a virulent pathogen that continues to cause significant morbidity and mortality in the antimicrobial era (1). Infection of a vascular catheter by this organism may cause dramatic illness, with bloodstream infection and hematogenous spread to other sites resulting in serious secondary infections such as osteomyelitis, epidural abscess, and endocarditis. Patients with relatively minor predisposing illness occasionally succumb to such lethal infection.

PATHOGENESIS

Most vascular catheter-related infections of short-term catheters appear to derive from cutaneous flora entering the catheter tract and moving distally along the exterior of the catheter to reach the bloodstream (2–5). Experiments in a guinea pig model suggested that such migration can occur rapidly, perhaps by capillary action once microbes are present at the catheter–skin interface in sufficient numbers (6). For long-term catheters, intraluminal spread from a contaminated hub appears to be a more important mode of infection (5,7,8). Electron microscopy of a *S. aureus*-infected catheter shows cocci 1 μ in diameter clumped in an extensive amorphous matrix on the surface of the catheter (9).

Catheter composition appears to be an important factor in the pathogenesis of infection, since modern teflon and polyurethane catheters are associated with extremely low rates of catheter infection, compared to the polyvinyl chloride catheters used previously (10–13). Studies of the adherence of different microbial species to various catheter materials have shown significantly greater adherence to polyvinyl chloride catheters than to teflon catheters (14). An animal model of *S. aureus* catheter infections found that silicone catheters could be infected with a lower inoculum than polyurethane, teflon, or polyvinyl chloride catheters during the first two days after insertion (15).

The efficiency of phagocytes operating in the vicinity of different catheter materials may also be important, as one study has shown impairment of the respiratory burst of polymorphonuclear neutrophils in the presence of polyvinyl chloride, teflon, and siliconized latex catheters or their eluates. Such impairment was not demonstrated with polyurethane catheters (16). A chemotactic defect has been demonstrated in patients receiving interleukin-2, who appear to have a higher risk for *S. aureus* infection of catheters (17). Impaired bactericidal activity of polymorphonuclear neutrophils has also been documented in patients with AIDS (18), who also have a higher rate of *S. aureus* catheter infections.

Fibronectin appears to be more active than fibrin or fibrinogen in promoting adherence of *S. aureus* to catheter surfaces (19). Polyurethane catheters removed from patients showed significantly less adherence of *S. aureus* ($p < 0.01$) and contained significantly less fibronectin than polyvinyl chloride or Hickman catheters (19). Another study found that polyvinyl chloride catheters bound significantly more fibronectin than heparin-bonded polyurethane catheters, but also found that *S. aureus* bound significantly more to heparin-bonded polyurethane than to the polyvinyl chloride catheters if fibronectin was not present in vitro (20). Thrombospondin, a glycoprotein stored in platelets, also appears to promote adherence of *S. aureus* to catheter surfaces (21,22).

S. aureus and *Candida albicans* appear to be more likely to cause infection of a catheter once colonization has occurred, compared to other colonizing microbes. For catheters growing at least 100 CFU on quantitative culture of the catheter tip, *S. aureus* resulted in bloodstream infection in 69% of cases, compared to 75% for *C. albicans*, 38% for *Staphylococcus epidermidis*, and 41% for *Enterococcus faecalis* (23). *S. aureus* was also more likely to result in purulence at the catheter site than other microbes (40% of cases of *S. aureus* colonization vs 10% of cases of colonization with other microbes, $p = .007$) (23). *S. aureus* produces a variety of enzymes and toxins that may contribute to this enhanced virulence, such as catalase, hyaluronidase, nuclease, β-lactamase, toxic shock syndrome toxin, enterotoxin, staphylococcal superantigens, α-toxin, β-toxin, γ-toxin, δ-toxin, and leukocidin (24). When introduced into subcutaneous tissue in the presence of a foreign body such as a silk suture, the mean infectious dose is tremendously reduced (25).

INCIDENCE

The incidence of primary bloodstream infection in hospitals reporting data to the National Nosocomial Infection Surveillance (NNIS) program overseen by the Centers for Disease Control and Prevention (CDC) from 1980 to 1989 was 0.28 per 100 discharges (26). The same rate was documented in a 1-year prospective study in a Danish university hospital (27). Laboratory-confirmed bloodstream infection was diagnosed in 122 (0.11%) of 107,382 patients in five community hospitals in Sydney, Australia, during a 1-year period (28). A university hospital in Atlanta reported that both community-acquired and nosocomial *S. aureus* bloodstream infection had increased significantly during a recent decade, and that an important part of this increase was related to vascular catheters (29).

The incidence of primary bloodstream infection due to *S. aureus* in NNIS hospitals increased significantly during the decade of the 1980s (26). The rate also increased significantly in each of the four types of reporting hospitals. Large teaching hospitals reported a 176% increase (95% confidence interval, 72% to 343%), from 4/10,000 discharges in 1980 to 1.13/1000 discharges in 1989. Small teaching hospitals reported a 122% increase (95% CI, 58%–211%) during the same period, small nonteaching hospitals reported a 283% increase (95% CI, 139%–514%), and large nonteaching hospitals reported a 272% increase (95% CI, 115%–544%).

During the next decade, data from hospital-wide surveillance stopped being reported by the NNIS system, but primary bloodstream infections in ICUs reporting data to the NNIS system declined by 31% to 44% in different types of participating ICUs (30).

Fifteen to 20% of endemic nosocomial bloodstream infections are due to *S. aureus*, which accounts for 8% of epidemics of nosocomial bloodstream infection (31). In one study, approximately one-third of endemic nosocomial bloodstream infections appeared to be related to indwelling catheters, with vascular catheters accounting for a large majority of these infections (32). One-third to one-half of all *S. aureus* nosocomial bacteremias have been due to vascular catheters (33,34).

A recent study of nosocomial endocarditis, which excluded cases related to prosthetic valves, found that *S. aureus* accounted for 62% of cases. Causation was related to vascular catheters in 86% of cases (35).

MORTALITY

The virulence of *S. aureus* has been recognized in many studies of catheter-related infections (4,36–44). A review of 25 studies of catheter-related *S. aureus* bacteremia found that 24% of patients suffered an infectious complication (95% CI, 19.9%–28.1%) (45). Overall, 59 of 177 patients in these 25 studies died (33.3%, 95% CI, 26.4%–40.2%) (45). Almost half of the deaths in these studies were attributed to the catheter infection by the authors of the individual studies (14.8%, 95% CI, 10.8%–18.8%) (45).

A meta-analysis of the case fatality rate associated with catheter-related infections, which included 187 studies and 3569 catheter infections, found an overall case fatality rate of 14.0% (95% CI, 12.4%–15.6%) (46). The authors of the individual studies attributed death to the catheter infection in 2.7% (95% CI, 2.0%–3.4%) of cases, accounting for approximately 19% of all of the deaths in these studies. For cases of *S. aureus* catheter infection included in this meta-analysis, the overall case fatality rate was 18.2%. Death was attributed to the catheter infection in 11.1% of cases, accounting for 61% of the deaths. The proportion of deaths attributed to catheter infection was significantly higher for *S. aureus* than for other etiologic agents (odds ratio = 3.81, 95% CI, 2.70–5.41). A prospective epidemiologic study in a Danish hospital demonstrated a case fatality rate of 38% for nosocomial bacteremia overall, but the case fatality rate for *S. aureus* was 65%, with 25% being attributed to the infection (27). A recent study from an English hospital reported no deaths in 50 cases of *S. aureus* catheter-related bacteremia among hemodialysis patients (47).

A recent meta-analysis summarized the results of many studies of the mortality associated with methicillin-resistant *S. aureus* (MRSA), as opposed to methicillin-susceptible *S. aureus* (MSSA) bacteremia. It found that there was significantly higher mortality with MRSA after adjusting for comorbidity and severity of illness (OR = 1.93, 95% CI = 1.54–2.42, p < 0.001) (48).

RISK FACTORS

The risk of bloodstream infection in patients with a vascular catheter is related to the type of catheter, with modern peripheral venous catheters being associated with extremely low rates of infection and central venous catheters accounting for up to 90% of such infections (49). An increased risk for *S. aureus* infection of central venous catheters has been described for several patient groups. Patients with end stage renal disease requiring hemodialysis or peritoneal dialysis have long been recognized as being at higher risk of *S. aureus* catheter infections. Almost all of the higher risk occurs in patients who are nasal carriers of *S. aureus* (50,51).

In one study, *S. aureus* nasal carriage was associated with a threefold higher risk of *S. aureus* bacteremia; *S. aureus* colonization of skin at the catheter site was associated with a 26-fold higher risk of *S. aureus* bacteremia (52).

In one study of patients undergoing chronic ambulatory peritoneal dialysis (CAPD), patients with diabetes mellitus were significantly more likely to be carriers of *S. aureus* (77% versus 36%) (53). Catheter exit site infections were four times more frequent among carriers than noncarriers (0.4 episodes per patient year versus 0.1 per patient year, $p = 0.012$). A separate study of CAPD patients found only a modest increase in infections among diabetic patients (1.4 per patient year versus 1.2 per patient year) and concluded that diabetes was not an important risk factor for catheter infection in these patients. A third study of patients undergoing CAPD followed 30 patients for 13 months, with periodic cultures for *S. aureus* carriage (50). *S. aureus* accounted for 8 of 25 episodes of peritonitis and 12 of 20 episodes of exit site infection during the study, and patients with nasal colonization were at higher risk of infection than noncarriers (50). In a fourth study regarding peritoneal dialysis-related infections, 26% of 378 exit site swabs grew microbes, and 25 (25%) of 99 positive cultures grew *S. aureus* (54).

In a study of patients undergoing hemodialysis, nasal carriage of *S. aureus* was associated with a higher rate of bacteremia (0.095 per patient year versus 0.0417 per patient year), but the presence of diabetes was an even more important risk factor (relative risk = $11.4, p = 0.004$). The presence of a central venous catheter was a significant predictor of bacteremia (RR = $14.3, p = 0.002$) (55).

Therapy with interleukin-2 has been shown to increase the risk of staphylococcal catheter-related bacteremia (56). A dose gradient was demonstrated for increasing exposure to interleukin-2, with no bacteremias being documented during 320 catheter days before therapy, 18% of patients becoming infected during 343 catheter days of low-dose therapy, and 38% of patients becoming infected during 96 catheter days of high-dose therapy ($p = 0.01$). Another study found that 19% of interleukin-2-treated patients developed sepsis, compared to 2.8% of patients receiving total parenteral nutrition, 4.1% of patients in the surgical intensive care unit, and 1.9% of patients with solid tumors. *S. aureus* was the etiologic agent in 13 of 20 episodes of sepsis. *S. aureus* colonization significantly increased the risk of *S. aureus* infection (RR = $6.3, 95\%$ CI, $2.8–14.5, p < 0.001$). Skin desquamation at the catheter site also significantly increased the risk (RR = $2.0, 95\%$ CI, $1.3–3.1$). The simultaneous occurrence of *S. aureus* colonization and desquamation at the catheter site was associated with a relative risk of 14.5 for *S. aureus* bacteremia (95% CI, $4.1–50.9$) (57). A third study found sepsis in 9% of patients receiving interleukin-2 without antibiotic prophylaxis. In that study, *S. aureus* accounted for 7 of 8 episodes of sepsis (58).

Human immunodeficiency virus infection appears to be another risk factor for *S. aureus* infection. In one study excluding patients with a history of intravenous drug abuse or lymphedema, the incidence of *S. aureus* bacteremia in a population of patients with AIDS or AIDS-related complex was 5.4 per 1000 patient years, and 73% of cases were catheter-related (59). In another study, *S. aureus* accounted for 24% of catheter-related infections in AIDS patients, compared to 16% in other immunocompromised patients (60). A third study found that the most frequent etiologic agent causing nosocomial infections among patients with HIV infection was *S. aureus*, which was responsible for 27.6% of cases, followed by *Pseudomonas aeruginosa* (13.8%) and *Enterobacter cloacae* (13.8%) (61).

CLINICAL MANIFESTATIONS

Central venous catheter-related bloodstream infection is most often manifested by fever alone, with up to 70% of cases showing no local inflammation at the catheter site (62). A study of catheter-related *S. aureus* bloodstream infection found fever in all of 21 cases, with a mean temperature of 39.6°C (range, 37.8–41.1) (36). The clinical onset was described as "dramatic," with sudden high temperature and often rigors. Those with bacteremia due to a peripheral catheter usually had cellulitis at the catheter site, often with a purulent exudate. Eighty-one percent of patients had leukocytosis ranging as high as 31,000/mm^3. Two chronically leukopenic patients showed an increase above their baseline count associated with a left shift (i.e., an increasing percentage of immature polymorphonuclear neutrophils). The mean number of positive blood cultures per patient was 3.7 (range, 1–7). Although rare with modern peripheral venous catheters, a recent case report described a patient with *S. aureus* infection of a peripheral venous catheter that progressed to suppurative phlebitis complicated by lethal endocarditis (63). By contrast, most patients with inflammation at the site of a peripheral venous catheter appear to have only a bland physicochemical phlebitis that is unrelated to infection (64) and does not occur more frequently in *S. aureus* carriers (65).

Infectious complications have generally occurred in at least one-quarter of cases of catheter-related *S. aureus* bacteremia (45,47). Perhaps the most important complication to consider is endocarditis, because of the frequent lack of specific signs (66–68) and because short-course therapy for bacteremia with up to two weeks of antibiotics will often fail if endocarditis is present. One recent study found that 8 (16%) of 50 cases of hemodialysis catheter-related *S. aureus* bacteremia were complicated by endocarditis (47). Another recent study found that 16 (23%) of 69 patients with catheter-related *S. aureus* bacteremia became complicated by endocarditis (69).

A recent review of studies of short-course therapy of catheter-related *S. aureus* bacteremia found that 6.1% relapsed after therapy, usually with endocarditis or a metastatic infection such as epidural abscess (45). Most such relapses have occurred within 9 weeks (70). A more recent study reported that 2 of 21 patients receiving short-course therapy relapsed. Both of the relapses were noted to occur among 3 patients receiving less than 10 days of therapy (71). Adding this experience to the pooled experience with short-course therapy from 11 previous studies would yield 10 relapses among 153 patients (6.5%) (45). If the 3 patients receiving less than 10 days of therapy are excluded, the pooled rate would be 8 relapses among 150 patients (5.3%).

The classical manifestations of endocarditis—such as new or changing murmur, splenomegaly, and embolic lesions—are each present in only a minority of cases (72). Nolan and Beatty therefore attempted to develop criteria for differentiating patients with *S. aureus* bacteremia from those with endocarditis (70). Community acquisition, lack of an obvious primary site of infection, and presence of metastatic sequelae (e.g., intraabdominal, renal, or cerebral abscess) were each associated with a high risk for endocarditis in their study. By contrast, only 2 of the 26 cases of *S. aureus* endocarditis that they studied had an obvious primary site of infection, which was acquired in the hospital and had no metastatic sequelae (70). A lower risk of endocarditis among nosocomial cases was also found in several other studies (37,73,74). These data conflict with those of the study cited above, which found that endocarditis was as common with nosocomial catheter-related *S. aureus* bacteremia as it was with community-acquired noncatheter-related *S. aureus* bacteremia (69). However, the same investigators recently presented data providing at least partial confirmation of the other studies: Complicated *S. aureus* bacteremia was reported to occur less often with community-acquired than with hospital- or healthcare-associated *S. aureus* bacteremia (75). Another group of investigators recently reported that 21% of community-acquired *S. aureus* bacteremia was complicated by endocarditis, compared with 5% of hospital-acquired *S. aureus* bacteremia and 12% of hemodialysis-associated *S. aureus* bacteremia (76).

Criteria for diagnosing infective endocarditis using echocardiography have been published (77). According to this scheme, a definite diagnosis can be made by either pathological or clinical criteria. The pathological diagnosis requires culture of an organism from a vegetation, or histologic confirmation of a vegetation or intracardiac abscess. The clinical criteria include major and minor criteria, and a definite diagnosis would require the presence of two major criteria, one major and three minor criteria, or five minor criteria. The major criteria include blood culture results suggestive of endocarditis—because of either the species involved or the continuousness of the positive cultures—and evidence of endocardial involvement by echocardiography, such as (a) intracardiac mass on valve or supporting structure, (b) abscess, or (c) new partial dehiscence of the prosthetic valve or new valvular regurgitation. Minor criteria include a predisposing heart condition, fever ($>38\,^\circ$C), valvular phenomena (e.g., emboli or mycotic aneurysms), immunologic phenomena (e.g., Osler's nodes or Roth spots), microbiologic evidence (e.g., blood cultures showing a pathogen not meeting major criteria or a serologic test consistent with endocarditis), and echocardiographic evidence suggestive of endocarditis but not meeting major criteria. It should be noted that a recent study from the same institution that developed these criteria for diagnosing endocarditis found that transthoracic echocardiography had a sensitivity of only 27% when compared with routine usage of transesophageal echocardiography (TEE) in all cases of *S. aureus* bacteremia in which TEE was not contraindicated (69).

Other manifestations of catheter-related *S. aureus* infections have included such diverse presentations as sternoclavicular arthritis and clavicular osteomyelitis after *S. aureus* infection of a subclavian catheter (78); mycotic aneurysms and osteomyelitis after umbilical artery catheterization in a neonate (79); endarteritis with pseudoaneurysm, septic arthritis, osteomyelitis, and distal emboli after femoral artery catheterization (71,80,81); psoas abscess and discitis after femoral vein catheterization for hemodialysis (82); and an infected atrial thrombus following placement of a right atrial catheter (83). Most reported cases of infected pseudoaneurysm have involved *S. aureus* infection (84–88).

A self-limited, sterile reactive arthritis has been reported as a rare complication following catheter-related *S. aureus* bacteremia in HLA-B27 negative patients (89).

The persistence of high-grade bacteremia despite antibiotic therapy and removal of the catheter suggests the presence of septic phlebitis (90). Septic phlebitis related to a peripheral catheter may be associated with local inflammation and induration overlying the vein, but this is not present in all cases. With central venous catheters, septic phlebitis is usually not associated with local signs of inflammation nor with clinical signs of venous obstruction, which are present in only a minority of radiographically documented cases. Deep venous thrombosis in such cases may be documented by venography, sonography, or CT scan.

Thirty cases were included in a recent review of published cases of spinal epidural abscess following epidural catheterization. Of these, 19 (63%) were due to *S. aureus* (91). Nine (90%) of 10 had persistent neurologic deficit after thoracic epidural abscess, compared to only 3 (20%) of 15 after lumbar epidural abscess.

THERAPY

Catheter-related bloodstream infection has generally been treated with one to two weeks of therapy for most etiologic agents. For *S. aureus*, however, there has been concern about the risk of complicating endocarditis, and until recently many have routinely treated the condition for at least four weeks (92–94). During the past two decades, several studies have suggested that the risk of complicating endocarditis is sufficiently low (i.e., <10% of cases) that short-course therapy (10 to 14 days) is safe for patients with apparently uncomplicated catheter-related bacteremia (37,39,70,71,95–97). A meta-analysis of 11 studies of short-course therapy found a relapse rate of 6.1% (95% CI, 2.0%–10.2%). Two studies found that most relapses after short-course therapy occurred when therapy lasted less than 10 days (39,71).

A more recent study reported that only 1 (5%) of 21 patients completing prolonged therapy for *S. aureus* endocarditis relapsed, compared to 12 (18%) of 67 who had a negative TEE and thus presumably received short-course therapy (although the duration of therapy was not reported) (69). None of the 12 relapses in that study was endocarditis; they all involved deep *S. aureus* tissue infection at other sites. More recent data from the same investigators have suggested that patients with continuing fever at 72 hours; positive blood cultures drawn on days 2–4; a higher number of positive blood cultures; and/or failure to remove an infected source were significantly associated with complicated *S. aureus* bacteremia (75). The authors suggested that such patients should be carefully evaluated for metastatic sites of infection and should probably not receive short-course antibiotic therapy.

Delayed removal of the catheter has been associated with persistence of *S. aureus* bacteremia (71) or higher mortality in several observational studies (38,98,99). A retrospective study of *S. aureus* infections of Hickman catheters reported that failure to remove the catheter was associated with a worse outcome (38). Of 37 evaluable episodes of *S. aureus* bacteremia, 22 were cured with catheter removal plus antibiotics, whereas 8 of the 15 patients whose catheters were not removed were cured with antibiotics and 7 failed antibiotic therapy (4 relapses and 3 deaths due to progressive catheter-related sepsis) (38). Another retrospective study concluded that failure to remove an infected catheter was related to higher mortality among 25 patients with MRSA bacteremia, 13 (52%) of whom died (99).

A fourth observational study found that 13 (56%) of 23 patients from whom an infected catheter was not removed suffered relapse or died due to *S. aureus* infection, and 80% of the patients whose catheters were not removed were hemodialysis patients (98). The authors reported that failure to replace the catheter was the most important reason for treatment failure, according to a logistic regression analysis (98). By contrast, a fifth and more recent observational study reported on 50 cases of *S. aureus* CRBSI in hemodialysis patients, none of whom died even though the catheter was not removed in 19 episodes (47). All 8 documented episodes of endocarditis or deep *S. aureus* infection at another site appeared to relate to the spread of infection during the intitial bacteremia, rather than to relapse and subsequent bacteremia from the site of an unchanged catheter. Two of the 8 had their catheters removed at the time of admission, three had their catheters removed during the first day, one during the second day, and one on the fourth day after admission (47).

Fever or bacteremia persisting more than 3 days after catheter removal was associated with an increased risk of endocarditis in one study, suggesting the need for a longer course of therapy in such patients (39). Placement of a central catheter tip into the right atrium or into the pulmonary artery has also been related to an increased risk for development of endocarditis, presumably due to trauma to endocardial surfaces caused by the catheter, followed by seeding of these roughened surfaces during subsequent bacteremia (100).

AIDS and AIDS-related complex have also been found to be adverse prognostic factors in catheter-related *S. aureus* bacteremia, as 6 (35%) of 17 patients relapsed with late metastatic complications after a mean of 18 days of antibiotic therapy (59). Some authors have recommended that patients with HIV infection who develop catheter-related *S. aureus* bloodstream infection should routinely receive a longer course of therapy, such as 3 to 4 weeks (101).

The drug of choice for treating *S. aureus* bacteremia has been a beta lactam to which the isolate is susceptible. For the rare penicillin-susceptible isolates, high-dose penicillin would be the drug of choice (e.g., 20 million units IV per day for an adult with normal renal function). For the majority of isolates that are penicillin-resistant, a penicillinase-resistant penicillin would be the choice (e.g., nafcillin 1.5 g IV every 4 hours, for an adult). In cases of penicillin allergy, a first-generation cephalosporin has frequently been used with success (e.g., cefazolin 100mg/kg/d intravenously, in 3 divided doses). For those unable to tolerate a beta lactam and those with methicillin-resistant *S. aureus*, vancomycin is the drug of choice (30mg/kg/d intravenously, in 2 divided doses). Because of its long half-life and consequent infrequent dosing, vancomycin should not be used as a drug of convenience for treating beta lactam-susceptible *S. aureus* infection in nonallergic patients. Such systematic overuse of vancomycin would add further pressure for selection of vancomycin resistance among organisms such as *Enterococcus faecium*, which has caused many nosocomial epidemics during the past decade (102). An additional concern with such overreliance on vancomycin for treatment of *S. aureus* bacteremia derives from several studies reporting higher failure rates and slower clearance of bacteremia in patients with *S. aureus* endocarditis treated with vancomycin (103–107).

Antibiotic lock therapy provides a new approach to treatment without removing the catheter, by infusing parenteral antibiotics through the catheter and then locking a high concentration into the catheter over a 12-hour period each night (108–116). Such therapy, usually given over a two-week period, has been successful in curing the infection and salvaging the infected catheter in 97% of patients requiring long-term vascular access with infections due to a variety of pathogens, including 12 cases of *S. aureus* infection (109,110). The success rate was only 43%, however, when this method was applied to infected subcutaneous ports in one study (108). The mean duration of follow-up without relapse in the study with 12 *S. aureus* cases was 20.5 months. These data suggest that uncomplicated, mild-to-moderate *S. aureus* infection of long-dwelling tunneled or hemodialysis catheters may be treated without catheter removal if infection is confined to the lumen of the catheter [i.e., in the absence of tunnel or exit site infection (117)]. Vancomycin has been shown to be stable in both total parenteral nutrition solutions and heparin solutions at room temperature for a 24-hour period, allowing for concurrent therapy during TPN infusion and/or for antibiotic lock with heparin overnight, if indicated (118).

Therapy of superficial catheter-related septic phlebitis has generally consisted of ligation and venectomy, coupled with antimicrobial therapy for 2 to 3 weeks. Incision and drainage with antibiotics, but without venectomy, has been reported to work in some cases. For central venous septic phlebitis, catheter removal and prolonged antibiotic therapy, coupled with anticoagulation, are necessary (119).

PREVENTION

Prevention of catheter-related *S. aureus* infection depends upon the principles used for prevention of catheter infections in general, which can prevent infections caused by all pathogens (120). In a randomized trial, placement of catheters using maximal barriers (cap, mask, sterile long-sleeved gown and gloves, and large drapes) was associated with a significantly lower rate of infection than when only a mask, sterile gloves, and a small drape were used (121). A cohort study found similar protection using the same barriers, except that a cap was not used (122). The importance of technique during insertion was additionally confirmed in a study by Armstrong et al., which found a significant association between catheter colonization and inexperience of the clinician inserting the catheter (123).

Site selection also may have an important effect, because subclavian vein placement has been associated with lower infection rates than internal jugular vein placement in some cohort studies (122,124). Two randomized trials have shown significantly higher rates of deep venous thrombosis and trends toward higher rates of catheter infections with femoral rather than with subclavian catheters (125,126).

Peripherally inserted central catheters have been associated with very low rates of infection, but they have been used primarily in outpatients (127,128). Only limited data are available for their use in hospitalized patients (129,130). Lower infection rates with this approach may be related to lower concentrations of resident bacteria on the arm than on the neck or chest (131,132).

Tunneling of catheters has been done partly to reduce the risk of catheter infection. Several studies have raised questions as to the effectiveness of tunneling for preventing infection (127,133,134), whereas others have suggested that it works (136–138). A recent CDC guideline recommended that hemodialysis catheters that will be used longer than 3 weeks should be cuffed. The guideline provided references to several observational studies, each of which involved tunneling of the cuffed catheters (120). Subcutaneous ports have been associated with significantly lower infection rates than those of tunneled catheters (139).

Dressing the catheter with povidone iodine ointment resulted in significant prevention of *S. aureus* bacteremia in a randomized trial involving subclavian dialysis catheters (140). An older study found no benefit with povidone iodine ointment, however, and further studies are needed (141). By contrast, use of polymyxin-neomycin-bacitracin ointment should be avoided on central venous catheters because of a fivefold increase in Candida colonization with this product (142). In a randomized controlled trial (RCT), mupirocin ointment applied to central venous catheter sites resulted in a reduction in the frequency of significant colonization of catheter tips—from 25% in controls receiving no antimicrobial ointment to 5% among those receiving mupirocin (143). In a second RCT, mupirocin applied to hemodialysis catheter sites was associated with prolonged catheter use, decreased *S. aureus* colonization of the catheter site, and decreased *S. aureus* bacteremia (144). The recent CDC guideline on preventing catheter infection did not recommend the use of mupirocin at the catheter site, because one study has suggested the possibility of development of mupirocin resistance among coagulase-negative staphylococci at the site (120).

Transparent dressings have been associated with a higher risk of infection in a randomized trial (145), and with a higher risk of significant colonization in a meta-analysis (146). A more recent trial found no difference in infection or colonization (147), but a subsequent trial by the same authors reported a significantly higher rate of colonization with transparent dressings, a result similar to that identified by the meta-analysis mentioned above (148). Further studies of transparent dressings are needed, especially considering their higher cost.

Antimicrobial catheters and catheter cuffs have been reported to exert significant protection against catheter-related bloodstream infection (142,149–152). Although antibiotic coating has been shown to work (153–156), concern has been expressed regarding the use of clinically current antibiotics for this purpose because of the potential for selecting antibiotic-resistant flora (152). Use of an antiseptic-impregnated catheter, which has also been shown to significantly reduce CRBSI (157), may obviate this concern because antiseptics are commonly used in large numbers of patients, without selection of resistance to clinically useful antibiotics (152). In multiple randomized trials, scheduled replacement of central venous catheters has proven ineffective in preventing catheter infection and should no longer be recommended (58,135,158–160). Scheduled replacement appears to significantly increase the risk of major mechanical complications if new site puncture is used, and paradoxically, to increase the rate of bloodstream infection if guidewire exchange is employed (160).

Multiple studies have suggested a benefit from using a special IV team to care for total parenteral nutrition catheters, compared to care by the regular ward team (161–164). A recent study showed benefit from the use of an IV team to care for peripheral IVs (165).

Specific prevention of *S. aureus* infection was demonstrated in a randomized trial of intravenous oxacillin prophylaxis in patients undergoing interleukin-2 therapy. By contrast, changing the catheter every 3 days was not effective in lowering the rate of infection in this trial (58). Prevention of *S. aureus* bacteremia has also been demonstrated among hemodialysis patients by weekly application of nasal creams containing mupirocin (166). Similar therapy using chlorhexidine and neomycin nasal cream has significantly reduced the risk of *S. aureus* peritonitis among CAPD patients colonized with *S. aureus* (167–169). In one study, this strategy led to a reduction from 28% to 13% ($p < 0.001$) in the number of CAPD catheters that had to be removed during a year because of infection (167). Application of mupirocin to the hemodialysis catheter site significantly prevented *S. aureus* bacteremia in another randomized trial (144). A randomized trial of intranasal application of mupirocin twice daily for five consecutive days every four weeks among peritoneal dialysis patients demonstrated a significant reduction of nasal carriage (10% versus 48%) as well as exit site infections (14 versus 44 in the placebo group, $p = 0.006$) (170).

Recent in vitro studies have suggested novel mechanisms for preventing catheter infection. One study showed that copper or silver/copper-coated catheters decrease adherence of *S. aureus* to teflon, polyvinyl chloride, and silicone rubber catheters (171). Similarly, a negatively charged direct electric current of 10 µA reduced *S. aureus* adherence to catheters, whereas a positively charged current had no effect (172). The use of a 20-µA current flowing through a silver wire wrapped helically around the proximal segment of catheters has resulted in lower rates of adherence of *S. aureus*, *S. epidermidis*, and *C. albicans* in vitro, and lower rates of colonization in an animal model, when compared to regular catheters and chlorhexidine-silver sulfadiazine-impregnated catheters (173). A minocycline-EDTA flush solution has been shown to have broad antimicrobial activity in vitro (174,175) and was successfully used to prevent catheter infection in three patients who required prolonged catheterization and had repeated bouts of catheter sepsis before use of the flush solution.

REFERENCES

1. Sheagren JN. *Staphylococcus aureus*: the persistent pathogen. N Engl J Med 1984; 310:1368–1373.
2. Maki DG, Stolz S. The epidemiology of central-venous catheter-related bloodstream infection (BSI) [abstr J47]. Programs and Abstracts of the 34th Interscience Conference of Antimicrobial Agents and Chemotherapy, Orlando, 1994.
3. Bjornson HS, Colley R, Bower RH, Duty VP, Schwartz-Fulton JT, Fisher JE. Association between microorganism growth at the catheter insertion site and colonization of the catheter in patients receiving total parenteral nutrition. Surgery 1982; 92:720–727.
4. Cheesborough JS, Finch RG, Burden RP. A prospective study of the mechanisms of infection associated with hemodialysis catheters. J Infect Dis 1986; 154:579–589.

5. Linares J, Sitges-Serra A, Garau J, Perez JL, Martin R. Pathogenesis of catheter sepsis: a prospective study with quantitative and semiquantitative cultures of catheter hub and segments. J Clin Micro 1985; 21:357–360.

6. Cooper CL, Schiller AL, Hopkins CC. Possible role of capillary action in pathogenesis of experimental catheter-associated dermal tunnel infections. J Clin Micro 1988; 26:8–12.

7. Moro ML, Vigano EF, Lepri AC. Risk factors for central venous catheter related infections in surgical and intensive care units. Infect Control Hosp Epidemiol 1994; 15:253–264.

8. Raad I, Costerton W, Sabharwal U, Sacilowski M, Anaissie E, Bodey C. Ultrastructural analysis of indwelling vascular catheters: a quantitative relationship between luminal colonization and duration of placement. J Infect Dis 1993; 168:400–407.

9. Marrie TJ, Costerton JW. Scanning and transmission electron microscopy of in situ bacterial colonization of intravenous and intraarterial catheters. J Clin Micro 1984; 19:687–693.

10. Tully JL, Griedland GH, Baldini LM, Goldmann DA. Complications of intravenous therapy with steel needles and Teflon catheters a comparative study. Am J Med 1981; 70:702–706.

11. Tager IB, Ginsberg MB, Ellis SE. An epidemiologic study of the risks associated with peripheral intravenous catheters. Am J Epidemiol 1983; 118:839–851.

12. Maki DG, Ringer M. Evaluation of dressing regimens for prevention of infection with peripheral intravenous catheters gauze, a transparent polyure-thane dressing, and an iodophor-transparent dressing. JAMA 1987; 258:2396–2403.

13. Garland JS, Nelson DB, Cheah TE, Hennes HH, Johnson TM. Infectious complications during peripheral intravenous therapy with Teflon catheters: a prospective study. Pediatric Infect Dis J 1998; 6:918–921.

14. Sheth NK, Rose HD, Franson TR, Buckmire FL, Sohnle PG. In vitro quantitative adherence of bacteria to intravascular catheters. J Surg Res 1983; 34:213–218.

15. Sherertz RJ, Carruth WA, Marosok RD, Espeland MA, Johnson RA, Solomon DD. Contribution of vascular catheter material to the pathogenesis of infection: the enhanced risk of silicone in vivo. J Biomed Mater Res 1995; 29:635–645.

16. Lopez-Lopez G, Pascual A, Perea EL. Effect of plastic catheters on the phagocytic activity of human polymorphonuclear leukocytes. Eur J Clin Micro Infect Dis 1990; 9:324–328.

17. Klempner MS, Noring R, Mier JW, Atkins MB. Acquired chemtactic defect in neutrophils from patients receiving interleukin-2 immunotherapy. N Engl J Med 1990; 322:959–965.

18. Murphy PM, Lane HC, Fauci AS, Gallin JI. Impairment of neutrophil bactericidal capacity in patients with AIDS. J Infect Dis 1988; 158:627–630.

19. Vaudaux P, Pittet D, Haeberli A. Fibronectin is more active than fibrin or fibrinogen in promoting *Staphylococcus aureus* adherence to inserted intra-vascular catheters. J Infect Dis 1993; 167:633–641.

20. Russell PB, Kline J, Yoder MC, Polin RA. Staphylococcal adherence to polyvinyl chloride and heparin-bonded polyurethane catheters in species dependent on and enhanced by fibronectin. J Clin Micro 1987; 25:1083–1087.

21. Herrmann M, Lai QJ, Albrecht RM, Mosher DF, Proctor RA. Adhesion of *Staphylococcus aureus* to surface-bound platelets: role of fibrinogen/fibrin and platelet integrins. J Infect Dis 1993; 167:312–322.

22. Herrmann M, Suchard SJ, Boxer LA, Waldvogel FA, Lew PD. Thrombospondin binds to *Staphylococcus aureus* and promotes staphylococcal adherence to surfaces. Infect Immun 1991; 59:279–288.

23. Sherertz RJ, Raad I, Belani A. Three year experience with sonicated vascular catheter cultures in a clinical microbiology laboratory. J Clin Micro 1990; 28:76–82.

24. Waldvogel FA. *Staphylococcus aureus* (including toxic shock syndrome). In: Mandell GL, Bennett JE, Dolin R, eds. Principles and Practice of Infectious Diseases. 4th ed. New York: Churchill Livingstone, 1995:1754–1777.

25. Elek SD, Conen PE. The virulence of *Staphylococcus pyogenes* for man: a study of the problems of wound infection. Br J Exp Patho 1961; 42:26–277.

26. Bannerjee SN, Emori TG, Culver DH. Secular trends in nosocomial primary bloodstream infections in the United States, 1980–1989. Am J Med 1991; 91(suppl 3B):87S–89S.

27. Eliasen K, Nielsen PB, Espersen E. A one-year survey of nosocomial bacteraemia at a Danish university hospital. J Hyg 1986; 97:471–478.

28. Gosbell IB, Newton PJ, Sullivan BE. Survey of blood cultures from five community hospitals in south-western Sydney, Australia. Australian and New Zealand Journal of Medicine 10-1-1999; 29(5):684–692.

29. Steinberg JP, Clark CC, Hackman BO. Nosocomial and community-acquired *Staphylococcus aureus* bacteremias from 1980 to 1993: impact of intravascular devices and methicillin resistance. Clinical Infectious Diseases 8-1-0096; 23(2 [2]):255–259.

30. Anonymous. Monitoring hospital-acquired infections to promote patient safety—United States, 1990–1999. MMWR 2000; 49:149–153.

31. Maki DG. Nosocomial bacteremia: a epidemiologic overview. Am J Med 1981; 70:719–732.

32. McGowan JE, Parrott PL, Duty VP. Nosocomial bacteremia. Potential for prevention of procedure-related cases. JAMA 1977; 237:2727–2729.

33. Libman H, Arbeit RD. Complications associated with *Staphylococcus aureus* bacteremia. Arch Intern Med 1984; 44:541–545.

34. Mylotte JM, McDermott C. *Staphylococcus aureus* bacteremia caused by infected intravenous catheters. Am J Infect Control 1987; 15:1–6.

35. Linares MP, Nunez FM, Cordero LL, Perereira SS, Romero PE, Moure CR. Nosocomial infective endocarditis in patients without prosthesis. Revista Clinica Espanola December 1997; 197(12):814–818.

36. Watanakunakorn C, Baird IM. *Staphylococcus aureus* bacteremia and endocarditis associated with a removable infected intravenous device. Am J Med 1977; 63:523–526.

37. Mylotte JM, McDermott C, Spooner JA. Prospective study of 114 consecutive episodes of *Staphylococcus aureus* bacteremia. Rev Infect Dis 1987; 9:891–907.

38. Dugdale DC, Ramsey PG. *Staphylococcus aureus* bacteremia in patients with Hickman catheters. Am J Med 1990; 89:137–141.

39. Raad I, Sabbagh MF. Optimal duration of therapy for catheter-related *Staphyhlococcus aureus* bacteremia: a study of 55 cases and review. Clin Infect Dis 1992; 14:75–82.

40. Rahal JJ, Chan YK, Johnson G. Relationship of staphylococcal tolerance, teichoic acid antibody, and serum bactericidal activity to therapeutic outcome in *Staphylococcus aureus* bacteremia. Am J Med 1986; 81:43–52.

41. Bentley DW, Lepper MR. Septicemia related to the indwelling venous catheter. JAMA 1968; 206:1749–1752.

42. Ryan JAJ, Abel RM, Abbott WM, Hopkins CC, Chesney TM, Colley R, Phillips K, Fischer JE. Catheter complications in total parenteral nutrition: a prospective study of 200 consecutive patients. N Engl J Med 1974; 290:757–761.

43. Bryan CS, Kirkhart B, Brenner ER. Staphylococcal bacteremia: current patterns in nonuniversity hospitals. South Med J 1984; 77:693–696.

44. Collignon PJ, Munro R, Sorrell TC. Systemic sepsis and intravenous devices. A prospective survey. Med J Aust 1984; 141:345–348.

45. Jernigan JA, Farr BM. Short-course therapy of catheter-related *Staphylococcus aureus* bacteremia: a meta-analysis. Annals of Internal Medicine 1993; 119(4):304–311.

46. Byers KE, Adal KA, Anglim AM, Farr BM. Case fatality rate for catheter-related bloodstream infections (CRBSI): a meta-analysis. Infect Control Hosp Epidemiol 1995; 16(Part 2, suppl):23.

47. Peacock SJ, Curtis N, Berendt AR, Bowler IC, Winearls CG, Maxwell P. Outcome following haemodialysis catheter-related *Staphylococcus aureus* bacteremia. J Hosp Infect 1999; 41(3):223–228.

48. Cosgrove S, Sakoulas G, Perencevich E, Schwaber M, Karchmer AW, Carmeli Y. Comparison of mortality with methicillin-resistant and methicillin susceptible *Staphylococcus aureus* (MSSA) bacteremia: a meta analysis. Clin Infect Dis 2003; 36:53–59.

49. Maki DG. Nosocomial bloodstream infections [abstr 3]. Third Decennial International Conference on Nosocomial Infections, Atlanta, GA, July 31–August 3, 1990.

50. Sewell CM, Calrridge L, Lacke C, Weinmna EJ, Young EJ. Staphylococcal nasal carriage and subsequent infection in peritoneal dialysis patients. JAMA 1982; 248:1493–1495.

51. Kreft B, Eckstein S, Kahl A, Frei U, Witte W, Trautmann M. Clinical and genetic analysis of *Staphylococcus aureus* nasal colonization and exit-site infection in patients undergoing peritoneal dialysis. Eur J Clin Micro Infect Dis 2001; 20(10):734–737.

52. Nielsen J, Ladefoged SD, Kolmos HJ. Nephrol dialysis transplant dialysis catheter-related septicaemia-focus on *Staphylococcus aureus* septicaemia. Nephrol Dial Transplant 1998; 13:2847–2852.

53. Luzar MA, Coles GA, Faller B, Slingeneyer A, Dah GD, Briat C, Wone C, Knefati Y, Kessler M, Peluso F. *Staphylococcus aureus* nasal carriage and infection in patients on continuous ambulatory peritoneal dialysis. N Engl J Med 1990; 322:505–509.

54. Kreft B, Ilic S, Zieburh W, Kahl A, Frei U, Sack K, Trautmann M. Adherence of *Staphylococcus aureus* isolated in peritoneal dialysis-related exit-site infections to HEp-2 cells and silicone peritoneal catheter materials. Nephrol Dial Transplant 1998; 13(12):3160–3164.

55. Roubicek C, Brunet UC, Mallet MN, Dussol B, Gonzales A, Andrieu D, Merzouk T, Jaber K, Berland Y. Nasal carriage of *Staphylococcus aureus*: prevalence in a hemodialysis center and effect on bacteremia. Nephrologie 1995; 16:229–232.

56. Richards JM, Gilewski TA, Vogelzang NJ. Association of interleukin-2 therapy with staphylococcal bacteremia. Cancer 1991; 67:1570–1575.

57. Snydman DR, Sullivan B, Gill M, Gould JA, Parkinson DR, Atkins MB. Nosocomial sepsis associated with interleukin-2. Ann Intern Med 1990; 112:1102–1107.

58. Bock SN, Lee RE, Fisher B, Rubin JT, Schwarzentruber DJ, Wei JP, Callender DP, Yang JC, Lotze MT, Pizzo PA. A prospective randomized trial evaluating prophylactic antibiotics to prevent triple-lumen catheter-related sepsis in patients treated with immunotherapy. J Clin Oncol 1990; 8:161–169.

59. Jacobson MA, Gellermann H, Chambers H. *Staphylococcus aureus* bacteremia and recurrent staphylococcal infection in patients with acquired immunodeficiency syndrome and AIDS related complex. Am J Med 1988; 85:172–176.

60. Skoutelis AT, Murphy RL, MacDonell KB, VonRoenn JH, Sterkel CD, Phair JP. Indwelling central venous catheter infections in patients with acquired immunodeficiency syndrome. J Acquired Immune Deficiency Syndromes, 1990, (3):335–342.

61. Frank U, Daschner FD, Schulgen G, Mills J. Incidence and epidemiology of nosocomial infections in patients infected with human immunodeficiency virus. Clin Infect Dis 1997; 25(2):318–320.

62. Pittet D, Chuard C, Rae AC, Auckenthaler R. Clinical diagnosis of central venous catheter line infections: a difficult job [abstr 453]. Programs and Abstracts of the 31st Interscience Conference of Antimicrobial Agents and Chemotherapy, Chicago, 1991.

63. Widmer A, Zimmerli W. Fatal peripheral catheter phlebitis. Schweizerische Medizinische Wochenschrift. Journal Suisse de Medecine 1988; 118:1053–1055.

64. Maki DG, Ringer M. Risk factors for infusion-related phlebitis with small peripheral venous catheters a randomized controlled trial. Ann Intern Med 1991; 114:845–854.

65. Lipsky BA, Peugeot RL, Boyko EJ, Kent DL. A prospective study of *Staphylococcus aureus* nasal colonization and intravenous therapy-related phlebitis. Arch Intern Med 1992; 152:2109–2112.

66. Hedstrom SA, Christensson B. *Staphylococcus aureus* septicaemia and endocarditis at the University Hospital in Lund 1976–1980. Scand J Infect Dis Suppl 1983; 41:38–48.

67. Watanakunakorn C, Tan JS. Diagnostic difficulties of staphylococcal endocarditis in geriatric patients. Geriatrics 1973; 28:168–173.

68. Watanakunakorn C, Tan JS, Phair JR. Some salient features of *Staphylococcus aureus* endocarditis. Am J Med 1973; 54:473–481.

69. Fowler VG, LI J, Corey GR, Boley J, Marr KA, Gopal AK, Kong LK, Gottlieb

G, Donovan CL, Sexton DJ, Ryan T. Role of echocardiography in evaluation of patients with *Staphylococcus aureus* bacteremia: experience in 103 patients. J Amer Coll Cardiol 1997; 30:1072–1078.

70. Nolan CM, Beaty HN. *Staphylococcus aureus* bacteremia. Current clinical patterns. Am J Med 1976; 60:495–500.

71. Malanoski GJ, Samore MM, Pefanis A, et al. *Staphylococcus aureus* bacteremia: minimal effective therapy and unusal infectious complications associated with arterial sheath catheters. Arch Intern Med 1995; 155:1161–1166.

72. Bayer AS, Scheld WM. Endocarditis and intravascular infections. In: Mandell CL, Bennett JE, Dolin R, eds. Principles and Practice of Infectious Diseases 5th ed. Philadelphia: Churchill Livingstone, 2000:857–902.

73. Bayer AS, Lam K, Ginzton L, Norman DC, Chiu CY, Ward JI. *Staphylococcus aureus* bacteremia. Clinical serologic, and echocardiographic findings in patients with and without endocarditis. Arch Intern Med 1987; 147:457–462.

74. Cooper R, Platt R. *Staphylococcus aureus* bacteremia in diabetic patients. Am J Med 1982; 73:658–662.

75. Fowler VG, Olsen MK, Corey GR, Woods CW, Reller LB, Cheng AC, Dudley T, Oddone EZ. Clinical identifiers of *Staphylococcus aureus* bacteremia. Arch Int Med 2003; 163:2066–2072.

76. Chang FY, MacDonald BE, Peacock JE, Musher DM, Triplett P, Mylotte J, O'Donell A, Wagener MM, Yu VL. A prospective multicenter study of *S. aureus* bacteremia: incidence of endocarditis, risk factors for mortality, and clinical impact of methicillin resistance. Medicine 2003; 82:322–332.

77. Durack DT, Lukes AS, Bright DK, Service DE. New criteria for diagnosis of infective endocarditis: Utilization of specific echocardiographic findings. Am J Med 1994; 96:200–209.

78. Moreno-Guillen S, Eiros-Bouza JM, Espinosa-Parra EJ, Fernandez-Guerero ML, Rivera MT. Osteoarticular infections associated with catheterization of the subclavian vein. Enfermedades Infecciosas y Microbiologia Clinica 1991; 9:33–34.

79. Lim MO, Gresham EL, Franken EA, Leake RD. Osteomyelitis as a complication of umbilical artery catheterization. Am J Dis Child 1977; 131:142–144.

80. Frazee BW, Flaherty JP. Septic endarteritis of the femoral artery following angioplasty (Review). Rev Infect Dis 1991; 13:620–623.

81. Culver DA, Chua J, Rehm SJ, Whitlow P, Hertzer NR. Arterial infection and *Staphylococcus aureus* bacteremia after transfemoral cannulation for percutaneous carotid angioplasty and stenting. Journal of Vascular Surgery 2002; 35(3):576–579.

82. Kikuchi S, Muro K, Yoh K, Iwabuchi S, Tomida C, Yamaguchi N, Kobayashi M, Nagase S, Aoyagi K, Koyama A. Two cases of psoas abscess with discitis by methicillin-resitant *Staphylococcus aureus* as a complication of femoral-vein catheterization for haemodialysis. Nephrol Dial Transplant 1999; 14(5):1279–1281.

83. Horner SM, Bell JA, Swanton AH. Infected right atrial thrombus-an important but rare complication of central venous lines. Eur Heart J 1993; 14:138–140.

84. Soderstrom CA, Wasserman DH, Ranson KJ, Caplan ES, Cowley RA.

Infected false femoral artery aneurysms secondary to monitoring catheters. A Cardiovasc Surg 1983; 24:63–68.

85. Arnow PM, Costas CO. Delayed rupture of the radial artery caused by catheter-related sepsis. Rev Infect Dis 1988; 10:1035–1037.

86. Cohen A, Reyes R, Kirk M, Fulks RM. Osler's nodes, pseudoaneurysm formation and sepsis complicating percutaneous radial artery cannulation. Crit Care Med 1984; 12:1078–1079.

87. Falk PS, Scuderei PE, Sherertz RJ, Motsinger SM. Infected radial artery pseudo-aneurysms occurring after percutaneous radial artery cannulation. Chest 1992; 101:490–495.

88. Fanning WL, Aronsom M. Osler node, Janeway lesions and splinter hemmorrhages. Arch Dermatol 1977; 113:648–649.

89. Siam AR, Hammoudeh M. *Staphylococcus aureus* triggered reactive arthritis. Ann Rheumatic Dis 1995; 54:131–133.

90. Farr BM. Nonendocardial vascular infections. In: Hoeprich PD, Jordanb MC, Roanld AR, eds. Infectious Diseases. Philadelphia: J.B. Lippincott, 1994:1248–1258.

91. Okano K, Kondo H, Tsuchiya R, Naruke T, Sato M, Yokoyama R. Spinal epidural abscess associated with epidural catheterization: report of a case and a review of the literature. Japanese journal of Clinical Oncology 1999; 29(1):49–52.

92. Rabinovich S, Smith IM, January LE. The changing patterns of bacterial endocarditis. Med Clin North Am 1968; 52:1091–1101.

93. Lerner PI, Weinstein L. Infective endocarditis in the antibiotic era. N Eng J Med 1966; 274:388–393.

94. Hamburger M. Treatment of bacterial endocarditis. Mod Treat 1964; 1:1003–1015.

95. Iannini PB, Crossley K. Therapy of *Staphylococcus aureus* bacteremia associated with a removable focus of infection. Ann Intern Med 1976; 84:558–560.

96. Bayer AS, Tillman DB, Concepcion N, Guze LB. Clinical value of teichoic acid antibody titers in the diagnosis and management of the staphylococcemias. West J Med 1980; 132:294–300.

97. Ehni WF, Reller LB. Short-course therapy for catheter-associated *Staphylococcus aureus* bacteremia. Arch Intern Med 1989; 149:533–536.

98. Fowler VG, Sanders LL, Sexton DJ. Outcome of *Staphylococcus aureus* bacteremia according to compliance with recommendations of infectious diseases specialist: experience with 244 patients. Clin Infect Dis 1998; 27:478–486.

99. Cheong I, Samsudin LM, Law GH. Methicillin-resistant *Staphylococcus aureus* bacteremia at a tertiary teaching hospital. British Journal of Clinical Practice 1996; 50(5):237–239.

100. Sasaki TM, Panke TW, Dorethy JF, Lindberg RB, Pruirt BA. The relationship of central venous and pulmonary artery catheter position to acute right-sided endocarditis in severe thermal injury. J Trauma 1979; 19:740–743.

101. Mortara LA, Bayer AS. *Staphylococcus aureus* bacteremia and endocarditis. Infect Dis Clin North Am 1993; 7:53–68.

102. HICPAC. Recommendations for preventing the spread of vancomycin resistance. Hospital Infection Control Practices Advisory Committee (HICPAC). Infect Control Hosp Epidemiol 1995; 16:105–113.

103. Hartstein AI, Mulligan ME, Morthland VH, Kwok RY. Recurrent *Staphylococcus aureus* bacteria. J Clin Micro 1992; 30:670–674.

104. Markowitz N, Quinn EL, Saravolatz LD. Trimethoprim-sulfamethoxazole compared to vancomycin for the treatment of *Staphylococcus aureus* infection. Ann Intern Med 1992; 117:390–398.

105. Levine DP, Fromm BS, Reddy BR. Slow response to vancomycin or vancomycin plus rifampin therapy among patients with methicillin-resistant *Staphylcoccus aureus*. Ann Intern Med 1991; 115:674–680.

106. Small PM, Chambers HF. Vancomycin for *Staphylococcus aureus* endocarditis in intravenous drug abusers. Antimicrob Agents Chemother 1990; 34:1227–1231.

107. Chambers HF, Miller RT, Newman MD. Right-sided *Staphylococcus aureus* endocarditis in intravenous drug abusers: two-week combination therapy. Ann Intern Med 1988; 109:619–624.

108. Longuet P, Douard MC, Arlet G. Venous access port-related bacteremia in patients with acquired immunodeficiency syndrome or cancer: the reservoir as a diagnostic and therapeutic tool. Clin Infect Dis 2001; 32:1776–1783.

109. Krzywda EA, Gotoff RA, Andris DA, Marciniak TF, Edmiston CE, Quebbeman EJ. Antibiotic lock treatment (ALT): impact on catheter salvage and cost savings [abstr J4]. Programs and Abstracts of the 35th Interscience Conference of Antimicrobial Agents and Chemotherapy, San Francisco, 1995.

110. Capdevila JA, Segarra A, Planes AM, Gasser I, Gavalda J, Pahissa A. Long term follow-up of patients with catheter related sepsis (CRS) treated without catheter removal [abstr J3]. Programs and Abstracts of the 35th Interscience Conference of Antimicrobial Agents and Chemotherapy, San Francisco, 1995.

111. Messing B, Peitra-Cohen S, Debure A, Beliah M, Bernier JJ. Antibiotic-lock technique: a new approach to optimal therapy for catheter-related sepsis in home-parenteral nutrition patients. JPEN 1988; 12:185–189.

112. Gaillard JL, Merlino R, Pajot N, Goulet O, Fauchere JL, Ricour C, Veron M. Conventional and nonconventional modes of vancomycin administration to decontaminate the internal surface of catheters colonized with coagulase-negative staphylococci. JPEN 1990; 14:593–597.

113. Arnow PM, Kushner R. Malassezia furfur catheter infection cured with antibiotic lock therapy [letter]. Am J Med 1982; 90:128–130.

114. Douard MC, Arlet G, Leverger G, Paulien R, Waintrop C, Clementi E, Eurin B. Quantitative blood cultures for diagnosis and management of catheter-related sepsis in pediatric hematology and oncology patients. Intens Care Med 1991; 17:30–35.

115. Elian JC, Frappaz D, Ros A, Gay JP, Guichard D, Dorche G, Aubert G, Boutielle M, Ollaguier M, Freycon F. Study of serum kinetics of vancomycin during the "antibiotic-lock" technique. Arch Fr Pediatr 1992; 49:357–360.

116. Cowan CE. Antibiotic lock technique. J Intravenous Nurs 1992; 15:283–287.

117. Mermel LA, Farr BM, Sherertz RJ, Raad II, O'Grady N, Harris JS, Craven DE. Guidelines for the management of intravascular catheter-related infection. Clin Infect Dis 2001; 32:1249–1272.

118. Yao JD, Arkin CF, Karchmer AW. Vancomycin stability in heparin and total parenteral nutrition solutions: novel approach to therapy of central venous catheter-related infections. JPEN 1992; 16:268–274.
119. Verghese A, Widrich WC, Arbeit RD. Central venous septic thrombophlebitis—the role of medical therapy. Medicine 1985; 64:394–400.
120. O'Grady N, Alexander M, Dellinger E, Gerberding JL, Heard SO, Maki DG, Masur H, McCormick RD, Mermel LA, Pearson ML, Raad II, Randolph A, Weinstein RA. Guidelines for the Prevention of Intravascular Catheter-Related Infections. Infect Control Hosp Epidemiol 2002; 23(12): 759–769.
121. Raad I, Hohn DC, Gilbreath BJ, Suleiman N, Hill LA, Bruso PA, Marts K, Mansfield PF, Bodey GP. Prevention of central venous catheter related infections by using maximal sterile barrier precautions during insertion. Infect Control Hosp Epidemiol 1994; 15(4 Pt 1):231–238.
122. Mermel LA, McCormick RD, Springman SR, Maki DG. The pathogenesis and epidemiology of catheter related infection with pulmonary artery Swan-Ganz catheters:a prospective study utilizing molecular subtyping. Am J Med 1991; 91(suppl 3B):197S–205S.
123. Armstrong CW, Mayhall CG, Miller KB, Newsome HH Jr, Sugerman HJ, Dalton HP, Hall GO, Gennings C. Prospective study of catheter replacement and other risk factors of infection of hyperalimentation catheters. J Infect Dis 1986; 154:808–816.
124. Richet H, Hubert B, Nitemberg G, Andrenant A, Buu-Hoi A, Ourbak P, Gulicier C, Veron M, Boisiron A, Bourier AM. Prospective multicenter study of vascular catheter. Related complications and risk factors for positive patients. J Clin Micro 1990; 28:2520–2525.
125. Merrer J, De Jonghe B, Bernard MD, Golliot F, Lefrant JY, Raffy B, Barre E, Rigaud JP, Casciani D, Misset B, Bosquet C, Outin H, Brun-Buisson C, Nitenberg G. Complications of femoral and subclavian venous catheterization in critically ill patients: A randomized controlled trial. JAMA 2001; 286(6):700–707.
126. Trottier SJ, Veremakis C, O'Brien J, Auer Al. Femoral Deep Vein thrombosis associated with central venous catheterization: Results from a prospective, randomized trial. Crit Care Med 1995; 23(1):52–59.
127. Raad I, Davis S, Becker M, Hohn D, Houston D, Umphrey J, Bodey GP. Low infection rate and long durability of nontunnelled silastic catheters. Arch Intern Med 1993; 153:1791–1796.
128. Tice AD, Bonstell HP, Marsh PK, Craven PC, McEniry DW, Harding S. Peripherally inserted central venous catheters for outpatient intravenous antibiotic therapy. Infect Dis Clin Pract 1993; 2:186–190.
129. Linblad B, Wolff T. Infectious complications of percutaneously inserted central venous catheters. Acta Anaesthesiol Scand 1985; 29:587–589.
130. Bottino J, Mecredie K, Grosehel DHM, Lawson M. Long-term intravenous therapy with peripherally inserted silicone elastomer central venous catheters in patients with malignant diseases. Cancer 1979; 43:1937–1943.
131. Maki DG. Marked differences in skin colonization of insertion sites for central venous, arterial and peripheral IV catheters. The major reason for differing

risks of catheter-related infection? [abstr 712]. Programs and Abstracts of the 30th Interscience Conference of Antimicrobial Agents and Chemotherapy, Atlanta, GA, 1990.

132. Noble WC. Dispersal of skin microorganisms. Br J Dermatol 1975; 93:477–485.

133. Andrivet P, Bacquer A, Vu Ngoc C, Ferme C, Letinier JY, Gautier H, Gallet CB, Brun-Buisson C. Lack of clinical benefit from subcutaneous tunnel insertion of central venous catheters in immunocompromised patients. Clin Infect Dis 1994; 18:199–206.

134. Guichard I, Nitemberg G, Abitbol JL, Andreemont A, Leclercq B, Escudier B. Tunnelled versus non-tunnelled catheters for parenteral nutrition in an intensive care unit: a controlled prospective study of catheter related sepsis. Clin Nutr 1986; 5(suppl 1):169.

135. Powell C, Kudsk KA, Kulich PA, Mandelbaum JA, Fabri PJ. Effect of frequent guidewire changes on triple-lumen catheter sepsis. JPEN 1988; 12: 462–464.

136. Nahum E, Levy I, Katz J, Samra Z, Ashkenazi S, Ben-Ari J, Schonfeld T, Dagan O. Efficacy of subcutaneous tunneling for prevention of bacterial colonization of femoral central venous catheters in critically ill children. Pediatric Infect Dis J 2002;21(11):1000–1004.

137. Timsit J, Bruneel F, Cheval C, Mamzer MF, Garrouste-Orgeas M, Wolff M, Misset B, Chevret S, Regnier B, Carlet J. Use of tunneled femoral catheters to prevent catheter-related infection: A randomized, controlled trial. Ann Intern Med 1999; 130(9):729–735.

138. Timsit J, Sebille V, Farkas JC, Misset B, Martin JB, Chevret S, Carlet J. Effect of subcutaneous tunneling on internal jugular catheter-related sepsis in critically ill patients: a prospective randomized multicenter study. JAMA 1996; 276(17):1416–1420.

139. Howell PB, Walters PE, Donowitz GR, Farr BM. Risk factors for infection of adult patients with cancer who have tunnelled central venous catheters. Cancer 1995; 75(6):1367–1375.

140. Levin A, Mason AJ, Jindal KK, Fong IW, Goldstein MB. Prevention of hemodialysis subclavian vein catheter infections by topical povidone iodine. Kidney Int 1991; 40:934–938.

141. Prager RL, Silva J. Colonization of central venous catheters. South Med J 1984; 77:458–461.

142. Flowers RH, Schwenzer RJ, Kopel RJ, Fisch MJ, Tucker SI, Farr BM. Efficacy of an attachable subcutaneous cuff for the prevention of intravascular catheter-related infection: a randomized controlled trial. JAMA 1989; 261(6):878–883.

143. Hill RLR, Fisher AP, Ware RJ, Wilson S, Casewell MW. Mupirocin for the reduction of colonization of internal jugular cannulae- randomized controlled trial. J Hosp Infect 1990; 15(311):321.

144. Sesso R, Barbosa D, Leme IL, Sader H, Canziani ME, Manfredi S, Draibe S, Pignatari AC. *Staphylococcus aureus* prophylaxis in hemodialysis patient using central venous catheter: effect of mupirocin ointment. Journal of the American Society of Nephrology 1998; 9(6):1085–1092.

145. Conly JM, Grieves K, Peters B. A prospective, randomized study comparing

transparent and dry gauze dressings for central venous catheters. J Infect Dis 1989; 159:310–319.

146. Hoffman KK, Weber DJ, Samsa GP, Rutala WA. Transparent polyurethane film as an intravenous catheter dressing: a meta-analysis of the infection risks. JAMA 1992; 267(15):2072–2076.

147. Maki DG, Stolz SM, Wheeler SJ, Mermel LA. A prospective, randomized trial of gauze and two polyurethane dressings for site care of pulmonary artery catheters: implications for catheter management. Crit Care Med 1994; 22:1729–1737.

148. Maki DG, Mermel L, Martin M, Knasinski V, Berry D. A highly-semipermeable polyurethane dressing does not increase the risk of CVC-related BSI: a prospective, multicenter, investigator-blinded trial [abstr J64]. Programs and Abstracts of the 36th Interscience Conference of Antimicrobial Agents and Chemotherapy, New Orleans, Louisiana, 1996.

149. Romano G, Berti M, Goldstein BP, Borghi A. Efficacy of a central venous catheter (Hydrocath) loaded with teicoplanin in preventing subcutaneous staphylococcal infection in the mouse. Int J Med Microbiol Virol Parasitol Infect Dis 1993; 279:426–433.

150. Maki DG, Cobb L, Garman JK, Shapiro JM, Ringer M, Helgerson RB. An attachable silver-impregnated cuff for prevention of infection with central venous catheters: a prospective randomized multicenter trial. Am J Med 1988; 85:307–314.

151. Clemence MA, Anglim AM, Jernigan JA, Adal KA, Titus MG, Duani DK, Farr BM. A study of prevention of catheter related bloodstream infection with an antiseptic impregnated catheter [abstr J199]. Programs and Abstracts of the 34th Interscience Conference on Antimicrobial Agents and Chemotherapy, Orlando FL, October 4–7, 1994.

152. Maki DG, Wheeler S, Stolz SM, Mermel LA. Prevention of central venous catheter-related bloodstream infection by use of an antiseptic-impregnated catheter. A randomized, controlled trial. Ann Intern Med 1997; 127(4): 257–266.

153. Kamal GD, Pfalier MA, Remple LE, Jebsom PJR. Reduced intravascular catheter infection by antibiotic bonding. JAMA 1991; 265:2364–2368.

154. Trooskin SZ, Donetz AP, Harvey HA, Greco RS. Prevention of catheter sepsis by antibiotic bonding. Surgery 1985; 97:547–551.

155. Sherertz RJ, Carruth WA, Hampton AA, Byron MP, Solomon DD. Efficacy of antibiotic-coated catheters in preventing subcutaneous *Staphylococcus aureus* infection in rabbits. J Infect Dis 1993; 167:98–106.

156. Darouiche HO, Raad I, Heard SO, Thornby JI, Wenker OC, Gabrielli A, Berg J, Khardori N, Hanna H, Hachem R, Harris RL, Mayhall G. A comparison of two antimicrobial-impregnated central venous catheters. N Eng J Med 1999; 340:1–8.

157. Veenstra DL, Saint S, Saha S, Lumley T, Sullivan SD. Efficacy of antiseptic-impregnated catheters in preventing catheter-related bloodstream infection: a meta-analysis. JAMA 1999; 281:261–267.

158. Uldall PR, Merchant N, Woods F, Yarworski U, Vas S. Changing subclavian haemodialysis cannulas to reduce infection. Lancet 1981; 1:1373.

159. Eyer S, Brummitt C, Crossley K, Siegel H, Cerra F. Catheter-related sepsis: a

prospective, randomized study of three methods of long-term catheter maintenance. Crit Care Med 1990; 18(1073):1079.

160. Cobb DK, High KP, Sawyer RG, Sable CA, Adams RB, Lindley DA, Pruett TL, Schwenzer K, Farr BM. A controlled trial of scheduled replacement of central venous and pulmonary-artery catheters. N Engl J Med 1992; 327(15): 1062–1068.

161. Faubion WC, Wesley JR, Khalidi N, Silvi J. Total parenteral nutrition catheter sepsis: impact of the team approach. J Parenteral Enteral Nutr 1986; 10:642–645.

162. Freeman JB, Lemire A, Maclean LD. Intravenous alimentation and septicemia. Surg Gynecol Obstet 1972; 135:708–712.

163. Nehme AE. Nutritional support of the hospitalized patient. The team concept. JAMA 1980; 243:1906–1908.

164. Nelson DB, Kien CL, Mohr B, Frank S, Davis SD. Dressing changes by specialized personnel reduce infection rates in patients receiving central venous parenteral nutrition. JPEN 1986; 10:220–222.

165. Soifer NE, Borzak S, Edlin BR, Weinstein RA. Prevention of peripheral venous catheter complications with an intravenous therapy team: a randomized controlled trial. Arch Intern Med 1998 March 9; 158(5):473–478.

166. Boelaert JR, Van Landuyt HW, De Baere YA, Gheyle DW, Daneels RF, Schurgers ML, Matthys EG, Gordts BZ. Epidemiology and revention or *Staphylococcus aureus* infections during hemodialysis [review]. Nephrologie 1994; 15:157–161.

167. Wilson AP, Scott GM, Lewis C, Neild G, Rudge C. Audit of infection in continuous ambulatory peritoneal dialysis. J Hosp Infect 1994; 28:264–271.

168. Ludiam H, McCann M. The prevention of infection with *Staphylococcus aureus* in continuous ambulatory peritoneal dialysis. J Hosp Infect 1991; 17:325–326.

169. Ludlam HA, Young AE, Berry AJ, Phillips I. The prevention of infection with *Staphylococcus aureus* in continuous ambulatory peritoneal dialysis. J Hosp Infect 1989; 14:293–301.

170. Anonymous. Nasal mupirocin prevents *Staphylococcus aureus* exit-site infection during peritoneal dialysis. Mupirocin Study Group. Journal of the American Society of Nephrology 1996; 7(11):2403–2408.

171. McLean RJ, Hussain AA, Sayer M, Vincent PS, Hughes DJ, Smith TJ. Antibacterial activity of multilayer silver-copper surface films on catheter material. Can J Microbiol 1993; 39:895–899.

172. Liu WK, Tebbs SE, Byrne PO, Elliott TS. The effects of electric current on bacteria colonizing intravenous catheters. J Infect 1993; 27(261):269.

173. Raad I, Zermeno A, Dumo M, Bodey GP. In vitro antimicrobial efficacy of silver iontophoretic catheter. Biometrics 1996; 17(11):1055–1059.

174. Raad I, Hachem R, Tcholakian RK, Sherertz R. Efficacy of minocycline and EDTA lock solution in preventing catheter-related bacteremia, septic phlebitis, and endocarditis in rabbits. Antimicrob Agents Chemother 2002; 43(2):327–332.

175. Chatzinikolaou I, Zipf TF, Hanna HA, Umphrey J, Roberts WM, Sherertz R, Hachem R, Raad I. Minocycline-ethylenediaminetetraacetate lock solution for the prevention of implantable port infections in children with cancer. Clin Infect Dis 2003; 36(1):116–119.

7

Catheter-Related Infections Caused by Coagulase-Negative Staphylococci

Mathias Herrmann and Georg Peters

Institute of Medical Microbiology and Hygiene
University of Saarland Hospital
Homburg/Saar and
Institute of Medical Microbiology
University of Muenster
Muenster, Germany

INTRODUCTION

Coagulase-negative staphylococci (CoNS), particularly *Staphylococcus epidermidis*, are the species most frequently isolated from infections associated with the use of vascular catheters. The propensity of these species to cause invasive disease, frequently manifestating as primary bacteremia, has for a long time been a conundrum in modern medicine: In contrast to their highly pathogenic coagulase-positive counterpart, *Staphylococcus aureus*, for a long time CoNS have been considered avirulent microorganisms that form a major component of the cutaneous microflora. Since the 1980s, however, it has been recognized that these organisms are readily able to colonize and infect various devices used for diagnostic and therapeutic procedures such as intravascular catheters, cerebrospinal fluid shunts, prosthetic heart valves, orthopedic devices, pacemakers, peritoneal dialysis catheters, vascular grafts, and ventricular assist devices (1). In fact, CoNS are now the leading organism for nosocomial bacteremia (2), and it is suggested that most of these cases are a consequence of infection of intravascular catheters. Bacteremia due to CoNS is associated with considerable hospital expenditures, morbidity, and also an increased mortality rate (3–5), yet treatment options are increasingly narrowed by emerging resistance against previously active antimicrobials (6). Over the last decades, important insight into the pathogenesis of these low-virulence microorganisms has been gained, particularly with respect to their interaction with a polymer surface, and it has now become clear that the intimate multifactorial interaction with the artificial surface is the basis for the role of these organisms in catheter-related infection (7). However, at this time it is not possible to translate the enhanced understanding of the pathogenic mechanisms in preventive or prophylactic measures specifically directed against this group of microorganisms, and additional efforts have to be made to introduce innovative, pathogen-directed strategies in clinical application.

The following chapter reviews our current state of knowledge on several aspects of the biology and clinical implications of catheter-associated infections due to CoNS.

PATHOGENESIS

With CoNS being a resident organism of the skin and mucous membranes of both patient and medical personnel, it is generally thought that these sources are the most common origin for infection of indwelling catheters (8). Additional sources for catheter colonization and infection may include the bloodstream or intravenous fluids. In particular, the bloodstream may cause hematogenous seeding with CoNS, as exposure to unrelated bacteremia is a strong risk factor for catheter-related infection in ICU patients (9). This patient group may be particularly prone to short-term, clinically inapparent bacteremia, but CoNS bacteremia appears to be frequent even in healthy persons. In addition to bacteremia, the severity of the underlying disease and subsequently the frequency and invasiveness of disease-related interventions have been demonstrated to be independent risk factors (10), whereas others (such as the duration of catheterization or hospitalization) appear to be cofactors for catheter-related infections rather than independent risk factors. However, while these more general aspects of the formal pathogenesis (discussed in detail in Chapter 2) are applicable to catheter infections caused by CoNS, several particular aspects of the biology of CoNS contributing to pathogenicity merit further discussion (Fig. 1).

After the discovery that catheters and implants are a frequent source of sepsis and infections due to CoNS, various materials used in biomedicine were analyzed with respect to their susceptibility to CoNS colonization, and it became clear that CoNS are able to attach to a wide range of materials such as thermoplastic polyurethane, silicone elastomer, ungrafted or grafted polyurethane, and teflon (11). Soon it was recognized that the basic pathogenetic events resulting in CoNS catheter-related infections consist of a two-step process: adherence to the surface and accumulation with slime and biofilm

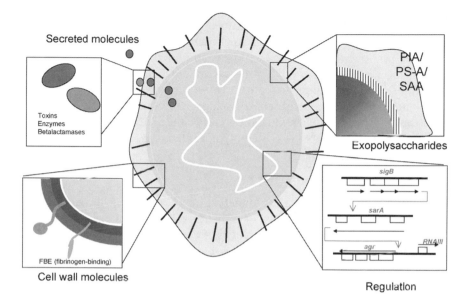

Figure 1 Structure–function relationship of coagulase-negative staphylococci. CoNS provide several types of pathogenicity and virulence factors. Among these, secreted molecules with matrix- and tissue-degrading activity as well as a cell wall adhesin with fibrinogen-binding activity are present. Several factors contribute to biofilm formation: The polysaccharide intercellular adhesin (PIA) [which is structurally and closely homologous to the polysaccharide adhesin (PS/A) and the slime-associated antigen (SAA)] plays a major role by mediating cell–cell interaction and formation of a mature biofilm (see also Figure 3). Additional factors such as the accumulation-associated protein (AAP) appear to be involved in biofilm formation; their role is yet to be established. The expression of various of these virulence factors is coordinated by a global regulator system consisting of *sigB*, *sarA*, and *agr*. The respective contribution of these and putative additional regulators to bacterial adaptation as well as their interaction are only partially resolved.

production on the surface. Tests have been developed to determine the ability of CoNS to adhere to polymers and/or to form biofilm (12,13), and various earlier studies with clinical isolates have supported this concept (14–19). Both steps depend on bacterial and surface properties that are in turn greatly conditioned by spatial and temporal determinants (20). For example, the surface properties of the extracutaneous portion of an inserted catheter is largely different from the intravascular portion, the composition of protein-aceous and cellular elements deposited on the intravascular catheter surface depends on the time of insertion, and even the microbial surface character-istics differ as a function of the localization of the organism on the skin or in the vessel milieu. Therefore, the factors contributing to catheter colonization by CoNS cannot be viewed independently of these conditions, and it has to be acknowledged that most in vitro experiments studying the adherence or accumulation phenomena have employed simplified surface conditions that do not correspond to the subtle physical or biochemical surface gradients encountered in indwelling catheters. However, over the last few years, examination of singular factors contributing to the complex events ultimately resulting in catheter colonization have greatly enhanced our understanding of the pathogenicity of CoNS in these polymer infections.

Adherence to Polymer Surfaces

The first step in the colonization or infection of a polymer device is the—probably irreversible—adherence of a bacterial cell to the polymer surface (21–24). CoNS may attach to surfaces through nonspecific and specific interactions (Fig. 2). In saline, buffer, or other nutrient- and protein-free media, the main nonspecific forces mediating attachment are electrostatic and hydrophobic interactions (23,24). The DLVO theory (termed according to its first describers Derjaguin & Landau and Vervey & Overbeek) regards adhesion as a balance between van der Waals attraction and electrostatic repulsion; using sophisticated optical trap methods, its validity for attachment of colloidal, bacterial-sized particles has been demonstrated (25). According to the thermodynamic model, adherence is the net result of all active forces and is dependent on the surface properties of both the bacterial cell and the polymer in a given liquid environment. In general, the more hydrophobic strains adhere more strongly to hydrophobic polymers than hydrophilic strains. Finally, attachment of most Gram-positive microorganisms is greatly promoted on positively charged polymers, owing to the overall negative bacterial surface charge and is strongly reduced on negatively charged polymers due to repulsion.

In CoNS, contributive factors to most of these mechanisms have been identified. Almost all CoNS strains are able to attach to unadsorbed polymer surfaces, albeit at different quantitative levels (22,26). A number of specific CoNS factors contributing to this attachment have been described. The large staphylococcal surface proteins SSP-1 and SSP-2 have been identified and antigenically characterized (27,28), yet these findings may be restricted to one *S. epidermidis* isolate, and neither the molecular characterization of the proteins nor the attachment-contributive mechanisms have been elucidated. Using transposon mutagenesis (29), the gene encoding the surface-associated autolysin AtlE of *S. epidermidis* O-47 that mediates primary attachment of bacterial cells to a polymer surface has been cloned and sequenced (30). This molecule is proteolytically processed and comprises an amidase and a glucoaminidase domain, as well as three central repetitive sequences. Loss of this protein results in a significantly reduced surface hydrophobicity, but at present it is not clear whether specific domains such as the central repeat

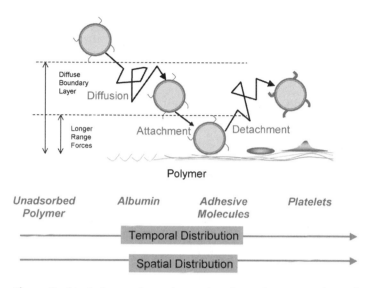

Figure 2 Staphylococcal attachment is a dynamic process. According to the laws of mass transport, particles in a colloidal fluid will be moved toward a surface by Brownian motion forces or directed flow. After surpassing repulsive forces governed by physicochemical interactions in the surface vicinity, they will ultimately attach through nonspecific or specific (macromolecule-mediated) interactions. Attachment is irreversible in many cases, but in the presence of shear rates or other forces, single organisms or clusters may also detach, particularly if multiple cells accumulate on the surface, ultimately resulting in bacteremia. The conditions resulting in catheter colonization vary as a function of time (duration of catheter insertion; adsorption of adhesive blood factors) and localization of the respective catheter portion (extra-cutaneous, transcutaneous, endovascular portion).

region or the overall modification of the physicochemical surface character-istics contribute to this effect.

Aside from proteins, a polysaccharide designated as polysaccharide/adhesin (PS/A) has been associated with initial adherence in vitro (31). This polysaccharide, which is identical or at least highly homologous to the polysaccharide intercellular adhesin (PIA) (see later discussion in this chapter), has also been shown to be involved in virulence in select animal models (32–34). In addition to these factors, cell wall properties also contrib-ute to primary attachment to unadsorbed polymers. The overall negative staphylococcal surface charge is due to the fact that the teichoic acids con-tain fewer positively charged D-alanine residues than negatively charged phosphate groups (35). Accordingly, a mutant deficient in D-alanine esters displays reduced attachment to polystyrene (36). The mutant has been con-structed in an *S. aureus* background, but it is conceivable that similar condi-tions are also operative in CoNS.

If polymer surfaces are in contact with colloidal fluids such as serum or blood plasma, proteins such as albumin are immediately adsorbed to the surface, resulting in a major change of the physicochemical surface characteristics (37,38). In fact, many physical forces contributing to nonspecific adhesion such as hydrophobic interaction are greatly reduced after this surface modification, and when tested in vitro, adhesion of CoNS to hydrophobic polymer surfaces is often largely diminished compared to adhesion to unadsorbed surfaces (39). In noncolloidal buffer systems, even preadsorption of adhesive proteins may rather reduce adhesion of CoNS compared to adhesion to unadsorbed plastic, probably due to the aforementioned modification of physicochemical interaction (40).

Compared to attachment to unadsorbed polymers in a physiological colloidal milieu, however, surface adsorption with certain adhesive proteins generally promotes adhesion greatly, as numerous in vitro studies have shown. Fibrin deposits on catheter material may promote bacterial colonization (41–43), and thrombus formation on a catheter has been identified as a major risk factor for device infection (44). Extracellular matrix proteins such as fibrinogen (45), fibronectin (46), laminin (47), collagen (48), thrombospondin (49), and vitronectin have been shown to bind to *S. aureus* and to promote adhesion of *S. aureus* to solid surfaces (50), most importantly via specific adhesins of the microbial surface components recognizing adhesive matrix molecules (MSCRAMM) type of molecule (51). In contrast, CoNS lack most of the MSCRAMM type of adhesins. Nevertheless, in a physiological milieu, several matrix molecules bind to CoNS and promote attachment. In contrast to *S. aureus*, only limited information is available on the nature and genetic organization of adhesins on *S. epidermidis*-recognizing extracellular matrix proteins. A fibrinogen-binding protein homologous to the MSCRAMM family of cell wall proteins has been identified in *S. epidermidis* (52). This molecule has been termed Fbe. A mutant deficient in Fbe production displays reduced attachment to fibrinogen-coated surfaces (53), and the use of anti-Fbe-antibodies interferes with attachment to immobilized fibrinogen (54). SdrG, another *S. epidermidis* adhesin of the MSCRAMM family, interacts with the Bβ-chain of fibrinogen (55). While fibronectin has been shown to promote adhesion of a large number of *S. epidermidis* strains to polymer surfaces in vitro (50) and fibronectin in vivo adsorbed on catheter material does also promote adhesion of *S. epidermidis* strain RP62A (56), a fibronectin-binding adhesin in CoNS has remained elusive. More recently, work with purified teichoic acid from *S. epidermidis* has shown that this cell wall constituent may contain site(s) active in recognition of surface-adsorbed fibronectin by *S. epidermidis* (57). Most recently, using phage display, a fibrinonectin-binding protein from *S. epidermidis* (Embp) has been identified (58). Further characterization of its role using deletion mutants in appropriate test systems and information on the presence of this protein in various *S. epidermidis* isolates and non-*S. epidermidis* CoNS species are warranted. Finally, it has been demonstrated that not only *S. aureus* but also *S. epidermidis* may interact with immobilized platelets (59). This is likely due to specific, albeit unresolved, mechanisms (20) that may also involve the expression of CoNS exopolysaccharides (60). While CoNS may adhere to polymeric surfaces due to physicochemical binding forces, specific ligand–adhesin-type mechanisms may involve certain extracellular matrix and plasma proteins. This interaction may even occur in complex cooperative binding events.

Accumulation on Polymer Surfaces, Production of Extracellular Slime, and Biofilm Formation

The rapid process of primary adherence is followed by a more time-consuming step, namely, the accumulation on the polymer surface. Biofilm formation has been studied in great detail allowing researchers to establish the typical growth patterns of CoNS on polymer surfaces (Fig. 3).

Morphological investigations on various types of intravascular catheters using scanning electron microscopy (SEM) and transmission electron microscopy (TEM) gained the first insight into the pathogenesis of these infections. In a stationary in vitro catheter-colonization model it could be demonstrated that CoNS organisms adhere to the polymer surface independently of the presence of surface irregularities (61,62). With increasing incubation time, microcolonies and finally multiple cell layers are formed on the polymer surface. Starting with an incubation time of about 12 h, the adherent cells become covered by a thin film of material that steadily increases in thickness. Most of the attached cells are then covered by this slime matrix produced by the staphylococci. These observations could subsequently be confirmed on various other ex vivo materials (63–65). Thus, from these early studies, it could be shown that staphylococci are able to adhere to and grow on polymer surfaces. In the course of surface colonization, they produce an extracellular slime substance in which they become entirely embedded, and a biofilm is produced. The morphology of this surface colonization is identical both in vivo and in vitro, suggesting similar mechanisms. These observations lead to the hypothesis that the slime matrix or biofilm, respectively, may protect the embedded staphylococci against host response mechanisms as well as against antibiotics (66).

These morphological studies show that *S. epidermidis* forms multiple cell layers on the polymer surface; the cells in these layers are enveloped and protected by copious amounts of an amorphous slimy material. The slime substance is not a capsule but loosely associated with the staphylococcal cells. If plasma or serum is present during an experiment or in vivo, host serum proteins may also be involved in the build-up of this matrix. The slimy material is so prominent upon morphological examination that it has been attributed a pathogenic role in polymer infection since its discovery. The nature of its composition, however, has remained elusive for a prolonged

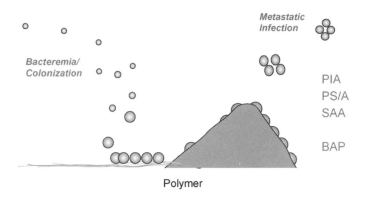

Accumulation

Figure 3 Staphylococcal accumulation on artificial surfaces results in manifest biofilm formation. After primary attachment, coagulase-negative staphylococci form intercell interactions, express an exopolysaccharide [mainly consisting of an atypical β-1,6-linked *N*-acetyiglucosamine (PIA)], and ultimately form mature biofilms with multiple consequences on the efficacy of local host defense mechanisms and antimicrobial activity (see text). Other (protein) factors associated with biofilm production such as the accumulation-associated protein (AAP) have been identified; the mechanisms of their action is unresolved.

period, as contamination with medium-derived compounds has impeded its chemical analysis (67,68), and until 1996, reports on the chemical composition of the slime were conflicting. Mack et al. identified a polysaccharide antigen from *S. epidermidis* strain 1457 induced by glucose whose expression paralleled CoNS accumulation (69). Subsequently, approaches using transposon mutants deficient in this antigen (70) and biochemical characterizations (71) allowed for the identification of highly similar polysaccharides in CoNS presenting a unique structure composed of β-1,6-linked *N*-acetylglucosamine residues. According to the attributed function, this polysaccharide was named polysaccharide intercellular adhesin (PIA). Pier and colleagues have isolated a galactose-rich capsular polysaccharide adhesin (PS/A) from *S. epidermidis* RP62A that mediates attachment to polymer silastic catheter tubings (72). Antibodies against this antigen block adherence, stabilize its structure, and can be used for protection (73). The similarity or identity of PS/A and PIA has been an issue of debate; more recently, it has been proven that PS/A is at least closely related to PIA, as it is also a 1,6-linked *N*-acetylglucosamine (74). Furthermore, the slime-associated antigen, originally described by Christensen et al. (75), appears also to be antigenically and biochemically highly similar when compared with PIA (76).

    The genetic basis of the expression of PIA has been resolved by the identification of the *icaADBC* locus (77,78). *icaA* contains the *N*-acetylglucosaminyltransferase activity, and *icaC* allows for expression of long-chain polymers essential for antigenicity and biofilm formation. PIA expression represents a factor contributing to *S. epidermidis* pathogenicity, as in a mouse foreign-body infection model, a PIA-negative mutant was shown to be significantly less virulent compared to wildtype (79). Expression of PIA may also be modified by an insertional element, IS256, into the *icaADBC* gene cluster (80,81). On the other hand, additional *icaADBC*-independent factors appear to be operative for functional biofilm expression (82). Elucidation of the *icaADBC* gene cluster allowed for identification of PIA analogues [termed poly-*N*-succinyl glucosamine (PNSG)] also in *S. aureus* (83,84). As it has now been shown that this analogue is not succinylated, it has been renamed poly-*N*-acetylglucosamine (PNAG)(74). Again, PNAG is strongly chemically related to PIA. It is intriguing that both *S. aureus* and *S. epidermidis* appear to express a family of highly related antigens allowing for cell–cell interaction and resulting in accumulative growth both on artificial and on biological substrates.

However, besides PIA, other factors seem to be necessary for intercellular adherence and biofilm formation. Detailed examination of an adhesion-positive, accumulation-negative CoNS mutant revealed the lack of a 140-kDa protein in the mutant. Consequently, a putative function of this 140-kDa protein in the accumulation process of the wildtype was therefore attributed (85). Subsequent studies demonstrated that the antibodies raised against the 140-kDa antigen [now referred to as accumulation-associated antigen, (AAP)] could block biofilm formation, and that in a panel of clinical *S. epidermidis* isolates, the presence of the antigen positively correlated with biofilm formation (86). Meanwhile, AAP has been cloned and sequenced, and complementation studies are under way to determine the mechanism of its involvement in the accumulation process. In *S. aureus*, a biofilm-associated protein (BAP) has been described, albeit mainly observed in nonhuman (dairy) isolates (87). This molecule interferes with the interaction of *S. aureus* with extracellular matrix molecules (88). A BAP-analogue nucleotide sequence has been identified in *S. epidermidis* strain RP62A (Tormo et al., unpublished; GenBank accession # AY028618); the mechanisms and its role in pathogenicity have to be determined.

Biofilm formation—PIA-dependent and -independent—appears to be controlled by global gene regulators in *S. epidermidis*. Global gene regulators control the concerted expression of various adaptive and virulence factors in staphylococci via complex regulatory networks that are only partially understood, particularly in CoNS. One regulator that has attracted considerable scientific attention is the alternative sigma factor σ^B regulating gene expression upon environmental stress. The respective gene, *sigB*, is also linked to the expression of PIA conferred by icaADBC (84,89,90), but in one study a *sigB* deletion mutant did not show alterations in biofilm formation (91). Another global regulator that is well investigated in *S. aureus* is the accessory gene regulator *agr*. The role of this regulator is also increasingly understood in

S. epidermidis. Interestingly, *agr* encodes a two-component system as well as its autoinducing ligand (92). As *agr* is autoinduced by an extracellular ligand, it represents a sensor of population density, and the autoinducing peptide pheromones (containing a cyclic thiolactone residue) may confer cross-species inhibiting properties (93). Thus, in a complex milieu such as in biofilms, staphylococci may sense the bacterial population characteristics and accordingly adapt the global regulation of effector genes, a mechanism termed quorum sensing. In addition to the aforementioned pheromones, heptapeptides disrupting quorum-sensing mechanisms have been described (94). While these observations led to exciting hypotheses of bacterial interference mediated by bacterial quorum sensing, recent evidence from in vivo studies in humans of *agr* alleles of nasal colonizing isolates suggests a more important role of biological coselection of certain genetic backgrounds associated with a given *agr* genotype (95). Finally, a homologue of the *sarA* regulator, which in *S. aureus* carries multiple regulatory functions on cell wall adhesin expression and *agr* activation, is also found in *S. epidermidis*; however, the interpromoter region of this *sarA* gene differs from its *S. aureus* counterpart, possibly suggesting target gene differences and a disparate pattern for *sar* activation (96).

Insight into these regulatory phenomenona may ultimately result in practical approaches for alternative treatment strategies. For example, salicylic acid, the primary metabolite of aspirin, has been shown to exert profound effects on biofilm formation (97). Most recently, it has been shown that salicylic acid mediates a downregulation of staphylococcal *agr* and another regulator, *sar* (98). This mechanism may contribute to eradication of biofilm-forming *S. epidermidis* by a combination therapy consisting of salicylic acid and vancomycin (99).

Additional Important Virulence Factors in CoNS Catheter Infections

The clinical experience with polymer-associated staphyloccocal infections clearly shows that the host seems to be unable, in many cases, to handle the infection and in particular to eliminate the staphyloccoci from the infected polymer device (100,101). Opsonization and subsequent phagocytosis by polymorphonuclear neutrophils (PMN) and macrophages are the major response mechanisms of the human host against staphyloccoci. Therefore, several investigations have addressed the question of whether surface-grown staphyloccoci resist opsonophagocytosis and whether extracellular slime and biofilm production may contribute to this resistance.

Nearly all experimental data available have been derived using *S. epidermidis* and crude extracellular slime substance (ESS) produced by *S. epidermidis* in chemically defined and contaminant-free medium. These data have demonstrated that ESS elicits a significant chemotactic response but also a decreased responsiveness to known chemotactic stimuli in human PMN (102–104). PMN preincubated with ESS also showed enhanced adherence to plastic wells and a decrease in chemiluminescence response, whereas PMN degranulation was enhanced. Furthermore, ESS interfered with bacterial opsonization with the extracellular slime substance acting as a physical barrier for the deposition of complement or IgG on the cell surface (19,105). Taken together, these effects may effectively lead to a decreased ability for intracellular killing of CoNS by PMN. In addition, the interference of *S. epidermidis* ESS with PMN function may even be enhanced by the negative effects of the polymer itself on PMN function (106). *S. epidermidis* ESS seems also to interfere with other host defense mechanisms such as T-cell proliferation, T-cell surface antigen presentation patterns, and NK cell activity (107–111).

Another fact based on clinical experience is that antibacterial chemotherapy is often not able to cure catheter-associated staphylococcal infections despite the use of antibiotics with proven in vitro acitivity (112). It has been postulated that staphylococci growing on a polymer surface and embedded in a biofilm matrix consisting of ESS may be protected against the action of administered antibiotics. Using various approaches, this concept could generally be experimentally confirmed (12,113–116). These experimental findings could at least partially explain the clinical experience of antibiotic failure in cases of catheter-associated CoNS infections. Surface-grown CoNS probably exhibit a special type of surface growth-associated phenotypic resistance that does not appear in liquid growth.

Several extracellular enzymes secreted from CoNS have been reported to have matrix- or tissue-degrading activity. Among these are a metalloprotease with elastase activity (117), a serine protease (epiP) (118,119), several lipases (120,121), and a putative nuclease analogue. With completion of the genome data of *S. epidermidis*, additional enzymes are expected to be identified. In contrast, the presence of genes encoding for toxin production in CoNS has been a long matter of debate. More recently, it has been shown that the genes encoding toxic shock syndrome toxin 1, exfoliative toxins, and classical enterotoxins were absent in a large collection of isolates belonging to various CoNS species (122). Therefore, it has to be assumed that toxin-mediated disease, particularly disease mediated by the superantigen activity of certain toxins produced by *S. aureus*, is not relevant in catheter-related infections caused by human CoNS isolates.

MICROBIOLOGY

Coagulase-negative staphylococci are members of the family of Micrococcaceae. These Gram-positive, cluster-forming microorganisms are differentiated from *S. aureus* primarily by the lack of the exoenzyme coagulase (which in

S. aureus forms fibrin by activation of thrombin). Additional markers used in the clinical microbiology workup to differentiate *S. aureus* from CoNS are the lack of the immunoglobulin G (IgG)-binding protein A (Spa) as well as the lack of certain cell wall adhesins recognizing matrix and plasma molecules such as the clumping factor (Clf). Moreover, CoNS do not possess certain capsular polysaccharides (Cps) specific for *S. aureus* such as the type 5/8 Cps associated with *S. aureus* invasive disease. Accordingly, for diagnostic purposes, the group of CoNS is differentiated from *S. aureus* using rabbit plasma and performing either the slide clumping test or the tube coagulase test. Several rapid commercial latex agglutination tests examining the presence of Clf, Spa, and Cps are also available. In addition, biochemical reactions (e.g., mannitol fermentation) may allow lab technicians to distinguish between *S. aureus* and CoNS. With the use of nucleic acid amplification techniques, additional markers such as the gene for the *S. aureus* thermonuclease (alone or in conjunction with other markers such as the *coa* gene) have been used for rapid discrimination of CoNS.

CoNS have been subdivided into 32 species; 15 of these species have been associated with human disease. Biochemical characterization has been the mainstay for species identification since the first identification scheme by Kloos and Schleifer (123), and miniaturized biochemical panels are now available for use in manual, semiautomatic, or automatic identification systems. Most CoNS involved in polymer-associated infections belong to the *S. epidermidis* group (*S. epidermidis sensu stricto, Staphylococcus hominis, Staphylococcus haemolyticus, Staphylococcus warneri, Staphylococcus capitis*). Within the *S. epidermidis* group, *S. epidermidis sensu stricto* accounts for about two-thirds of all strains (124). This observation reflects the situation present in the normal human microflora and is also known from other coagulase-negative staphylococcal infections, for instance, in immunocompromised patients. In addition to members of the *S. epidermidis* group, *Staphylococcus schleiferi* and particularly *Staphylococcus lugdunensis* (125) have also been implicated with clinical disease. *Staphylococcus saprophyticus* (126) is an infrequent pathogen in urinary tract infections; it does not play a particular role in endovascular device-associated infections.

To address the question whether a given CoNS isolate (e.g., from a catheter tip or the exit site) is to be regarded as the cause of a systemic infection, typing methods have been used. Conventional methods including antibiotic resistance profiles, biochemical reaction patterns, and phage typing are often of limited value in differentiating isolates. Plasmid profiling and sodium dodecyl sulphate polyacrylamide gel electrophoresis (SDS-PAGE) patterns of extracellular proteins have been more successfully used for epidemiological studies or other purposes (127,128), but some strains are not typeable using these assays. Modern genomic methods with a high discriminatory power include arbitrarily primed polymerase chain reaction (PCR) (129) and pulsed-field gel electrophoresis (130). All these methods have been shown to be extremely useful for revealing epidemiological or etiological links associated with CoNS infections (131,132), but they are of limited value in distinguishing catheter-associated from commensal CoNS strains.

CoNS from nosocomial infections, particularly *S. epidermidis*, are typically resistant to multiple antimicrobials, particularly to β-lactams. While almost all CoNS produce penicillinase, most clinical isolates are resistant to penicillinase-resistant penicillins as well as to all other β-lactams due to expression of *mecA* analogues conferring resistance to methicillin by production of a penicillin-binding protein (PBP2a or PBP2′) with reduced affinity to β-lactams. In fact, on the basis of homology studies it has been suggested that the *mecA* gene in *S. aureus* arose from a *mecA* analogue in *Staphylococcus sciuri* (133). In addition, many clinical CoNS isolates are resistant to macrolides, chloramphenicol, tetracyclines, fluorquinolones, aminoglycosides, and cotrimoxazol. Finally, CoNS species were the first staphylococci with reduced susceptibility to glycopeptides such as vancomycin (134).

EPIDEMIOLOGY

Based upon the data from an enormous amount of case reports and clinical studies extensively reviewed elsewhere (135), there is no doubt that staphylococci are the most frequently isolated organisms involved in polymer-associated infections. Furthermore, it is obvious that coagulase-negative staphylococci (CoNS) generally predominate over *S. aureus*, especially in infections associated with intravascular catheters. Approximately 30–40% of central venous catheter-related infections are caused by coagulase-negative staphylococcal species (136,137); other authors report that *S. epidermidis* accounts for up to 75% of the cultured microorganisms (138). This proportion is irrespective of the type of catheter and includes long-term-implanted as well as short-term-inserted catheters, Swan-Ganz catheters, catheters used for specific purposes such as plasmapheresis or hemodialysis, or hyperalimentation catheters, which have all been shown to yield CoNS, particularly *S. epidermidis*, as the leading microorganism (138). CoNS have also been increasingly isolated from the blood of hospitalized patients; again, this increase is thought to be in large part due to an increase in line-associated CoNS infections (2,139).

CLINICAL MANIFESTATIONS

From the clinical point of view, one can examine staphylococcal catheter-associated infections according to their onset, i.e., the time of the first clinical manifestation of disease: early-onset infections occur within days or weeks after implantation (Hickman-Broviac) or insertion (Sheldon, Swan-Ganz, central venous catheter) of an intravascular catheter. In these cases, the inoculation of the pathogen takes place at the time of the respective procedure, and late-onset infections occur after a much longer interval of several weeks or even months, and according to some authors, even as long as six months later. Late-onset infections may be caused by true late hematogenous infection, but the inoculation of the pathogen may also occur at the time of surgical or nonsurgical insertion of the catheter, followed by a long latent phase.

Fever is a frequent sign for CoNS bacteremia, but even in the case of bacteremia only a moderate elevation of the temperature usually occurs. Additional signs of sepsis such as chills, hypotension and shock, hyperventilation and respiratory failure, and gastrointestinal and neurological symptoms would be more suggestive of infusate-related Gram-negative bacteremia (140). In fact, device-associated infections, particularly those caused by low-virulence organisms such as CoNS, are characterized by a paucity of specific symptoms pointing toward the catheter as the source of infection (141). Moreover, local signs of superficial inflammation may be unspecific (142), and only approximately 50% of patients with CoNS catheter infections exhibit local signs of inflammation such as redness, warmth, tenderness, or purulence at the catheter exit site (141). Clinical signs of spreading cellulitis around the subcutaneous tunnel tract of long-term catheters may be more indicative of pathogens other than CoNS. Thus, in the absence of a purulent exit site [a sign that is highly indicative of catheter infection (143)], the catheter can only be suspected as the origin of infection, and a microbiological examination has to be performed to confirm or exclude this diagnosis. The long-lasting nature of the infection is a further characteristic of CoNS infections, especially if the infected device is not removed. In these cases, other signs of chronic infection such as anemia or splenomegaly may appear. In fatal cases, multiple micro-abscesses can be found during autopsy in parenchymatous organs, especially in the spleen, liver, and lung.

DIAGNOSIS

Local infection of the intraluminal catheter segment (tip) is usually asserted by culture of the removed catheter portion. CoNS species can be isolated from 8–40% of removed catheters (141), but only a small percentage of these catheters will become the source for catheter-related bacteremia. Thus, the application of (semi)quantitative catheter culture techniques, described in Chapter 3, to identify catheters as being contaminated in contrast to colonized or locally infected (the latter being more frequently associated with bacteremia) (144–146) is both appropriate and necessary if CoNS are suspected as the cause for a nosocomial bloodstream infection.

Whereas the definitive diagnosis of catheter-related sepsis is based on the recovery of the same organism on the catheter segments and in the blood together with corresponding clinical symptoms, several studies have shown that between 70 and 90% of catheters removed for suspicion of catheter-related bacteremia were not infected and, in fact, could have been maintained (8,136,147). As the placement of a new catheter carries significant risks (148) and elevated costs, and as routine catheter exchanges without clinical or microbiological evidence for a bloodstream infection are not indicated (149), noninvasive methods including rapid techniques (150), quantitative hemo-cultures drawn both peripherically and through the implicated catheter (151,152), and the combined use of superficial hub and skin cultures have been developed to prove or rule out catheter infection with the catheter maintained (see Chapter 3). More recently, differential time to positivity of blood cultures drawn in parallel through a peripheral vein and a suspected catheter has been successfully employed (153,154) for indirect identification of the catheter as the source of nosocomial bacteremia. In most instances, however, catheter-related bacteremia caused by CoNS is suspected due to one or several positive conventional blood cultures in a patient with vascular access and fever. Yet, isolation of commensal skin organisms such as CoNS from a peripheral blood culture may reflect a contamination rather than true bacteremia (155). Thus, it has been proposed that more than one blood culture yielding the same species should be required to establish the diagnosis of true bacteremia (156). In addition, modern typing techniques may be useful for proof of identity of the isolates, particularly if a precious catheter such as a Broviac-Hickman or a Port catheter is suspected for infection (157). Previously, in the presence of bacteremia, it was deemed necessary to remove the implicated catheter both as a therapeutic and diagnostic measure yielding the intravascular catheter as the most reliable specimen segment. However, as single blood cultures positive for CoNS may not necessarily be due to an infected intravascular catheter, this finding should rather prompt additional culture attempts rather than catheter removal.

MANAGEMENT/THERAPY

If infection is suspected either because of local signs of infection with or without positive superficial cultures or because of fever and/or positive blood cultures, several aspects have to be considered for optimal management: (i) the type and severity of infection (exit-site infection, deep tunnel infection, or systemic catheter-related bacteremia), (ii) the type of underlying disease, and (iii) the necessity or at least the interest to maintain the catheter.

Taken together, the results from the various studies amount to the following approach to a patient with suspected or proven catheter-related infection due to CoNS. Local exit-site inflammation usually does not require catheter ablation and can be treated with local care (158). Purulent tunnel infections are usually an indication for catheter removal (158). However, in patients with catheter-related bacteremia due to CoNS, a catheter-conserving approach can be successfully employed (in >80% of the cases) (147,159). This now more generally accepted approach carries a 20% chance that bacteremia will recur, whereas only a 3% risk of recurrence is present when the catheter is removed (160). Catheter salvage has been also successfully employed in pediatric patients (161,162). Therefore, in the case of CoNS bacteremia suspected to be catheter-related, different approaches may feasible; the choice of either of the following alternatives depends on the individual patient situation and the diagnostic possibilities provided by the clinical microbiology laboratory:

1. In the case of severe disease or of underlying severe immunodeficiency (such as the pediatric neonatal or the neutropenic host), the suspect catheter should be removed, preferably after application of an antibiotic dose through the device before insertion of a new catheter at a new site. The same approach may be used for patients with risk factors for endovascular CoNS infections, such as patients with endovascular grafts. It is generally recommended to treat catheter-related bloodstream infections systemically with appropriate antibiotics. This also applies for bloodstream infection caused by CoNS, although the risk of a complicated course and the emergence of infectious sequelae is considerably lower compared with *S. aureus* bloodstream infections. The duration of therapy is debated; most experts opt for a 5–7-day course, usually with a glycopeptide antibiotic (163,164). Experimental compounds against *S. epidermidis* have been developed (165) and new antimicrobials with activity against CoNS have been introduced into clinical practice (166,167). Furthermore, the use of established alternatives in combination with other antistaphylococcal substances has been evaluated (168). However, at this point, their specific value in catheter-related bacteremia has not been established, and they should be retained for infections with organisms resistant to standard therapeutic approaches. At any rate, upon presence of CoNS bacteremia, the need for further vascular catheterization should be reevaluated and unnecessary vascular accesses should be removed and cultured.

2. If the catheter is valuable, it may be maintained, and exit-site and hub cultures as well as additional quantitative blood cultures may help to estimate the probability of establishing catheter-related bacteremia. In the case of isolation of CoNS from the blood and suspicion of its relatedness to an infected catheter, systemic therapy may be initiated even without these diagnostic procedures, since the cure rate of a CoNS-infected catheter by systemic antimicrobials is high. Alternatively, the catheter may be treated using the antibiotic-lock technique (169). Of course, the catheter must be dispensable for at least several hours. Multiple-lumen catheters may be cured using a rotative lock technique. If the clinical situation does not

improve, or if blood cultures remain positive, the removal of the catheter is imperative. Techniques to exchange the catheter over a guidewire have been employed for various catheter types (170), but they have become less popular because of the risks of embolization or of seeding of microorganisms to the new catheter (171,172), as well as the cumbersome nature of the technique.

Over the past few years, the previously uniform therapeutic approach to the patient with CoNS vascular catheter infection has become considerably nuanced. This implies new diagnostic and therapeutic challenges both for the clinician and the clinical microbiology laboratory, but it helps to optimize treatment of patients who rely on increasingly sophisticated vascular access devices for monitoring and therapy.

PREVENTION AND CONTROL

Preventive measures to reduce catheter-related infections caused by CoNS employ the same principles as those established for the prevention of catheter-related infections in general. Therefore, the aspects discussed in Chapter 5 also apply for the prevention of catheter infections caused by CoNS. Scrupulous adherence to the measures proposed in the published guidelines (137) and avoidance of systemic antibiotic prophylaxis are the mainstays in the prevention of CoNS catheter infections.

Whereas a number of strategies involving modification of catheter surfaces have been employed to interfere with bacterial colonization and prevent subsequent infection such as antimicrobial or antiadhesive impregnation and coatings [e.g., using silver-impregnated cuffs, heparin, or antimicrobial agents (173–175)], comparably little information is available describing specific interference with known staphylococcal pathogenicity factors for prevention of catheter-associated infections. Lack of the fibrinogen-binding protein Fbe confers reduced attachment to fibrinogen-coated catheter materials (53). Antibodies directed against PS/A protect animals from catheter-related bacteremia (32). Anti-Aap antibodies prevent biofilm formation of *S. epidermidis* in vitro (86). However, none of these or other observations have yet been translated into a practical approach to prevent staphylococcal catheter infections in humans. Thus, further research targeting CoNS catheter colonization is necessary to develop novel preventive strategies without employing antimicrobials or antiseptics that may carry the risk of selection of resistant isolates.

IX. SUMMARY AND CONCLUSION

Coagulase-negative staphylococci represent the major organism associated with catheter-related infections. The importance of this group of pathogens in primary nosocomial bloodstream infections cannot be overemphasized. In clinical practice, the differentiation between true CoNS bacteremia from contamination remains a challenge; however, the role of these microorganisms as true pathogens is undoubtable. This fact has greatly spurred research on pathogenic mechanisms of CoNS resulting in important advances of our understanding of artificial surface colonization and host defense mechanisms. Refined diagnostic procedures to identify the catheter as a source for bacteremia and an individualized approach for treatment have enlarged our spectrum of options in the handling of patients with suspected or proven catheter-related bacteremia. Technical advances and guidelines for catheter insertion and care have also contributed to the control of primary CoNS bacteremia. On the other hand, in most instances, clinical CoNS isolates are highly resistant, and the mainstay of therapy, glycopeptides, has been recently challenged by the emergence of isolates with reduced susceptibility. In addition, the placement of a vascular access with increasingly sophisticated catheters is indispensable in most hospitalized patients. This challenge has been coined by Dennis Maki as "Devices versus Nature" (176). The need to translate the exciting results of 25 years of insightful research on the biology of these pathogens into applicable preventive and therapeutic strategies is more present than ever.

ACKNOWLEDGMENTS

The authors gratefully acknowledge grant support by the Deutsche Forschungsgemeinschaft (DFG priority programmes 1047 and 1130, DFG collaborative research centers 293 and 492), the University of Saarland, and the Medical Faculty of the University of Muenster.

REFERENCES

1. Vuong C, Otto M. *Staphylococcus epidermidis* infections. Microbes Infect 2002; 4:481–489.
2. Schaberg DR, Culver DH, Gaynes RP. Major trends in the microbial etiology of nosocomial infection. Am J Med 1991; 91(suppl 3B):72S–75S.
3. Finkelstein R, Fusman R, Oren I, Kassis I, Hashman N. Clinical and epidemiologic significance of coagulase-negative staphylococci bacteremia in a tertiary care university Israeli hospital. Am J Infect Control 2002; 30:21–25.
4. Lark RL, Chenoweth C, Saint S, Zemencuk JK, Lipsky BA, Plorde JJ. Four year prospective evaluation of nosocomial bacteremia: epidemiology, microbiology, and patient outcome. Diagn Microbiol Infect Dis 2000; 38:131–140.
5. Thylefors JD, Harbarth S, Pittet D. Increasing bacteremia due to coagulase-negative staphylococci: fiction or reality? Infect Control Hosp Epidemiol 1998; 19:581–589.
6. Raad I, Alrahwan A, Rolston K. *Staphylococcus epidermidis*: emerging resistance and need for alternative agents. Clin Infect Dis 1998; 26:1182–1187.

7. Dunne WM Jr. Bacterial adhesion: seen any good biofilms lately? Clin Microbiol Rev 2002; 15:155–166.
8. Maki DG. Infections due to infusion therapy. In: Bennett JV, Brachman PS, eds. Hospital Infections. Boston: Little, Brown, 1992:849–898.
9. Safdar N, Kluger DM, Maki DG. A review of risk factors for catheter-related bloodstream infection caused by percutaneously inserted, noncuffed central venous catheters: implications for preventive strategies. Medicine (Baltimore) 2002; 81:466–479.
10. Henderson DK. Intravascular device-asociated infection: current concepts and controversies. Infect Surg 1988; 7:365–371.
11. Götz F, Peters G. Colonization of medical devices by coagulase-negative staphylococci. In: Waldvogel FA, Bisno AL, eds. Infections Associated With Indwelling Devices. Washington, D.C.: ASM Press, 2000:55–88.
12. Peters G, Schumacher-Perdreau F, Jansen B, Bey M, Pulverer G. Biology of *Staphylococcus epidermidis* extracellular slime. In: Pulverer G, Quie PG, Peters G, eds. Pathogenicity and clinical significance of coagulase-negative staphylococci. Stuttgart, New York: Gustav Fischer Verlag, 1987:15–32.
13. Christensen GD, Simpson WA, Younger JJ, Baddour LM, Barrett FF, Melton DM, Beachey EH. Adherence of coagulase-negative staphylococci to plastic tissue culture plates: a quantitative model for the adherence of staphylococci to medical devices. J Clin Microbiol 1985; 22:996–1006.
14. Davenport DS, Masanari RM, Pfaller MA, Balc MJ, Streed SA, Hierholzer WJ Jr. Usefulness of a test for slime production as a marker for clinically significant infections with coagulase-negative staphylococci. J Infect Dis 1986; 153:332–339.
15. Deighton MA, Balkau B. Adherence measured by microtiter assay as a virulence marker for *Staphylococcus epidermidis* infections. J Clin Microbiol 1990; 28:2442–2447.
16. Diaz-Mitoma F, Harding GKM, Hoban DJ, Roberts RS, Low DE. Clinical significance for slime production in ventriculoperitoneal shunt infections caused by coagulase-negative staphylococci. J Infect Dis 1987; 156:555–560.
17. Ishak MA, Gröschel DGM, Mandell GL, Wenzel RP. Association of slime with pathogenicity of coagulase-negative staphylocci causing nosocomial septicemia. J Clin Microbiol 1985; 22:1025–1029.
18. Kotilainen P. Association of coagulase-negative staphylococcal slime production and adherence with the development and outcome of adult septicemias. J Clin Microbiol 1990; 28:2779–2785.
19. Kristinsson KG, Spencer RC, Brown CB. Clinical importance of production of slime by coagulase-negative staphylococci in chronic ambulatory peritoneal dialysis. J Clin Pathol 1986; 39:117–118.
20. Anderson JM, Marchant RE. Biomaterials: factors favoring colonization and infection. In: Waldvogel FA, Bisno AL, eds. Infections Associated with Indwelling Medical Devices. Washington, D.C.: ASM Press, 2000:89–109.
21. Dankert J, Hogt AH, Feijen J. Biomedical polymers: Bacterial adhesion, colonization and infection. In: Williams DF, ed. Critical Reviews in Biocompatibility. Boca Raton: CRC Press, 1986:219–301.
22. Espersen F, Wilkinson BJ, Gahrn-Hansen B, Thamdrup Rosdahl V, Clemensen I. Attachment of staphylococci to silicone catheters in vitro. APMIS 1990; 98:471–478.

23. Hogt AH, Dankert J, Hulstaert CE, Feijen J. Cell surface characteristics of coagulase-negative staphylococci and their adherence to fluorinated poly(etylenepropylene). Infect Immun 1986; 51:294–301.

24. Jansen B, Peters G, Pulverer G. Mechanisms and clinical relevance of bacterial adhesion to polymers. J Biomat Appl 1988; 2:520–543.

25. Clapp AR, Ruta AG, Dickinson RB. Three-dimensional optical trapping and evanescent wave light scattering for direct measurement of long range forces between a colloidal particle and a surface. Rev Sci Instrum 1999; 70:2627–2636.

26. Pascual A, Fleer A, Westerdaal NAC, Verhoef J. Modulation of adherence of coagulase-negative staphylococci to teflon catheters in vitro. Eur J Clin Microbiol Infect Dis 1986; 5:518–522.

27. Timmermann CP, Fleer A, Besnier JM, de Graaf L, Cremers F, Verhoef J. Characterization of a proteinaceous adhesion of *Staphylococcus epidermidis* which mediates attachment to polystyrene. Infect Immun 1991; 59:4187–4192.

28. Veenstra GJC, Cremers FFM, Van Dijk H, Fleer A. Ultrastructural organization and regulation of a biomaterial adhesin of *Staphylococcus epidermidis*. J Bacteriol 1996; 178:537–541.

29. Heilmann C, Gerke C, Perdreau-Remington F, Götz F. Characterization of Tn917 insertion mutants of *Staphylococcus epidermidis* affected in biofilm formation. Infect Immun 1996; 64:277–282.

30. Heilmann C, Hussain M, Peters G, Götz F. Evidence for autolysin-mediated primary attachment of *Staphylococcus epidermidis* to a polystyrene surface. Mol Microbiol 1997; 24:1013–1024.

31. Muller E, Hübner J, Guttierez N, Takeda S, Goldman DA, Pier GD. Isolation and characterization of transposon mutants of *Staphylococcus epidermidis* deficient in capsular polysaccharide/adhesin and slime. Infect Immun 1993; 61:551–558.

32. Kojima Y, Tojo M, Goldmann DA, Tosteson TD, Pier GB. Antibody to the capsular polysaccharide/adhesin protects rabbits against catheter-related bacteremia due to coagulase-negative staphylococci. J Infect Dis 1990; 162:435–441.

33. Takeda J, Pier GB, Kojima Y, Tojo M, Muller E, Tosteson TD, Goldman DA. Protection against endocarditis due to *Staphylococcus epidermidis* by immunization with capsular polysaccharide/adhesin. Circulation 1991; 84:2539–2546.

34. Shiro H, Muller E, Guttierez N, Boisot S, Grout M, Tosteson TD, Goldmann D, Pier GB. Transposon mutants of *Staphylococcus epidermidis* deficient in elaboration of capsular polysaccharide/adhesin and slime are avirulent in a rabbit model of endocarditis. J Infect Dis 1994; 169:1042–1049.

35. Peschel A, Otto M, Jack RW, Kalbacher H, Jung G, Gotz F. Inactivation of the dlt operon in *Staphylococcus aureus* confers sensitivity to defensins, protegrins, and other antimicrobial peptides. J Biol Chem 1999; 274:8405–8410.

36. Gross M, Cramton SE, Gotz F, Peschel A. Key role of teichoic acid net charge in *Staphylococcus aureus* colonization of artificial surfaces. Infect Immun 2001; 69:3423–3426.

37. Cottonaro CN, Roohk HV, Shimizu G, Sperling DR. Quantitation and characterization of competitive protein binding to polymers. Transactions of the American Society for Artificial Organs 1981; 27:391–395.

38. Kochwa S, Litwak RS, Rosenfield RE, Leonard EF. Blood elements at foreign surfaces: a biochemical approach to the study of the adsorption of plasma proteins. Ann NY Acad Sci 1977; 283:37–49.
39. Vaudaux PE, Waldvogel FA, Morgenthaler JJ, Nydegger UE. Adsorption of fibronectin onto polymethylmethacrylate and promotion of *Staphylococcus aureus* adherence. Infect Immun 1984; 45:768–774.
40. Muller E, Takeda S, Goldman DA, Pier GB. Blood proteins do not promote adherence of coagulase-negative staphylococci to biomaterials. Infect Immun 1991; 59:3323–3326.
41. Peters WR, Bush WH Jr, McIntyre RD, Hill LD. The development of fibrin sheath on indwelling venous catheters. Surg Gynecol Obstet 1973; 137:43–47.
42. Francois P, Schrenzel J, Stoerman-Chopard C, Favre H, Herrmann M, Foster TJ, Lew DP, Vaudaux PE. Identification of plasma proteins adsorbed on hemodialysis tubing promoting *Staphylococcus aureus* adhesion. J Lab Clin Med 1999; 135:32–42.
43. Mehall JR, Saltzman DA, Jackson RJ, Smith SD. Fibrin sheath enhances central venous catheter infection. Crit Care Med 2002; 30:908–912.
44. Stillman RM, Soliman F, Garcia L, Sawyer PN. Etiology of catheter-associated sepsis. Correlation with thrombogenicity. Arch Surg 1977; 112: 1497–1499.
45. Hawiger J, Hammond DK, Timmons S. Human fibrinogen possesses binding site for staphylococci on Aa and Bb polypeptide chains. Nature 1975; 258:643–645.
46. Kuusela P. Fibronectin binding to *Staphylococcus aureus*. Nature 1978; 276:718–720.
47. Lopes JD, dos Reis M, Brentani RR. Presence of laminin receptors in *Staphylococcus aureus*. Science 1985; 229:275–277.
48. Paulsson M, Wadström T. Vitronectin and type-I collagen binding by *Staphylococcus aureus* and coagulase-negative staphylococci. FEMS Microbiol Immunol 1990; 65:55–62.
49. Herrmann M, Suchard SJ, Boxer LA, Waldvogel FA, Lew PD. Thrombospondin binds to *Staphylococcus aureus* and promotes staphylococcal adherence to surfaces. Infect Immun 1991; 59:279–288.
50. Herrmann M, Vaudaux PE, Pittet D, Auckenthaler R, Lew PD, Schumacher-Perdreau F, Peters G, Waldvogel FA. Fibronectin, fibrinogen, and laminin act as mediators of adherence of clinical staphylococcal isolates to foreign material. J Infect Dis 1988; 158:693–701.
51. Foster TJ, Höök M. Surface protein adhesins of *Staphylococcus aureus*. Trends Microbiol 1998; 6:484–488.
52. Nilsson M, Frykberg L, Flock JI, Pei L, Lindberg M, Guss B. A fibrinogen-binding protein of *Staphylococcus epidermidis*. Infect Immun 1998; 66:2666–2673.
53. Pei L, Flock JI. Lack of fbe, the gene for a fibrinogen-binding protein from *Staphylococcus epidermidis*, reduces its adherence to fibrinogen coated surfaces. Microb Pathog 2001; 31:185–193.
54. Pei L, Flock JI. Functional study of antibodies against a fibrogenin-binding protein in *Staphylococcus epidermidis* adherence to polyethylene catheters. J Infect Dis 2001; 184:52–55.

55. Davis SL, Gurusiddappa S, McCrea KW, Perkins S, Hook M. SdrG, a fibrinogen-binding bacterial adhesin of the microbial surface components recognizing adhesive matrix molecules subfamily from *Staphylococcus epidermidis*, targets the thrombin cleavage site in the Bbeta chain. J Biol Chem 2001; 276:27799–27805.

56. Vaudaux PE, Pittet D, Haeberli A, Huggler E, Nydegger UE, Lew PD, Waldvogel FA. Host factors selectively increase staphylococcal adherence on inserted catheters: a role for fibronectin and fibrinogen/fibrin. J Infect Dis 1989; 160:865–875.

57. Hussain M, Heilmann C, Peters G, Herrmann M. Teichoic acid enhances adhesion of *Staphylococcus epidermidis* to immobilized fibronectin. Microb Pathog 2001; 31:261–270.

58. Williams RJ, Henderson B, Sharp LJ, Nair SP. Identification of a fibronectin-binding protein from *Staphylococcus epidermidis*. Infect Immun 2002; 70:6805–6810.

59. Wang IW, Anderson JM, Marchant RE. *Staphylococcus epidermidis* adhesion to hydrophobic biomedical polymer is mediated by platelets. J Infect Dis 1993; 167:329–336.

60. Sapatnekar S, Kieswetter KM, Merritt K, Anderson JM, Cahalan L, Verhoeven M, Hendriks M, Fouache B, Cahalan P. Blood–biomaterial interactions in a flow system in the presence of bacteria: effect of protein adsorption. J Biomed Mater Res 1995; 29:247–256.

61. Peters G, Locci R, Pulverer G. Adherence and growth of coagulase-negative staphylococci on surfaces of intravenous catheters. J Infect Dis 1982; 146:479–482.

62. Peters G, Saborowski F, Locci R, Pulverer G. Investigations on staphylococci infection of transvenous endocardial pacemaker electrodes. Am Heart J 1984; 108:359–365.

63. Marrie TJ, Nelligan J, Costerton JW. A scanning and transmission electron microscope study of an infected pacemaker lead. Circulation 1982; 66:1339–1341.

64. Marrie TJ, Costerton JW. Scanning and transmission electron microscopy of in situ bacterial colonization of intravenous and intraarterial catheters. J Clin Microbiol 1984; 19:687–693.

65. Peters G, Locci R, Pulverer G. Microbial colonization of prosthetic devices. II. Scanning electron microscopy of naturally infected intravenous catheters. Zbl Bakt Hyg I Abt Orig B 1981; 173:293–299.

66. Peters G. Adherence and proliferation of bacteria on artificial surfaces. In: Jackson GG, Schlumberger HD, Zeiler HJ, eds. Perspectives in Antiinfective Therapy. Braunschweig, Wiesbaden: Friedrich Vieweg & Sohn, 1988:209–215.

67. Hussain M, Hastings JGM, White PJ. Isolation and composition of the extracellular slime made by coagulase-negative staphylococci in a chemically defined medium. J Infect Dis 1991; 163:534–541.

68. Drewry DT, Galbraith L, Wilkinson BJ, Wilkinson SG. Staphylococcal slime: a cautionary tale. J Clin Microbiol 1990; 28:1292–1296.

69. Mack D, Siemssen N, Laufs R. Parallel induction by glucose of adherence and a polysaccharide antigen specific for plastic-adherent *Staphylococcus epidermidis*. Infect Immun 1992; 60:2048–2057.

70. Mack D, Nedelmann M, Krokotsch A, Schwarzkopf A, Heesemann J, Laufs R. Characterization of transposon mutants of biofilm-producing *Staphylococcus epidermidis* impaired in the accumulative phase of biofilm production: Genetic identification of a hexosamine-containing polysaccharide intercellular adhesin. Infect Immun 1994; 62:3244–3253.

71. Mack D, Fischer W, Krokotsch A, Leopold K, Hartmann R, Egge H, Laufs R. The intercellular adhesin involved in biofilm accumulation of *Staphylococcus epidermidis* is a linear β-1,6-linked glucosaminoglycan: purification and structural analysis. J Bacteriol 1996; 178:175–183.

72. Tojo M, Yamashita DA, Goldman DA, Pier GD. Isolation and characterization of a capsular polysaccharide adhesin from *Staphylococcus epidermidis*. J Infect Dis 1988; 157:713–722.

73. Kojima Y, Tojo M, Goldmann DA, Tosteson TD, Pier GB. Antibody to the capsular polysaccharide/adhesin protects rabbits against catheter-related bacteremia due to coagulase-negative staphylococci. J Infect Dis 1990; 162:435–441.

74. Maira-Litran T, Kropec A, Abeygunawardana C, Joyce J, Mark G III, Goldmann DA, Pier GB. Immunochemical Properties of the Staphylococcal Poly-*N*-Acetylglucosamine Surface Polysaccharide. Infect Immun 2002; 70:4433–4440.

75. Christensen GD, Barker LP, Mawhinney TP, Baddour LM, Simpson WA. Identification of an antigenic marker of slime production for *Staphylococcus epidermidis*. Infect Immun 1990; 58:2906–2911.

76. Baldassari L, Donelli G, Gelosia A, Voglino MC, Simpson AW, Christensen GD. Purification and characterization of the staphylococcal slime-associated antigen and its occurrence among *Staphylococcus epidermidis* clinical isolates. Infect Immun 1996; 64:3410–3415.

77. Heilmann C, Schweitzer O, Gerke C, Vanittanakom N, Mack D, Götz F. Molecular basis of intercellular adhesion in the biofilm-forming *Staphylococcus epidermidis*. Mol Microbiol 1996; 20:1083–1091.

78. Gerke C, Kraft A, Süssmuth R, Schweitzer O, Götz F. Characterization of the *N*-acetylglucosaminyltransferase activity involved in the biosynthesis of the *Staphylococcus epidermidis* polysaccharide intercellular adhesin. J Biol Chem 1998; 273:18586–18593.

79. Rupp ME, Ulphani JS, Fey PD, Bartscht K, Mack D. Characterization of the importance of polysaccharide intercellular adhesin/hemagglutinin of *Staphylococcus epidermidis* in the pathogenesis of biomaterial-based infection in a mouse foreign body infection model. Infect Immun 1999; 67:2627–2632.

80. Ziebuhr W, Krimmer V, Rachid S, Lossner I, Gotz F, Hacker J. A novel mechanism of phase variation of virulence in *Staphylococcus epidermidis*: evidence for control of the polysaccharide intercellular adhesin synthesis by alternating insertion and excision of the insertion sequence element IS256. Mol Microbiol 1999; 32:345–356.

81. Loessner I, Dietrich K, Dittrich D, Hacker J, Ziebuhr W. Transposase-dependent formation of circular IS256 derivatives in *Staphylococcus epidermidis* and *Staphylococcus aureus*. J Bacteriol 2002; 184:4709–4714.

82. Dobinsky S, Kiel K, Rohde H, Bartscht K, Knobloch JK, Horstkotte MA, Mack D. Glucose-related dissociation between icaADBC transcription and biofilm expression by *Staphylococcus epidermidis*: evidence for an additional

factor required for polysaccharide intercellular adhesin synthesis. J Bacteriol 2003; 185:2879–2886.

83. McKenney D, Pouliot KL, Wang Y, Murthy V, Ulrich M, Doring G, Lee JC, Goldmann DA, Pier GB. Broadly protective vaccine for *Staphylococcus aureus* based on an in vivo-expressed antigen. Science 1999; 284:1523–1527.

84. Cramton SE, Ulrich M, Gotz F, Doring G. Anaerobic conditions induce expression of polysaccharide intercellular adhesin in *Staphylococcus aureus* and *Staphylococcus epidermidis*. Infect Immun 2001; 69:4079–4085.

85. Schumacher-Perdreau F, Heilmann C, Peters G, Götz F, Pulverer G. Comparative analysis of a biofilm forming *Staphylococcus epidermidis* strain and its adhesion-positive, accumulation-negative isogenic mutant. FEMS Microbiol Lett 1994; 117:71–78.

86. Hussain M, Herrmann M, von Eiff C, Perdreau-Remington F, Peters G. A 140-kilodalton extracellular protein is essential for the accumulation of *Staphylococcus epidermidis* strains on surfaces. Infect Immun 1997; 65:519–524.

87. Cucarella C, Solano C, Valle J, Amorena B, Lasa I, Penades JR. Bap, a *Staphylococcus aureus* surface protein involved in biofilm formation. J Bacteriol 2001; 183:2888–2896.

88. Cucarella C, Tormo MA, Knecht E, Amorena B, Lasa I, Foster TJ, Penades JR. Expression of the Biofilm-Associated Protein Interferes with Host Protein Receptors of *Staphylococcus aureus* and Alters the Infective Process. Infect Immun 2002; 70:3180–3186.

89. Knobloch JK, Bartscht K, Sabottke A, Rohde H, Feucht HH, Mack D. Biofilm formation by *Staphylococcus epidermidis* depends on functional RsbU, an activator of the sigB operon: differential activation mechanisms due to ethanol and salt stress. J Bacteriol 2001; 183:2624–2633.

90. Rachid S, Cho S, Ohlsen K, Hacker J, Ziebuhr W. Induction of *Staphylococcus epidermidis* biofilm formation by environmental factors: the possible involvement of the alternative transcription factor sigB. Adv Exp Med Biol 2000; 485:159–166.

91. Kies S, Otto M, Vuong C, Gotz F. Identification of the sigB operon in *Staphylococcus epidermidis*: construction and characterization of a sigB deletion mutant. Infect Immun 2001; 69:7933–7936.

92. Novick RP. Autoinduction and signal transduction in the regulation of staphylococcal virulence. Mol Microbiol 2003; 48:1429–1449.

93. Otto M, Echner H, Voelter W, Gotz F. Pheromone cross-inhibition between *Staphylococcus aureus* and *Staphylococcus epidermidis*. Infect Immun 2001; 69:1957–1960.

94. Balaban N, Giacometti A, Cirioni O, Gov Y, Ghiselli R, Mocchegiani F, Viticchi C, Del Prete MS, Saba V, Scalise G, Dell'Acqua G. Use of the quorum-sensing inhibitor RNAIII-inhibiting peptide to prevent biofilm formation in vivo by drug-resistant *Staphylococcus epidermidis*. J Infect Dis 2003; 187:625–630.

95. Lina G, Boutite F, Tristan A, Bes M, Etienne J, Vandenesch F. Bacterial competition for human nasal cavity colonization: role of staphylococcal agr alleles. Appl Environ Microbiol 2003; 69:18–23.

96. Fluckiger U, Wolz C, Cheung AL. Characterization of a sar homolog of *Staphylococcus epidermidis*. Infect Immun 1998; 66:2871–2878.

97. Muller E, Al Attar J, Wolff AG, Farber BF. Mechanism of salicylate-

mediated inhibition of biofilm in *Staphylococcus epidermidis*. J Infect Dis 1998; 177:501–503.

98. Bayer AS, Cheung AL, Kupferwasser LI, Yeaman MR. The Nonsteroidal Anti-Inflammatory Drugs (NSAIDs), Salicylic Acid and Diclofenac, Down-modulate Both Sar- and Agr-Dependent Genes in *Staphylococcus aureus* (SA). General Meeting of the American Society for Microbiology [abstr].

99. Polonio RE, Mermel LA, Paquette GE, Sperry JF. Eradication of biofilm-forming *Staphylococcus epidermidis* (RP62A) by a combination of sodium salicylate and vancomycin. Antimicrob Agents Chemother 2001; 45:3262–3266.

100. Quie PG, Belani KK. Coagulase-negative staphylococcal adherence and persistence. J Infect Dis 1987; 156:543–547.

101. Sugarman B, Young EJ. Infections Associated with Prosthetic devices. Boca Raton: CRC Press, 1984.

102. Johnson GM, Carparas LS, Peters G. Slime production enhances resistance of *Staphylococcus epidermidis* to phagocytic killing: Interference with opsonization and oxidative burst. Ped Res 1989; 25:181A.

103. Johnson GM, Lee PE, Regelmann WE, Gray ED, Peters G, Quie PG. Interference with granulocyte function by *Staphylococcus epidermidis* slime. Infect Immun 1986; 54:13–20.

104. Johnson CM, Regelmann WE, Gray ED, Peters G, Quie PG. Staphylococcal slime and host-defenses—Effects on polymorphonuclear granulocytes. In: Pulverer G, Quie PG, Peters G, eds. Pathogenicity and Clinical Significance of Coagulase-Negative Staphylococci. Stuttgart, New York: Gustav Fischer Verlag, 1987:33–44.

105. Regelmann WE, Gray ED, Thomas P, Peters G. *Staphylococcus epidermidis* slime effects on bacterial opsonization and PMN Leucocyte function. Ped Res 1984; 18(part 2):1131.

106. Zimmerli W, Lew PD, Waldvogel FA. Pathogenesis of foreign body infection. Evidence for a local granulocyte defec. J Clin Invest 1984; 73:1191–1200.

107. Peters G, Gray ED, Johnson GM. Immunomodulating properties of extracellular slime substance. In: Bisno AL, Waldvogel FA, eds. Infections Associated with Indwelling Medical Devices. Washington, DC: American Society for Microbiology, 1989:61–74.

108. Gray ED, Peters G, Verstegen M, Regelmann WE. Effect of extracellular slime substance from *Staphylococcus epidermidis* on the human cellular immune response. Lancet 1984; 365–367.

109. Gray ED, Regelmann WE, Peters G. Staphylococcal slime and host defenses—Effects on lymphocytes and immune function. In: Pulverer G, Quie PG, Peters G, eds. Pathogenicity and Clinical Significance of Coagulase-Negative Staphylococci. Stuttgart, New York: Gustav Fischer Verlag, 1987:45–54.

110. Stout RD, Ferguson KP, Yi-Ning L, Lambe DW. Staphylococcal eopolysaccharides inhibit lymphocyte proliferative responses by activation of monocyte proliferative responses by activation of monocyte prostaglandin production. Infect Immun 1992; 60:922–927.

111. Stout RD, Miller AR, Lambe DW. Staphylococcal glycocalix activates macrophage prostaglandin E2 and interleukin 1 production and modulates tumor necrosis factor a and nitric oxide production. Infect Immun 1994; 62:4160–4166.

112. Herrmann M, Lew PD. Foreign body infections: From intravenous catheters to hip prosthesis. In: Vincent JL, ed. Update in Intensive Care and Emergencey Medicine 10. Update 1990. Berlin: Springer-Verlag, 1990:53–60.

113. Elliott TS, D'Abrera VC, Dutton S. The effect of antibiotics on bacterial colonisation of vascular cannulae in a novel in-vitro model. J Med Microbiol 1988; 26:229–235.

114. Evans RC, Holmes CJ. Effect of vancomycin hydrochloride on *Staphylococcus epidermidis* biofilm associated with silicone elastomer. Antimicrob Agents Chemother 1987; 31:889–894.

115. Sheth NK, Franson TR, Sohnle PG. Influence of bacterial adherence to intravascular catheters on in vitro antibiotic susceptibility. Lancet 1985; II: 1266–1268.

116. Christina AG, Hobgood CD, Webb LX, Myrvik QN. Adhesive Colonization of biomaterials and antibiotic resistance. Biomaterials 1987; 8:423–426.

117. Teufel P, Gotz F. Characterization of an extracellular metalloprotease with elastase activity from *Staphylococcus epidermidis*. J Bacteriol 1993; 175:4218–4224.

118. Schnell N, Engelke G, Augustin J, Rosenstein R, Ungermann V, Gotz F, Entian KD. Analysis of genes involved in the biosynthesis of antibiotic epidermin. Eur J Biochem 1992; 204:57–68.

119. Peschel A, Augustin J, Kupke T, Stevanovic S, Gotz F. Regulation of epidermin biosynthetic genes by EpiQ. Mol Microbiol 1993; 9:31–39.

120. Farrell AM, Foster TJ, Holland KT. Molecular analysis and expression of the lipase of *Staphylococcus epidermidis*. J Gen Microbiol 1993; 139(Pt 2):267–277.

121. Rosenstein R, Gotz F. Staphylococcal lipases: biochemical and molecular characterization. Biochimie 2000; 82:1005–1014.

122. Becker K, Haverkamper G, von Eiff C, Roth R, Peters G. Survey of staphylococcal enterotoxin genes, exfoliative toxin genes, and toxic shock syndrome toxin 1 gene in non-*Staphylococcus aureus* species. Eur J Clin Microbiol Infect Dis 2001; 20:407–409.

123. Kloos WE, Schleifer KH. Simplified scheme for routine identification of human *Staphylococcus* species. J Clin Microbiol 1975; 1:82–88.

124. Peters G, Schumacher-Perdreau F, Pulverer G. Adherence of coagulase-negative staphylococci to polymers. Medical Microbiology. London: Academic Press, 1986:209–226.

125. Vandenesch F, Etienne J, Reverdy ME, Eykyn SJ. Endocarditis due to *Staphylococcus lugdunensis*: report of 11 cases and review. Clin Infect Dis 1993; 17:871–876.

126. Hell W, Meyer HG, Gatermann SG. Cloning of aas, a gene encoding a *Staphylococcus saprophyticus* surface protein with adhesive and autolytic properties. Mol Microbiol 1998; 29:871–881.

127. Christensen GD, Parisi JT, Bisno AL, Simpson WA, Beachey EH. Characterization of clinically significant strains of coagulase-negative staphylococci. J Clin Microbiol 1983; 18:258–269.

128. Schumacher-Perdreau F, Jansen B, Peters G, Pulverer G. Typing of coagulase-negative staphylococci isolated from foreign body infections. Eur J Clin Microbiol Infect Dis 1988; 7:270–273.

129. van Belkum A, Kluytmans J, van Leeuwen W, Bax R, Quint W, Peters E,

Fluit A, Vandenbroucke-Grauls C, van den Brule A, Koeleman H, Melchers W, Meis J, Elaichouni A, Vaneechoutte M, Moonens F, Maes N, Struelens M, Tenover F, Verbrugh H. Multicenter evaluation of arbitrarily primed PCR for typing of *Staphylococcus aureus* strains. J Clin Microbiol 1995; 33:1537–1547.

130. Goering RV. The application of pulsed field gel electrophoresis to analysis of the global dissemination of methicillin-resistant *Staphylococcus aureus*. In: Brun-Buisson C, Casewell MW, El Solh N, Régnier B, eds. Methicillin Resistant Staphylococci. Paris: Flammarion Médecine-Sciences, 1995:76–81.

131. Jansen B, Hartmann C, Schumacher-Perdreau F, Peters G. Late onset endophthalmitis associated with intraocular lens: a case of molecularly proved *Staphylococcus epidermidis* aetiology. Brit J Ophthalmol 1991; 75:440–441.

132. Perdreau-Remington F, Stefanik D, Peters G, Ludwig C, Rütt R, Wenzel R, Pulverer G. Microbial ecology of explanted prosthetic hips: A four year prospective study of 52 patients with "aseptic" prosthetic joint loosening. Eur J Clin Microbiol Infect Dis 1996; 15:160–165.

133. Wu S, Piscitelli C, de Lencastre H, Tomasz A. Tracking the evolutionary origin of the methicillin resistance gene: cloning and sequencing of a homologue of mecA from a methicillin susceptible strain of *Staphylococcus sciuri*. Microb Drug Resist 1996; 2:435–441.

134. Schwalbe RS, Stapelton JT, Gilligan PH. Emergence of vancomycin resistance in coagulase-negative staphylococci. N Engl J Med 1987; 316:927–931.

135. Kloos WE, Bannerman TE. Update on clinical significance of coagulase-negative staphylococci. Clin Microbiol Rev 1994; 7:117–140.

136. Widmer AF. IV-Related infections. In: Wenzel RPB, ed. Prevention and Control of Nosocomial Infections. Philadelphia: Williams and Wilkins, 1993:556–579.

137. O'Grady NP, Alexander M, Dellinger EP, Gerberding JL, Heard SO, Maki DG, Masur H, McCormick RD, Mermel LA, Pearson ML, Raad II, Randolph A, Weinstein RA, Healthcare Infection Control Practices Advisory Committee. Guidelines for the prevention of intravascular catheter-related infections. Centers for Disease Control and Prevention. MMWR Recomm Rep 2002; 51:1–29.

138. Archer GL. *Staphylococcus epidermidis* and other coagulase-negative staphylococci. In: Mandell GL, Bennett JE, Dolin R, eds. Principles and Practice of Infectious Diseases. Philadelphia: Churchill Livingstone, 2000:2092–2100.

139. Edmond MB, Wallace SE, McClish DK, Pfaller MA, Jones RN, Wenzel RP. Nosocomial bloodstream infections in United States hospitals: a three-year analysis. Clin Infect Dis 1999; 29:239–244.

140. Maki DG. Infections caused by intravascular devices used for infusion therapy: Pathogenesis, prevention, and management. In: Bisno AL, Waldvogel FA, eds. Infections Associated with Indwelling Medical Devices. Washington, D.C.: American Society for Microbiology, 1994:155–212.

141. Rupp ME, Archer GL. Coagulase-negative staphylococci: pathogens associated with medical progress. Clin Infect Dis 1994; 19:231–245.

142. Moyer MA, Edwards LD, Farley L. Comparative culture methods on 101 intravenous catheters. Routine semiquantitative, and blood cultures. Arch Intern Med 1983; 143:66–69.

143. Armstrong CW, Mayhall G, Miller KB, Newsome HH Jr, Sugerman HJ, Dalton HP, Hall GO, Hunsberger S. Clinical predictors of infection of central venous catheters used for total parenteral nutrition. Infect Control Hosp Epidemiol 1990; 11:71–78.

144. Maki DG, Weise CE, Sarafin HW. A semiquantitative culture method for identifying intravenous-catheter infection. N Engl J Med 1977; 296:1305.

145. Brun-Buisson C, Abrouk F, Legrand P, Huet Y, Larabi S, Rapin M. Diagnosis of central venous catheter-related sepsis: critical level of quantitative tip cultures. Arch Intern Med 1987; 147, 873–877.

146. Sherertz RJ, Raad II, Belani A, Koo LC, Rand KH, Pickett DL, Straub SA, Fauerbach LL. Three-year experience with sonicated vascular catheter cultures in a clinical microbiology laboratory. J Clin Microbiol 1990; 28:76–82.

147. Raad II, Bodey GP. Infectious complications of indwelling vascular catheters. Clin Infect Dis 1992; 15:197–208.

148. Cobb DK, High KP, Sawyer RG, Sable CA, Adams RB, Lindley DA, Pruett TL, Schwenzer KJ, Farr BM. A controlled trial of scheduled replacement of central venous and pulmonary-artery catheters. N Engl J Med 1992; 327:1062–1068.

149. Cook D, Randolph A, Kernerman P, Cupido C, King D, Soukup C, Brun-Buisson C. Central venous catheter replacement strategies: a systematic review of the literature. Crit Care Med 1997; 25:1417–1424.

150. Rushforth JA, Hoy CM, Kite P, Puntis JW. Rapid diagnosis of central venous catheter sepsis. Lancet 1993; 342:402–403.

151. Fan ST, Teoh-Tchan CH, Lau KF. Evaluation of central venous catheter sepsis by differential quantitative blood cultures. Eur J Clin Microbiol Infect Dis 1989; 8:142–144.

152. Flynn PM, Shenep JL, Barret FF. Differential quantitation with a commercial blood culture tube for diagnosis of catheter-related infection. J Clin Microbiol 1988; 26:1045–1046.

153. Blot F, Nitenberg G, Chachaty E, Raynard B, Germann N, Antoun S, Laplanche A, Brun-Buisson C, Tancrede C. Diagnosis of catheter-related bacteraemia: a prospective comparison of the time to positivity of hub-blood versus peripheral-blood cultures. Lancet 1999; 354:1071–1077.

154. Seifert H, Cornely O, Seggewiss K, Decker M, Stefanik D, Wisplinghoff H, Fatkenheuer G. Bloodstream infection in neutropenic cancer patients related to short-term nontunnelled catheters determined by quantitative blood cultures, differential time to positivity, and molecular epidemiological typing with pulsed-field gel electrophoresis. J Clin Microbiol 2003; 41:118–123.

155. Kirchoff LV, Sheagren JN. Epidemiology and clinical significance of blood cultures positive for coagulase-negative staphylococcus. Infect Control 1985; 6:479–486.

156. Garner JS, Jarvis WR, Emori TG, Horan TC, Hughes JM. CDC definition for nosocomial infections. Am J Infect Control 1988; 16:128–140.

157. Maslow JN, Slutsky AM, Arbeit R. Application of pulsed-field gel electrophoresis to molecular epidemiology. In: Persing DH, Smith TF, Tenover FC, White TJ, eds. Diagnostic Molecular Microbiology: Principles and Applications. Washington, D.C.: American Society for Microbiology, 1993:563–572.

158. Benezra D, Kiehn TE, Gold JW, Brown AE, Turnbull AD, Armstrong D. Prospective study of infections in indwelling central venous catheters using quantitative blood cultures. Am J Med 1988; 85(4):495–498.

159. Karmochkine M, Brunet F, Lanore JJ, Belghit M, Mira JP, Dhainaut JF, Monsallier JF. Recovery from staphylococcal septicaemia in neutropenic patients without removal of the previously inserted central venous catheter. Eur J Med 1993; 2(3):143–147.

160. Raad I, Davis S, Khan A, Tarrand J, Elting L, Bodey GP. Impact of central venous catheter removal on the recurrence of catheter-related coagulase-negative staphylococcal bacteremia. Infect Control Hosp Epidemiol 1992; 13(4):215–221.

161. Flynn PM, Shenep JL, Stokes DC, Barrett FF. In situ management of confirmed central venous catheter-related bacteremia. Pediatr Infect Dis J 1987; 6:729–734.

162. Rubin LG, Shih S, Shende A, Karayalcin G, Lanzkowsky P. Cure of implantable venous port-associated bloodstream infections in pediatric hematology–oncology patients without catheter removal. Clin Infect Dis 1999; 29:102–105.

163. Hampton AA, Sherertz RJ. Vascular-access infections in hospitalized patients. Surg Clin North Am 1988; 68:57–71.

164. Raad I. Intravascular-catheter-related infections. Lancet 1998; 351:893–898.

165. Kiri N, Archer G, Climo MW. Combinations of lysostaphin with beta-lactams are synergistic against oxacillin-resistant *Staphylococcus epidermidis*. Antimicrob Agents Chemother 2002; 46:2017–2020.

166. Giacometti A, Cirioni O, Ghiselli R, Orlando F, Mocchegiani F, Riva A, Del Prete MS, Saba V, Scalise G. Efficacy of quinupristin–dalfopristin in preventing vascular graft infection due to *Staphylococcus epidermidis* with intermediate resistance to glycopeptides. Antimicrob Agents Chemother 2002; 46:2885–2888.

167. John MA, Pletch C, Hussain Z. In vitro activity of quinupristin/dalfopristin, linezolid, telithromycin and comparator antimicrobial agents against 13 species of coagulase-negative staphylococci. J Antimicrob Chemother 2002; 50:933–938.

168. Grif K, Dierich MP, Pfaller K, Miglioli PA, Allerberger F. In vitro activity of fosfomycin in combination with various antistaphylococcal substances. J Antimicrob Chemother 2001; 48:209–217.

169. Messing B, Peitra-Cohen S, Debure A, Beliah M, Bernier J-J. Antibiotic-lock technique: A new approach to optimal therapy for catheter-related sepsis in home-parenteral nutrition patients. J Parenter Enteral Nutr 1988; 12:185–189.

170. Carlisle EJ, Blake PG, McCarthy F, Vas S, Uldall R. Septicemia in long-term jugular hemodialysis catheters: eradicating infection by changing the catheter over a guidewire. Int J Artif Organs 1991; 14:150–153.

171. Pettigrew RA, Lang SD, Haydock DA, Parry BR, Bremner DA, Hill GL. Catheter-related sepsis in patients on intravenous nutrition: a prospective study of quantitative catheter cultures and guidewire changes for suspected sepsis. Br J Surg 1985; 72:52–55.

172. Johnson CW, Miller DL, Ognibene FP. Acute pulmonary emboli associated

with guidewire change of a central venous catheter. Intensive Care Med 1991; 17:115–117.

173. Veenstra DL, Saint S, Saha S, Lumley T, Sullivan SD. Efficacy of antiseptic-impregnated central venous catheters in preventing catheter-related blood-stream infection: a meta-analysis. JAMA 1999; 281:261–267.

174. Appelgren P, Ransjo U, Bindslev L, Espersen F, Larm O. Surface heparin-ization of central venous catheters reduces microbial colonization in vitro and in vivo: results from a prospective, randomized trial. Crit Care Med 1996; 24:1482–1489.

175. Darouiche RO, Raad II, Heard SO, Thornby JI, Wenker OC, Gabrielli A, Berg J, Khardori N, Hanna H, Hachem R, Harris RL, Mayhall G. A comparison of two antimicrobial-impregnated central venous catheters. Catheter Study Group. N Engl J Med 1999; 340:1–8.

176. Maki DG. Risk factors for nosocomial infection in intensive care. 'Devices vs Nature' and goals for the next decade. Arch Intern Med 1989; 149:30–35.

8

Intravascular Catheter-Related Infections Due to Gram-Negative Bacilli

Harald Seifert

Institute for Medical Microbiology, Immunology and Hygiene
University of Cologne
Cologne, Germany

INTRODUCTION

The past two decades have witnessed a marked change in the distribution of pathogens reported to cause nosocomial bloodstream infections (BSI) (1–4). There was a constant increase in the proportion of Gram-positive versus Gram-negative organisms implicated in nosocomial BSI, and this shift was mainly due to significant increases of infections with coagulase-negative staphylococci (CoNS), *Staphylococcus aureus*, and enterococci (3,5,6). These organisms currently account for between 40% and more than 60% of the recovered bloodstream pathogens (1–4). A considerable part of these infections is associated with the increasing use of intravascular catheters.

Bloodstream infection caused by aerobic Gram-negative bacilli has received less attention in the recent literature (7). Little is known, in particular, about the impact of Gram-negative bacilli associated with device-related infections. This also holds true with regard to the factors involved in the pathogenesis of intravascular catheter-related infections (CRI), since the vast majority of studies investigating the pathogenesis of foreign-body infections have focused on Gram-positive organisms (8).

There is an ever-increasing number of Gram-negative species causing infections related to indwelling devices (9). This chapter attempts to summarize the current knowledge of Gram-negative microorganisms as a cause of CRI, their contribution to infections due to specific devices, as well as specific considerations regarding the pathogenesis and management of CRI related to Gram-negative bacilli. It focuses on intravascular catheter-related infections caused by three major groups of Gram-negative organisms: (a) members of the family Enterobacteriaceae, (b) *Pseudomonas aeruginosa*, and (c) *Acinetobacter* spp. CRI caused by other Gram-negative organisms, such as rare Enterobacteriaceae, nonaeruginosa pseudomonads, and other nonfermenting Gram-negative bacilli, is covered in the chapter on Miscellaneous Organisms in this book.

EPIDEMIOLOGY

General Aspects: Source of Data

Because very few studies have specifically addressed the issues related to CRI caused by Gram-negative bacilli, it is rather difficult to obtain the necessary data from the literature. Various studies have analyzed the epidemiology of BSI in different settings and in different types of hospitals (1,4,10–12). Other investigators have focused on nosocomial bacteremia (3,13,14); polymicrobial bacteremia (15,16); bacteremia in specific patient populations, such as cancer patients (6,9,17–19), bone marrow transplant patients (20), HIV-infected patients (21,22), patients on hemodialysis (23), pediatric patients (24,25), critically ill patients (14,26–29), and burn patients (30–32); on bacteremia of unknown origin (33); and on BSI caused by Gram-negative organisms in general (7,34,35) or by specific Gram-negative pathogens such as *Acinetobacter* spp. (36,37), Enterobacteriaceae (38–42), and *P. aeruginosa* (43–48). Information regarding CRI caused by Gram-negative bacilli may also be derived from retrospective or prospective studies that specifically address device-related infections (17,49–53). Both approaches, however, have major limitations. The various reports on bacteremia and BSI in different epidemiological settings provide information on the epidemiology of the microorganisms involved, patient characteristics, and mortality, and often also include the presumed sources or portals of entry of the bacteremia. However, the vast majority of these retrospective case series have not employed stringent definitions and microbiological methods to accurately identify a device as the cause of bacteremia. If a pathogen is recovered from the bloodstream but not concomitantly from a distant site, including an indwelling vascular catheter, bacteremia is usually considered to be of unknown origin. This may lead to an underestimation of catheter-related BSI, because catheters are often removed—but not always cultured—if signs and symptoms of sepsis evolve.

Prospective clinical studies of CRI that have addressed different issues—such as different types of catheters and catheter design (51,54–56), antimicrobial bonding (57–59), different types of dressings (60), and the consequences (61) and the prevention of these infections (62–64)—also suffer from the different definitions and microbiological methods used by different investigators (52,53). In addition, device-related infections due to Gram-negative bacilli have only rarely been analyzed separately with regard to their specific contribution to morbidity and mortality, as well as to their specific management problems, and the reported numbers of these infections are usually too small to allow for statistical evaluation. Consequently, the data presented in this chapter that are obtained from different types of studies published over a period as long as two decades may aid in coping with the special problem posed by CRI caused by Gram-negative bacilli. However, prospective clinical studies are needed that address the specific issues related to these infections in more detail.

Catheter-Related Bacteremia Caused by Gram-Negative Organisms

Kreger et al. evaluated 612 episodes of Gram-negative bacteremia over a 10-year period from 1965 to 1974 (34). The urinary tract was the most frequent source of bacteremia, and *E. coli* was the most frequent etiologic agent. The source of bacteremia remained unknown in 30% of the cases, but intravascular catheters were not implicated. Bryan and coworkers studied 1186 episodes of Gram-negative bacteremia over a five-year period from 1977 to 1981 (35). Again, intravascular devices as a source of bacteremia were not evaluated. In a study of 500 episodes of clinically significant bacteremia and fungemia conducted by Weinstein and colleagues (11), Gram-negative bacteremia arose mainly from genitourinary, respiratory, and gastrointestinal sources. An intravascular catheter was the source of bacteremia in only 5 episodes (2%), but a portal of entry could not be identified in nearly one-third of the episodes.

In more recent series, 30–40% of all bacteremias were caused by members of the family Enterobacteriaceae or by *P. aeruginosa* and related genera (10,12). In a three-year study of positive blood cultures, Roberts et al. found 1504 isolates from 1244 episodes of clinically significant bacteremia, and 727 of these (47%) were Gram-negative bacilli (12). The urinary tract was the most frequent portal of entry, accounting for 16% of episodes. An intravascular catheter was considered the source of bacteremia in 8%, and the source remained unknown for another 9%. The proportion of Gram-negative bacilli causing CRI is not reported. Mortality for cases of bacteremia from intravascular sources was 20%. Similar results were reported from Geerdes et al. (10). Among 980 episodes of both community- and hospital-acquired clinically significant bacteremia, 159 (16%) were related to intravascular devices, and 10% of these were caused by Gram-negative organisms. More recently, among 9519 bacterial pathogens associated with both community and nosocomial bloodstream infections in the United States, Canada, and Latin America (SENTRY Antimicrobial Surveillance Program, 1997), 43.8% were Gram-negative, and 5 of the 10 predominant organisms were Gram-negative. *Escherichia coli, Klebsiella* spp., *P. aeruguinosa, Enterobacter* spp., and *Acinetobacter* spp. were the most frequently isolated organisms (4). Conversely, among 10,617 episodes of nosocomial bacteremia detected during a study period of three years at 49 hospitals in the United States, Edmond and colleagues found only 23% Gram-negative isolates (3). Unfortunately, neither study provides data as to the origins of BSI.

The incidence and causative agents of intravascular device-related infections may vary considerably with the patient population studied and the methods and definitions employed. Using strict criteria, Kiehn and Armstrong investigated the spectrum of organisms causing 933 episodes of bacteremia and fungemia associated with surgically implanted intravascular devices in immunocompromised patients (9). Fifty percent of bacteremic episodes in these patients were vascular access-related, and 46% of these were caused by Gram-negative organisms. Among the major organism groups, the percentages of septic episodes that were device-related were 44% for Enterobacteriaceae and 69% for *P. aeruginosa*. In a recent study of the incidence of bacteremia in organ transplant patients, Gram-negative bacilli constituted 47% of the pathogens found in 125 cases of clinically significant bacteremia. The most common portals of entry were the abdominal site (18%) and the urinary tract (15%). Only 6% of bacteremia cases were attributed to intravascular catheters, whereas the source was unidentified in 38% (65).

Bacteremia is reported to be polymicrobial in 6–14% of cases and in that form it is most often associated with increased mortality (66,67). In a recent review extending over a period of 17 years, polymicrobial bacteremia caused by Gram-negative bacilli most commonly occurred in intraabdominal, urinary tract, and wound infections, whereas catheters were the presumed source of infection in only 3–5% of cases (66,67). Conversely, in a prospective study of polymicrobial bacteremia in ICU patients that employed adequate microbiologic methods to detect catheter-related bacteremia, intravascular devices (43%) were the most common source of polymicrobial bacteremia (15). Catheter replacement in patients who develop polymicrobial bacteremia was therefore suggested by the authors. The association of polymicrobial BSI with CRI was also noted by Martino et al. (68).

Infections Caused by Gram-Negative Bacilli Related to Specific Devices

The incidence and etiological organisms of intravascular device-related infections may be strongly influenced by the type and intended use of the device. The rate of infections related to different intravascular devices may range from < 0.2% for small peripheral catheters to >50% for central venous catheters (CVCs) used in burn patients (30,69). Infections related to specific devices are dealt with in the respective chapters of this book. In this chapter, the incidence of Gram-negative bacilli as causative agents of CRI is summarized for different types of intravascular catheters.

Devices Used for Short-Term Vascular Access

Peripheral Intravenous Catheters: The lowest rates of infection are now with small peripheral intravenous catheters. The risk for bacteremia due to these devices is very low (< 0.2%). Gram-negative bacteria are rarely implicated and usually range in frequency between 0 and 4% (70–73). In a prospective study by Richet and coworkers, however, 28% of the pathogens isolated from peripheral catheters were Gram-negative bacilli (49).

Nontunneled Central Venous Catheters: Nontunneled, percutaneously inserted CVCs are the most commonly used central catheters and account for the majority of catheter-related bloodstream infections. Prospective studies investigating the epidemiology, associated risk factors, and means for prevention of infections related to these devices have found rates of catheter-related BSI in the range of 3–5% (63,74,75).

In a prospective study, Gil and colleagues found Gram-negative organisms in 22 of 41 (54%) colonized catheters and in 6 of 11 (55%) associated bacteremias (51). Other investigators reported Gram-negative bacilli implicated in CRI to range between 12 and 42% (49,50,74–76). *P. aeruginosa, Enterobacter* spp., *S. marcescens, K. pneumoniae*, and *Acinetobacter* spp. were the organisms most frequently encountered among Gram-negative isolates. Gowardman et al. reported an incidence of 3.98 catheter-related bloodstream infection (CRBSI) per 1000 catheter-days among 400 ICU patients with nontunnelled CVCs, 25% of which were caused by Gram-negative bacteria (77). In a prospective survey to determine the rate of CRBSI among cases of primary BSI in febrile neutropenic cancer patients with short-term, nontunnelled catheters, quantitative paired blood cultures from central venous catheter (CVC) and peripheral vein, and Bactec™ blood culture bottles were obtained to determine the differential time to positivity (DTP) (53). Eighteen of 49 episodes of primary BSI (37%) were CRBSI, and 31 (63%) were BSI with an unknown portal of entry. Among the organisms recovered, 27% were Gram-negative. The results of several studies are summarized in Table 1.

Pulmonary Artery (PA) Catheters: Flow-directed Swan-Ganz pulmonary artery (PA) catheters are widely used for hemodynamic monitoring of critically ill patients. The infectious complications of PA catheters have been reviewed extensively by Mermel and Maki (78). The incidence of PA catheter-related BSI has been estimated to be in the range of

Table 1 Frequency of Gram-Negative Organisms Associated with Short-Term CVCs, Compiled from Several Studies

Study	Haslett, 1988 (76)	Yeung, 1988 (75)	Gil, 1989 (51)	Eyer, 1990 (74)	Richet, 1990 (49)	Sherertz, 1990 (50)	Seifert, 2003 (53)
Total no. of isolates reported	76	42	41	43	123	1032	22
				No (%) of isolates			
Organism							
Gram-Negative bacilli	17 (22)	5 (12)	22 (54)	18 (42)	32 (26)	287 (28)	6 (27)
Escherichia coli [a]	0	0	1 (5)	1 (6)	0	40 (14)	1 (17)
Enterobacter spp.	5 (29)	0	2 (10)	6 (33)	2 (6)	45 (16)	1 (17)
Klebsiella spp.	2 (12)	2 (40)	3 (14)	3 (17)	5 (16)	18 (6)	1 (17)
Serratia spp.	1 (6)	1 (20)	4 (19)	0	2 (6)	19 (7)	0
Pseudomonas aeruginosa	5 (29)	0	6 (29)	4 (22)	13 (41)	143 (50)	1 (17)
Acinetobacter spp.	4 (24)	1 (20)	4 (19)	1 (5)	4 (13)	12 (4)	0
Stenotrophomonas maltophilia	0	0	0	0	0	0	2 (34)

[a] Percent of Gram-negative isolates.

one case of bacteremia per 100 catheters. CoNS were recovered from more than half of the colonized catheters, but from only one-third of catheter-related BSI. Gram-negative enteric bacilli were recovered from 20% of colonized catheters but from only 11% of associated BSI, whereas *P. aeruginosa* accounted for 5% of colonized catheters and 5% of catheter-related BSI. In a prospective observational study, Kac et al. reported an incidence of 17.7 colonized catheters and 0.93 cases of BSI per 1000 catheter days among 164 pulmonary artery catheters. Colonization was caused by Gram-negative rods in 48% (79).

Arterial Catheters: Arterial pressure monitoring has become indispensible in modern hospital care, predominantly for ICU patients. In a prospective study of 130 arterial catheters used for hemodynamic monitoring, 23 (18%) produced local infection and five (3.8%) produced associated BSI (80). *Candida* spp. (31%), Gram-negative bacilli (17%), and enterococci (17%) predominated in these infections; three of five bacteremias (60%) were due to Enterobacteriaceae. With more frequent replacement of the monitoring system, the risk of endemic BSI associated with arterial catheters used for hemodynamic monitoring has more recently been estimated to be in the range of 1% (69). One specific feature of these devices is that they have frequently been associated with epidemic BSI. Donowitz et al. investigated an outbreak of *S. marcescens* bacteremia and demonstrated the presence of the epidemic organism on all in-use transducer heads (81). The authors postulated transmission of bacteria from the hands of hospital personnel into the fluid column of the device during manipulation of the system. Beck-Sagué and Jarvis reviewed 24 outbreaks of nosocomial BSI investigated by the Centers for Disease Control (82). Intravascular pressure-monitoring devices were implicated as the source of infection in eight outbreaks (33%); seven of these were due to Gram-negative bacilli. In all outbreaks, improperly disinfected reusable transducers served as reservoirs. More recently, however, CRBSI was not observed in a surveillance study of 807 intra-arterial catheters placed for cancer chemotherapy (83), and only 9 cases (0.15%) of CRBSI were detected among 7470 patients who underwent cardiac surgery and required radial arterial pressure monitoring. One of these cases was caused by a Gram-negative rod, *E. cloacae* (84).

Devices Used for Long-Term Vascular Access

Tunneled Central Venous Catheters: Surgically implanted silicone elastomer catheters—including Hickmans, Broviacs, Groshongs, and Quintons—have revolutionized the management of patients requiring prolonged central venous access, particularly for chemotherapy, parenteral nutrition (TEP), and hemodialysis. The risk of infection caused by these catheters is significantly lower than that reported with use of nontunneled catheters and has been estimated to be in the range of 0.2% bacteremias per 100 catheter-days (85,86).

Decker and Edwards reviewed 13 studies of BSIs associated with Broviac catheters in pediatric patients and found Gram-negative bacilli as the etiologic agents in 28%, with *Klebsiella* spp., *E.coli*, and *Enterobacter* spp. as predominating organisms (87). Local infections such as exit-site and tunnel infections in these patients were even more frequently caused by Gram-negative rods (41% of all organisms recovered). In adult patients with surgically implanted CVCs of the Hickman/Broviac type, the frequency of Gram-negative bacteria involved in catheter-related BSI ranged from 26 to 55% (17,88–90). The results of several studies are summarized in Table 2. Gram-negative bacilli were also responsible for 12 of 23 (52%) exit-site infections and for 12 of 20 (60%) tunnel infections reported by Benezra et al. (88). *P. aeruginosa* was the most common isolate (44%) from exit-site infections reported by Johnson et al. (90). It was suggested that one reason for the predominance of waterborne organisms such as *P. aeruginosa* may have been related to the fact that patients were not restricted from bathing or swimming.

More recently, Jean et al. conducted a prospective study to assess the incidence of CRBSI in 129 tunneled hemodialysis catheters (91). Among 56 episodes of bacteremia accounting for an incidence of 1.1 per 1000 catheter-days, 12 cases (21%) were caused by Gram-negative bacteria, with *S. marcescens* (n = 6), *P. aeruguinosa* (n = 4), and *E. coli* (n = 2) recovered most frequently. In another recent multicenter survey conducted in Canadian neonatal intensive care units, the incidence of nosocomial BSI was 7.2 per 1000 umbilical catheter-days, 13.1 per 1000 percutaneous catheter-days, and 12.1 per 1000 Broviac catheter-days, with 8.7%, 3.4%, and 11.3% of infections, respectively, caused by Gram-negative rods (24). Among 51 episodes of CRBSI in bone marrow transplant recipients reported by Elishoov et al., 50% were caused by Gram-negative pathogens (55).

Totally Implantable Intravascular Devices (TIDs): Surgically implanted subcutaneous ports have the lowest reported rates of catheter-related BSI among long-term catheters (17,92). In one of the largest prospective studies of the infectious complications associated with long-term vascular access devices, involving 1431 cancer patients, Groeger et al. (17) demonstrated a risk of 0.21 infections per 1000 device days for TIDs versus 2.8 for catheters. The predominant organisms isolated in catheter-related bacteremia were Gram-negative bacilli (55%), whereas in port-related bacteremia, Gram-positive cocci (65%) were recovered more frequently than Gram-negative organisms (21%).

In a prospective survey to compare the time to positivity of hub versus peripherally obtained blood cultures for the diagnosis of catheter-related bacteremia, Blot et al. observed 9 of 17 cases (53%) of CRBSI caused by

Table 2 Frequency of Gram-Negative Organisms Associated with Long-Term Catheters, Compiled from Several Studies

Number (%) of isolates recovered from bacteremia (I) or local (exit-site or tunnel) infection (II)

Study	Johnson, 1986 (90)		Benezra, 1988 (88)		Decker,[a] 1988 (87)		Groeger, 1993 (17)		Rotstein, 1995 (89)	
	I	II	I	II	I	II	I	II	I	II
Total no. of isolates reported	47	27	37	43	326	100	346	60	148	99
Gram-negative bacilli	19 (40)	15 (56)	18 (49)	25 (58)	91 (28)	41 (41)	191 (55)	12 (20)	38 (26)	16 (16)
Escherichia coli[b]	4 (21)	0	0	0	16 (18)	5 (12)			11 (29)	3 (19)
Enterobacter spp.	4 (21)	1 (7)	7 (39)	0	12 (13)	5 (12)			5 (13)	2 (13)
Klebsiella spp.	2 (11)	0	0	0	16 (18)	9 (22)			4 (11)	1 (6)
Serratia spp.	0	0	0	0	1 (1)	0			2 (5)	1 (6)
Pseudomonas aeruginosa	3 (16)	12 (80)	8 (44)	23 (92)	10 (11)	16 (39)	23 (12)		9 (24)	7 (44)
Acinetobacter spp.	3 (16)	1 (7)	3 (17)	0	9 (10)	5 (12)			3 (8)	0

[a] Compiles 13 studies.
[b] Percent of Gram-negative isolates.

Gram-negative bacteria; the majority of patients had either totally implanted ports or tunneled catheters (52). Flynn and collegues observed a high rate of recurrence of CRBSI with a totally implantable central venous catheter in children with cancer (56). Using quantitative blood cultures, 6 of 21 organisms (29%) recovered from 21 cases of BSI related to TIDs and 109 of 187 organisms (58%) recovered from 151 cases of CRBSI related to Hickman/ Broviac catheters were Gram-negative bacilli.

Bloodstream Infections Caused by Contamination of Infusate or Blood Products

Bacterial Contamination of Infusate

Although less frequently than from infection of the percutaneous catheter tract or from a contaminated catheter hub, device-related BSI may also arise from contamination of infusate—parenteral fluid, blood products, or intravenous medications. In fact, cases of infusion-related bacteremia may be falsely attributed to the intravascular cannula due to failure to culture the infusate (70).

Infusion-related sepsis has been reviewed extensively by Maki (13,69). Bacteria may be introduced either during manufacture of the infusate (intrinsic contamination) or during its preparation and administration in the hospital (extrinsic contamination). The pathogens implicated in the vast majority of nosocomial bacteremias related to contaminated infusate have been Gram-negative bacilli. This may, at least in part, be due to the different growth properties of specific microorganisms in parenteral fluids (see Section on "Pathogenesis"). Whereas contaminated infusate is a rare cause of endemic, infusion-related infection with most intravascular devices, it is well-documented as a common cause of epidemic nosocomial bacteremia (13,69). In fact, nosocomial BSI caused by specific Gram-negative organisms such as *Enterobacter* spp—particularly *E. cloacae* and *E. agglomerans*—*S. marcescens*, and *Burkholderia* (*Pseudomonas*) *cepacia* that are able to multiply at room temperature in the solution involved points toward contaminated fluid as a possible source, and, if observed repeatedly, should prompt an in-depth epidemiological evaluation.

The problem and reported causes of epidemic infusion-related bacteremia due to intrinsic contamination of infusate—now exceedingly rare as a consequence of improved quality control standards—have been reviewed in detail by Maki (70). All of the outbreaks reported from U.S. and European hospitals, some of which have reached a nationwide scope, have involved Gram-negative bacilli (70,93). The largest outbreak of this kind occurred in 1970–1971 and involved 378 patients in 25 U.S. hospitals. It was ultimately traced to contamination of the closures of unopened infusion bottles with *E. cloacae* and *E. agglomerans* during the manufacturing process (94). More recently, outbreaks of *Pseudomonas* bacteremia and pseudobacteremia due to intrinsic contamination of 10% povidone iodine, a widely used skin antiseptic, have been reported (95).

Most epidemics of infusion-related bacteremia, however, have originated from a common source of extrinsic contamination in the hospital, such as the use of contaminated disinfectants, repeated use of contaminated multidose medication vials (96), or improper sterilization of medical equipment, in particular of transducers used for arterial pressure monitoring (81,97,98). There have been more than 30 epidemics of nosocomial BSI traced to contaminated fluid within the administration set of arterial pressure monitoring devices. Again, the majority of these outbreaks (90%) were caused by Gram-negative bacteria, most frequently *S. marcescens*, *Enterobacter* spp., and *B. cepacia* (97). It has been speculated that the major reason for the predominance of Gram-negative bacilli in these epidemics may be the specific growth properties of these organisms in heparinized saline and glucose-containing solutions. In many outbreaks, the hospital reservoir and the mode of transmission of the epidemic organism could not be determined, but the pathogen was found on the hands of health care workers involved in the care of patients receiving infusion therapy. In a recent report from the Centers for Disease Control (CDC), multiple outbreaks of nosocomial BSI that occurred in seven U.S. hospitals were linked to contamination of an intravenous anesthetic, propofol (99). Among 49 case patients identified, 10 (20%) acquired BSI due to Gram-negative pathogens: *Enterobacter agglomerans* and *S. marcescens*. Similarly, Ostrowsky and colleagues described an outbreak of *S. marcescens* bacteremia that was traced to a contaminated narcotic and involved 26 patients. Continuous infusion of fentanyl had been given to patients by a respiratory therapist who was found to have manipulated the fentanyl infusions, and whose hair samples tested positive for fentanyl (100).

Bacterial Contamination of Blood Products

Bacterial infections transmitted by contaminated blood or blood products have been rare, but they may be associated with severe morbidity, often culminating in septic shock and death. Various sources of contamination have been suggested, such as preexisting infection of the donor or bacterial invasion of the blood product during collection, preparation, and storage (101). A wide spectrum of bacteria have been implicated, but aerobic Gram-negative rods were the organisms most commonly involved (61%), with *Pseudomonas* spp. accounting for 28% of episodes. Transfusion-related sepsis due to *Yersinia enterocolitica* was associated with diarrheal illness of the donor (102), whereas an outbreak of *Salmonella* sepsis from platelet transfusions was traced to a hematogenous carrier of *Salmonella* cholera-suis (103). Cold-growing (psychrophilic) bacteria such as *Yersinia* spp., *P. fluorescens*, and *Flavobacterium* spp. may play an important role in the contamination of blood products, because once introduced even in small numbers they may grow to massive numbers during storage of whole blood at 4°C (104). In contrast, platelets are stored at room temperature and may become contaminated with bacteria such as *Enterobacter* spp. that grow well at 25°C to 37°C (105). In a recent review of transfusion-related sepsis, it is speculated that transfusion-related sepsis will eventually disappear as a consequence of the recent Food and Drug Administration (FDA) approval of culture methods for platelet bacterial testing and the promulgation of accreditation standards by the College of American Pathologists and American Association of Blood Banks to limit and detect platelet bacterial contamination (106).

CATHETER-RELATED INFECTIONS CAUSED BY SPECIFIC GRAM-NEGATIVE ORGANISMS

Enterobacteriaceae

The various members of the family Enterobacteriaceae, taken together, constitute the largest group of Gram-negative organisms involved in all types of nosocomial infections, including BSI and catheter-associated infections (17,78), and they clearly predominate over *P. aeruginosa* and other non-fermenting Gram-negative rods (107). If the different species are considered separately, *E. coli*, *Enterobacter* spp., *Klebsiella* spp., and *Serratia* spp. are the leading causes of nosocomial BSI, whereas *Citrobacter* spp., *Proteus* spp., *Morganella morganii*, and *Salmonella* spp. are only rarely encountered (3,7,10,11,35,68,107). Rare enterobacterial species that have been implicated in CRI include *Enterobacter amnigenus*, *Kluyvera cryocrescens*, and *Serratia odorifera*, and they are covered in the chapter on Miscellaneous Organisms in this book.

Escherichia coli

E. coli is the most common cause of enterobacterial bacteremia, ranging in frequency from 31 to 47% of all Gram-negative bacteremias, and is predominantly associated with urinary tract infections (7,12,34,38,107). In light of the frequency with which *E. coli* is isolated from the bloodstream, it may be surprising that *E. coli* is an exceptionally rare cause of intravascular device-associated BSI. Gransden and coworkers reviewed 861 cases of *E. coli* bacteremia observed during an 18-year survey (38). In more than half of all cases (57%), bacteremia originated in the urinary tract, but *E. coli* was never encountered infecting an intravenous line. Bodey and colleagues, in a similar series of *E. coli* bacteremia in cancer patients, identified a catheter as the source of infection in only 1% (108). In prospective studies of catheter-related infections, *E. coli* is recovered less often than other Enterobacteriaceae. The frequency of *E. coli* among Gram-negative infections associated with tunneled CVCs ranges from 10 to 26% (7,52,55,56,87–90), whereas nontunneled CVCs are rarely infected (0–14%) (49–51,53,74,76,77).

Enterobacter spp.

Enterobacter bacteremia is usually nosocomial and accounts for 5 to 16% of reported Gram-negative BSIs (7,11,12,34,35,109,110). In their large series of *Enterobacter* bacteremia in a cancer hospital, including 281 patients, Bodey and colleagues could identify a portal of entry in only 28%, and only two infections (<1%) were considered catheter-related (111). In contrast, the biliary tract (18%) and central venous catheters (15%) were the most common sources of *Enterobacter* bacteremia among 33 pediatric patients reviewed by Gallagher (39). Chow and coworkers prospectively studied 129 patients with *Enterobacter* bacteremia. An abdominal source was the most common portal of entry (39%), followed by the urinary tract (13%) and intravascular catheters (11%) (110). Of special importance is the rapid development of resistance to cephalosporin antibiotics by *Enterobacter* (110).

Enterobacter spp., and *E. cloacae* in particular, are among the most common Gram-negative organisms involved in CRI, rivaled only by *Klebsiella* spp. and *P. aeruginosa*. *Enterobacter* spp. constituted 12 to 39% of Gram-negative bacteria isolated from infections associated with long-term CVCs of the Hickman/Broviac type (9,55,56,87–90). *Enterobacter* spp. were also frequently found causing infections associated with short-term CVCs, ranging from 6 to 33% among Gram-negative organisms (49–51,53,74,76). *Enterobacter* is rarely, if ever, recovered from infections related to small peripheral venous catheters (31,49), pulmonary artery catheters (78,79), and arterial catheters (80,84,97).

Another characteristic feature of *Enterobacter* is its association with epidemics of bacteremia caused by contaminated intravenous products (16,99,100,105). *Enterobacter* spp. are among the leading causes of epidemic nosocomial bacteremia, accounting for 9 of 97 epidemics reviewed by Maki (13). *Enterobacter* spp. were also involved in 5 of 23 nosocomial epidemics (22%) of bloodstream infection traced to arterial pressure monitoring that were reviewed by Mermel and Maki (97).

Klebsiella spp.

Microorganisms of the genus *Klebsiella* are one of the leading causes (11–19%) of Gram-negative rod bacteremia, ranking second only to *E. coli* (7,11,12,34,36). *Klebsiella* bacteremia is most often a nosocomial disease with a strong association with septic shock (40). In an analysis of 100 episodes of *Klebsiella* bacteremia, García de la Torre et al. demonstrated that the most frequent portals of entry were the urinary, respiratory, and biliary tracts, whereas only four cases (4%) were considered catheter-related (40). Similarly, 13% of nosocomial *Klebsiella* bacteremia cases reported by Blot et al. were associated with contaminated central venous catheters in critically ill patients

(112). Conversely, among 92 episodes of *K. pneumoniae* BSI described by Pena et al., 43% were considered catheter-related (113).

Klebsiella spp. have been implicated in intravascular device-associated infections with frequency similar to *Enterobacter* spp. *K. pneumonia* usually predominates over *K. oxytoca*. *Klebsiella* spp. constituted 6 to 17% of Gram-negative bacteria isolated from infections associated with nontunneled CVCs (49–51,53,74,76), and they were also recovered from 11 to 23% of infections related to tunneled long-term CVCs that were caused by Gram-negative organisms (9,55,56,87,89,90). A *Klebsiella* species was the only Gram-negative organism found to be responsible for catheter-related sepsis associated with short peripheral catheters (71), although these organisms are exceptionally rare in these infections (49).

Klebsiella spp. were also implicated—although less frequently than *Enterobacter* spp. and *Serratia* spp.—in nosocomial outbreaks associated with pressure transducers used for arterial pressure monitoring (82,97), as well as in epidemic nosocomial bacteremia related to contaminated infusate (13). More recently, Pena et al. reported on a significant association between intravascular CRBSI and isolation of ESBL-producing *K. pneumoniae* (113).

Serratia spp.

Serratia bacteremia is hospital-acquired in nearly all instances and tends to be associated with especially long durations of hospitalization. *Serratia* spp. constitute between 2 and 6% of bacteremia cases in large surveys of Gram-negative bacteremia (7,11,12,34,36). In recent reviews of *Serratia* bacteremia, the respiratory tract, urinary tract, and surgical wounds served as the most important portals of entry. Catheters were implicated as the origin of infection in only 2–9% (41,114). Like *Enterobacter* spp., these organisms are often multidrug resistant.

Serratia spp. are considerably less often involved in CRI and catheter-related BSI than *Enterobacter* spp. and *Klebsiella* spp., ranging in frequency between 1 and 19% of all Gram-negative organisms recovered from infections associated with nontunneled CVCs (42,49–51,53,74,76) as well as long-term tunneled CVCs (9,87,89–91). However, *Serratia* spp. are among the organisms that should suggest the possibility of a contaminated infusion product if identified as a clear cause of device-associated bacteremia. *S. marcescens* accounted for 6 of 23 reported outbreaks (26%) of infection related to arterial pressure monitoring (97) and was the causative agent of nosocomial epidemic BSIs associated with a contaminated infusate (13,99,100).

Pseudomonas aeruginosa

P. aeruginosa is a ubiquitous organism that has been isolated from water, soil, and plants. It is also a frequent colonizer of human skin and mucous membranes, especially in hospitalized patients. The capability of *P. aerugi-*

nosa to withstand adverse environmental conditions may have contributed to its role as a successful nosocomial pathogen. Hospital reservoirs of *P. aeruginosa* infection have included respiratory equipment, humidifiers, fluids for intravascular administration, ophthalmic solutions, soap, sinks, and disinfectants (115).

Baltch recently gave a comprehensive historical review of the published literature on *P. aeruginosa* bacteremia (116). This bacteremia is predominantly nosocomial and typically occurs among patients with severe underlying disease. *P. aeruginosa* accounts for 8–17% of Gram-negative bacteremia cases in large series (7,10–12,35) and has been ranked sixth among the pathogens causing nosocomial BSI in critical care unit patients reported to the CDC (107).

The urinary tract, the respiratory tract, and the skin appear to be the most common portals of entry for *P. aeruginosa* into the bloodstream. In their review of 108 cases of *P. aeruginosa* bacteremia, Flick and Cluff found the respiratory tract (20%) and the urinary tract (19%) to be the major sources, followed by intravascular catheters (15%) and the skin (11%) (117). In the largest series of *P. aeruginosa* bacteremia reported to date, Bodey et al. could not identify the portal of entry in the majority of cases. *P. aeruginosa* was cultured concomitantly from an intravascular catheter in only five cases (1%) (43). In more recent reports, the rate of catheter-related BSI among cases of *P. aeruginosa* bacteremia ranged between 7% and 14% (44,45,48,118,119).

P. aeruginosa is among the predominant Gram-negative organisms causing CRI associated with various types of intravascular catheters, such as tunneled CVCs (9,17,52,55,56,88–91), nontunneled CVCs (49–51,53,74,76), small peripheral venous catheters (31,49), and pulmonary artery catheters (78), ranging in frequency from 10 to 50% of all Gram-negative isolates. Not surprisingly, these organisms appear to play a predominant role as etiologic agents of CRIs in burn patients (30,120,121).

Whereas *P. aeruginosa* bacteremia has appeared to decrease in cancer patients in recent years (9), this infection is on the increase in patients with AIDS (122–124). Roilides and coworkers reviewed 13 bacteremias and 25 nonbacteremic infections caused by *Pseudomonas* spp. in children infected with HIV (123). Central venous catheter-related infections were most frequent and accounted for 10 of 13 bacteremias and 10 of 25 nonbacteremic infections. *P. aeruginosa* was the most common pathogen. Nelson et al. found 19 episodes of *Pseudomonas* bacteremia among 584 adult patients with AIDS (124). Association with central venous catheters in 11 of 19 cases (58%) and the high mortality caused by CVC-unrelated bacteremias and in those patients whose central line was not removed was noted. Many investigators have noted the extremely high rate of mortality associated with hospital-acquired *P. aeruginosa* infections, which may range between 50 and 80% (34,35,45,117) but has appeared to decrease in the more recent past, probably due to the introduction of antipseudomonal betalactam antibiotics (43,119).

Mortality is most pronounced in bacteremia secondary to respiratory tract infection and skin/soft tissue infections (45,116,118), but it appears to be considerably lower in catheter-related infections (43,125) and as low as 9% in patients with AIDS (123).

Acinetobacter Species

Until recently, the genus *Acinetobacter* comprised a single species, *A. calcoaceticus*, and two subspecies or biovars, *A. calcoaceticus* var. *lwoffii* and *A. calcoaceticus* var. *anitratus*. Following extensive taxonomic reorganization of the genus (126), at least 32 (genomic) species are currently recognized, including the named species *A. baumannii*, *A. calcoaceticus*, *A. haemolyticus*, *A. johnsonii*, *A. junii*, *A. lwoffii*, *A. parvus*, *A. radioresistens*, *A. schindleri*, and *A. ursingii*.

In recent years, *Acinetobacter* species have emerged as clinically important pathogens. Although the organisms are widely prevalent in nature, most human infections are hospital-acquired, with *A. baumannii* being the predominant species.

Acinetobacter baumannii

Nosocomial *A. baumannii* infections—such as respiratory tract infections, urinary tract infections, meningitis, and bacteremia—mainly affect patients with severe underlying illnesses in the ICU (36,37,98,127,128). *Acinetobacter* spp. account for 1 to 6% of Gram-negative bloodstream isolates in large surveys of bacteremia (7,10–12), with considerable regional differences. In 1991, at the Institute for Medical Microbiology, Immunology and Hygiene, (University of Cologne, Germany), *Acinetobacter* spp. were among the top five organisms isolated from blood cultures, and among Gram-negative pathogens were second only to *E. coli*.

A substantial part of *A. baumannii* bacteremia cases represent catheter-related infections that usually carry a more favorable prognosis. The association of *Acinetobacter* bacteremia with indwelling vascular access devices has been reported in early reviews dating to the early 1960s (129). As reviewed by Seifert and colleagues (36), the rate of catheter-related infections among BSI caused by *Acinetobacter* spp. varied considerably (8–90%) in more recent reports (36,37,98,130,131). Rolston et al. (130) noted an increase in the number of *A. calcoaceticus* septicemia cases in cancer patients that paralleled the increasing use of intravascular catheters over a period of ten years. Beck-Sagué and coworkers (98) described an outbreak of *A. baumannii* infections that was traced to contaminated pressure transducers and involved 75 patients. In the largest survey of *A. baumannii* bacteremia reported to date (36), intravascular catheters were the major portal of entry and accounted for 39 of 87 (45%) bacteremia cases, followed by respiratory tract infections (31%) and skin and soft tissue infections (4%). The overall mortality was 44%, ranging from 21%

in patients with catheter-related BSI to 100% in patients with pneumonia. However, according to a recent survey of *A. baumannii* bacteremia in critically ill patients, the reported attributable mortality rate was only 8%, and 7% of cases were considered catheter-related (128).

In large prospective studies, *Acinetobacter* spp. were among the major organisms causing CRI. They accounted for 7 to 12% of Gram-negative bacteria isolated from infections associated with long-term CVCs of the Hickman/Broviac type (9,87,89,90). With similar frequency ranging from 4 to 24%, they were associated with infections of short-term CVCs due to Gram-negative organisms, in particular in patients with burns (30–32,76,121). Siegman-Igra et al. (127) reported 25 cases of nosocomial *Acinetobacter* meningitis secondary to invasive neurosurgical procedures. The majority of infections were associated with indwelling ventriculostomy tubes (52%) or CSF fistulae (28%). Galvao et al. (132) reported 23 cases of *Acinetobacter* peritonitis in chronic peritoneal dialysis. *Acinetobacter* represented the second most common Gram-negative pathogen in CAPD peritonitis, and was nearly as frequent as *Pseudomonas*. Catheter removal for cure of the infection was only rarely indicated.

Most of the early studies and many of the more recent studies were not based on the current taxonomy of the genus *Acinetobacter*, or did not use appropriate methods to unambiguously identify the intravascular catheter as the portal of entry in *Acinetobacter* BSI. Therefore, bacteremia cases and CRI due to *A. baumannii* and to other *Acinetobacter* species have never been clearly separated. In fact, the clinical significance of *A. baumannii* and its propensity to cause device-related bacteremia is clearly different from that of other *Acinetobacter* spp., as will be pointed out in the next section.

Acinetobacter spp. Other Than *Acinetobacter baumannii*

The clinical importance and hospital epidemiology of *Acinetobacter* spp. other than *A. baumannii* (formerly *A. calcoaceticus* var. *lwoffii*) are less well understood. These organisms are considered part of the normal flora of the human skin and mucous membranes and have only rarely been implicated in human disease. However, rare cases of meningitis, endocarditis, and bacteremia have been described (130,133–136).

Nosocomial bacteremia due to these organisms is mostly sporadic and almost exclusively related to intravascular devices (137). Seifert and colleagues recently reviewed 55 episodes of true bacteremia caused by *Acinetobacter* spp. other than *A. baumannii* that ocurred in 53 patients during a study period of 18 months (134). *Acinetobacter* spp. were not recovered from any other specimen obtained for culture in these patients, except from catheter tips. The most frequently isolated species were *A. johnsonii* (n = 14), *Acinetobacter* species 3 (n = 12), and *A. lwoffii* (n = 10). These species are also the most common *Acinetobacter* spp. isolated from the skin of healthy volunteers and hospitalized patients (138). Other *Acinetobacter* spp. (*A. junii*, *A. haemoly-*

ticus, Acinetobacter species 6, 10, and 12) were only rarely recovered from blood specimens. The clinical presentation was usually benign, and all but four patients (93%) were cured. Using strict criteria, fifty episodes (90.9%) of *Acinetobacter* bacteremia were considered definite or probably catheter-related. Only six patients showed clinical signs of exit-site infection. One episode of meningitis following neurosurgery was felt to be related to an indwelling ventricular catheter.

The main differences regarding predisposing factors, epidemiologic features, and clinical characteristics of CRBSI caused by *A. baumannii* and *Acinetobacter* spp. other than *A. baumannii*, have been reviewed in detail by Seifert (139).

PATHOGENESIS

The complex pathogenesis of CRI is reviewed by Sherertz in another chapter of this book. However, nearly all in vitro and animal studies investigating the pathogenesis of infections related to intravascular devices have focused on Gram-positive organisms, in particular coagulase-negative staphylococci and *S. aureus*, as well as *Candida* spp. (8). Little is known about the specific factors involved in the pathogenesis of CRI due to Gram-negative organisms.

It is widely accepted that the largest proportion of catheter-related BSIs derive from the cutaneous flora at the insertion site or from contamination of the catheter hub (69). As demonstrated earlier, enteric Gram-negative rods— if compared with Gram-positive bacteria—are implicated less frequently in catheter-related infections, especially those associated with peripheral and nontunneled CVCs. This may be partly explained by the fact that Gram-negative bacteria, with the exception of *Acinetobacter* spp., are not part of the resident human skin flora. However, with prolonged hospitalization, patients are increasingly colonized with nosocomial pathogens, namely *P. aeruginosa*, *Enterobacter*, and *Klebsiella* spp., especially in areas with high endemic transmission, such as ICUs. In a prospective surveillance study, we recently showed that during a nosocomial outbreak due to *A. baumannii* in a surgical ICU, 74% of patients hospitalized for more than 72 hours were colonized with the epidemic strain after a mean ICU stay of four days (140). Respiratory tract colonization was usually demonstrated initially and followed by colo- nization of various body surface sites. The skin of the subclavian region, the area most commonly used for the insertion of CVCs, showed the highest colonization rates, followed by the axilla, groin, and antecubital fossa. Thus, in the epidemiological setting described here, nosocomial Gram-negative pathogens may colonize intravascular catheters in a way similar to that of the common Gram-positive bacteria that are usually present on human skin.

The properties that cause adherence of staphylococci to intravascular catheters play a predominant role in the pathogenesis of device-related infections due to CoNS. Usually, Gram-negative bacteria adhere less readily to polymer surfaces than CoNS, with the exception of *P. aeruginosa* and *Acinetobacter* spp. (141). Scanning electron microscope studies revealed that colonization of polyurethane catheters with different *Acinetobacter* spp. occurred in a similar time frame and to an extent comparable to CoNS (author's unpublished observation).

Like most environmental bacteria, *P. aeruginosa* lives predominantly in biofilms adherent to available surfaces, from which it periodically releases planktonic (free-swimming) cells. *P. aeruginosa* possesses a tremendous array of virulence factors that have been excellently reviewed by Woods and Vasil (142). As observed with CoNS, growth in biofilms protects *P. aeruginosa* cells from antibacterial factors produced by the host as well as from antibiotics, and may account for the survival and extended persistence of the bacteria on foreign devices. *P. aeruginosa* embedded in thick biofilm has been seen on a variety of transcutaneous medical devices such as vascular catheters (143), peritoneal catheters (144), and urinary catheters (145). It has been suggested that polymer catheters made of PVC or silicone may favor survival and growth of *P. aeruginosa* (146).

Other mechanisms, such as the invasion of bacteria from contaminated parenteral fluid, are only rarely involved in CRBSI caused by staphylococci (71) but, as demonstrated earlier, they may play an important role in the pathogenesis of CRBSI caused by Gram-negative bacteria. The contribution of hematogenous seeding of the catheter tip from remote unrelated sites of infection to catheter colonization and sepsis has only rarely been demonstrated (69). In patients with hematological disorders, however, especially in those with altered mucosal barriers following cytotoxic chemotherapy, there may be translocation of endogenous gut bacteria to the catheter (147). Groeger and coworkers suggested that this mechanism may explain the fact that device-related bacteremia in cancer patients was caused predominantly by Gram-negative enteric bacilli (17).

The different growth properties of microbial pathogens in parenteral fluids may also play an important role. Although microbial growth in most solutions used for parenteral administration is rather poor, different infusion fluids may support the growth of specific organisms. Parenteral nutrition solutions are excellent substrates for the growth of certain microorganisms. Goldmann and coworkers demonstrated that *K. pneumoniae* and *S. marcescens* grew exuberantly in peptone containing casein hydrolysate–dextrose solution, whereas other bacteria tested, such as *S. aureus*, *E. coli*, and *P. mirabilis,* grew more slowly and *P. aeruginosa* slowly died (148). Distilled water may allow the proliferation of *B. cepacia* (149), *Acinetobacter*, and *Serratia* spp. (69). Glucose-containing solutions (5% dextrose in water) support the growth of *Klebsiella* spp., *Enterobacter* spp., *Serratia* spp., and *B. cepacia*, whereas *E. coli*, *Proteus* spp., and *P. aeruginosa* gradually loose viability (150). Sodium chloride solutions may support the growth of many Gram-negative bacteria. These solutions, however, usually do not allow growth of Gram-positive bacteria. Lipid emulsions, in contrast, allow rapid multiplication of nearly all microorganisms (151).

COMPLICATIONS

Arnow and coworkers recently assessed the consequences of intravascular catheter sepsis in 94 patients with 102 episodes of CRBSI due to percutane-ously inserted catheters (61). Major complications occurred in 33 (32%) of the episodes and included septic shock (12 episodes), sustained sepsis (12), suppurative thrombophlebitis (7), metastatic infection (2), endocarditis (2), and arteritis (2). The risk of major complications was highest in catheter-related BSI caused by *Candida* spp. (64%), *P. aeruginosa* (50%), and *S. aureus* (38%), followed by Gram-negative enteric bacilli (20%).

Suppurative thrombophlebitis, defined as the presence of intraluminal pus, is an inflammation of the vein wall due to the presence of microorganisms and is frequently associated with thrombosis and sustained bacteremia (151a). Suppurative thrombophlebitis is the most serious form of catheter-related infection and is particularly frequent in burn and trauma patients (152). In recent years, most cases of septic thrombophlebitis have been due to Gram-negative bacteria. Garrison and coworkers reviewed 29 cases of septic thrombophlebitis over a seven-year period (153). Gram-negative enteric bacilli, especially *Enterobacter* and *Klebsiella* spp., were the causative agents in 21 cases (72%), followed by *S. aureus* (24%). Similar results were reported by Johnson and coworkers, who noted a correlation between the isolation of enteric organisms (Gram-negative rods and enterococci) from the inflamed veins and recent abdominal surgery (154). Surgical intervention with excision of the inflamed vein is considered the treatment of choice for suppurative thrombophlebitis. For catheter-related central vein suppurative thrombo-phlebitis, the recommended approach is catheter removal, anticoagulation with heparin, and prolonged antibiotic therapy (155).

Infective endocarditis is another serious complication of CRI. Gouello et al. recently reviewed 22 patients with nosocomial endocarditis (156). Intravascular devices were the source of bacteremia resulting in endocarditis in 11 (50%) of these cases. Nosocomial endocarditis was due predominantly to *S. aureus* and CoNS, whereas only two episodes were due to a Gram-negative pathogen, *P. aeruginosa*.

MANAGEMENT

The management of device-related infection depends on the type of catheter, the underlying illness of the patient, the infecting microorganism, and the type of infection (157), and is covered in the respective chapters elsewhere in this book. This section attempts to summarize the currently recommended approaches to the management of intravascular device-related infection caused specifically by Gram-negative organisms.

Although the infection of CVCs may be successfully treated without catheter removal, it is common practice to remove and culture a short-term, percutaneous, noncuffed intravascular catheter that is suspected of being infected, irrespective of the pathogen cultured (157,158). This holds true also for peripheral catheters, pulmonary artery catheters, and arterial catheters used for hemodynamic monitoring. As outlined in a recently published guideline for the management of catheter infections, systemic antibiotic therapy for 10–14 days is recommended for cases of Gram-negative BSI related to removable central venous catheters (157). However, prospective studies to support this approach are lacking. Antibiotic therapy should be based on in vitro suceptibility of the infecting pathogen, but the superiority of a specific class of antibiotics in the treatment of Gram-negative device-related BSI has not been demonstrated.

Uncomplicated BSI associated with surgically implanted Hickman or Broviac catheters usually responds to intravenous antibiotic therapy with the catheter left in place, particularly if antibiotic lock therapy is instituted. Most investigators did not observe that the type of pathogen was an important factor in curing patients with catheter-related bacteremia without removal of the catheter (56,86,90,159). Of 172 episodes of CRBSI reported by Flynn and colleagues, 149 (87%) were successfully treated with intravenous antimicrobial therapy and without catheter removal initially (56). However, there were eight cases of recurrent bacteremia (44%) in 18 patients with totally implantable catheters that had remained in place, as opposed to 10 recurrences (8%) among 131 patients with Hickman/Broviac catheters that were not removed initially. Among 16 cases of BSI related to Hickman/Broviac catheters caused by *E. cloacae* and treated with antibiotics alone, only one case of recurrence (6%) was observed 94 days after initial recovery of the organism. Similarly, two recurrences (18%) were observed among 11 cases of *P. aeruguinosa* CRBSI after 21 and 105 days, respectively. Of the eight recurrences associated with infected totally implantable catheters, two were due to Gram-negative pathogens.

In contrast, Rotstein and associates demonstrated that fungal or Gram-negative pathogens were most predictive of catheter removal (89). Twenty-five (24%) of 103 Hickman catheter-related infections due to Gram-positive organisms resulted in catheter removal, in contrast to 13 (52%) of 25 infections caused by Gram-negative bacilli. Certain organisms such as *S. aureus*, *Bacillus* spp., *Corynebacterium jeikeium*, yeasts, and atypical mycobacteria have been traditionally considered to be difficult to eradicate and may require catheter removal. Mermel and colleagues have recommended that uncomplicated BSI related to tunneled central venous catheters or totally implantable ports may be treated with systemic and antibiotic lock therapy for 14 days. Complicated cases of CRBSI such as those associated with tunnel infection or port abscess, in contrast, require catheter removal combined with systemic antibiotics for 14 days (157).

Various reports have demonstrated that catheter-related BSI, including those caused by enteric Gram-negative bacilli, can be cured with intravenous antibiotics administered over the infected catheter (56,86,87,125,159). More recently, a new technique to treat central venous catheter infection has been proposed. Called the antibiotic lock technique, it involves instillation of a highly concentrated antimicrobial agent into the catheter lumen, where it remains in place for 12 hours. Successful management of CRI with this technique, including infections caused by Gram-negative organisms, has been documented (160–162). In a similar protocol, Rao et al. successfully treated Broviac catheter infection caused by Gram-negative bacilli with 8-hourly instillation of 1 ml of heparinized amikacin solution (163). Capdevila et al. prospectively studied 36 chronic renal failure patients who had 13 episodes of CRBSI (164). Vancomycin and/or ciprofloxacin were administered in a 4-hour continuous infusion, at a concentration of 100 µg/ml, into each catheter lumen between two dialysis sessions. All episodes in which *S. epidermidis* and *P. aeruguinosa* accounted for 77% of the isolates were successfully treated without catheter removal.

Gascon and colleagues recently described the successful catheter salvage in a hemodialysis patient with CRBSI caused by *P. aeruguinosa*, using IV aztreonam and oral clarithromycin after initial therapy with ceftazidim and amikacin had failed to eradicate the organism (165). Clarithromycin was administered in an attempt to destroy the *Pseudomonas* biofilm. Krishnasami et al. (23) prospectively analyzed the efficacy of an antibiotic lock protocol, consisting of vancomycin (5 mg/ml), gentamicin (4 mg/ml), and cefazolin (10 mg/ml) combined with systemic intravenous antibiotic therapy administered for three weeks in patients with dialysis catheter-related bacteremia. Catheter salvage occurred in 40 of 62 patients (64.5%). The bacteriological success rate was similar for Gram-positive (64%) and Gram-negative pathogens (59%). However, serious complications occurred in 11 patients, including septic shock (5 patients), septic arthritis (1), and endocarditis (3). Six of the infections resulting in serious complications were caused by Gram-negative bacilli. The antibiotic lock technique was recently reviewed extensively by Carratalà (166).

Catheter removal was significantly associated with survival in patients with bacteremia caused by *A. baumannii*, whereas appropriate antimicrobial therapy was not (36). The occurrence of multiresistant strains often limits therapeutic options (167). *Acinetobacter* spp. other than *A. baumannii*, in contrast, are usually susceptible to most antimicrobial agents, and successful management of bacteremia due to these organisms in one series included catheter removal in 45 cases (82%) and appropriate antimicrobial therapy in 34 cases (62%). Seven patients were successfully treated with the catheter left in place (134).

The management of catheter-related infections caused by *Pseudomonas* is less clear. Whereas some reseachers have found *P. aeruginosa* among the organisms that more frequently have required catheter removal (89), others have not documented a correlation between specific Gram-negative organisms and failure to eradicate these organisms from an infected catheter left in place (56,125,168). Elting and Bodey reviewed their experience with catheter-related bacteremia caused by *S. maltophilia* and nonaeruginosa Pseudomonas spp. (169). They noted a high rate of treatment failure and recurrence when the catheter was not removed, whereas all patients whose catheters were removed were cured. Similar observations were made by Nelson et al. in patients with catheter-related *P. aeruginosa* bacteremia associated with HIV (124). Conversely, 13 of 20 catheter-related *P. aeruginosa* infections (65%) reported by Roilides et al. (123) were successfully treated with appropriate antibiotics without removal of the involved catheter. Prompt initiation of appropriate therapy, usually administered as a combination of an antipseudomonal betalactam and an aminoglycoside, is considered crucial to improve survival.

Whereas exit-site infections usually can be treated with antibiotics and local care without removal of the catheter (87,90), management with the catheter left in place is probably less successful in tunnel infections that require catheter removal if not responding promptly to intravenous antibiotics (88,170). This may be especially true if these infections are caused by *P. aeruginosa*. Of the 20 tunnel infections reported by Benezra and associates (88), only five were successfully treated with antibiotics, and the other 15 required catheter removal for cure. Eleven of the cases requiring catheter removal were caused by *P. aeruginosa*.

CONCLUSION

Although less often implicated than Gram-positive organisms, Gram-negative bacilli, in particular members of the family Enterobacteriaceae, *P. aeruginosa*, and *Acinetobacter* spp., account for up to one-third of infections associated with most intravascular devices. Rates as high as 50% have been observed in catheter-related BSI, as well as in exit-site and tunnel infections due to these organisms, if surgically implanted catheters are involved. Of particular importance is the propensity of certain Gram-negative organisms to cause infections associated with bacterial contamination of infusate and contamination of blood products, probably due to the specific growth properties of Gram-negative bacilli in various infusion fluids. These organisms have also been implicated in the majority of hospital outbreaks of infusion-related bacteremia.

Factors involved in the pathogenesis of CRI associated with Gram-negative bacilli have only rarely been investigated. As with CoNS, the adherence properties and the formation of biofilm of certain Gram-negative organisms, such as *P. aeruginosa* and *Acinetobacter* spp., may play an important role in the pathogenesis of these infections.

The treatment of CRI due to Gram-negative organisms is usually not different from the general recommendations regarding the management of infections associated with intravascular devices, although this question has not been specifically addressed in prospective clinical trials. Treatment of Gram-negative infections associated with surgically implanted catheters, including antibiotic lock therapy, has been equally successful as with Gram-positive organisms. Possible complications such as sustained bacteremia and suppurative thrombophlebitis, which is most often caused by Gram-negative organisms, have to be considered. There is evidence, however, that CRI due to *P. aeruginosa* usually requires catheter removal for cure.

REFERENCES

1. Banerjee SN, Emori TG, Culver DH, Gaynes RP, Jarvis WR, Horan T, Edwards JR, Tolson J, Henderson T, Martone WJ. Secular trends in nosocomial primary bloodstream infections in the United States, 1980–1989. Am J Med 1991; 91(suppl 3B):86S–89S.
2. Schaberg DR, Culver DH, Gaynes RP. Major trends in the microbial etiology of nosocomial infection. Am J Med 1991; 91(suppl 3B):72S–75S.
3. Edmond MB, Wallace SE, McClish DK, Pfaller MA, Jones RN, Wenzel RP. Nosocomial bloodstream infections in United States hospitals: a three-year analysis. Clin Infect Dis 1999; 29:239–244.
4. Diekema DJ, Beekmann SE, Chapin KC, Morel KA, Munson E, Doern GV. Epidemiology and outcome of nosocomial and community-onset bloodstream infection. J Clin Microbiol 2003; 41:3655–3660.
5. Patterson JE, Sweeney AH, Simms M, Carley N, Mangi R, Sabetta J, Lyons RW. An analysis of 110 serious enterococcal infections. Epidemiology, antibiotic susceptibility, and outcome. Medicine (Baltimore) 1995; 74:191–200.
6. Wisplinghoff H, Seifert H, Wenzel RP, Edmond MB. Current trends in the epidemiology of nosocomial bloodstream infections in patients with hematological malignancies and solid neoplasms in hospitals in the United States. Clin Infect Dis 2003; 36:1103–1110.
7. Diekema DJ, Pfaller MA, Jones RN, Doern GV, Winokur PL, Gales AC, Sader HS, Kugler K, Beach M. Survey of bloodstream infections due to gram-negative bacilli: frequency of occurrence and antimicrobial susceptibility of isolates collected in the United States, Canada, and Latin America for the SENTRY Antimicrobial Surveillance Program, 1997. Clin Infect Dis 1999; 29:595–607.
8. Goldmann DA, Pier GB. Pathogenesis of infections related to intravascular catheterization. Clin Microbiol Rev 1993; 6:176–192.
9. Kiehn TE, Armstrong D. Changes in the spectrum of organisms causing bacteremia and fungemia in immunocompromised patients due to venous access devices. Eur J Clin Microbiol Infect Dis 1990; 9:869–872.

10. Geerdes HF, Ziegler D, Lode H, Hund M, Loehr A, Fangmann W, Wagner J. Septicemia in 980 patients at a university hospital in Berlin: prospective studies during 3 selected years between 1979 and 1989. Clin Infect Dis 1992; 15:991–1002.

11. Weinstein MP, Reller LB, Murphy JR, Lichtenstein KA. The clinical significance of positive blood cultures: a comprehensive analysis of 500 episodes of bacteremia and fungemia in adults. 1. Laboratory and epidemiologic observations. Rev Infect Dis 1983; 5:35–53.

12. Roberts FJ, Geere IW, Coldman A. A three-year study of positive blood cultures, with emphasis on prognosis. Rev Infect Dis 1991; 13:34–46.

13. Maki DG. Nosocomial bacteremia. An epidemiologic overview. Am J Med 1981; 70:719–732.

14. Smith RL, Meixler SM, Simberkoff MS. Excess mortality in critically ill patients with nosocomial bloodstream infections. Chest 1991; 100:164–167.

15. Rello J, Quintana E, Mirelis B, Gurgui M, Net A, Prats G. Polymicrobial bacteremia in critically ill patients. Intensive Care Med 1993; 19:22–25.

16. Archibald LK, Ramos M, Arduino MJ, Aguero SM, Deseda C, Banerjee S, Jarvis WR. *Enterobacter cloacae* and *Pseudomonas aeruginosa* polymicrobial bloodstream infections traced to extrinsic contamination of a dextrose multidose vial. J Pediatr 1998; 133:640–644.

17. Groeger JS, Lucas AB, Thaler HT, Friedlander-Klar H, Brown AE, Kiehn TE, Armstrong D. Infectious morbidity associated with long-term use of venous access devices in patients with cancer. Ann Intern Med 1993; 119:1168–1174.

18. Velasco E, Byington R, Martins CA, Schirmer M, Dias LM, Goncalves VM. Prospective evaluation of the epidemiology, microbiology, and outcome of bloodstream infections in hematologic patients in a single cancer center. Eur J Clin Microbiol Infect Dis 2003; 22:137–143.

19. Gonzalez-Barca E, Fernandez-Sevilla A, Carratala J, Granena A, Gudiol F. Prospective study of 288 episodes of bacteremia in neutropenic cancer patients in a single institution. Eur J Clin Microbiol Infect Dis 1996; 15:291–296.

20. Collin BA, Leather HL, Wingard JR, Ramphal R. Evolution, incidence, and susceptibility of bacterial bloodstream isolates from 519 bone marrow transplant patients. Clin Infect Dis 2001; 33:947–953.

21. Vidal F, Mensa J, Martinez JA, Almela M, Marco F, Gatell JM, Richart C, Soriano E, Jimenez de Anta MT. *Pseudomonas aeruginosa* bacteremia in patients infected with human immunodeficiency virus type 1. Eur J Clin Microbiol Infect Dis 1999; 18:473–477.

22. Nicastri E, Petrosillo N, Viale P, Ippolito G. Catheter-related bloodstream infections in HIV-infected patients. Ann N Y Acad Sci 2001; 946:274–290.

23. Krishnasami Z, Carlton D, Bimbo L, Taylor ME, Balkovetz DF, Barker J, Allon M. Management of hemodialysis catheter-related bacteremia with an adjunctive antibiotic lock solution. Kidney Int 2002; 61:1136–1142.

24. Chien LY, Macnab Y, Aziz K, Andrews W, McMillan DD, Lee SK. Canadian Neonatal Network. Variations in central venous catheter-related infection risks among Canadian neonatal intensive care units. Pediatr Infect Dis J 2002; 21:505–511.

25. Wisplinghoff H, Seifert H, Tallent SM, Bischoff T, Wenzel RP, Edmond MB. Nosocomial bloodstream infections in pediatric patients in United States hospitals: epidemiology, clinical features and susceptibilities. Pediatr Infect Dis J 2003; 22:686–691.

26. Digiovine B, Chenoweth C, Watts C, Higgins M. The attributable mortality and costs of primary nosocomial bloodstream infections in the intensive care unit. Am J Respir Crit Care Med 1999; 160:976–981.

27. Rello J, Ochagavia A, Sabanes E, Roque M, Mariscal D, Reynaga E, Valles J. Evaluation of outcome of intravenous catheter-related infections in critically ill patients. Am J Respir Crit Care Med 2000; 162:1027–1030.

28. Renaud B, Brun-Buisson C, ICU-Bacteremia Study Group. Outcomes of primary and catheter-related bacteremia. A cohort and case-control study in critically ill patients. Am J Respir Crit Care Med 2001; 163:1584–1590.

29. Rosenthal VD, Guzman S, Orellano PW. Nosocomial infections in medical-surgical intensive care units in Argentina: attributable mortality and length of stay. Am J Infect Control 2003; 31:291–295.

30. Franceschi D, Gerding RL, Philips G, Fratianne RB. Risk factors associated with intravascular catheter infections in burned patients: a prospective, randomized study. J Trauma 1989; 29:811–816.

31. Maki DG, Jarrett F, Sarafin HW. A semiquantitative culture method for identification of catheter-related infection in the burn patient. IV. Growth microbial pathogens in fluids for intravenous infusions. J Surg Res 1977; 22:513–520.

32. Santucci SG, Gobara S, Santos CR, Fontana C, Levin AS. Infections in a burn intensive care unit: experience of seven years. J Hosp Infect 2003; 53: 6–13.

33. Leibovici L, Konisberger H, Pitlik SD, Samra Z, Drucker M. Bacteremia and fungemia of unknown origin in adults. Clin Infect Dis 1992; 14:436–443.

34. Kreger BE, Craven DE, Carling PC, McCabe WR. Gram-negative bacteremia. III. Reassessment of etiology, epidemiology and ecology in 612 patients. Am J Med 1980; 68:332–343.

35. Bryan CS, Reynolds KL, Brenner ER. Analysis of 1,186 Episodes of gram-negative bacteremia in non-university hospitals: The effects of antimicrobial therapy. Rev Infect Dis 1983; 5:629–638.

36. Seifert H, Strate A, Pulverer G. Nosocomial bacteremia due to *Acinetobacter baumannii*: clinical features, epidemiology, and predictors of mortality. Medicine (Baltimore) 1995; 74:340–349.

37. Cisneros JM, Reyes MJ, Pachon J, Becerril B, Caballero FJ, García-Garmendia JL, Ortiz C, Cobacho AR, Bacteremia due to *Acinetobacter baumannii*: epidemiology, clinical findings, and prognostic features.

38. Gransden WR, Eykyn SJ, Phillips I, Rowe B. Bacteremia due to *Escherichia coli*: a study of 861 episodes. Rev Infect Dis 1990; 12:1008–1018.

39. Gallagher PG. *Enterobacter* bacteremia in pediatric patients. Rev Infect Dis 1990; 12:808–812.

40. García de la Torre M, Romero-Vivas J, Martínez-Beltrán J, Guerrero A, Meseguer M, Bouza E. *Klebsiella* bacteremia: an analysis of 100 episodes. Rev Infect Dis 1985; 7:143–150.

41. Bouza E, García de la Torre M, Erice A, Cercenado E, Loza E, Rodriguez-Créixems M. *Serratia* bacteremia. Diagn Microbiol Infect Dis 1987; 7:237–247.

42. Choi SH, Kim YS, Chung JW, Kim TH, Choo EJ, Kim MN, Kim BN, Kim NJ, Woo JH, Ryu J. *Serratia* bacteremia in a large university hospital: trends in antibiotic resistance during 10 years and implications for antibiotic use. Infect Control Hosp Epidemiol 2002; 23:740–747.

43. Bodey GP, Jadeja L, Elting L. *Pseudomonas* bacteremia: Retrospective analysis of 410 episodes. Arch Intern Med 1985; 145:1621–1629.

44. Vazquez F, Mendoza MC, Villar MH, Vindel A, Mendez FJ. Characteristics of *Pseudomonas aeruginosa* strains causing septicemia in a Spanish hospital 1981–1990. Eur J Clin Microbiol Infect Dis 1992; 11:698–703.

45. Bisbe J, Gatell JM, Puig J, Mallolas J, Martinez JA, Jimenez de Anta MT, Soriano E. *Pseudomonas aeruginosa* bacteremia: univariate and multivariate analyses of factors influencing the prognosis in 133 episodes. Rev Infect Dis 1988; 10:629–635.

46. Kuikka A, Sivonen A, Emelianova A, Valtonen VV. Prognostic factors associated with improved outcome of *Escherichia coli* bacteremia in a Finnish university hospital. Eur J Clin Microbiol Infect Dis 1997; 16:125–134.

47. Grisaru-Soen G, Lerner-Geva L, Keller N, Berger H, Passwell JH, Barzilai A. *Pseudomonas aeruginosa* bacteremia in children: analysis of trends in prevalence, antibiotic resistance and prognostic factors. Pediatr Infect Dis J 2000; 19:959–963.

48. Blot S, Vandewoude K, Hoste E, Colardyn F. Reappraisal of attributable mortality in critically ill patients with nosocomial bacteraemia involving *Pseudomonas aeruginosa*. J Hosp Infect 2003; 53:18–24.

49. Richet H, Hubert B, Nitemberg G, Andremont A, Buu-Hoi A, Ourbak P, Galicier C, Veron M, Boisivon A, Bouvier AM, Ricome JC, Wolff MA, Pean Y, Berardi-Grassias L, Bourdain JL, Hautefort B, Laaban JP, Tillant D. Prospective multicenter study of vascular-catheter-related complications and risk factors for positive central-catheter cultures in intensive care unit patients. J Clin Microbiol 1990; 28:2520–2525.

50. Sherertz RJ, Raad II, Belani A, Koo LC, Rand KH, Pickett DL, Straub SA, Fauerbach LL. Three-year experience with sonicated vascular catheter cultures in a clinical microbiology laboratory. J Clin Microbiol 1990; 28:76–82.

51. Gil RT, Kruse JA, Thill-Baharozian MC, Carlson RW. Triple-vs single-lumen central venous catheters. A prospective study in a critically ill population. Arch Intern Med 1989; 149:1139–1143.

52. Blot F, Nitenberg G, Chachaty E, Raynard B, Germann N, Antoun S, Laplanche A, Brun-Buisson C, Tancrede C. Diagnosis of catheter-related bacteremia: a prospective comparison of the time to positivity of hub-blood versus peripheral-blood cultures. Lancet 1999; 354:1071–1077.

53. Seifert H, Cornely O, Seggewiss K, Decker M, Stefanik D, Wisplinghoff H, Fatkenheuer G. Bloodstream infection in neutropenic cancer patients related to short-term nontunnelled catheters determined by quantitative blood cultures, differential time to positivity, and molecular epidemiological typing with pulsed-field gel electrophoresis. J Clin Microbiol 2003; 41:118–123.

54. Castagnola E, Garaventa A, Viscoli C, Carrega G, Nantron M, Molinari C, Moroni C, Giacchino R. Changing pattern of pathogens causing broviac catheter-related bacteraemias in children with cancer. J Hosp Infect 1995; 29:129–133.

55. Elishoov H, Or R, Strauss N, Engelhard D. Nosocomial colonization, septicemia, and Hickman/Broviac catheter-related infections in bone marrow transplant recipients. A 5-year prospective study. Medicine (Baltimore) 1998; 77:83–101.

56. Flynn PM, Willis B, Gaur AH, Shenep JL. Catheter design influences recurrence of catheter-related bloodstream infection in children with cancer. J Clin Oncol 2003; 21:3520–3525.

57. Kamal GD, Pfaller MA, Rempe LE, Jebson PJ. Reduced intravascular catheter infections by antibiotic bonding. A prospective, randomized, controlled trial. JAMA 1991; 265:2364–2368.

58. Darouiche RO, Raad II, Heard SO, Thornby JI, Wenker OC, Gabrielli A, Berg J, Khardori N, Hanna H, Hachem R, Harris RL, Mayhall G. Catheter Study Group. A comparison of two antimicrobial-impregnated central venous catheters. N Engl J Med 1999; 340:1–8.

59. Ranucci M, Isgro G, Giomarelli PP, Pavesi M, Luzzani A, Cattabriga I, Carli M, Giomi P, Compostella A, Digito A, Mangani V, Silvestri V, Mondelli E. Catheter Related Infection Trial (CRIT) Group. Impact of oligon central venous catheters on catheter colonization and catheter-related bloodstream infection. Crit Care Med 2003; 31:52–59.

60. Hoffmann KK, Western SA, Kaiser DL, Wenzel RP, Groschel DH. Bacterial colonization and phlebitis-associated risk with transparent polyurethane film for peripheral intravenous site dressings. Am J Infect Control 1988; 16:101–106.

61. Arnow PM, Quimosing EM, Beach M. Consequences of intravascular catheter sepsis. Clin Infect Dis 1993; 16:778–784.

62. Maki DG, Ringer M, Alvarado CJ. Prospective randomised trial of povidon-iodone, alcohol, and chlorhexidine for prevention of infection associated with central venous and arterial catheters. Lancet 1991; 338:339–343.

63. Flowers RH, Schwenzer KJ, Kopel RF, Fisch MJ, Tucker SI, Farr BM. Efficacy of an attachable subcutaneous cuff for the prevention of intravascular catheter-related infection. JAMA 1989; 261:878–883.

64. O'Grady NP, Alexander M, Dellinger EP, Gerberding JL, Heard SO, Maki DG, Masur H, McCormick RD, Mermel LA, Pearson ML, Raad II, Randolph A, Weinstein RA. Healthcare Infection Control Practices Advisory Committee. Guidelines for the prevention of intravascular catheter-related infections. Infect Control Hosp Epidemiol 2002; 23:759–769.

65. Wagener MM, Yu VL. Bacteremia in transplant recipients: a prospective study of demographics, etiologic agents, risk factors, and outcomes. Am J Infect Control 1992; 20:239–247.

66. Weinstein MP, Reller LB, Murphy JR. Clinical importance of polymicrobial bacteremia. Diagn Microbiol Infect Dis 1986; 5:185–196.

67. Reuben AG, Musher DM, Hamill RJ, Broucke I. Polymicrobial bacteremia: clinical and microbiologic patterns. Rev Infect Dis 1989; 11:161–183.

68. Martino R, Gomez L, Pericas R, Salazar R, Sola C, Sierra J, Garau J. Bacteraemia caused by non-glucose-fermenting Gram-negative bacilli and *Aeromonas* species in patients with haematological malignancies and solid tumours. Eur J Clin Microbiol Infect Dis 2000; 19:320–323.

69. Maki DG. Infections caused by intravascular devices. In: Bisno AL, Waldvogel FA, eds. Infections Associated with Indwelling Medical Devices. 2d ed. Washington: ASM Press, 1994:155–212.

70. Maki DG, Mermel L. Infections due to infusion therapy. In: Bennet JV, Brachman PS, eds. Hospital Infections. 4th ed. Philadelphia: Lippincott-Raven, 1998:689–724.

71. Maki DG, Weise CE, Sarafin HW. A semiquantitative culture method for identifying intravenous-catheter-related infection. N Engl J Med 1977; 296: 1305–1309.

72. Maki DG, Ringer M. Risk factors for infusion-related phlebitis with small peripheral venous catheters. A randomized controlled trial. Ann Intern Med 1991; 114:845–854.

73. Bregenzer T, Conen D, Sakmann P, Widmer AF. Is routine replacement of peripheral intravenous catheters necessary? Arch Intern Med 1998; 158:151–156.

74. Eyer S, Brummitt C, Crossley K, Siegel R, Cerra F. Catheter-related sepsis: prospective randomized study of three methods of long-term catheter maintenance. Crit Care Med 1990; 18:1073–1079.

75. Yeung C, May J, Hughes R. Infection rate for single lumen v triple lumen subclavian catheters. Infect Control Hosp Epidemiol 1988; 9:154–158.

76. Haslett TM, Isenberg HD, Hilton E, Tucci V, Kay BG, Vellozzi EM. Microbiology of indwelling central intravascular catheters. J Clin Microbiol 1988; 26:696–701.

77. Gowardman JR, Montgomery C, Thirlwell S, Shewan J, Idema A, Larsen PD, Havill JH. Central venous catheter-related bloodstream infections: an analysis of incidence and risk factors in a cohort of 400 patients. Intensive Care Med 1998; 24:1034–1039.

78. Mermel LA, Maki DG. Infectious complications of Swan-Ganz pulmonary artery catheters. Pathogenesis, epidemiology, prevention, and management. Am J Respir Crit Care Med 1994; 149:1020–1036.

79. Kac G, Durain E, Amrein C, Herisson E, Fiemeyer A, Buu-Hoi A. Colonization and infection of pulmonary artery catheter in cardiac surgery patients: epidemiology and multivariate analysis of risk factors. Crit Care Med 2001; 29:971–975.

80. Band JD, Maki DG. Infections caused by arterial catheters used for hemodynamic monitoring. Am J Med 1979; 67:735–741.

81. Donowitz LG, Marsik FJ, Hoyt JW, Wenzel RP. *Serratia marcescens* bacteremia from contaminated pressure transducers. JAMA 1979; 242:1749–1751.

82. Beck-Sagué CM, Jarvis WR. Epidemic bloodstream infections associated with pressure transducers: a persistent problem. Infect Control Hosp Epidemiol 1989; 10:54–59.

83. Raad I, Abi-Said D, Carrasco CH, Umphrey J, Hill LA. The risk of infection

associated with intra-arterial catheters for cancer chemotherapy. Infect Control Hosp Epidemiol 1998; 19:640–642.

84. El-Hamamsy I, Durrleman N, Stevens LM, Leung TK, Theoret S, Carrier M, Perrault LP. Incidence and outcome of radial artery infections following cardiac surgery. Ann Thorac Surg 2003; 76:801–804.

85. Press OW, Ramsey PG, Larson EB, Fefer A, Hickman RO. Hickman catheter infections in patients with malignancies. Medicine-Baltimore 1984; 63:189–200.

86. Weightman NC, Simpson EM, Speller DC, Mott MG, Oakhill A. Bacteraemia related to indwelling central venous catheters: prevention, diagnosis and treatment. Eur J Clin Microbiol Infect Dis 1988; 7:125–129.

87. Decker MD, Edwards KM. Central venous catheter infections. Pediatr Clin North Am 1988; 35:579–612.

88. Benezra D, Kiehn TE, Gold JW, Brown AE, Turnbull AD, Armstrong D. Prospective study of infections in indwelling central venous catheters using quantitative blood cultures. Am J Med 1988; 85:495–498.

89. Rotstein C, Brock L, Roberts RS. The incidence of first Hickman catheter-related infection and predictors of catheter removal in cancer patients. Infect Control Hosp Epidemiol 1995; 16:451–458.

90. Johnson PR, Decker MD, Edwards KM, Schaffner W, Wright PF. Frequency of broviac catheter infections in pediatric oncology patients. J Infect Dis 1986; 154:570–578.

91. Jean G, Charra B, Chazot C, Vanel T, Terrat JC, Hurot JM, Laurent G. Risk factor analysis for long-term tunneled dialysis catheter-related bacteremias. Nephron 2002; 91:399–405.

92. Mueller BU, Skelton J, Callender DP, Marshall D, Gress J, Longo D, Norton J, Rubin M, Venzon D, Pizzo PA. A prospective randomized trial comparing the infectious and noninfectious complications of an externalized catheter versus a subcutaneously implanted device in cancer patients. J Clin Oncol 1992; 10:1943–1948.

93. Matsaniotis NS, Syriopoulou VP, Theodoridou MC, Tzanetou KG, Mostrou GI. *Enterobacter* sepsis in infants and children due to contaminated intravenous fluids. Infect Control 1984; 5:471–477.

94. Maki DG, Rhame FS, Mackel DC, Bennett JV. Nationwide epidemic of septicemia caused by contaminated intravenous products. I. Epidemiologic and clinical features. Am J Med 1976; 60:471–485.

95. Jarvis WR. Nosocomial outbreaks: the Centers for Disease Control's Hospital Infections Program experience, 1980–1990. Epidemiology Branch, Hospital Infections Program. Am J Med 1991; 91(suppl 3B):101S–106S.

96. Jarvis WR, Highsmith AK, Allen JR, Haley RW. Polymicrobial bacteremia associated with lipid emulsion in a neonatal intensive care unit. Pediatr Infect Dis 1983; 2:203–208.

97. Mermel LA, Maki DG. Epidemic bloodstream infections from hemodynamic pressure monitoring: signs of the times. Infect Control Hosp Epidemiol 1989; 10:47–53.

98. Beck-Sagué CM, Jarvis WR, Brook JH, Culver DH, Potts A, Gay E, Shotts BW, Hill B, Anderson RL, Weinstein MP. Epidemic bacteremia due to

Acinetobacter baumannii in five intensive care units. Am J Epidemiol 1990; 132:723–733.

99. Bennett SN, McNeil MM, Bland LA, Arduino MJ, Villarino ME, Perrotta DM, Burwen DR, Welbel SF, Pegues DA, Stroud L, Zeitz PS, Jarvis WR. Postoperative infections traced to contamination of an intravenous anesthetic, propofol. N Engl J Med 1995; 333:147–154.

100. Ostrowsky BE, Whitener C, Bredenberg HK, Carson LA, Holt S, Hutwagner L, Arduino MJ, Jarvis WR. *Serratia marcescens* bacteremia traced to an infused narcotic. N Engl J Med 2002; 346:1529–1537.

101. Morduchowicz G, Pitlik SD, Huminer D, Alkan M, Drucker M, Rosenfeld JB, Block CS. Transfusion reactions due to bacterial contamination of blood and blood products. Rev Infect Dis 1991; 13:307–314.

102. Bufill JA, Ritch PS. *Yersinia enterocolitica* serotype 0:3 sepsis after blood transfusion. N Engl J Med 1989; 320:810.

103. Rhame FS, Root RK, MacLowry JD, Dadisman TA, Bennett JV. *Salmonella* septicaemia from platelet transfusions. Study of an outbreak traced to a hematogenous carrier of *Salmonella* cholerae-suis. Ann Intern Med 1973; 78:633–641.

104. Murray AE, Bartzokas CA, Shepherd AJN, Roberts FM. Blood transfusion-associated *Pseudomonas fluorescens* septicaemia: is this an increasing problem? J Hosp Infect 1987; 9:243–248.

105. Buchholz DH, Young VM, Friedman NR, Reilly JA, Mardiney MR Jr. Bacterial proliferation in platelet products stored at room temperature. Transfusion-induced *Enterobacter* sepsis. N Engl J Med 1971; 285:429–433.

106. Palavecino E, Yomtovian R. Risk and prevention of transfusion-related sepsis. Curr Opin Hematol 2003; 10:434–439.

107. Jarvis WR, Martone WJ. Predominant pathogens in hospital infections. J Antimicrob Chemother 1992; 29(suppl A):19–24.

108. Bodey GP, Elting L, Kassamali H, Lim BP. *Escherichia coli* bacteremia in cancer patients. Am J Med 1986; 81(suppl 1A):85–95.

109. Bouza E, Garcia de la Torre G, Erice A, Loza E, Diaz-Borrego JM, Buzón L. *Enterobacter* bacteremia. An analysis of 50 episodes. Arch Intern Med 1985; 145:1024–1027.

110. Chow JW, Fine MJ, Shlaes DM, Quinn JP, Hooper DC, Johnson MP, Ramphal R, Wagener MM, Miyashiro DK, Yu VL. *Enterobacter* bacteremia: clinical features and emergence of antibiotic resistance during therapy. Ann Intern Med 1991; 115:585–590.

111. Bodey GP, Elting LS, Rodriguez S. Bacteremia caused by *Enterobacter*: 15 years of experience in a cancer hospital. Rev Infect Dis 1991; 13:550–558.

112. Blot SI, Vandewoude KH, Colardyn FA. Clinical impact of nosocomial *Klebsiella* bacteremia in critically ill patients. Eur J Clin Microbiol Infect Dis 2002; 21:471–473.

113. Pena C, Pujol M, Ardanuy C, Ricart A, Pallares R, Linares J, Ariza J, Gudiol F. An outbreak of hospital-acquired *Klebsiella pneumoniae* bacteraemia, including strains producing extended-spectrum beta-lactamase. J Hosp Infect 2001; 47:53–59.

114. Saito H, Elting L, Bodey GP, Berkey P. *Serratia* bacteremia: review of 118 cases. Rev Infect Dis 1989; 11:912–920.

115. Pollack M. *Pseudomonas aeruginosa.* In: Mandell GL, Douglas RG, Bennett J, eds. Principles and pratice of infectious diseases. 4th ed. New York: Churchill Livingstone, 1995:1980–2003.

116. Baltch AL. *Pseudomonas aeruginosa* bacteremia. In: Baltch AL, Smith RP, eds. *Pseudomonas aeruginosa* infections and treatment. New York: Marcel Decker, 1994:73–128.

117. Flick MR, Cluff LE. *Pseudomonas* bacteremia. Review of 108 cases. Am J Med 1976; 60:501–508.

118. Mallolas J, Gatell JM, Miró JM, Marco F, Bisbe J, Jiménez de Anta MT, Soriano E. Analysis of prognostic factors in 274 consecutive episodes of *Pseudomonas aeruginosa* bacteremia. Antibiot Chemother 1991; 44:106–114.

119. Hilf M, Yu VL, Sharp J, Zuravleff JJ, Korvick JA, Muder RR. Antibiotic therapy for *Pseudomonas aeruginosa* bacteremia: outcome correlations in a prospective study of 200 patients. Am J Med 1989; 87:540–546.

120. McManus AT, Mason AD, McManus WF, Pruitt BA. Twenty-five year review of *Pseudomonas aeruginosa* bacteremia in a burn center. Eur J Clin Microbiol 1985; 4:219–223.

121. Lesseva M. Central venous catheter-related bacteraemia in burn patients. Scand J Infect Dis 1998; 30:585–589.

122. Fichtenbaum CJ, Woeltje KF, Powderly WG. Serious *Pseudomonas aeruginosa* infections in patients infected with human immunodeficiency virus: a case-control study. Clin Infect Dis 1994; 19:417–422.

123. Roilides E, Butler KM, Husson RN, Mueller BU, Lewis LL, Pizzo PA. Pseudomonas infections in children with human immunodeficiency virus infection. Pediatr Infect Dis J 1992; 11:547–553.

124. Nelson MR, Shanson DC, Barter GJ, Hawkins DA, Garrard BG. *Pseudomonas septicaemia* associated with HIV. AIDS 1991; 5:761–763.

125. Rizzari C, Palamone G, Corbetta A, Uderzo C, Vigano EF, Codecasa G. Central venous catheter-related infections in pediatric hematology-oncology patients: role of home and hospital management. Pediatr Hematol Oncol 1992; 9:115–123.

126. Bouvet PJ, Grimont PA. Taxonomy of the genus *Acinetobacter* with the recognition of *Acinetobacter baumannii* sp. nov., *Acinetobacter haemolyticus* sp. nov., *Acinetobacter johnsonii* sp. nov., and *Acinetobacter junii* sp. nov. and emended descriptions of *Acinetobacter calcoaceticus* and *Acinetobacter lwoffii*. Int J Syst Bacteriol 1986; 36:228–240.

127. Siegman-Igra Y, Bar-Yosef S, Gorea A, Avram J. Nosocomial Acinetobacter meningitis secondary to invasive procedures: report of 25 cases and review. Clin Infect Dis 1993; 17:843–849.

128. Blot S, Vandewoude K, Colardyn F. Nosocomial bacteremia involving *Acinetobacter baumannii* in critically ill patients: a matched cohort study. Intensive Care Med 2003; 29:471–475.

129. Daly AK, Postic B, Kass EH. Infections due to organisms of the genus Herella. Arch Int Med 1962; 110:86–91.

130. Rolston K, Guan Z, Bodey GP, Elting L. *Acinetobacter calcoaceticus* septicemia in patients with cancer. South Med J 1985; 78:647–651.

131. Tilley PAG, Roberts FJ. Bacteremia with *Acinetobacter* species: risk factors and prognosis in different clinical settings. Clin Infect Dis 1994; 18:896–900.

132. Galvao C, Swartz R, Rocher L, Reynolds J, Starmann B, Wilson D. *Acinetobacter* peritonitis during chronic peritoneal dialysis. Am J Kidney Dis 1989; 14:101–104.

133. Reindersma P, Nohlmans L, Korten JJ. *Acinetobacter*, an infrequent cause of community acquired bacterial meningitis. Clin Neurol Neurosurg 1993; 95:71–73.

134. Seifert H, Strate A, Pulverer G. Bacteremia due to *Acinetobacter* species other than Acinetobacter baumannii. Infection 1994; 22:379–385.

135. Weinberger I, Davidson E, Rotenberg Z, Fuchs J, Agmon J. Prosthetic valve endocarditis caused by *Acinetobacter calcoaceticus* subsp. *lwoffii*. J Clin Microbiol 1987; 25:955–957.

136. Linde HJ, Hahn J, Holler E, Reischl U, Lehn N. Septicemia due to *Acinetobacter junii*. J Clin Microbiol 2002; 40:2696–2697.

137. Seifert H, Strate A, Schulze A, Pulverer G. Vascular catheter-related bloodstream infections due to *Acinetobacter johnsonii* (formerly *A. calcoaceticus* var. *lwoffii*): report of 13 cases. Clin Infect Dis 1993; 17:632–636.

138. Seifert H, Dijkshoorn L, Gerner-Smidt P, Pelzer N, Tjernberg I, Vaneechoutte M. The distribution of *Acinetobacter* species on human skin: comparison of phenotypic and genotypic identification methods. J Clin Microbiol 1997; 35:2819–2825.

139. Seifert H. *Acinetobacter* species as a cause of catheter-related infections. Zbl Bakt 1995; 283:161–168.

140. Seifert H, Schulze A, Hofmann R, Pulverer G. Skin and mucous membrane colonization is an important source of nosocomial *Acinetobacter baumannii* infection: a prospective surveillance study. 7th International Congress for Infectious Diseases, Hongkong, June 10–13, 1996, Abstract # 10656.

141. Peters G, Locci R, Pulverer G. Microbial colonization of prosthetic devices. II. Scanning electron microscopy of naturally infected intravenous catheters. Zbl Bakt 1981; 173:293–299.

142. Woods DE, Vasil ML. Pathogenesis of *Pseudomonas aeruginosa* infections. In: Baltch AL, Smith RP, eds. *Pseudomonas aeruginosa* infections and treatment. New York: Marcel Dekker, 1994:21–50.

143. Kowalewska-Grochowska K, Richards R, Moysa GL, Lam K, Costerton JW, King EG. Guidewire catheter change in central venous catheter biofilm formation in a burn population. Chest 1991; 100:1090–1095.

144. Dasgupta MK, Costerton JW. Significance of biofilm adherent bacterial microcolonies on Tenckhoff catheters in CAPD patients. Blood Purif 1989; 7:144–155.

145. Nickel JC, Downey JA, Costerton JW. Ultrastructural study of microbiologic colonization of urinary catheters. Urology 1989; 34:284–291.

146. Martínez-Martínez L, Pascual A, Perea EJ. Effect of three plastic catheters on survival and growth of *Pseudomonas aeruginosa*. J Hosp Infect 1990; 16:311–318.

147. Tancrede CH, Andremont AO. Bacterial translocation and Gram-negative bacteremia in patients having hematological malignancies. J Infect Dis 1985; 15:99–103.

148. Goldmann DA, Martin WT, Worthington JW. Growth of bacteria and fungi in total parenteral nutrition solutions. Am J Surg 1973; 126:314–318.

149. Carson L, Favero M, Bond W, Petersen NJ. Morphological biochemical and growth characteristics of Pseudomonas cepacia from distilled water. Appl Microbiol 1973; 25:476–483.

150. Maki DG, Martin WT. Nationwide epidemic of septicemia caused by contaminated infusion products. IV. Growth of microbial pathogens in fluids for intravenous infusion. J Infect Dis 1975; 131:267–272.

151. Crocker KS, Noga R, Filibeck DJ, Krey SH, Markovic M, Steffee WP. Microbial growth comparisons of five commercial parenteral lipid emulsions. JPEN J Parenter Enteral Nutr 1984; 8:391–395.

151a. Andes DR, Urban AW, Acher CW, Maki DG. Septic thrombosis of the basilic, axillary, and subclavian veins caused by a peripherally inserted central venous catheter. Am J Med 1998; 105:446–450.

152. Gillespie P, Siddiqui H, Clarke J. Cannula related suppurative thrombophlebitis in the burned patient. Burns 2000; 26:200–204.

153. Garrison RN, Richardson JD, Fry DE. Catheter-associated septic thrombophlebitis. South Med J 1982; 75:917–919.

154. Johnson RA, Zajac RA, Evans ME. Suppurative thrombophlebitis: correlation between pathogen and underlying disease. Infect Control 1986; 7:582–585.

155. Topiel MS, Bryan RT, Kessler CM, Simon GL. Case report: treatment of silastic catheter-induced central vein septic thrombophlebitis. Am J Med Sci 1986; 291:425–428.

156. Gouello JP, Asfar P, Brenet O, Kouatchet A, Berthelot G, Alquier P. Nosocomial endocarditis in the intensive care unit: an analysis of 22 cases. Crit Care Med 2000; 28:377–382.

157. Mermel LA, Farr BM, Sherertz RJ, Raad II, O'Grady N, Harris JS, Craven DE. Infectious Diseases Society of America; American College of Critical Care Medicine; Society for Healthcare Epidemiology of America. Guidelines for the management of intravascular catheter-related infections. Clin Infect Dis 2001; 32:1249–1272.

158. Raad II, Bodey GP. Infectious complications of indwelling vascular catheters. Clin Infect Dis 1992; 15:197–210.

159. Wang EEL, Prober CG, Ford-Jones L, Gold R. The management of central intravenous catheter infections. Pediatr Infect Dis 1984; 3:110–113.

160. Johnson DC, Johnson FL, Goldman S. Preliminary results treating persistent central venous catheter infections with the antibiotic lock technique in pediatric patients. Pediatr Infect Dis J 1994; 13:930–931.

161. Benoit JL, Carandang G, Sitrin M, Arnow PM. Intraluminal antibiotic treatment of central venous catheter infections in patients receiving parenteral nutrition at home. Clin Infect Dis 1995; 21:1286–1288.

162. Krzywda EA, Andris DA, Edmiston CE, Quebbeman EJ. Treatment of Hickman catheter sepsis using antibiotic lock technique. Infect Control Hosp Epidemiol 1995; 16:596–598.

163. Rao JS, O'Meara A, Harvey T, Breatnach F. A new approach to the management of Broviac catheter infection. J Hosp Infect 1992; 22:109–116.

164. Capdevila JA, Segarra A, Planes AM, Ramirez-Arellano M, Pahissa A, Piera L, Martinez-Vazquez JM. Successful treatment of haemodialysis catheter-related sepsis without catheter removal. Nephrol Dial Transplant 1993; 8: 231–234.

165. Gascon A, Iglesias E, Zabala S, Belvis JJ. Catheter salvage in a patient on hemodialysis with a catheter-related bacteremia by *Pseudomonas aeruginosa*. Usefulness of clarithromycin. Am J Nephrol 2000; 20:496–497.

166. Carratala J. The antibiotic-lock technique for therapy of 'highly needed' infected catheters. Clin Microbiol Infect 2002; 8:282–289.

167. Seifert H, Baginski R, Schulze A, Pulverer G. Antimicrobial susceptibility of *Acinetobacter* species. Antimicrob Agents Chemother 1993; 37:750–753.

168. Flynn PM, Shenep JL, Stokes DC, Barrett FF. In situ management of confirmed central venous catheter-related bacteremia. Pediatr Infect Dis J 1987; 6:729–734.

169. Elting LS, Bodey GP. Septicemia due to *Xanthomonas* species and non-aeruginosa *Pseudomonas* species: increasing incidence of catheter-related infections. Medicine (Baltimore) 1990; 69:296–306.

170. Hiemenz J, Skelton J, Pizzo PA. Perspective on the management of catheter-related infections in cancer patients. Pediatr Infect Dis 1986; 5:6–11.

9

Fungal Infections of Catheters

Sergio B. Wey and Arnaldo L. Colombo
São Paulo Federal Medical School
São Paulo, Brazil

INTRODUCTION

The past three decades have witnessed major changes in hospital populations and in the technology used in healthcare. As a result, there has been an improvement in patient survival; some of these patients are highly susceptible to infection. These patients often have diseases and complications that require the use of invasive techniques for both monitoring and treatment. Fungi are pathogens that can take advantage of these procedures, especially in the compromised host.

Multiple studies from various hospitals have reported an increased rate of nosocomial fungal infections. Bloodstream infections (BSI) are one of the most serious hospital-acquired infections and many are caused by the use of vascular catheters, which are widely used in hospitals for monitoring and intravenous therapy, especially in intensive care units.

Several factors interfere with an analysis of fungal infections caused by indwelling intravascular catheters. One is the widely differing criteria used to define fungal infection or colonization of vascular catheters. Another is that the vast majority of published articles do not differentiate between the different etiologic agents involved in such infections. Many studies do not specify catheter type or whether the catheter had been in use on a short- or long-term basis. To complicate matters further, different populations of patients with a variety of different intravascular catheters are analyzed together.

The incidence of nosocomial bloodstream infection has ranged from 1.2 to 13.9 per 1000 hospital admissions, and from 0.3 to 2.02 per 1000 days of care (1). Primary nosocomial candidemia rates ranged from 2.8 per 10,000 discharges in nonteaching hospitals to 6.1 per 10,000 discharges in large teaching hospitals in 1989, according to data collected by the National Nosocomial Infections Surveillance (NNIS) program (2). This represented a fivefold increase over the period 1980–1989. Beck-Sagué and coworkers (3) analyzed data collected by the NNIS program from 115 hospitals from January 1980 to December 1990. During this time, 30,477 nosocomial fungal infections were reported. The nosocomial fungal infection rate at the facilities increased from 2.0 infections per 1000 patients discharged in 1980 to 3.8 in 1990, while cases of nosocomial fungemia rose from 1.0 to 4.9 per 10,000 patients discharged. The proportion of nosocomial infections reported by all hospitals due to fungal pathogens at all major sites of infection rose from 6% in 1980 to 10.4% in 1990, and the proportion of nosocomial bloodstream infection that was fungal increased from 5.4 to 9.9%. The proportion of bloodstream infections due to fungal pathogens varied depending on patient care characteristics. Patients who had a central intravascular catheter were more than three times as likely to have a fungus isolated as were patients with bloodstream infection who did not have such a catheter ($P < 0.001$).

Central line-associated bloodstream infection rates have varied among different types of intensive care units (ICUs). Device-associated bloodstream infections have accounted for more than 90% of the bloodstream infections reported to the NNIS (4). In a prospective study of five hospitals in Germany and Switzerland, Daschner and colleagues (5) reported that nosocomial bloodstream infections accounted for 14.2 to 28.8% of all nosocomial infections occurring in the ICUs.

Most of the species of microorganisms causing primary nosocomial bloodstream infections at NNIS hospitals did not change significantly from 1975 to 1983 (4). In 1975, *Candida* spp. did not appear on the list of the 10 leading pathogens, but in 1983, it was the seventh most common pathogen, representing 5.6% of cases. *Candida* accounted for 7.8% of cases for the period 1986–1989, and was the fourth most common etiologic agent in primary bloodstream infections. Morrison and colleagues (6), using a state-wide surveillance network in Virginia, found that coagulase-negative staphylococcus and *Candida* spp. were the only pathogens that demonstrated statistically significant increases in bloodstream infection rates over the period 1978–1984. Fungi accounted for 6% of bloodstream infections in a neonatal intensive care unit between 1976 and 1978, and 13% of bloodstream infections in the same unit between 1979 and 1981 (7).

Another study describes the trends in antifungal use and the epidemiology of nosocomial yeast infection between 1987–1988 and 1993–1994. Rates of yeast infections increased threefold in the medical and surgical intensive care units, reaching rates in 1993–1994 of 6.95 and 5.25/1000 patient days, respectively. The rate of bloodstream infections increased from 0.044/ 1000 patient days to 0.098 (8). During the same period, the incidence of candidemia increased fivefold in medical centers having more than 500 beds and 2.2-fold in those with fewer than 200 beds. *Candida* was responsible for 7.2% of bloodstream infections (10.2% in ICUs), preceded by enterococci, *Staphylococcus aureus* and coagulase-negative staphylococci (3). Over the past two decades, *Candida* species have become the fourth most common cause of bloodstream infections among patients in intensive care units (9). A 20-fold increase in the rate of candidemia was reported in a single institution where nosocomial infections were prospectively surveyed from 1981 through 1990 (10). However, recent data suggest that this incidence may be stable in some other institutions (11).

Mortality due to fungal nosocomial bloodstream infection is significant. Miller and Wenzel (12), studying 385 episodes of nosocomial bloodstream infections, found that the presence of *Candida* spp. and *Pseudomonas* spp. were independent predictors of death. An NNIS analysis (3) showed that patients with fungemia were more likely to die during hospitalization [954 (29%) of 3256] than were patients with bloodstream infection due to non-fungal pathogens [5594 (17%) of 3882; relative risk (RR), 1.8; 95% confidence interval (CI), 1.7–1.9; $P < 0.001$].

A relationship between candidemia and indwelling vascular catheters has been recognized for decades. In 1962, Louria et al. (13) reported that 23 of the 29 patients who developed systemic candidiasis had indwelling vascular catheters. In four of these patients, cultures from the skin around apparently uninfected cutdown sites, taken at the onset of fungemia, grew species of *Candida* that were identical to those found in the blood.

Fungi can cause important infection in long-term intravascular catheters such as Hickman and Broviac-tunneled catheter and subcutaneous ports. Between January 1982 and December 1983, King and coworkers (14) studied 335 Broviac catheters placed in 270 infants and children. Laboratory-confirmed bloodstream infection occurred on 77 occasions (23%), an average of one episode for every 434 days of catheter use. Eighty-three bacterial isolates (94%) and five fungal isolates were recovered from blood culture. The fungemias involved two patients with *Candida* spp. and three patients with *Malassezia furfur*.

Uderzo et al. (15) studied infectious and mechanical complications occurring with long-term central venous catheters in children with hematological malignancies who underwent bone marrow transplantation. *Pseudomonas* and *Candida* species were more commonly isolated in hospital-managed patients, whereas coagulase-negative staphylococci were more frequently isolated in domiciliary infections.

Colombo et al. (16) analyzed 145 consecutive patients with fungemia. The majority of cases had received broad spectrum antibiotics before the onset of candidemia. Nonalbicans species accounted for 63% of all episodes.

The species most frequently causing candidemia were *Candida albicans* (37%), *Candida parapsilosis* (25%), and *Candida tropicalis* (24%). The overall crude case fatality rate was 50%.

In summary, it seems likely that during the past decade, the overall incidence of nosocomial fungemia has continued to increase, with most cases involving *Candida* species and many such infections being related to the use of intravascular catheters.

PATHOGENESIS

The pathogenesis of fungal infections due to intravascular devices may be infusion-related or cannula-related. Infusion-related sepsis is very rare, but the lack of awareness of the problem can contribute to underreporting by health care workers (17–19).

The infusate can be contaminated during manufacture (intrinsic contamination) or during preparation and administration in the hospital (extrinsic contamination) (17). There are several reports of fungemias secondary to the contamination of parenteral formulations (20–22).

There is a strong relationship between *C. parapsilosis* fungemia or systemic infection and hyperalimentation using intravascular devices (23). The adherence of *C. parapsilosis* to plastic materials exceeds that of *C. albicans*. The capability of *C. parapsilosis* isolates to proliferate and produce large amounts of slime in glucose-containing solutions may help to understand their ability to adhere to plastic material and cause catheter-related fungemia (23–26).

Another example of a systemic yeast infection specifically related to catheter use is *M. furfur*. Fungemia due to *M. furfur*, which does not involve the gastrointestinal tract, almost invariably has an intravascular line as a portal of entry. This organism proliferates in fat emulsions and has been particularly associated with catheter-related fungemias in pediatric patients undergoing hyperalimentation (18,27). Occlusion of catheter and adhesion of the central venous catheter to the wall of the vein has been reported in association with *M. furfur* infection (28,29).

Central venous catheters, particularly long-term catheters, are the intravascular devices most likely to cause infection (17). The source of catheter-related bacteremia has been investigated by several authors and is still a controversial subject. The skin surrounding the insertion site can be a source of the fungus and, as a consequence, of catheter-related infections. Other investigators have highlighted the hub as an important source of catheter-related bloodstream infection (17,30–32). Raad et al. (33) found that luminal colonization increases progressively with duration of catheterization and that in short-term central venous catheters, the skin was the main source of extraluminal catheter colonization; in long-term vascular catheters (>30 days), colonization is predominantly luminal.

Despite the paucity of published studies on the pathogenesis of catheter-related fungemia, it seems reasonable to discuss mechanisms of fungal infection according to the models that have been proposed to explain catheter-related bacteremia. Thus far, suboptimal site care during insertion and thereafter by health care workers and skin colonization appear to be potential sources for fungal infections. Once the organism reaches the catheter, it adheres to and propagates on the surface of the catheter or the surrounding fibrin clot. However, it is important to note that the data used to support the cutaneous source of candidemia is surprisingly incomplete. Indeed, there is no single study that supports the skin hypothesis on the basis of density and sequence of candidal colonization or by using molecular-relatedness studies (34).

Fungi can be found colonizing the site of catheter insertion and the subcutaneous tract created by the catheter in patients with infected intravascular devices (35,36). This is an indication that catheter-related fungemia can be the result of invasion of yeast at the site of catheter insertion and along the subcutaneous tract created by the catheter. It is likely that the administration of broad-spectrum antibiotics plays a role in eradicating endogenous competing flora and promoting overgrowth of yeast in the skin area surrounding the catheter entry site. Polymyxin-neomycin-bacitracin ointment placed at the catheter exit site results in a 50% decrease in the frequency of bacterial colonization, but a fivefold increase in fungal colonization of the catheter (37), and has been associated with an increased risk of catheter-related candidiasis in some studies (38). In addition, underlying diseases can contribute to local yeast catheter wound colonization and infection (39).

Another possibility is yeast colonization of the hub through contact of the device with the patient's skin flora or the hands of health care personnel, with subsequent entry of fungi into the catheter lumen at the time of catheterization and migration along the luminal surface to the intravascular portion of the device. In support of this hypothesis is the observation of an adherent biofilm, including hyphal elements, on the luminal surface of long-term intravascular catheters removed from patients who had developed *Candida* spp. fungemia (40,41).

Finally, hematogenous seeding of vascular catheters following secondary fungemia could cause catheter colonization and persistence of infection. According to Anaisse et al. (42), this phenomena is not frequent, but it may be more common for *Candida* spp. than for other microorganisms causing catheter-related bloodstream infections (17). There is an increasing evidence, in neutropenic patients, that the gut may be a prominent source of candidemia, especially if they have mucositis. It has been postulated that circulating yeast attach to the intravascular catheter, thus creating a continuous focus of seeding into the bloodstream (18). Infected indwelling intravenous devices are often the source of persistent infection in cancer patients, although in patients with extensive gastrointestinal tract mucosal excoriation, the endogenous flora may serve as a reservoir. Persistent granulocytopenia, recent insertion of an intravascular catheter, and prior broad-spectrum antibiotic therapy are common predisposing factors for breakthrough fungal infection (43).

Primary cutaneous aspergillosis has been reported as a cause of infection at the cutaneous catheter exit site. In this clinical situation, the source of infection appears to be the adhesive tape or arm boards (44–47). Other molds have been associated with infections related to intravascular devices, such as *Paecilomyces* spp. and *Fusarium* spp. (48,49).

Candida species can be a cause of suppurative peripheral thrombophlebitis. According to Walsh et al., the pathogenesis of this infection appears to be the result of preceding candidal colonization of the skin and inadequate intravenous site care in susceptible patients, permitting candidal infection of the catheter wound and progression to the venous wall. Additionally, candidemia from other sites could cause colonization of the catheter with subsequent candidal trombophlebitis (50).

After colonization of the catheter, microbial factors and host immunity play a role in the progression to fungemia and clinical sepsis (39).

DIAGNOSIS

Gram staining and cultures must be performed from pus obtained from any superficial or subcutaneously infected site that is related to the use of peripheral or central venous lines. In cases of suppurative peripheral thrombophlebitis, histopathology and culture of the removed segment of thrombosed vein is usually very helpful in diagnosing the causative agent (51,52).

Several methods have been described for the diagnosis of vascular catheter-related septicemia (53–55). Unfortunately, the accuracy of these methods for correctly identifying catheter-related fungal infections has not been demonstrated. A semiquantitative roll plate culture method and several quantitative methods that permit culture of the internal surface of catheters have been applied to the diagnosis of catheter-related septicemia (56,57). However, the original data obtained in these studies were related to bacterial and not fungal infections. As a consequence, there is not a validated "gold standard" for diagnosing catheter-related fungemia.

Khatib et al. (58) published data from a retrospective study in which 3544 intravascular catheters had been cultured by a semiquantitative culture technique (SQC). *Candida* species were present in 80 catheters. The authors found a high rate of SQC-positive specimens among patients with invasive candidiasis, but also found that many colonized catheters were not associated with corresponding clinical illness.

Telenti et al. (59), studying the relationship between quantitative data from peripheral blood cultures and source of infection, found a good correlation between high-grade candidemia (>25 colony-forming units (cfu)/10 ml of blood) and an intravascular source of fungemia. Of 48 episodes of high-grade fungemia, 43 (90%) were associated with an infected intravascular device. However, it is important to note that the authors used Maki's criteria as the gold standard to classify episodes of candidemia that were associated with an intravascular device (53).

Available culture methods are associated with low sensitivity for recognition of systemic candidiasis. New diagnostic approaches have been used to identify and monitor the course of patients with disseminated candidiasis. These methods include the detection of cell wall mannan, cytoplasmic antigens similar to *Candida* enolase antigens, and specific metabolites such as D-arabinitol. Another possibility is the detection of *Candida* spp.-specific genomes by polymerase chain reaction. All of these methods are currently under development and investigation, and are not routinely available in clinical microbiology laboratories (60).

EPIDEMIOLOGY AND RISK FACTORS

Previous studies have identified several risk factors for the development of nosocomial fungemia. Among the clinical characteristics that most consistently increase this risk are neutropenia, use of broad-spectrum antibiotics, hyperalimentation, antecedent surgery (especially abdominal surgery), and indwelling catheters (18). In 1967, Ellis and Spivack (61) described a series of 12 patients with disseminated candidemia; all had intravenous catheters in place and *Candida* was recovered from three of the catheters. In the same year, Louria et al. (62) presented a series of seven patients with fungemia due to yeasts other than *C. albicans*. All patients had intravascular catheters. Vic-Dupont, Coulaud, and Delrieu (63) found that intravascular catheters were the source for 16 out of 30 cases of candidemia. Between 1969 and 1970, Williams et al. (64) published a review of 27 cases of *Candida* septicemia; 25 of the patients had indwelling central venous catheters. More significantly, the authors found that 89% of these 25 patients had developed positive cultures after the central venous line had been in place for two weeks.

Long-term, indwelling, central venous catheters have facilitated the care of patients with cancer, but local and systemic infections remain a major cause of morbidity and catheter failure. Fungal infections have complicated the management of patients with these catheters for many years. In 1979, Hickman et al. (65) published an article showing *Candida* spp. and *Nocardia* spp. colonization of Broviac catheters in bone marrow transplant recipients.

Lecciones and colleagues (18) reviewed a total of 155 episodes of fungemia associated with an indwelling central catheter that had developed in 149 inpatients with cancer during a 10-year period (January 1979 to December 1988). The majority of the patients had lymphoma or solid tumors, and most episodes of fungemia were associated with neutropenia, the use of broad-spectrum antibiotics, and/or hyperalimentation. Many patients had received chemotherapy or undergone surgery (usually abdominal) within the month preceding the diagnosis of fungemia. Ninety-eight percent of fungemic episodes were caused by *Candida* spp., with *C. albicans* accounting for approximately three-fourths of cases and *C. tropicalis* accounting for 13%. One episode of *M. furfur* and one of *Saccharomyces cerevisiae* fungemia were also found. Eighty percent of infected catheters were short-term catheters.

Moro and coworkers (22) observed 623 episodes of central venous catheterization among 607 patients admitted to intensive care units. Overall, 58 catheter-related infections were recorded (9.3/100 catheters): 47 were local infections (7.5/100 catheters) and 11 were septicemias (1.8/100). *Candida albicans* represented three (5.9%) of the local infections and *Candida* spp. were responsible for five episodes of catheter-related sepsis. The authors found that colonization with *Candida* species was frequently associated with systemic infections.

Franceschi et al. (66) studied the risk factors associated with intravascular catheter infections in burn patients. They analyzed 101 intravascular catheter sites from 89 patients. The overall incidence of colonized catheters was 25.7% (>15 cfu). The most frequent organisms recovered from the colonized tips were *Pseudomonas* spp. (30.7%), coagulase-negative *Staphylococcus* (27%), and *C. albicans* (27%). The incidence of catheter colonization was inversely correlated with the distance of the catheter insertion from the site of the burn. A stepwise, logistic, multivariate analysis showed cutaneous colonization at the insertion site, at the time of catheter removal, to be a significant risk factor for catheter colonization.

Siegman-Igra et al. identified 110 patients (126 episodes) with catheter-related bloodstream infection during 1986 in a medical center in Israel. Gram-positive and Gram-negative bacteria shared equal parts among the 145 blood isolates. *S. aureus* was the most common species (43/145, 30%). *Candida* species was found to be responsible for 8% of intravascular catheter-related infection. Fungal isolates were more common among tunnelled catheter infections than among others (6/18, 33% vs. 5/108, 5%, $P < 0.001$) (67).

Wey and colleagues (68) studied risk factors for nosocomial candidemia in 88 patients who had at least one blood culture positive for *Candida* spp. These patients were pair-matched using six criteria: age, period at risk, primary diagnosis, surgery, date of admission, and sex. Using a stepwise, logistic, regression analysis, four independent variables were selected that predicted the acquisition of nosocomial candidemia. These were the number of antibiotics received before infection, prior use of a Hickman catheter, isolation of *Candida* spp. from other body sites, and prior hemodialysis. Bross et al. (69) studied adult patients without leukemia who acquired nosocomial candidemia. Each patient was matched to a control based on medical specialty and duration of hospitalization up to the first *Candida* spp.-positive blood culture. Seven risk factors were identified through a logistic regression and include: prior antibiotic use, candiduria, central catheter use, and azotemia. Karanabis et al. (70) compared 30 cancer patients with candidemia with 58 controls. The multivariate logistic model showed the following independent risk factors for candidemia: positive peripheral cultures for *Candida* spp. ($P = 0.002$), central catheterization ($P = 0.03$), and neutropenia ($P = 0.05$). These last three studies reached similar conclusions about the use of central lines and antibiotics as risk factors for candidemia.

Groeger and colleagues (71) followed 1430 cancer patients who had undergone long-term treatment with venous access devices for at least 500 days. Fungi were responsible for 11 (3.3%) of the bloodstream infections that were related to tunneled catheters, and in one (3.5%) of the infections related to subcutaneous ports. The fungi cultured were: *C. parapsilosis* (5), *C. albicans* (2), *Rhodotorula rubra* (1), *M. furfur* (1), *Torulopsis glabrata* (1), *Alternaria* spp. (1), and *Aspergillus niger* (1).

An important risk factor for infection/colonization of an indwelling intravascular catheter by a fungus is the use of total parenteral nutrition (TPN). This therapeutic measure has been associated with an appreciable risk of sepsis, with fungal sepsis being an especially serious complication (72). The incidence of catheter-associated bacteremia in patients receiving TPN ranges from 0 to 14% with an average of 3 to 5%. *Candida* species are the usual fungal isolates. *Malassezia furfur* is a rare but serious infection, associated with TPN in young children (73). A case of catheter-related infection caused by *Malassezia sympodialis* was described in a patient after total gastrectomy for a gastric cancer (74). The patient was receiving central venous hyperalimentation.

Data from NNIS between 1980 and 1990 (2) show that patients with bloodstream infections receiving total parenteral nutrition or those in intensive care units were more likely to develop fungemia (15.6 and 11.0%, respectively) than those not receiving total parenteral nutrition (6.4%) or not in intensive care units (8.1%). When parenteral nutrition was controlled for, central intravascular catheterization was significantly associated with fungemia. Among patients with central intravascular catheters receiving total parenteral nutrition who developed bloodstream infections, those in intensive care units were still somewhat more likely to have fungemia (RR, 1.2; 95% CI, 1.1–1.4).

Outbreak of *C. parapsilosis* fungemia has been traced to contaminated vacuum pumps used to prepare parenteral nutrition solutions, central intravascular pressure monitoring, and use of parenteral nutrition in immunocompromised hosts (2). Solomon et al. (21) described an outbreak of *C. parapsilosis* bloodstream infection in patients receiving parenteral nutrition. Epidemiologic investigation showed an association with the use of an electrically powered vacuum pump to assist parenteral nutrition. Cultures from the vacuum pump showed heavy growth of *C. parapsilosis* from multiple sites. Laboratory investigation demonstrated that sterile solutions could be contaminated by the vacuum pump. Use of the vacuum pump was stopped, and no further cases occurred. *Candida parapsilosis* was also responsible for nosocomial fungemia in eight infants in a neonatal intensive care unit. A case-control study compared the cases with 29 weight-matched controls. Logistic regression analysis indicated that the risk factors for candidemia were duration of umbilical artery catheterization, duration of parenteral nutrition, and estimated gestational age. Parenteral nutrition therapy was often administered through the umbilical artery catheter, which was also used for monitoring arterial pressure. The transducer domes thus contained parenteral nutrition fluid. Transducers were usually disinfected with alcohol. Laboratory investigation showed that the heads of 6 of 11 blood pressure transducers in use and one of four transducers in storage after cleaning were culture-positive for *C. parapsilosis*. After control measures were instituted, no further cases occurred (75).

Ruiz-Diez et al. (76) analyzed nine preterm infants admitted to the neonatal intensive care unit between March 1993 and August 1994. The infants were infected with or colonized by *C. albicans*. A total of 36 isolates (including isolates from catheters and parenteral nutrition) were examined for molecular relatedness by PCR fingerprinting and restriction fragment length polymorphism analysis. They were able to identify eight different profiles. A strain with one of these profiles was present in three patients and in their respective catheters. Patients infected with or colonized by this isolate profile were clustered in time. The authors concluded that *C. albicans* was most commonly producing long-term colonization, although horizontal transmission probably due to catheters also occurred.

McKinnon et al. (77) analyzed the risk factors for *Candida* infection in surgical intensive care units. A total of 301 consecutively admitted patients were analyzed for five or more days. The most frequent risk factors were presence of peripheral and central intravenous catheters, bladder catheters, mechanical ventilation, and lack of enteral or intravenous nutrition.

Kac et al. (78) assessed the incidence and etiology of colonization and infection of pulmonary artery catheters inserted in cardiac surgery patients admitted at a 17-bed cardiac surgery intensive care between May 1997 and May 1998. Of 164 pulmonary artery catheters inserted in 157 patients, 19 (11.6%) and 1 (0.6%) were associated with colonization (mean duration of catheterization, 7.5 days) and bacteremia, respectively. The incidence was 17.7 and 0.93 episodes per 1000 catheterization-days, respectively. *Candida albicans* caused 4% of pulmonary artery catheter colonization. Gram-positive cocci and Gram-negative rods represented 48% each. From multivariate analysis, more than four days of catheterization was the single variable associated with a significantly increased risk of pulmonary artery catheter colonization [odds ratio (OR), 9.81; 95% CI, 1.23–77.5, $P = 0.03$].

The National Epidemiology of Mycosis Survey (NEMIS) was a prospective, multicenter study conducted at six geographically dispersed academic medical centers to examine rates of and risk factors for the development of candidal BSI among patients in surgical and neonatal ICUs (from October 1993 to November 1995). During the study period, 42 candidal BSIs developed among the 4276 admitted patients (9.82 candidal BSIs per 1000 admissions). *Candida* species accounted for 9.2% of the total number of BSIs ($N = 458$). More than half of the *Candida* isolates recovered from blood were nonalbicans species. The mortality rate was significantly higher among patients who developed candidal BSI than among other patients (41 vs. 8%; OR, 7.52; 95% IC, 3.9–14.6; $P < 0.001$). Of 42 patients who developed candidal BSIs, 41 had a central venous catheter in place during their ICU stay prior to the development of infection. Among these 41 patients, the rate of candidal BSIs was 1.23 per 1000 patient-days, versus 0.11 per 1000 patient-days among patients who did not have a CVC in place (RR, 8.1, 95% IC, 1.1–59.6; $P = 0.04$). A multivariate model that included only patients who underwent surgery ($N = 3201$) identified an association between increased risk of candidal BSI and having had a triple-lumen catheter placed (RR = 5.4, 95% IC, 1.2–23.6; $P = 0,03$) (9).

CLINICAL SYNDROMES AND AGENTS

Unfortunately, there are no characteristic clinical signs and symptoms to indicate a diagnosis of disseminated fungal disease. There is the possibility that infected or colonized catheters may seed organisms to various body sites, resulting in a great variety of clinical presentations, depending on the affected organs. For example, when *Candida* is disseminated, multiple organs are usually affected, especially including the kidney, brain, myocardium, and eye.

Candida species are the most common fungi isolated from intravascular catheters. Horn and Conway (79) documented four cases of candidemia related to fully implantable venous access systems in patients with cystic fibrosis. These cases were successfully treated, but removal of the venous access device was necessary in each case. Tchekmedyian et al. (41) described a case of a patient with acute nonlymphocytic leukemia who developed *Staphylococcus epidermidis* bacteremia and candidemia after maintenance chemotherapy. The patient also developed an infected abdominal aortic aneurysm. The same organisms were cultured from the aneurysm as from the Hickman catheter. This suggests that the Hickman catheter was the source of the candidemia and that it may well have caused the infection in the aneurysm.

Fungal thrombophlebitis is a major concern for those with indwelling intravascular catheters. Both peripheral and deep vascular structures can be involved, as well as the venous and arterial sides of the circulation (80). *Candida* species are not usually considered a cause of suppurative peripheral thrombophlebitis. Walsh et al. (50) described seven cases of suppurative peripheral thrombophlebitis during a 15-month period. They defined candidal peripheral thrombophlebitis by the following criteria: **(a)** clinical evidence of venous catheter-associated thrombophlebitis manifested by warmth, tenderness, erythema, palpable cord, and/or suppuration at the percutaneous catheter puncture site, and **(b)** microbiological evidence of *Candida* spp., demonstrated by culture in resected vein specimens or pus expressed from the intravenous catheter puncture site. The median duration of hospitalization until development of candidal peripheral thrombophlebitis was 27 days, and subjects had a median age of 64 years. All patients were admitted to the surgical service and had underlying diseases, including cancer in three, diabetes mellitus in three, and ethanol abuse in two. All but one patient underwent surgery. None of the patients was receiving corticosteroids, cytotoxic therapy, or parenteral hyperalimentation at the time the thrombophlebitis developed. All patients had concomitant infections and all had received antibiotics for at least two weeks before candidal thrombophlebitis was diagnosed. Five of the seven patients had had candidal colonization of urine, sputum, or wounds preceding their phlebitis. Gram stain and culture of expressed pus in three patients showed only *Candida* species. Five patients had veins resected surgically that were grossly purulent; all five grew *Candida* species. *C. albicans* was present in five patients, *C. tropicalis* in one, and *C. lipolytica* in another. Four had candidemia, but none had ocular or cutaneous manifestations of systemic candidiasis.

Fry et al. (81) found 32 episodes of septic thrombophlebitis in 143 patients who had had an intravascular device. *Candida* spp. was isolated in two of them. In no case was it necessary to excise veins in the absence of local signs of infection and inflammation at the venous access site. None of the cases was related to central venous catheters.

Fungal infections of long-term catheters are difficult to differentiate clinically from bacterial infections. When nonpurulent erythematous lesions progress to radial necrotic lesions at the exit site of the catheter, *Aspergillus* infection should be suspected (46). If there is purulent discharge at the exit site, the pus should be examined microscopically and cultured.

Fungal infection can also affect the pocket of fully implantable devices. Such infections may be present with local inflammation, including erythema and necrosis over the reservoir. *Aspergillus* spp. are not often found in vascular catheters, but Allo et al. described nine cases of primary cutaneous aspergillosis at the entry site of Hickman catheters in immunocompromised patients (46). All patients had underlying hematologic cancer and the Hickman catheter had been placed to provide venous access for chemotherapy, hyperalimentation, or both. Clinical signs of infection included erythema, induration, and cutaneous or subcutaneuous necrosis at the point of entry into the subclavian vein, in the subcutaneous tunnel, or at the exit site from the skin. Diagnosis was confirmed by positive wound culture for *Aspergillus flavus* in all but one patient.

Tan and colleagues (48) reported the case of an 18-month-old white male baby with obstructive uropathy, secondary to embryonal rhabdomyosarcoma group III involving the bladder and prostate. A tunnelled, central venous catheter (Hickman) was inserted at the time of the tumor biopsy, but removed three months later after the patient developed a catheter-associated chest wall abscess and sepsis due to *Klebsiella pneumoniae*. A fully implantable central venous catheter Portcath was therefore inserted one month later to allow chemotherapy to continue. The blood cultures obtained from the Portcath and peripheral vein were positive for the same mold, subsequently identified as *Paecilomyces lilacinus*. The catheter was removed and amphotericin B was initiated. The patient was discharged without further clinical evidence of infection.

Right atrial thrombosis is a potentially lethal complication associated with central venous catheters, which are now used in nearly 70% of all patients in pediatric intensive care units (82). Paut el al. (83) reported a case of right atrial septic thrombosis due to catheter-related fungal sepsis in a young trauma victim. A nine-year-old boy with "multiple trauma" was submitted to surgery, received cefamandol for five days, and a CVC was inserted on the second day post-trauma, to allow total parenteral nutrition. The patient improved, but on day 12, sepsis developed and was treated empirically with antibiotics. On day 14, blood specimens, as well as the catheter tip, proved positive for *C. albicans* and amphotericin and five flucytosine were initiated. On day 17, candidal endophthalmitis was diagnosed, and a large right atrial mass was confirmed by two-dimensional echocardiography. The patient was submitted to surgery and a mass containing fungi was removed. The patient improved and was discharged from the intensive care unit on day 36.

The compromised host is especially susceptible to infection due to uncommon microorganisms. Sycova-Milá et al. (84) reported a case of *Trichosporon capitatum* catheter-associated fungemia, which followed a severe clinical course in a compromised host and was successfully treated with amphotericin B plus flucytosine. The yeast was found in both blood and catheter cultures. Kiehn and coworkers (85) reported 23 patients between 1985 and 1989 who had catheter-related *Rhodotorula* sepsis. All 23 had indwelling central venous catheters that had been in place from one to 22 months (average, 9.3 months). Blood was drawn from both the catheter and a peripheral source, but only one patient had a peripheral blood culture positive for *Rhodotorula* spp. Colony counts of yeast from the catheter cultures often exceeded 100 (15 patients) and even 1000 (seven patients) cfu/ml of blood.

The incidence of *Fusarium* spp. infection is increasing, especially among compromised patients. Disseminated fusariosis is an uncommon disease, and the reasons for the increasing incidence are multiple. Important factors include the use of intensive chemotherapeutic regimens for the treatment of malignancies and bone marrow transplant recipients, the empirical use of broad-spectrum antibiotics, the early use of amphotericin B in febrile neutropenic patients, and the increasing number of patients with impaired mucosal or skin barriers due to underlying malignancy or chemotherapy. Ammari et al. (86) described the case of a 13-year-old boy with acute promyelocytic leukemia, in remission, who had a catheter-related *Fusarium solani* fungemia and pulmonary infection. The patient had many factors that predisposed him to opportunistic infection, including underlying malignancy, immunosuppressive chemotherapy, and an indwelling central venous line. The blood cultures obtained by venopucture and through the Broviac catheter were positive for *F. solani*.

Malassezia furfur is the etiologic agent of tinea versicolor and is considered a benign agent. However, some reports from the literature suggest a strong correlation between *M. furfur* sepsis and the use of intravascular catheters. It was cultured from the lumen of 32% of catheters removed from infants over one week of age in a neonatal intensive care unit (87). Two of these patients also had clinical evidence of systemic infection.

CONTROL MEASURES

Nosocomial infections have become increasingly more difficult to prevent and manage. The most important infection control measures for the prevention of fungal colonization of indwelling intravascular catheters are quite similar to those recommended for bacterial infections, which have been outlined elsewhere in this text. However, some peculiarities of fungal complications should be addressed.

An intravascular catheter is probably the most important removable source of *Candida* spp. in the bloodstream of both adults and children.

Flowers et al. (37) performed a randomized controlled trial in order to evaluate the efficacy of an attachable subcutaneous cuff to prevent central vascular catheter-related infection among patients receiving intensive care. All catheters were dressed with polyantibiotic ointment containing polymyxin, neomycin, and bacitracin. They found that catheters with cuffs were associated with less frequent bloodstream infection compared with controls (0 vs. 13%). However, an unexpectedly large proportion (75%) of catheter infections were due to *C. albicans*. This may have been due in part to the use of polyantibiotic ointment, as suggested by a pooled analysis of previous trials that demonstrated increased *Candida* colonization in catheters in which the ointment had been used.

Several studies have evaluated the effect of an antiseptic-impregnated central venous catheter for prevention of catheter-related infection in intensive care unit patients. Sheng et al. compared a catheter impregnated with chlorhexidine and silver sulfadiazine to a catheter made of polyurethane (control). The antiseptic catheters were less likely to be colonized by microorganisms, but there was no significant difference between both groups in catheter-related infections [0.9 versus 4.9 infections per 100 catheters; relative risk 0.17 (95% CI, 0.03 to 1.15); $P = 0.07$]. Gram-positive cocci and fungi were more likely to colonize in the standard polyurethane catheters ($P = 0.06$ and 0.04 compared to antiseptic catheters, respectively). Two patients in the control group died directly due to catheter-related candidemia (88).

Candidal peripheral thrombophlebitis can be prevented by vigorous skin preparation, site care, and routine rotation of peripheral intravenous catheter sites every 48 to 72 hours (50). Other infection control measures to prevent candidal peripheral thrombophlebitis include limiting the spectrum and duration of antimicrobial therapy to specific culture-defined organisms, short time intervals, and meticulous care of intravenous sites. New scientific approaches are needed to help establish better techniques for catheter management.

THERAPY

The aim of this chapter is not so much to address the use of specific antifungal agents as to outline some general therapeutic measures. Whether the infected catheter should always be removed is polemical. The major problem with candidemia or fungemia is determining which patients have tissue invasion and thus require antifungal therapy, and which can be treated by simply removing the catheter. Whereas most bacterial infections of long-term CVC can be cured without removal of the catheter, the same is not true of fungal catheter infections. There have been occasional reports of fungal infection associated with long-term CVCs that were cured with antifungal therapy alone. But the overwhelming experience of fungal infection (usually with *Candida* species) associated with the use of the long-term CVC is that the catheter must be removed for resolution of the infection to occur (89).

The decision to remove the catheter must be made on an individual basis because many case-specific and patient-specific factors prevent ironclad recommendations. Removal of the catheter system is indicated for the following situations: documented *Candida* or fungal catheter-associated infection, tunnel infection, or persistent bloodstream infections after the third day of appropriate intravenous antimicrobial therapy (90).

Most authors have concluded that it is prudent to remove any catheter and treat the patient with intravenous amphotericin B when catheter infection is due to *Candida* spp. or *Aspergillus* spp. Patients with fungal infections of their catheters should be monitored for dissemination. *Aspergillus* mainly disseminates to the lung, whereas *Candida* has a predilection for the eye, necessitating frequent funduscopic examinations (91).

Kiehn at al. (85) studied 23 patients who had had catheter-related *Rhodotorula* sepsis. Thirteen were treated with antifungal therapy and removal of the catheter while five patients received antifungal therapy alone and another five had the catheter removed without antifungal therapy. All patients survived the fungemic episode and experienced no recurrence.

Allo et al. (46) treated nine cases of primary cutaneous aspergillosis at Hickman catheter sites. The treatment consisted of intravenous amphotericin B, oral flucytosine, and local wound care. Three patients recovered completely without operative debridement, and three more recovered after operative debridement and delayed grafting. Two patients died of disseminated aspergillosis, and one died of unrelated causes while still recovering from primary cutaneous aspergillosis. Successful treatment required resolution of aplasia or leukopenia, catheter removal, systemic treatment with amphotericin B, and local wound care.

Treatment of peripheral candidal thrombophlebitis includes removal of the peripheral venous catheter. Walsh et al. (50) documented a cluster of seven cases of peripheral candidal thrombophlebitis, all of which resolved. Three patients received systemic therapy (amphotericin B), two received topical care, and five underwent venous resection.

In the past, catheter-related candidiasis has been managed in some cases by simply removing the catheter. Many patients were cured by this approach, but the attributable mortality of candidemia has been estimated at 38% (68). Fourteen percent of nonneutropenic patients developed endophthalmitis in one study (38). Most authorities recommend amphotericin B for therapy of neutropenic patients with candidiasis. For nonneutropenic patients, fluconazole 400 mg qd and amphotericin B 0.6 mg/kg/day were equivalent in a randomized trial (38). Catheter infection was believed responsible for 72% of cases of candidiasis. Most authorities recommend removal of catheters infected with *Candida* (91).

There are no data in the literature to guide clinicians regarding the use of antimicrobial therapy for patients whose catheter tip cultures reveal significant growth in the absence of culture-proven bacteremia or fungemia. In this setting, a febrile patient with valvular heart disease or a patient with neutropenia (absolute neutrophil count, 1000 cells/ml), whose catheter tip culture reveals significant growth of *S. aureus* or *C. albicans* by means of semiquantitative (>15 cfu) or quantitative ($>10^2$ cfu) culture should be followed closely for signs of infection, and some experts would administer a short course (5–7 days) of antibiotics (92).

The removal of all central venous catheters from all patients with candidemia is considered to be standard care. However, this practice is not always possible, and it is associated with significant cost and potential complications. The physician's decision regarding catheter removal is probably as important as the choice of drug therapy. Catheter removal has been proposed as part of the standard therapeutic approach. The largest difference appears to be that between neutropenic and nonneutropenic patients.

In nonneutropenic patients, catheter removal has repeatedly been correlated with more rapid clearance of the bloodstream and/or better prognosis (93–95). Anaissie et al. retrospectively evaluated the impact of central venous catheter removal on the outcome of 416 candidemic cancer patients (93). When catheter exchange was examined in relationship to the time of initiation of antifungal therapy, complete catheter exchange did improve outcome slightly. Becoming or remaining neutropenic, APACHE III score, and the presence of documented visceral dissemination were much more important than catheter exchange in predicting outcome.

Nguyen et al. (96) evaluated prospectively 427 consecutive episodes of candidemia as part of a multicenter observational study. From this group, 82 neutropenic patients had evaluable catheter data. Of these patients, there was significantly lower mortality among those who had their catheters removed (11 vs. 29%, $P < 0.045$).

Nucci and Anaissie performed a computerized MEDLINE database search to evaluate the effect of CVC removal on the outcome of patients with candidemia (97). Appropriate articles included in the research were those published from January 1966 through December 2000 in any language. The keywords used were "candidemia," "catheter," and "outcome." Abstracts presented from 1987 through 2000 at the yearly meetings of the American Society for Microbiology, the Infectious Diseases Society of America, and the Society for Healthcare Epidemiology of America were also reviewed. The authors selected studies that evaluated catheter removal as a prognostic factor (of mortality) in candidemia, performed a multivariate analysis, and included in this analysis any severity of illness score that had been validated as a predictor of death. Two-hundred-and-three articles on candidemia were identified. Only four studies met all initial criteria. Two of those showed removal to be marginally effective (98,99), one article found removal of the catheter to be ineffective (100), and one study found removal to be effective (101). No study was found that had as its primary endpoint the evaluation of vascular catheter removal in patients with candidemia.

In a retrospective study conducted in an Italian tertiary care hospital, the incidence of nosocomial candidemia was evaluated. Over a six-year period (1992–1997), a total of 189 episodes of candidemia occurred in 189 patients, accounting for an average incidence of 1.14 episodes per 10,000 patient-days per year. *Candida albicans* was the most frequent isolated pathogen, accounting for 54% of fungal isolates, followed by *C. parapsilosis* (23%), *Candida glabrata* (7%), *C. tropicalis* (5%), and others. Seventy-one (58%) of the 123 valuable patients with central venous catheters underwent line removal; 51 of them had catheter-related candidemia. The 30-day crude mortality rate was 45%. Adequate antifungal therapy and central line removal independently reduced the high mortality of the disease (99).

Practice guidelines for treatment of candidiasis published in 2000 recommend removal of existing intravascular catheters for patients with candidemia or acute hematogenously disseminated candidiasis, especially in nonneutropenic patients (102).

The most recent published guidelines for management of intravascular catheter-related infections (from the Infectious Diseases Society of America, the American College of Critical Care Medicine, and the Society for Healthcare Epidemiology of America) also recommend removal of existing intravascular catheters for patients with catheter-related candidemia (92).

Antifungal therapy is necessary in all cases of vascular catheter-related candidemia because patients with catheter-associated candidemia who were treated with catheter removal but without systemic antifungal therapy have developed complications such as vertebral osteomyelitis and endophthalmitis, resulting in permanent loss of vision (92). Amphotericin B is recommended for suspected catheter-related candidemia in patients who are hemodynamically unstable or who have received prolonged fluconazole therapy. Patients who are hemodynamically stable and who have not had recent therapy with fluconazole, or those known to have a fluconazole-susceptible organism, can be treated with fluconazole instead of amphotericin B (92). Catheter-related *Candida krusei* infections should be treated with amphotericin B. Tunneled CVCs or implantable devices should be removed in the presence of documented catheter-related fungemia (92).

Attempting to salvage infected tunneled CVCs or implantable devices is not recommended because salvage rates with systemic fungal therapy and antibiotic lock therapy for *Candida* species have been in the 30% range (92).

For septic thrombosis of the great central vein due to *Candida* species, a prolonged course of amphotericin B therapy has been shown to be effective and is recommended; fluconazole can be used if the strain is susceptible.

Treatment of catheter-related bloodstream infection due to *M. furfur* includes discontinuation of intralipids and removal of intravascular catheters. Patients with catheter-related *M. furfur* fungemia should be treated with amphotericin B (92).

REFERENCES

1. Hamory BH. Nosocomial bloodstream and intravascular device-related infections. In: Wenzel RP, ed. Prevention and Control of Nosocomial Infections. Baltimore: Williams & Wilkins, 1987:283–319.
2. Banerjee SN, Emori TG, Culver DH, Gaynes RP, Horan TC, Edwards JR, Jarvis WR, Tolson JS, Henderson TS, Martone WJ. Secular trends in nosocomial primary bloodstream infections in the United States, 1980–1989. National Nosocomial Infections Surveillance System. Am J Med 1991; 91:86S–89S.
3. Beck-Sagué CM, Jarvis R and the National Nosocomial Infections Surveillance System. Secular trends in the epidemiology of nosocomial fungal infections in the United States, 1980–1990. J Inf Dis 1993; 167:1247–1251.
4. Pittet D. Nosocomial bloodstream infections. In: Wenzel RP, ed. Prevention and control of nosocomial infections. Baltimore: Williams & Wilkins, 1993:512–555.
5. Daschner FD, Frey P, Wolff G, Baumann PC, Suter P. Nosocomial infections in intensive care wards: a multicenter prospective study. Intensive Care Med 1982; 8:5–9.
6. Morrison AJ Jr, Freer CV, Searcy MA, Landry SM, Wenzel RP. Nosocomial bloodstream infections: secular trends in a statewide surveillance program in Virginia. Infect Control 1986; 7:550–553.
7. Donowitz LG, Haley CE, Gregory WW, Wenzel RP. Neonatal intensive care

unit bacteremia: emergence of gram-positive bacteria as major pathogens. Am J Infect Control 1987; 15:141–147.

8. Berrouane YF, Herwaldt LA, Pfaller MA. Trends in antifungal use and epidemiology of nosocomial yeast infections in a university hospital. J Clin Microbiol 1999; 37(3):531–537.

9. Blumberg HM, Jarvis WR, Soucie M, Edwards JE, Patterson JE, Pfaller MA, Rangel-frausto MS, Rinaldi MG, Saiman L, Wiblin RT, Wenzel RP and the NEMIS Study Group. Risk factors for candidal bloodstream infections in surgical intensive care unit patients: the NEMIS prospective multicenter study. Clin Infect Dis 2001; 33:177–186.

10. Pittet D, Wenzel RP. Nosocomial bloodstream infections: secular trends in rates, mortality, and contribution total hospital deaths. Arch Intern Med 1995; 155:1177–1184.

11. Garbino J, Rohner P, King T. Frequency, mortality and risk factors of candidemia at a tertiary care hospital. Crit Care 2000; 4(suppl):S50S.

12. Miller PJ, Wenzel RP. Etiologic organisms as independent predictors of death and morbidity associated with bloodstream infections. J Infect Dis 1987; 156, 471–477.

13. Louria DB, Stiff DP, Bennett B. Disseminated moniliasis in the adult. Medicine 1962; 41:317–333.

14. King DR, Komer M, Hoffman J, Ginn-Pease ME, Stanley ME, Powell D, Harmel RP Jr. Broviac catheter sepsis: the natural history of an iatrogenic infection. J Pediat Surg 1985; 20:728–733.

15. Uderzo C, D'Angelo P, Rizzari C, Vigano EF, Rovelli A, Gornati G, Codecasa G, Locasciulli A, Masera G. Central venous catheter-related complications after bone marrow transplantation in children with hematological malignancies. Bone Marrow Transplant 1992; 9:113–117.

16. Colombo AL, Nucci M, Salomão R, Branchini ML, RIchtman R, Derossi A, Wey SB. High rate of non-albicans candidemia in Brazilian tertiary care hospitals. Diagn Microbiol Infect Dis 1999; 34(4):281–286.

17. Maki DG. Pathogenesis, prevention and management of infections due to intravascular devices used for infusion therapy. In: Bisno AL, Waldvogel FA, eds. Infections Associated with Indwelling Medical Devices. Washington DC: American Society for Microbiology, 1989:161–177.

18. Lecciones JA, Lee JW, Navarro EE, Witebsky FG, Marshall D, Steinberg SM, Pizzo PA, Walsh TJ. Vascular catheter-associated fungemia in patients with cancer: analysis of 155 episodes. Clin Infect Dis 1992; 14:875–883.

19. Curry CR, Quie PG. Fungal septicemia in patients receiving parenteral hyperalimentation. N Engl J Med 1971; 285:1221–1225.

20. Plouffe JF, Brown DG, Silva J, Eck T, Stricof RL, Fekety R. Nosocomial outbreak of *Candida parapsilosis* fungemia related to intravenous infusions. Arch Intern Med 1977; 137:1686–1689.

21. Solomon SL, Khabbaz RF, Parker RH, Anderson RL, Gerathy MA, Furman RM, Martone WJ. An outbreak of *Candida parapsilosis* bloodstream infections in patients receiving parenteral nutrition. J Infect Dis 1984; 149(1):98–102.

22. Moro ML, Maffei C, Manso E, Morace G, Polonelli L, Biavasco F. Nosocomial outbreak of systemic candidosis associated with parenteral nutrition. Infect Control Hosp Epidemiol 1990; 11(1):27–35.

23. Weems JJ. *Candida parapsilosis*: epidemiology, pathogenicity, clinical manifestations, and antimicrobial susceptibility. Clin Infect Dis 1992; 14:756–766.

24. Branchini ML, Pfaller MA, Rhine-Chalberg J, Frempong T, Isenberg HD. Genotypic variation and slime production among blood and catheter isolates of *Candida parapsilosis*. J Clin Microbiol 1994; 32(2):452–456.

25. Pfaller MA, Messer SA, Hollis RJ. Variations in DNA subtype, antifungal susceptibility, and slime production among clinical isolates of *Candida parapsilosis*. Diagn Microbiol Infect Dis 1995; 21:9–14.

26. Critchley IA, Douglas LJ. Differential adhesion of pathogenic *Candida* species to epithelial and inert surfaces. FEMS Microbiol Lett 1985; 28:199–203.

27. Marcon MJ, Powell DA. Human infections due to *Malassezia* spp. Clin Microb Rev 1992; 5(2):101–119.

28. Kim EH, Cohen RS, Ramachandram P, Glasscock GF. Adhesion of percutaneously inserted silastic central venous lines to the vein wall associated with *Malassezia furfur* infection. J Parent Enter Nutr 1993; 17(5):458–460.

29. Azimi PH, Levernier K, Lefrak LM, Petru AM, Barrett T, Schenck H, Sandhu AJ, Duritz G, Valesco M. *Malassezia furfur*: a cause of occlusion of percutaneous central venous catheters in infants in the intensive care nursery. Pediatr Infect Dis J 1988; 7:100–103.

30. Sitges-Serra A, Puig P, Linares J, Perez JL, Jaurrieta E, Corente L. Hub colonization as the initial step in an outbbreak of catheter-related sepsis due to coagulase-negative staphylococci during parenteral nutrition. J Parenter Ent Nutr 1984; 8:668–672.

31. Linares J, Sitges-Serra A, Garau J, Perez JL, Martin R. Pathogenesis of catheter sepsis: a prospective study with quantitative and semiquantitative cultures of catheter hub and segments. J Clin Microb 1985; 21:357–360.

32. Cooper GL, Hopkins CC. Rapid diagnosis of intravascular catheter-associated infection by direct gram staining of catheter segments. N Engl J Med 1985; 312:1142–1147.

33. Raad II, Costeron W, Sabharwal U, Sacilowski M, Anaissie E, Bodey GP. Ultrastructural analysis of indwelling vascular catheters: a quantitative relationship between luminal colonization and duration of placement. J Infect Dis 1993; 168:400–407.

34. Nucci M, Anaissie E. Revisiting the source of candidemia: skin or gut? Clin Infect Dis 2001; 33(12):1959–1967.

35. Bjornson HS, Colley R, Bower RH, Duty VP, Schwatz-Fulton JT, Fisher JE. Association between microorganism growth at the catheter insertion site and colonization of the catheter in patients receiving total parenteral nutrition. Surgery 1982; 92(4):720–727.

36. McGeer A, Righer J. Improving our ability to diagnose infections associated with central venous catheters: value of Gram's staining and culture of entry site swabs. CMAJ 1987; 137:1009–1021.

37. Flowers RH III, Schwenzer KJ, Kopel RF, Fisch MJ, Tucker SI, Farr BM. Efficacy of an attachable subcutaneous cuff for the prevention of intravascular catheter-related infection. A randomized, controlled trial. JAMA 1989; 261:878–883.

38. Rex JH, Bennett JE, Sugar AM, Pappas PG, Van der Horst CM, Edwards JE,

Washburn RG, Scheld WM, Karchmer AW, Dine AP. A randomized trial comparing fluconazole with amphotericin B for the treatment of candidemia in patients without neutropenia. N Engl J Med 1994; 331:1130–1225.

39. Wade JC. Epidemiology of *Candida* infections. In: Bodey GP, ed. Candidiasis: Pathogenesis, Diagnosis, and Treatment. New York: Raven Press, 1993:85–107.

40. Tenney JH, Moody MR, Newman KA, Schimpff SC, Wade JC, Costerton JW, Reed WP. Adherent microorganisms on lumenal surfaces of long-term intravenous catheters. Arch Intern Med 1986; 146:1949–1954.

41. Tchekmedyian NS, Newman K, Moody MR, Costerton JW, Aisner J, Schimpff SC, Reed WP. Case report: special studies of the Hickman catheter of a patient with recurrent bacteremia and candidemia. Am J Med Sciences 1986; 291(6):419–424.

42. Anaisse E, Samonis G, Kortoyianni D, Costerton J, Sabharwal V, Bodey G, Raad I. Role of catheter colonization and unfrequent hematogenous seeding catheter-related infections. Eur J Clin Microbiol Infect Dis 1995; 14:134–137.

43. Safdar A, Armstrong D. Infectious morbidity in critically ill patients with cancer. Critical Care Clinics 2001; 17(3):531–570.

44. Young RC, Bennett JE, Vogel CL, Carboni PR, DeVita VT. Aspergillosis: the spectrum of the disease in 98 patients. Medicine 1970; 49:147–173.

45. Khardori N, Hayat S, Rolston K, Bodey GP. Cutaneous *Rhizopus* and *Aspergillus* infections in five patients with cancer. Arch Dermatol 1989; 125.952–956.

46. Allo MD, Miller J, Townsend T, Tan C. Primary cutaneous aspergillosis associated with Hickman intravenous catheters. N England J Med 1987; 317:1105–1108.

47. Hunt SJ, Nagi C, Gross KG, Wong DS, Mathews WC. Primary cutaneous aspergillosis near central venous catheters in patients with the acquired immunodeficiency syndrome. Arch Dermatol 1992; 128:1229–1232.

48. Tan TQ, Ogden AK, Tillman J, Demmler GJ, Rinaldi MG. *Paecilomyces lilacinus* catheter-related fungemia in an immunocompromised pediatric patient. J Clin Microbiol 1992; 30(9):2479–2483.

49. Rabodonirina M, Piens MA, Monier MF, Guého E, Fière D, Mojon M. Fusarium infections in Immunocompromised patients: case reports and literature review. Eur J Clin Microbiol Infect Dis 1994; 13:152–161.

50. Walsh TJ, Bustamente CI, Vlahov HC. Standiford, Candidal suppurative peripheral thrombophlebitis: recognition, prevention, and management. Infect Control 1986; 7(1):16–22.

51. Torres-Rojas JR, Stratton CW, Sanders CV, Horsman TP, Hawley HB, Dascomb HE, Vial LF Jr. Candidal suppurative peripheral thrombophlebitis. Ann Intern Med 1982; 96:431–435.

52. Johnson A, Oppenhein D. Vascular catheter-related sepsis: dignosis and prevention. J Hosp Infect 1992; 20:67–78.

53. Maki DG, Weise CE, Sarafin HW. A semiquantitative culture method for identifying intravenous-catheter-related infection. N Engl J Med 1977; 296(23):1305–1309.

54. Cleri DJ, Corrado ML, Seligman SJ. Quantitative culture of intravenous catheters and other intravascular inserts. J Infect Dis 1980; 141:781–786.

55. Sherertz RJ, Raad II, Balani A, Koo LC, Rand KH, Pickett DI, Straub SP, Fauerbach LL. Three year experience with sonicated vascular catheter cultures in a clinical microbiology laboratory. J Clin Microb 1990; 28:76–82.

56. Brun-Buisson C, Abrouk F, Legrand P, Houet Y, Larabi S, Rapin M. Diagnosis of central venous catheter-related sepsis. Critical levels of quantitative tip cultures. Arch Intern Med 1987; 147:873–877.

57. Raad II, Sabbagh MF, Rand KH, Sherertz RJ. Quantitative tip culture methods and the diagnosis of central venous catheter-related infections. Diagn Microbiol Infect Dis 1992; 15:13–20.

58. Khatib R, Clark JF, Briski LE, Wilson FM. Relevance of culturing *Candida* species from intravascular catheters. J Clin Microb 1995; 33(6):1635–1637.

59. Telenti A, Steckelberg JM, Stockman L, Edson RS, Roberts GD. Quantitative blood cultures in candidemia. Mayo Clin Proc 1991; 66:1120–1123.

60. Walsh TJ, Pizzo PA. Laboratory diagnosis of candidiasis. In: Bodey GP, ed. Candidiasis: Pathogenesis, Diagnosis, and Treatment. New York: Raven Press, 1993:109–135.

61. Ellis CA, Spivack ML. The significance of candidemia. Ann Intern Med 1967; 67(3):511–522.

62. Louria DV, Blevins A, Armastrong D, Burdick R, Lieberman P. Arch Intern Med 1967; 119:247–252.

63. Vic-Dupont V, Coulaud JP, Delrieu F. Les septiémies a candida. Press Medicale 1968; 76:747–750.

64. Williams RJ, Chandler JG, Orloff MJ. *Candida* septicemia. Arch Surg 1971; 103:8–11.

65. Hickman RO, Buckner CD, Clift RA, Sanders JE, Stewart P, Thomas ED. A modified right atrial catheter for access to the venous system in marrow transplant recipients. Surg Gynecol Obstet 1979; 148:871–875.

66. Franceschi D, Gerding RL, Phillips G, Fratianne RB. Risk factors associated with intravascular catheter infections in burned patients: A prospective, randomized study. J Trauma 1989; 29:811–816.

67. Siegman-Igra Y, Golan H, Schwartz D, Cahaner Y, De-Mayo G, Orni-Wasserlauf R. Epidemiology of vascular catheter-related bloodstream infections in a large university hospital in Israel. Scand J Infect Dis 2000; 32(4):411–415.

68. Wey SB, Mori M, Pfaller MA, Woolson RF, Wenzel RP. Risk factors for hospital-acquired candidemia. A matched case-control study. Arch Intern Med 1989; 149:2349–2353.

69. Bross J, Talbot FH, Maislin G, Hurwitz S, Strom BL. Risk factors for nosocomial candidemia: a case-control study in adults without leukemia. Am J Med 1989; 87:614–620.

70. Karanabis A, Hill C, Leclercq B, Tancrede C, Baume D, Andremont A. Risk factors for candidemia in cancer patients: a case-control study. J Clin Microbiol 1988; 26:429–432.

71. Groeger JS, Lucas AB, Thaler HT, Friedlander-Klar H, Brown AE, Kiehn TE, Armstrong D. Infectious morbidity associated with long-term use of venous devices in patients with cancer. Ann Inter Med 1993; 119:1168–1174.

72. Armstrong CW, Mayhall CG, Miller KB, Newsome HH, Sugerman HJ,

Dalton HP, Hall GO, Hunsberger S. Clinical predictors of infections of central venous catheters used for total parenteral nutrition. Infect Control Hosp Epidemiol 1990; 11:71–78.

73. Dankner WM, Spector SA, Ferier J, Davis CE. *Malassezia* fungemia in neonates and adults: complication of hyperalimentation. Rev Infect Dis 1987; 9:743–753.

74. Kikuchi K, Fujishiro Y, Totsuka K, Seshimo A, Kameoka S, Makimura K, Yamaguchi H. A case of central venous catheter-related infection with *Malassezia sympodialis*. Nippon Ishinkin Gakkai Zasshi 2001; 42(4):220–222.

75. Solomon SL, Alexander H, Eley JW, Anderson RL, Goodpasture HC, Smart S, Furman RM, Martone WJ. Nosocomial fungemia in neonates associated with intravascular pressure-monitoring devices. Pediatr Infect Dis 1986; 5:680–685.

76. Ruiz-Diez B, Martinez V, Alvarez M, Rodriguez-Tudela JL, Martinez-Suarez JV. Molecular tracking of *Candida albicans* in a neonatal intensive care unit: long-term colonizations versus catheter-related infections. J Clin Microbiol 1997; 35(12):3032–3036.

77. McKinnon PS, Goff DA, Kern JW, Devlin JW, Barletta JF, Sierawski SJ, Mosenthal AC, Gore P, Ambegaonkar AJ, Lubowski TJ. Temporal assessment of *Candida* risk factors in the surgical intensive care unit. Arch Surg 2001; 136(12):1401–1408.

78. Kac G, Durain E, Amrein C, Herisson E, Fiemeyer A, Buu-Hoi A. Colonization and infection of pulmonary artery catheters in cardiac surgery patients: epidemiology and multivariate analysis of risk factors. Crit Care Med 2001; 29(5):971–975.

79. Horn CK, Conway SP. Candidemia: risk factors in patients with cystic fibrosis who have totally implantable venous access systems. J Infection 1993; 26:127–132.

80. Widmer AF. IV-related infections. In: Wenzel RP, ed. Prevention and control of nosocomial infections. Baltimore: Williams & Wilkins, 1993:556–579.

81. Fry DE, Fry RV, Borzotta AP. Nosocomial blood-borne infection secondary to intravascular devices. Am J Surg 1994; 167:268–272.

82. Bagwell CE, Marchildon MB. Mural thrombi in children: potentially lethal complication of central venous hyperalimentation. Crit Care Med 1989; 17:295–296.

83. Paut O, Kreitmann B, Silicani MA, Wernet F, Broin P, Viard L, Camboulives J. Successful treatment of fungal right atrial thrombosis complicating central venous catheterization in a critically ill child. Intensive Care Med 1992; 18:375–376.

84. Sycova-Milá Z, Sufliarshy J, Trupl J, Jasendská Z, Blahvá M, Kremery V Jr. Catheter-associated septicemia due to *Trichosporon capitatum*. J Hosp Infect 1992; 22:257–261.

85. Kiehn TE, Gorey E, Brown AE, Edwards FF, Armstrong D. Sepsis due to *Rhodotorula* related to use of indwelling central venous catheters. Clin Infect Dis 1992; 14:841–846.

86. Ammari LK, Puck JM, McGown KL. Catheter-related *Fusarium solani* fungemia and pulmonary infection in a patient with leukemia in remission. Clin Infec Dis 1993; 16:148–150.

87. Aschner JL, Punsalang A, Maniscalco WM, Menegus MA. Percutaneous central venous catheter colonization with *Malassezia furfur*: incidence and clinical significance. Pediatrics 1987; 80:535–539.

88. Sheng WH, Ko WJ, Wang JT, Chang SC, Hsueh PR, Luh KT. Evaluation of antiseptic-impregnated central venous catheters for prevention of catheter-related infection in intensive care unit patients. Diag Microbiol Infect Dis 2000; 38(1):1–5.

89. Clarke DE, Raffin TA. Infectious complications of indwelling long-term central venous catheters. Chest 1990; 97:966–972.

90. Press OW, Ramsey PG, Larson EB, Fefer A, Kickman RO. Hickman catheter infections in patients with malignancies. Medicine 1984; 63:189–200.

91. Mayhall G. Diagnosis and management of infections of implantable devices used of prolonged venous access. Curr Clin Top Infect Dis 1992; 12:83–110.

92. Mermel LA, Farr BM, Sherertz RJ, Raad II, O'Grady N, Harris JS, Craven DE. Guidelines for the management of intravascular catheter-related infections. Infect Control Hosp Epidemiol 2001; 22:222–242.

93. Anaissie EJ, Rex JH, Uzun O, Vartivarian S. Predictors of adverse outocome in cancer patients with candidemia. Am J Med 1998; 104:238–245.

94. Dato VM, Dajani AS. Candidemia in children with central venous catheters: role of catheter removal and amphotericin B therapy. Pediatr Infect Dis 1990; 8:309–314.

95. Rex JH, Bennett JE, Sugar AM, Pappas PG, Serody J, Edwards JE, Washburn RG, the NIAID mycoses study group, and the candidemia study group. Intravascular catheter exchanges and the duration of candidemia. Clin Infect Dis 1995; 21:994–996.

96. Nguyen MH, Peacock JE, Tanner DC, Morris AJ, Nguyen ML, Snydman DR, Wagener MM, Yu VL. Therapeutic approaches in patients with candidemia. Evaluation in a multicenter prospective, observational study. Arch Intern Med 1995; 155:2429–2435.

97. Nucci M, Anaissie E. Should vascular catheters be removed from all patients with candidemia? An evidence-based review. Clin Infec Dis 2002; 34:591–599.

98. Anaissie EJ, Rex JH, Uzum O, Vartivarian S. Predictors of adverse outcome in cancer patients with candidemia. Am J Med 1998; 104:238–245.

99. Luzzati R, Amalfitano G, Lazzarini L, Soldani F, Bellino S, Solbiati M, Danzi MC, Vento S, Todeschini G, Vivenza C, Concia E. Nosocomial candidemia in non-neutropenic patients at an Italian tertiary care hospital. Eur J Clin Microbiol Infect Dis 2000; 19(8):602–607.

100. Nucci M, Silveira MI, Spenctor N, et al. Risk factors for death among cancer patients with fungemia. Clin Infect Dis 1998; 27:107–111.

101. Nucci M, Colombo AL, Silveira F, Tichtmann R, Salomão R, Branchini ML, Spector L. Risk factors for death in patients with candidemia. Infect Control Hosp Epidemiol 1998; 19:846–850

102. Rex JH, Walsh TJ, Sobel JD, Filler SG, Pappas PG, Dismukes WE, Edwards JE. Practice guidelines for the treatment of candidiasis. Clin Infect Dis 2000; 30:662–678.

10

Miscellaneous Organisms

Tanja Schülin

University of Medical Centre St. Radboud, Radboud University Nijmegen, The Netherlands

Andreas Voss

University of Medical Centre St. Radboud, and Nijmegen University Centre of Infectious Diseases Nijmegen, The Netherlands

INTRODUCTION

At present, coagulase-negative staphylococci are still the most frequently isolated pathogens from patients with catheter-related infections (CRI). The increasing use of indwelling devices in an expanding population of immuno-compromised patients may be the most important explanation for why the list of microorganisms involved in catheter-related infections continues to expand, since nonpathogenic microorganisms from the patient's skin or the environment, formerly often classified as contaminants, may cause infections. The improved microbiological diagnostics, with the development of easy-to-use identification systems and especially the more widespread use of molecular methods such as automated DNA sequencing, may have furthermore led to the recognition of rare or even "new" pathogens. Novel approaches in catheter design and materials may help to reduce colonization with *Staphylococcus epidermidis* and other gram-positive cocci (1), but may not always help to prevent infections due to other, frequently saprophytic microorganisms.

This chapter reviews case reports and a small series of CRI due to miscellaneous bacterial pathogens, i.e., microorganisms that rarely cause infection, as well as common pathogens that do not usually cause catheter-related infections. At present, case reports of catheter-related infections due to miscellaneous organisms are still rare enough to be reported in the medical literature, but in the aforementioned situation, we might encounter these organisms on a regular basis.

PATHOGENESIS

Since most of the organisms described in this chapter are rarely encountered in human infections, knowledge regarding their pathogenesis is sparse. In general, they are thought to be of low pathogenicity, thus most likely causing infections in an immunocompromised patient population. Some of the bacteria, such as corynebacteria, various nonfermenting gram-negative rods (*Burkholderia* spp., *Rhizobium* spp., nonaeruginosa *Pseudomonas* spp.), and rapidly growing mycobacteria, may then become pathogenic by producing a mucoid biofilm on a foreign body of plastic material (2–4). Immunocompromised patients, such as hematology, transplant, and HIV patients, may be more likely to get infected by unusual pathogens due to their lack of cellular immunity and the frequent use of implanted intravascular devices.

MICROBIOLOGY

In contrast to the classical bacteria causing CRI, among the miscellaneous pathogens, gram-negative organisms predominate over gram-positive organisms. The gram-negative organisms are classified as: (a) nonfermenters, (b) *Pseudomonas* spp. and related genera, and (c) other gram-negative bacilli. All of these gram-negative bacteria are listed in Table 1. Gram-positive pathogens causing CRI may be divided into the following categories: (a) *Bacillus* spp. and other gram-positive rods, (b) *Corynebacterium* spp. and related organisms, (c) gram-positive cocci other than staphylococci, (d) actinomycetes, and (e) mycobacteria (Table 2). Rare fungal catheter-related infections such as those due to *Malassezia furfur* or *Acremonium* are discussed elsewhere in this book. The more common gram-negative organisms involved in CRI, such as Enterobacteriaceae, *Pseudomonas aeruginosa*, and *Acinetobacter* species, as well as CRI caused by rare Enterobacteriaceae such as *Enterobacter amnigenus* and *Klyvera cryocrescens* are covered in Chapter 8.

    Since frequent reclassifications and new names designated to bacterial genera may lead to confusions, the newest nomenclature was used for the purpose of this chapter, followed by the older names in brackets.

EPIDEMIOLOGY

In most surveillance reports in the literature, percentage of CRI with unusual pathogens is still reported to be fewer than 5% (5–7). At the Memorial Sloan-Kettering Cancer Center, the extensive use of vascular access devices and associated device-related sepsis has resulted in changes in the type of organisms causing bloodstream infections (8). The proportion of bacteremia caused by miscellaneous organisms increased from 12 to 19% in 1984 and 1988, respectively (Table 3). Castagnola et al. reported in 1997 that from 102 episodes of Broviac catheter infections in children receiving antineoplastic chemotherapy or bone marrow transplantation, seven occurred due to unusual pathogens (9).

Catheter-related infections can be caused by bacteria originating from endogenous or exogenous sources leading to infections with pathogens from the hospital environment or the patients' own flora. Furthermore, implanted devices that allow patients to move rather freely, e.g., in their homes, may also be prone to become infected from environmental sources (10).

CLINICAL MANIFESTATION AND THERAPEUTIC OPTIONS

Miscellaneous Gram-Negative Bacteria

Over the past decades, bacteremia caused by previously unknown or rare gram-negative bacteria has increasingly been recognized, mainly in neutropenic patients, HIV patients, and children with malignancies (9,11,12).

Pseudomonas Species and Related Genera

The taxonomy of *Pseudomonas* species and related genera has undergone major changes during the past two decades. Some of the microorganisms now belong to the genus *Burkholderia, Comamonas, Ralstonia, Sphingomonas,* or *Stenotrophomonas.*

Bacteremia due to *Stenotrophomonas* (*Xanthomonas*) *maltophilia* and nonaeruginosa *Pseudomonas* species is still rare, but may be increasing. At the M. D. Anderson Cancer Center, the rate of bacteremia due to these bacteria significantly increased from three cases per 10,000 admissions in 1974 to 14 cases per 10,000 admissions in 1986 (12). About 50% of these infections were caused by *S. maltophilia,* whereas *P. stutzeri* and *P. putida* each accounted for about 10%. Other species such as *Burkholderia* (*Pseudomonas*) *cepacia, C. testosteroni, P. fluorescens, P. vesicularis, R. picketti* or *S. paucimobilis* were seen occasionally. The most important predisposing factor in the immunocompromised patients was the presence of an indwelling central venous or arterial line that was in place for an average of three months before the onset of bacteremia and found in 83% of the patients. Catheters were proven to be the source of the infection in 57 of 83 patients (69%) in whom the portal of entry was identified. Ninety-five percent of these patients responded to therapy. It was shown that the removal of the central venous catheter resulted in a 100% cure rate, irrespective of the appropriateness of the antibiotic therapy. Recurrent catheter-related infections were seen in 29% of patients who had received appropriate antibiotics, but in whom the catheter or the site of catheter insertion (due to guidewire exchange) had not been changed. Thus,

Table 1 Miscellaneous Gram-Negative Bacteria Causing Catheter-Related Infection

Gram-negative bacteria	Species	Author/year/reference number
Pseudomonas species & related genera	*Burkholderia cepacia*	Pegues et al. 1993 (14)
		Yu et al. 1999 (130)
		Kaitwatcharachai et al. 2000 (131)
	CDC Group IV c-2	Arduino et al. 1993 (22)
	Chryseomonas luteola (CDC Group Ve-1)	Kostman et al. 1991 (23)
	Comamonas acidovorans	Castagnola et al. 1994 (15)
		Ender et al. 1996 (16)
	Comamonas testosteroni	Le Moal et al. 2001 (17)
	Ralstonia (*Pseudomonas*) *pickettii*	Raveh et al. 1993 (29)
	Methylobacterium extorquens	Poirier et al. 1988 (19)
		Kaye et al. 1992 (20)
	Pseudomonas fluorescens	Elting and Bodey 1990 (12)
	Pseudomonas (*Flavimonas*) *oryzihabitans* (CDC Group Ve-2)	Kostman et al. 1991(23)
		Conlu et al. 1992 (26)
		Marin et al. 2000 (27)
	Pseudomonas putida	Anaissie et al. 1987 (21)
	Pseudomonas stutzeri	Elting and Bodey 1990 (12)
	Roseomonas gilardii	Alcala et al. 1997 (30)
		Marin et al. 2001 (31)
	Sphingomonas (*Pseudomonas*) *paucimobilis*	Decker et al. 1992 (35)
		Salazar et al. 1995 (34)
		Hsueh et al. 1998 (32)
	Stenothrophomonas maltophilia	Elting and Bodey 1990 (12)
		Herrero Romero et al. 2000 (36)
		Friedman et al. 2002 (37)
		Ratnalingham et al. 2002 (38)
Nonfermenters (nonfermentative gram-negative rods)	*Achromobacter piechaudii*	Kay et al. 2001 (48)
	Achromobacter xylosoxidans (*Alcaligenes xylosoxidans*)	Legrand and Anaissie 1992 (44)
		Cieslak and Raszka 1993 (41)
		Ramos et al. 1996 (132)
		Duggan et al. 1996 (49)
		Knippschild et al. 1996 (46)
		Manfredi et al. 1997 (45)
		Hernandez et al. 1998 (47)

Table 1 Continued

Gram-negative bacteria	Species	Author/year/reference number
	Chryseobacterium (*Flavobacterium*) spp.	Stamm et al. 1975 (54)
		Sader et al. 1995 (58)
		Hsueh et al. 1996/1997 (56,57)
		Nulens et al. 2001 (55)
	Ochrobactrum anthropi (*Achromobacter*, CDC Group-Vd)	Cieslak et al. 1992 (40)
		Gransden and Eykyn 1992 (42)
		Kern et al. 1993 (39)
		Alnor et al. 1994 (51)
		Gill et al. 1997 (61)
		Yu et al. 1998 (60)
		Saavedra et al. 1999 (133)
		Stiakaki et al. 2002 (134)
	Rhizobium (*Agrobacterium*) spp.	Edmond et al. 1993 (50)
		Alnor et al. 1994 (51)
		Yu et al. 1997 (135)
Other gram-negative bacilli	*Aeromonas hydrophila*	Siddiqui et al. 1992 (63)
		Rello et al. 1993 (127)
		Martino et al. 2000 (128)
	Bordetella bronchiseptica	Qureshi et al. 1992 (65)
	Campylobacter spp.	Hsueh et al. 1997 (66)
	Kingella kingae	Goutzmanis et al. 1991 (68)
	Moraxella osloensis	Buchman et al. 1993 (69)

removal of the catheter and, if still necessary, insertion at a new site seem to be of utmost importance in successfully managing CRI due to these micro-organisms.

B. cepacia is widely distributed throughout the environment, especially water and soil. Outbreaks of infection have been reported as a result of exposure to contaminated povidone-iodine solutions, parenteral fluids, and invasive pressure-monitoring devices (13,14). After contact with a contaminated heparin flush solution, 15 patients with catheter-associated *B. cepacia* bacteremia were identified in a U.S. oncology center (14).

Comamonas acidovorans is ubiquitous in the environment, including soil and foodstuffs. Recently, a boy with non-Hodgkin's lymphoma was reported with *C. acidovorans* CRI (15). The child was admitted for treatment of a herpes simplex virus ocular infection and experienced symptoms of sepsis

Table 2 Miscellaneous Gram-Positive Bacteria Causing Catheter-Related Infection

Gram-positive bacteria	Species	Author/year
Gram-positive cocci	*Enterococcus casseliflavus*	Van Goethem et al. 1994 (72)
	Enterococcus faecalis	Patterson et al., 1995 (70)
	Enterococcus faecium	Patterson et al., 1995 (70)
	Enterococcus gallinarum	Patterson et al., 1995 (70)
	Kokuria kristinae	Basaglia et al. 2002 (75)
	Micrococcus luteus	Peces et al. 1997 (73)
	Pediococcus pentosaceus	Atkins et al. 1994 (76)
	Rothia (Stomatococcus) *mucilaginosus*	Ascher et al. 1991 (77)
Coryneforms & related organisms	*Brevibacterium epidermidis*	McCaughey and Damani 1991 (94)
	Corynebacterium afermentans	Dealler et al. 1993 (78)
		Kerr et al. 1993 (79)
	Corynebacterium amycolatum	Oteo et al. 2001 (80)
	Corynebacterium aquaticum	Moore and Norton 1995 (81)
		Vasseur et al. 1998 (82)
	Corynebacterium jeikeium	Riebel et al. 1986 (83)
		Fish and Danziger 1993 (84)
		Wang et al. 2001 (85)
	Corynebacterium minutissimum	Cavendish et al. 1994 (86)
		Rupp et al. 1998 (87)
	Corynebacterium striatum	Tumbarello et al. 1994 (88)
	Corynebacterium urealyticum	Soriano et al. 1993 (4)
		Wood and Pepe 1994 (89)
Other gram-positive bacteria	*Microbacterium* spp.	Campbell et al. 1994 (91)
	(*Aureobacterium* spp.,	Bizette et al. 1995 (90)
	Corynebacterium CDC group	Grove et al. 1999 (92)
	A-4/A-5, Microbacterium spp.)	Lau et al. 2002 (93)
	Lactobacillus rhamnosus	Carretto et al. 2001 (100)
	Listeria monocytogenes	Katner and Joiner 1989 (101)
		Fish and Danziger 1993 (84)
	Rothia dentocariosa	Nivar-Aristy et al. 1991 (106)
Actinomycetes	*Gordonia (Rhodococcus,* *Gordona) rubropertincta*	Buchman et al. 1992 (107)
	Gordonia (Rhodococcus, *Gordona) terrae*	Buchman et al. 1992 (107)
		Pham et al. 2003 (108)
	Nocardia asteroides	Rubin et al. 1987 (109)
	Nocardia nova	Miron et al. 1994 (110)
	Nocardia otitidis-caviarum	Lee et al. 1994 (111)
	Tsukamurella paurometabolum	Shapiro et al. 1992 (112)
		Lai 1993 (113)
	Tsukamurella pulmonis	Maertens et al. 1998 (114)

Table 2 Continued

Gram-positive bacteria	Species	Author/year
Mycobacteria	*Mycobacterium aurum*	Esteban et al. 1998 (122)
	Mycobacterium avium complex	Schelonka et al. 1994 (117)
		Dube and Sattler 1996 (136)
	Mycobacterium chelonae	Hsueh et al. 1998 (3)
	Mycobacterium fortuitum complex	Raad et al. 1991 (116)
		Suara et al. 2001 (137)
	Mycobacterium neoaurum	Davison et al. 1988 (118)
		Holland et al. 1994 (119)
		George and Schlesinger 1999 (120)
		Woo et al. 2000 (121)
	Mycobacterium septicum sp. nov.	Schinsky et al. 2000 (123)
	Mycobacterium smegmatis	Skiest and Levi 1998 (124)
	Rapidly-growing mycobacteria	Gaviria et al. 2000 (115)

Table 3 Microorganisms Causing Bacteremia at Memorial Sloan-Kettering Cancer Center

Organisms	No. (%) of episodes	
	1984 ($n = 64$)	1988 ($n = 190$)
Anaerobes	42 (8)	35 (4)
- *Bacteroides* spp.	21 (4)	18 (2)
- *Clostridium* spp.	14 (3)	16 (2)
- Others	7 (1)	1
Nonaeruginosa *Pseudomonas* spp.	3 (1)	59 (5)
- *P. fluorescens*		3 (0.5)
- *Stenotrophomonas* (*Pseudomonas*) *maltophilia*		32 (3)
- *P. putida*		14 (1.5)
Others	19 (3)	96 (10)
- *Aeromonas* spp.	2	2
- *Achromobacter* (*Alcaligenes*) spp.	0	3
- *Bacillus* spp.	3 (1)	26 (3)
- *Corynebacterium* spp.	8 (2)	45 (5)
- *Chryseobacterium* (*Flavobacter*) spp.	0	4
- *Haemophilus influenzae*	0	4
- *Listeria* spp.	5 (1)	5 (1)
- *Micrococcus* spp.	0	7 (1)
- *Vibrio* spp.	1	0

(From Ref. 8.)

during infusion therapy. Treatment with ceftazidime and vancomycin was started; amikacin was added the next day when *C. acidovorans* was recovered from blood cultures. Despite a clinical response, bacteremia persisted until the Broviac catheter was removed. In contrast, in 1996, Ender et al. reported a case of *C. acidovorans* bacteremia managed with the preservation of the catheter in a pediatric patient (16). *Comamonas testosteroni* was isolated from the blood of a woman with breast cancer (17). The bacteremia cleared after adapted antimicrobial treatment and catheter removal.

Methylobacterium extorquens was originally isolated from the surface of a leaf (18). Various synonyms have been used previously for *Methylobacterium* such as: *Pseudomonas mesophilica*, *Protaminobacter rubra*, *Pseudomonas methanolica*, *Vibrio extorquens*, and *Mycoplana rubra*. *M. extorquens* is a pink-pigmented, opportunistic pathogen of low virulence, causing CRI, fever, pulmonary infiltrates, ulcers, and uveitis. So far, 16 cases have been reported (19,20). Blood isolates were shown to be susceptible to TMP/SMZ, tetracycline, imipenem, ciprofloxacin, and aminoglycosides. The indolent nature of the infection might justify antibiotic treatment without removal of the catheter, even though this recommendation is based on the results of only three cases (19).

Pseudomonas putida is a ubiquitous environmental saprophyte found in soil, in water, and on plants. The organism may also be a part of the normal human oropharyngeal flora. In 1987, *P. putida* was described as a newly recognized pathogen causing bacteremia in cancer patients at the M. D. Anderson Hospital in Texas (21). Between 1980 and 1985, the organism was isolated from blood culture specimens of 15 patients, including five cases that were considered to have polymicrobial bacteremia. The bloodstream infection appeared to be catheter-related in three patients who had phlebitis, cellulitis, or both at the catheter insertion site. The increase in *P. putida* infections during the study period was paralleled by a similar increase in the number of intravascular devices. In cases of catheter-related bacteremia, removal of the catheter in addition to antimicrobial treatment, e.g., ceftazidime, ciprofloxacin, imipenem, or piperacillin, was necessary to control the infection.

Other genera related to *Pseudomonas* that are known to cause bacteremia include CDC Group IV c-2, *Chryseomonas luteola* (CDC Group VE-1), and *Pseudomonas* (formerly *Flavimonas*) *oryzihabitans*, also formerly known as CDC Group Ve-2 or *Chromobacterium typhiflavuum* (22–26). Reported cases are generally associated with the presence of prosthetic material or catheters in immunocompromised patients.

Pseudomonas oryzihabitans is a relatively avirulent, nonfermenting, gram-negative rod, and has been isolated from skin, wounds, sputum, urine, and blood, but was not classified as clinically significant until the first report of infection in 1977 (25). Since then, *P. oryzihabitans* has been reported to cause CAPD-related peritonitis, indwelling venous catheter-related infections, and occasionally bacteremia (23–26). Of 36 cases reported until 1993, 22 episodes of *P. oryzihabitans* sepsis came from one center (24). Most of the patients had significant underlying medical problems, especially malignancies, and the source of infection was unclear, since no environmental cultures or cultures from other body sites of infected patients yielded the organism. In a Spanish report, infection of a Hickman catheter in an AIDS patient could be traced to synthetic bath sponges (27). Cases of CRIs were successfully treated with TMP/SMZ and antipseudomonal antibiotics. With some exceptions, the majority of reviewed cases (81%) did not require the removal of the catheter to control bacteremia.

So far, *Pseudomonas putrefaciens* has not been reported to cause catheter-related bacteremia, but three patients were described with CAPD peritonitis, which was probably associated with the Tenckhoff catheter (28).

Catheter-related infections due to *Ralstonia pickettii* were reported for the first time by Raveh et al. (29), who described four cases, all of which were associated with long-term indwelling intravenous devices, such as Infuse-a-port™, Broviac, and Hickman catheters.

Roseomonas gilardii sp. nov. is a pink-pigmented, oxidative bacterium that has been infrequently isolated from clinical samples. Alcala et al. report a case of CRI due to this organism in an immunocompromised patient with an implanted catheter (30). The catheter was removed and the patient recovered after seven days of therapy with ciprofloxacin. Another case was recently reported from Italy (31).

Two cases of CRI due to *Sphingomonas paucimobilis* were reported by Hsueh et al. (32). Both patients were immunocompromised and only recovered after the removal of the catheters. Another four patients from Spain were cured after catheter removal (33,34). In contrast to these findings, Decker et al. (35) reported two cases of *S. paucimobilis* CRI, which were successfully treated without removal of the Groshong catheters. Of interest, one of the patients was treated with TMP/SMZ, since the strain was resistant to ceftazidime.

Catheter-related infections caused by *Stenotrophomonas maltophilia* is still rare and occurs mostly in immunocompromised hosts. Over a six-year period, only five bacteremia cases related to an intravascular device were reported from a Spanish hospital (36). Four patients received antibiotics, and all patients were cured after catheter removal. In another report, 45 episodes of *S. maltophilia* bacteremia were observed over a 10-year period from 1990 to 2001 (37). All patients were immunocompromised, and in 38 cases, the source of infection was an indwelling device. Catheter removal seems to be crucial, since 92 % of patients with catheter removal survived, whereas only 54% did without catheter removal. Two cases of CRI due to *S. maltophilia* were reported from cystic fibrosis patients with implanted catheters (38). The source of infection was not the patients' own flora, but most likely contamination occurred during home-handling of the catheter. For cure in both cases, the device had to be removed.

Nonfermenters (Nonfermentative gram-negative Rods)

In general, the group of nonfermentative gram-negative bacteria includes a variety of heterogeneous organisms. An overview on colonization or infections due to these organisms is complicated by the fact that they frequently have undergone taxonomic changes.

Nonfermentative, nonfastidious gram-negative bacilli, formerly classified as *Achromobacter* spp. or *Achromobacter*-like organisms, have been assigned among others to *Agrobacterium* spp., *Alcaligenes* spp., and *Ochrobactrum anthropi*. The organisms have been isolated from clinical specimens, the environment, and hospital water supplies. As far as the confusing taxonomy allows interpretation, it is only recently that these microorganisms have been recognized in humans as pathogens associated with intravascular catheter infections (39–42).

Infections, including catheter-associated bacteremia, due to *Achromobacter xylosoxidans*, subspecies *xylosoxidans* (formerly *Alcaligenes xylosoxidans* and *Alcaligenes denitrificans*, subspecies *xylosoxidans*), were observed in cancer patients (43,44), and in patients with AIDS (41,45). Despite resistance to aminoglycosides, the patients were successfully treated with a combination of ceftazidime and amikacin without removing the catheter. Infections occurring in neutropenic hematology patients were successfully treated with imipenem and catheter removal (46,47). One case of CRI due to *Achromobacter piechaudii* has been reported in a hematology patient (48). The antimicrobial resistance of *Achromobacter* spp. appears to be unpredictable, and the optimal therapeutic management is unknown. After reviewing the literature, Legrand and Anaissie (44) came to the conclusion that infections usually respond to therapy with TMP/SMZ or an appropriate β-lactam antibiotic. The use of multiple antibiotics [including combinations with aminoglycosides, which shows synergistic or additive effects in vitro (49)] has also been recommended, but whether the infected device has to be removed remains unclear.

Agrobacterium species are nonfermentative saprophytic bacilli, which are found in aqueous environments and appear to be nonindigenous to human beings. Until 1997, 25 cases of systemic infections had been reported. Infections were strongly related to the presence of foreign plastic material (50). *Rhizobium* (*Agrobacterium*) *radiobacter* may produce copious amounts of slime and form biofilms, characteristics that may enhance its pathogenic ability to cause infections in patients requiring intravenous access and peritoneal dialysis (2,51). Community-acquired CRI may arise through handling plants, as reported by Alnor et al. (51) and Hulse et al. (52). Restriction enzyme analysis of *Agrobacterium* isolates from eight patients of one hospital revealed unique patterns in each case, thus excluding a common nosocomial source (52). In patients with mucositis and breakdown of the gastrointestinal barrier, translocation of the organism from the patient's gut might be another possible source. Antimicrobial susceptibility is variable and treatment must be based on individual antimicrobial susceptibility results. Most cases responded to treatment only after removal of the indwelling device.

   Chryseobacterium meningosepticum and *C. indologenes* (formerly *Flavobacterium* spp.) are found in water and in the hospital environment. Bacteremia was shown to be related to the infusion of contaminated blood products (53). In 1973, *Chryseobacterium* bloodstream infections occurred in 14 ICU patients in a five-month period (54), and further investigation revealed a common in-hospital source of infection. Fever and positive blood cultures persisted in eight of 14 patients, despite antibiotic treatment. The symptoms resolved in five of six patients after the arterial catheter had been removed. No deaths were directly related to *Chryseobacterium* bacteremia. Catheter-related infections due to *C. indologenes* and *C. meningosepticum* have been reported recently (55–58). All infections occurred in severely immunocompromised patients. In one series, the deaths of five from 36 infected patients were directly attributable to *C. indologenes* infection (57). Despite variable antimicrobial susceptibility of strains that makes antibiotic treatment difficult, Hsueh et al. reported successful treatment of CRI without removal of the catheter in six of seven patients (56).

   The first case of bacteremia caused by *Ochrobactrum anthropi* (formerly *Achromobacter*, CDC group-Vd) was reported by Kish et al. in 1984 (59). Since then, other, mainly catheter-related, bacteremia cases have been published (39,40,42,51,60), one case in an immunocompetent host (61). In general, catheter-related infections by these species have been described in neutropenic cancer patients as well as in nonneutropenic patients. Hospital water supplies and translocation from the gut were discussed as possible sources. The extensive resistance of these microorganisms to a wide range of antimicrobial agents, including penicillins, cephalosporins, aminoglycosides, and antibiotic therapy failure in spite of in vitro susceptibility, makes management even more difficult (40,42). In general, the choice of antibiotic treatment seems to depend on the individual antibiogram, and removal of the catheter is probably necessary, despite the fact that in one publication, removal of the catheter alone seemed to clear infection (42).

Other gram-negative Bacilli

Aeromonas hydrophila is a facultative anaerobe, oxidase-positive, gram-negative rod, belonging to the family Vibrionaceae. *Aeromonas* spp. can be found in water, soil, and foodstuffs. *Aeromonas* spp. may cause wound infections, diarrheal disease, and extraintestinal infections such as meningitis, osteomyelitis, peritonitis, urinary tract infections, and bloodstream infections. So far, most cases of bacteremia have occurred in patients with hepatic or pancreatic diseases and leukemia. One case of *A. hydrophila* bacteremia was reported among a group of 15 patients with pulmonary artery catheter infections, described by Rello et al. (62). The strain probably originated from the IV system, since the catheter hubs were contaminated with the organism. Siddiqui et al. (63) published a case report of a 50-year-old patient who died of a myonecrosis. The gas gangrene-like presentation due to *A. hydrophila* followed the insertion of an IV catheter into the long saphenous vein.

Bordetella spp. cause infections in humans and animals. Whereas *B. pertussis* and *B. parapertussis* are restricted to humans, *B. bronchiseptica* mainly causes respiratory infections in animals (64). *B. bronchiseptica* bacteremia is extremely rare. So far, only one case of catheter-related bacteremia has been reported (65). At the time of infection, a 33-year-old patient with AIDS received ganciclovir maintenance treatment via an indwelling Broviac catheter. Several weeks after experiencing a CRI due to *Bacillus subtilis*, which was cured without removing the catheter, the patient presented with high fever and chills. *Achromobacter* spp. was isolated from blood cultures and the patient received imipenem. After two weeks of treatment, the patient was discharged with the Broviac catheter still in place. However, another episode of CRI occurred three weeks later. This time, *B. bronchiseptica* was isolated from blood cultures, and despite treatment with imipenem, bacteremia only cleared after the catheter was removed. The authors presumed that the initial identification as *Achromobacter* spp., done in a commercial laboratory, may have been incorrect, since *B. bronchiseptica* and *Achromobacter* spp. differ only by a few biochemical reactions and the susceptibility tests of the two isolates were very similar (susceptible to aminoglycosides, ciprofloxacin, and imipenem; resistant to penicillins and cephalosporins). The second episode of CRI may therefore represent a relapse. As a possible source of the infection, close contact to an animal vector (cat) was suggested.

Campylobacter spp. are recognized as a leading cause of diarrhea in humans. Hsueh et al. reported a cancer patient with a peritoneo-caval shunt, from whom *C. coli* was cultured from the blood and from parts of a dysfunctioning shunt catheter. The patient was treated with ciprofloxacin and the catheter remained in situ. Unfortunately, it was not reported if the patient recovered (66).

Haemophilus influenzae has not yet been reported to cause CRI, but by 1993, 27 CSF shunt infections have been published, including the case described by Wong et al. (67). The reported cases were treated with antibiotics alone and removal of the shunt was not necessary. The exact pathogenesis of these infections remains unclear, but seeding of bacteria to the meninges and the shunt in the presence of bacteremia seems to be the most probable cause.

Kingella kingae is another uncommon resident of the upper respiratory tract, which has been reported to cause CRI (68). This fastidious coccobacillus is part of the so-called HACEK group of microorganisms (*Haemophilus* spp., *Actinobacillus actinomycetemcomitans, Cardiobacterium hominis, Eikenella corrodens, Kingella* spp.), which are known to cause rare cases of endocarditis. *K. kingae* mainly causes bacteremia and osteomyelitis, and since the organism does not colonize the skin, CRI is probably secondary to systemic infection. Treatment with penicillins, cephalosporins, aminoglycosides, or TMP/SMZ is recommended (68).

Moraxella osloensis is a gram-negative, oxidase-positive, aerobic coccobacillus, which is considered to be a part of the normal resident respiratory tract flora and has only rarely been implicated as a human pathogen. The first report of central venous catheter infection was published in 1993 (69). A 71-year-old woman receiving long-term total parenteral nutrition for her short bowel syndrome and suffering from chronic sinusitis experienced a sudden-onset fever and rigors after flushing of her Hickman line. No signs of exit site infection were present, but multiple blood cultures drawn through the line grew *M. osloensis*. The authors supposed that the organism had been introduced into the bloodstream either directly from the sinuses or through contamination of catheter hubs with sinus secretions. Treatment with vancomycin and gentamicin was started for presumptive CRI. Clinical signs resolved within a day and the patient was discharged after four weeks of IV treatment. *Moraxella* spp. are usually susceptible in vitro to penicillin, cephalosporins, aminoglycosides, chloramphenicol, and erythromycin, and, as shown previously, treatment of CRI may be possible without removing the infected catheter.

Miscellaneous Gram-Positive Bacteria

Gram-Positive Cocci

During the past decade, the prevalence and importance of infections caused by enterococci increased significantly. In a prospective, observational study of 110 patients with serious enterococcal infections, such as endocarditis, bacteremia, cholangitis, pancreatitis, osteomyelitis, pneumonia, and empyema, catheter-related bacteremia was the single most common infection, accounting for 28% of all infections (70). In infants, all infections were catheter-related bacteremia. Overall, 78% of the enterococcal isolates were identified as *E. faecalis*, 20% as *E. faecium*, and 1% as *E. gallinarum* and *E. casseliflavus*, respectively. *E. faecium* was the most common species accounting for relapse. In one of these patients with CRI due to high-level, vancomycin-resistant *E. faecium*, bacteremia recurred after resistance to ciprofloxacin developed, which was the only antibiotic to which the strain was initially susceptible.

Enterococcus casseliflavus is a motile enterococcus, which forms yellow pigmented colonies on blood agar and accounts for less than 1% of all human enterococcal isolates (71). Recently, the organism was isolated from multiple blood cultures drawn through both lumina of a Hickman catheter inserted into a 19-year-old patient with leukemia (72). The girl developed fever of unknown origin during aplasia following remission-induction therapy and was treated empirically with penicillin, ceftazidime, and vancomycin. Once the organism's identity and susceptibility was known, treatment was switched to ampicillin and teicoplanin since *E. casseliflavus* is intrinsically resistant to low levels of vancomycin, and after 48 h treatment the patient became afebrile. Unfortunately, it was not reported whether the colonized Hickman line was removed.

Micrococcus spp. have been isolated from different clinical specimens. Relapsing bacteremia due to *Micrococcus luteus* was reported in a hemodialysis patient with a Perm-a-cath™ catheter (73) and in a child (74). *Micrococcus kristinae* has recently been reclassified in the new genus *Kocuria*. This bacterium has been described as causing recurrent bacteremia in a woman with ovarian cancer (75). After two courses of antibiotic therapy with various agents (glycopeptide, ciprofloxacin, and clindamycin), the CVC was removed during the third episode of antimicrobial treatment with no further recurrence of the infection.

Pediococcus spp. are ubiquitous, facultative, anaerobic Gram-positive cocci, which until recently, were considered clinically irrelevant. *Pediococcus* spp. are widely used in the food-processing industry and are normal inhabitants of the gastrointestinal flora. So far, only two of the eight *Pediococcus* spp. known have been reported to cause infections in humans, but with the ongoing attempts to improve the diagnosis of vancomycin-resistant gram-positive cocci, the isolation of these organisms from clinical specimens can be expected to increase. Atkins et al. (76) presented an infant who required a central venous catheter for total parenteral nutrition secondary to gastroschisis. The infant developed a polymicrobial catheter-related bacteremia due to *Klebsiella pneumoniae*, coagulase-negative staphylococci, and a nonhemolytic streptococcus, later identified as *P. pentosaceus*. Since the catheter became obstructed, it was removed and cure was achieved following treatment with vancomycin and amikacin. The recent recognition of *P. pentosaceus* as a pathogen is probably due to an improved diagnosis rather than an increase in frequency or virulence. Its intrinsic resistance to vancomycin may lead to complications, especially during the treatment of nosocomial infections for which glycopeptides are often empirically used.

Ascher et al. (77) described 10 cases of bacteremia due to *Rothia mucilaginosus* (formerly *Stomatococcus mucilaginosus*, *Staphylococcus salivarius*, or *Micrococcus mucilaginosus*) and reviewed eight other case reports of bacteremia due to this organism. Mucositis and catheter-related infections were among the most common clinical presentations, and bacteremia was frequently associated with risk factors such as intravenous drug abuse, cardiac valve disease, the presence of foreign bodies (especially indwelling vascular catheters), and an immunocompromised state. *R. mucilaginosus* is an organism of low virulence and is readily treatable with antibiotics, such as erythromycin, cefazolin, or vancomycin. Treatment of CRI or foreign body-related infections might be successful without removal of the device.

Corynebacterium Spp. and Related Genera

Corynebacterium spp. comprise an extremely varied genus of which only *Corynebacterium diphteriae, C. jeikeium,* and *C. urealyticum* are considered indisputable pathogens. Single cases of CRI due to various *Corynebacteria* have been described over recent years.

C. afermentans var. *afermentans* is a gram-positive rod, formerly referred to as *Corynebacterium* CDC group ANF-1. As other coryneform bacteria, the microorganism is part of the normal resident skin flora. Two case reports of intravenous line infections with this organism have been published in the literature (78,79). The authors of both reports concluded that the bacteremia in their patients was due to the corynebacterium, even though the organism was only isolated from blood cultures or the catheter tip, but not from both sites. In another patient with *C. afermentans* bacteremia, Kerr et al. (79) attributed the failure to isolate *C. afermentans* from the line to the use of vancomycin at the time the catheter was removed. Despite adequate antibiotic treatment, fever only resolved after the Hickman line was removed. Intravenous lines are a likely source of this organism since in vitro experiments show *C. afermentans* to grow in large numbers on the surface of intravenous lines [Dealler unpublished, in reply to (79)].

In 2001, three cases of bacteremia—including one case of CRI—due to *C. amycolatum* were presented by Oteo et al., all of them occurring in immunocompromised patients (80). Two cases involving *C. aquaticum* were reported in 1995 and 1998 (81,82). Infections due to *C. jeikeium* (group JK) are reported most frequently in neutropenic or otherwise immunocompromised patients, including AIDS patients, with central venous catheters in place (83,84). In 2001, Wang et al. reviewed charts of 53 bone marrow transplant recipients with Hickman catheters and *C. jeikeium* bacteremia (85). Ten patients underwent catheter removal with subsequent vancomycin therapy, and 41 patients were treated with vancomycin with the catheter left in place. Salvage of the intravascular catheter was successful in 38 of 41 (93%) patients. The percentage of recurrent bacteremia was the same with and without catheter removal. The authors concluded that in many patients with Hickman catheters, *C. jeikeium* bacteremia might be treated successfully with vancomycin, without removal of the catheter.

Cavendish et al. (86) reported a polymicrobial catheter-related bacteremia involving a multiresistant strain of *C. minutissimum,* isolated from blood cultures and the tip of a femoral central venous catheter, together with *C. jeikeium,* and *S. aureus.* All three microorganisms, including *C. minutissimum,* which is usually susceptible to penicillin, cephalosporins, doxycycline, and clindamycin, were only susceptible to vancomycin. It was suggested that the placement of the catheter through a skin lesion was responsible for the catheter colonization and subsequent infection (86). Another case of CRI due to *C. minutissimum* was presented in 1998 by Rupp et al. (87).

Until now, a total of five patients with systemic *C. striatum* infections have been described, including one patient with bacteremia. Tumbarello et al. (88) provided the first report of *C. striatum* bacteremia in a patient with AIDS, and believed that the presence of a central venous catheter was the cause of the infection.

C. urealyticum (formerly CDC group D2) is a skin commensal known to cause urinary tract infections but rarely bacteremia. A case of CRI due to *C. urealyticum* was recently reported in a neutropenic patient, who did not respond to empirical treatment with imipenem and vancomycin (89). The patient recovered only after removal of the Hickman catheter, which was shown to be heavily contaminated with *C. urealyticum*. Isolates from the catheter and the blood culture were resistant to aminoglycosides and β-lactam antibiotics, including imipenem, but susceptible to vancomycin. This report underscores the importance of removing any device that might be the source of infection due to a skin commensal when bacteremia persists despite apparently appropriate antibiotics.

Microbacterium spp., including *Aureobacterium* spp., bacteria formerly as known *Corynebacterium* CDC group A-4 and A-5 and *Microbacterium* spp., have been reported to cause catheter-related bacteremia (90–93). Of special interest is a case report of an 11-year-old patient with acute myeloblastic leukemia, who developed catheter-related sepsis caused by a vancomycin-resistant *Corynebacterium* CDC group A-5 (91). The natural habitat and clinical significance of this organism are unknown, but resistance to vancomycin, which is commonly used to treat CRI in neutropenic patients, may complicate empirical treatment. The boy was successfully treated with cefotaxime, without removal of the catheter. The other reported patients responded well to various antibiotics, including vancomycin, but the catheter had to be removed in most cases.

Brevibacterium epidermidis is part of the normal resident skin flora. Until 1991, no cases of *B. epidermidis* infections have been reported in humans. However, in 1992, a 40-year-old man receiving total parenteral nutrition developed a CRI with erythema at the subclavian insertion site. Peripheral blood cultures and a culture of the catheter tip yielded coryneform bacteria, later identified as *B. epidermidis* (94). As most of the other CRI caused by *Corynebacterium* species, the case also reflects the tendency of so-called nonpathogenic skin organisms to cause central venous catheter infections.

Bacillus Spp. and Other Gram-Positive Bacteria

Bacillus spp. are aerobic, gram-positive or gram-variable, spore-forming rods, which are found in decaying organic matter, dust, soil, and water. They are frequent culture contaminants and, with the exception of *Bacillus anthracis*, often not considered to be clinically significant when recovered from clinical specimens. *Bacillus* spp. have been occasionally reported to cause meningitis, pneumonia, and bacteremia (95). Bacteremia has been detected among IV drug abusers with endocarditis (95,96), and after administration of an oral preparation (Bactisubtil®) containing *Bacillus subtilis* spores to immunocompromised patients (97). However, *Bacillus* bacteremia seems to be mainly related to the use of IV devices (96). If *Bacillus* spp. are isolated from blood cultures of a patient with sepsis, IV devices should be considered as the most probable source. Indwelling vascular catheters should be promptly removed, especially among immunocompromised patients, and empirical antibiotic treatment should be started (98). Among nonimmuno-compromised patients, the clinical course is indolent and bacteremia may even be self-limiting. In this setting, antibiotic treatment should be delayed until the antibiotic susceptibility is known. Whereas most *Bacillus* spp. are susceptible to β-lactam antibiotics, *B. cereus* is frequently resistant. Imipenem, ciprofloxacin, and gentamicin are highly active, as is vancomycin, which is also bactericidal at the MIC (99). In a patient with AIDS, *B. subtilis* bacteremia resolved with vancomycin therapy without removing the indwelling Broviac catheter (97).

Lactobacillus rhamnosus is part of the normal human flora and very rarely causes infections. Carretto et al. report a case of CRI due to this organism in a patient who underwent single lung transplant (100). The patient was treated with ciprofloxacin.

Fish and Danziger (84) reported 4.8% of all pathogens causing bacteremia in HIV-infected patients to be *Listeria monocytogenes*. The authors did not describe whether these infections were catheter-related, but Katner and Joiner (101) reported an AIDS patient whose bacteremia was traced to an indwelling IV catheter. Among U.S. cancer patients, 1% of bacteremia cases were due to this organism (8). *L. monocytogenes* was furthermore shown to cause a ventriculo-peritoneal shunt infection in a patient with a brain tumor, who was successfully treated with TMP/SMZ after removal of the device (102).

Rothia dentocariosa is a coccal to rod-shaped, anaerobic bacterium morphologically resembling *Actinomyces*, *Corynebacterium*, and *Nocardia* spp. It is part of the normal oral and upper respiratory tract flora and in general is susceptible to penicillins, cephalosporins, erythromycin, vancomycin, aminoglycosides, chloramphenicol, and TMP/SMZ. However, susceptibility results are limited to a few isolates and were determined using different methods (103,104). Infections are rare, but range from periodontal inflammation (104) and other infections of the oral cavity to endocarditis with brain abscess (105). An infection due to *R. dentocariosa* associated with an intravascular device was reported in a 46-year-old diabetic suffering multiple postsurgery complications, including renal failure that required hemodialysis. During hospitalization, when the patient was treated with vancomycin and gentamicin for CRI, and during the first months after discharge, the arterio-venous shunt, despite being implicated as the source of the infection, was still used for vascular access without evidence of local or systemic infection (106).

Actinomycetes

Actinomycetes are aerobic, catalase-producing, branched filamentous bacteria. The organisms are ubiquitous, having been found on human and animal body surfaces, as well as in soil and plants.

Gordonia (*Gordona, Rhodococcus*) species are known to cause rare cases of skin and pulmonary infections. Buchman et al. (107) described two immunocompetent patients with long-term parenteral nutrition with CRI due to *G. rubropertincta* and *G. terrae*, respectively. It was assumed that the microorganisms gained access to the bloodstream through manipulation and contamination of home TPN catheters. Both cases were successfully treated with antimicrobial therapy, and removal of catheters does not seem necessary, even though this was done in one case. Five cases of CRI caused by *G. terrae* in nonneutropenic cancer patients were recently reported from the United States (108). All patients were successfully treated with antibiotics, with the require-ment of catheter removal for two patients who had signs of systemic infection.

Catheter-related bacteremia has been reported with three different *Nocardia* species (109–111). A Tenckhoff catheter-associated infection due to *N. asteroides* (109) in a CAPD patient and an implantable central venous catheter infection with *N. nova* (110) were both successfully treated with antibiotics and removal of the catheter. In one case report, Hickman catheter-related bacteremia caused by *N. otitidis-caviarum* in a bone marrow trans-plant patient was successfully treated without removing the catheter, after switching from vancomycin to imipenem treatment (111).

Tsukamurella paurometabolum (formerly *Corynebacterium paurometa-bolum, Gordona aurantiaca, Rhodococcus aurantiacus*) is a pleomorphic gram-positive bacillus, which is weakly acid-fast. Until the case reports of Shapiro et al. (112), only a handful of human infections had been published, and none included bacteremia. The authors described three cases of *T. paurometabolum* bacteremia related to long-term use of central venous catheters in cancer patients. In all cases, persistence of positive blood cultures during antibiotic therapy necessitated removal of the catheter. A detailed case report of one of the patients was published by Lai (113) a year later. In 1998, a case of catheter-related bacteremia caused by *T. pulmonis* was published by Maertens et al. (114). Also in that case, the Hickman catheter had to be removed to clear infection.

Mycobacteria

Mycobacteria are acid-fast, aerobic, nonmotile bacteria. At least 25 species are associated with the development of granulomatous infections in humans.

Twenty-three patients who had undergone hematopoietic stem cell transplant were reported with catheter-related infections caused by various rapidly growing mycobacteria by Gaviria et al. in 2000 (115). All patients received antimycobacterial chemotherapy with at least two agents over a period from 3–6 weeks; in 21 of them, the catheter had to be removed.

M. chelonae and *M. fortuitum* (the *M. fortuitum* complex) are rapidly growing, ubiquitous mycobacteria found in soil and water. Both mycobacteria have been identified as the cause of skin/soft-tissue abscesses, wound infections, pulmonary infections, keratitis, peritonitis, endocarditis, and bacteremia. Bacteremia occurred in association with prosthetic valves, sternal wounds, and reused hemodialyzers. Until 1991, 29 cases of CRI had been reported in the literature (116). The incidence was reported to follow the increasing use of central venous catheters, but in general was low (1.2 cases per year). None of the patients with CRI due to *M. fortuitum* complex showed signs of a disseminated cutaneous form of the infection, except at the catheter insertion site. Another indication that the infections in the described patients were strictly catheter-related rather than due to disseminated disease is that none of the patients died and even those who initially failed treatment recovered after catheter removal. In addition to appropriate antibiotics (TMP/SMZ or amikacin, depending on in vitro susceptibility), removal of the catheter is essential. Furthermore, in cases with tunnel infections, surgical excision of the infected tissue (skin and tunnel track) is recommended. Recurrent *M. chelonae* CRI was reported in 1998 by Hsueh et al. (3). The recovered strain grew in two different morphotypes and the mucoid strain adhered to plastic material. The catheter was removed and the patient was treated with clarithromycin, ciprofloxacin, and amikacin for two months and recovered.

In contrast to the localized infection caused by *M. fortuitum* complex, Schelonka et al. (117) described two cases of secondary catheter-related *M. avium* complex (MAC) infections in patients with disseminated disease. CRI was probably due to seeding of the catheter by hematogenous spread of MAC. Bloodstream infection was cleared only after removal of the catheter (Port-a-cath). The treatment included rifampin, ethambutol, amikacin, clarithromycin, clofazimine, and ciprofloxacin. The last three drugs were continued for 14 and 20 months, respectively. *Mycobacterium neoaurum* is a rapidly growing mycobacterium, primarily found in soil, besides being recovered from dust and water, that had not been described to cause infections in humans until Davison et al. (118) reported the isolation of *M. neoaurum* from the Hickman catheter of an immunocompromised patient. Six years later, Holland et al. (119) reported a bone marrow transplant recipient who suffered from bacteremia and insertion site infection due to *M. neoaurum* during aplasia. Despite rapid clinical response during treatment with ticaracillin/clavulanate and tobramycin, bacteremia persisted until the catheter was removed. Microbiological cultures of the tip indeed revealed *M. neoaurum*. In 1999, the first

Table 4 Alphabetic List, Natural Source, and Clinical Data of Miscellaneous Organisms Causing Catheter-Related Infections

Microorganism	Reference no.	Natural source	Clinical infections	Recommended antibiotics[a]	Catheter removal
Aeromonas hydrophila	(63,107)	Water sources, environment, food	CRI, cellulitis, bacteremia, UTI, endocarditis, osteomyelitis, peritonitis, meningitis, diarrhea	TMP/SMZ, ciprofloxacin, tetracycline, aminoglycosides, piperacillin, 2nd + 3rd gen. cephalosporins	
Acinetobacter spp.	(138,139)	Environment, normal human flora	CRI, bacteremia	No antibiotics given/ piperacillin, amoxicillin/ clavulanate, cefoperazone, netromycin	+
Agrobacterium (Rhizobium) spp.	(2,5,9,13, 50–52, 140–142)	Environment, water sources, plants	CRI, endocarditis, UTI, CRI, endocarditis, UTI, peritonitis, bacteremia	Ciprofloxacin, TMP/ SMZ, imipenem, aminoglycosides, latamoxcef, piperacillin	+
Achromobacter (Alcaligenes) spp.	(1,2,33,41,43,44, 46–49)	Water sources, hospital environment, human GI tract, soil	CRI, bacteremia, peritonitis, meningitis, pneumonia, endocarditis, pyelonephritis	TMP/SMZ, antipseudomonal-penicillins, ceftazidime, cefepime, imipenem, aminoglycosides	?/–/+

Organism	Ref.	Source	Infections	Antibiotics	
Bacillus spp.	(9,95–98)	Environment, water sources	CRI, meningitis, wound infection, pneumonia, bacteremia, osteomyelitis	Imipenem, vancomycin, ciprofloxacin, aminoglycosides, betalactam antibiotics, depending on species	+/−
Bordetella bronchiseptica	(65)	Animal (rarely human) respiratory tract	CRI, CAPD peritonitis, meningitis, pneumonia, endocarditis	Ciprofloxacin, imipenem, aminoglycosides	+
Brevibacterium spp.	(9,94)	Human skin	CRI (insertion site)	Penicillins, erythromycin, tetracycline, cephalosporins, aminoglycosides, vancomycin	?
Burkholderia cepacia	(12–14,21, 130,131,143)	Water sources, environment, food (onions), animal sources, hospital equipment, including disinfectants	CRI, pneumonia, UTI, meningitis, endocarditis, wound infection, arthritis	Ceftazidime, piperacilline, imipenem, TMP/SMZ, failure of antibiotic treatment without catheter removal	+
Campylobacter spp.	(66,144)	Animals, environment	CRI (peritoneal-caval shunt), bacteremia	Ciprofloxacin, netilmicin (cave: ciprofloxacin resistance!)	+
CDC Group IV 2-c	(22)	Water sources	CRI	Ciprofloxacin, imipenem, ceftazidime	+/−

Table 4 Continued

Microorganism	Reference no.	Natural source	Clinical infections	Recommended antibiotics[a]	Catheter removal
Chryseomonas luteola	(23)	Primarily human saprophyte, water sources	CRI, endocarditis, bacteremia	Ureidopenicillins, 3. gen. cephalosporins, aminoglycosides	+
Comamonas acidovorans	(15,16)	Water sources, environment, food	CRI, bacteremia	(not mentioned)	+
Comamonas testosteroni	(17)		CRI	Piperacillin/tazobactam	+
Corynebacterium afermentans	(78,79)	Human skin and mucous membranes	CRI, endocarditis, bacteremia	Glycopeptide, rifampin, aminoglycosides	+
Corynebacterium amycolatum	(80)	Human skin and mucous membranes	CRI, bacteremia, pneumonia, wound infection	(not mentioned)	?
Corynebacterium aquaticum	(81,82)	Environment, fresh water	CRI, bacteremia	(not mentioned)	?
Corynebacterium jeikeium	(83–85)	Human skin and mucous membranes	CRI, endocarditis, bacteremia, UTI, pneumonia, meningitis	Glycopeptide, doxycycline, rifampin	+/−
Corynebacterium minutissimum	(86,87)	Human skin and mucous membranes	CRI, erythrasma, endocarditis	Glycopeptide, cephalosporins, penicillin, erythromycin, clindamycin, doxycycline	?
Corynebacterium striatum	(88)	Human skin and mucous membranes, cattle	CRI, pneumonia, endocarditis, arthritis, wound infection, bacteremia	Glycopeptides, rifampin, aminoglycosides	+/?

Organism		Habitat	Infections	Treatment	
Corynebacterium urealyticum	(89)	Human skin and mucous membranes	CRI, UTI, endocarditis, bacteremia	Glycopeptides, rifampin, aminoglycosides	+
Enterococcus casseliflavus	(71)	Human GI-tract	CRI, bacteremia	Ampicillin, teicoplanin, (cave: vancomycin resistance!)	?
Enterococcus faecalis/ faecium	(70)	Human GI-tract	CRI, bacteremia, endocarditis, cholangitis, pancreatitis, pneumonia	Glycopeptides ampicillin (+ aminoglycoside)	?
Ewingella americana *Flavimonas oryzihabitans*	(145) (23–26)	Natural and hospital environment, water sources, human saprophyte	CRI, wound infection, CAPD peritonitis, abscess, bacteremia	TMP/SMZ, ureidopenicillins, 3. gen. cephalosporins, aminoglycosides, imipenem, ciprofloxacin	–/+
Flavobacterium (Chryseobacterium) spp.	(54–58)	Water sources, hospital environment	CRI, bacteremia	?; commonly multi-resistant	+
Gordona spp.	(107)	Environment	CRI, meningitis, (sternal) wound infections, pulmonary infections	TMP/SMZ, imipenem, 3rd gen. cephalosporins, amikacin, ciprofloxacin	–/+
Kingella kingae	(68)	Human respiratory tract	CRI, endocarditis, bacteremia, osteomyelitis, endophthalmitis	Penicillins. cephalosporins, TMP/SMZ, aminoglycosides, erythromycin	?

Table 4 Continued

Microorganism	Reference no.	Natural source	Clinical infections	Recommended antibiotics[a]	Catheter removal
Kocuria kristinae	(75)	Human skin and mucous membranes, soil, animals	CRI, bacteremia	Clindamycin, erythromycin, ciprofloxacin	+
Lactobacillus rhamnosus	(100)		CRI	Ciprofloxacin	
Listeria monocytogenes	(101,102)	Environment, water sources, food, human and animal GI-tract	CRI, endocarditis, CNS infections, including CSF-shunt infection	Penicillin + aminoglycosides, TMP/SMZ, erythromycin, tetracycline, rifampin	?
Methylobacterium extorquens	(19,20)	Plants, environment, water sources, air	CRI, RTI, peritonitis, skin ulcers, uveitis	TMP/SMZ, imipenem, ciprofloxacin, aminoglycosides, tetracycline	−
Microbacterium spp. (Coryneform CDC Group A-5)	(90–93)	Environment, water sources, plants, dairy products, sewage, human skin (?)	CRI, bacteremia, endocarditis, endophtalmitis, cellulitis, central nervous system infection	Vancomycin, penicillin, 3rd generation cephalosporins (vancomycin resistance)	+/?
Moraxella osloensis	(69)	Human respiratory tract	CRI, septic arthritis, meningitis, endocarditis	Penicillins, cephalosporins, aminoglycosides, erythromycin	−
Mycobacterium aurum	(122)	Environment, water sources	CRI, bacteremia	Clarithromycin, amikacin	−

Organism	Ref.	Source	Disease	Treatment	
Mycobacterium avium complex	(117,136)	Environment, water sources	CRI, bacteremia, endocarditis, RTI, abscesses, wound inf., peritonitis	Rifampin. ethambutol, amikacin, clarithromycin, clofazimine, ciprofloxacin	+
Mycobacterium chelonae	(3)	Environment, water sources	CRI	Clarithromycin, ciprofloxacin, amikacin	+
Mycobacterium fortuitum complex	(116,137)	Environment, water sources	CRI, bacteremia, endocarditis, RTI, abscesses, wound inf., peritonitis	Rifampin. ethambutol, amikacin, clarithromycin, clofazimine, ciprofloxacin	+
Mycobacterium neoaurum	(118–121)	Environment, water sources	CRI	(?)	+
Mycobacterium septicum sp. nov.	(123)	Environment, water sources	CRI, bacteremia	Erythromycin, vancomycin, tobramycin	+
Mycobacterium snaegmatis	(124)		CRI, bacteremia	Doxycycline, ciprofloxacin	+
Nocardia asteroides	(109)	Environment, animals, humans, plants	CRI, pulmonary abscess, CNS infection, mycetoma	Sulfonamides + tetracycline or aminoglycoside, minocycline, betalacetams	+/−
Nocardia nova	(110)	Environment, water sources	CRI, mycetoma	Sulfonamides + tetracycline or aminoglycosides, minocycline, betalacetams	+/−

Table 4 Continued

Microorganism	Reference no.	Natural source	Clinical infections	Recommended antibiotics[a]	Catheter removal
Nocardia otitidis-caviarum	(111)	Environment, water sources	CRI, mycetoma	Imipenem, sulfonamides + tetracycline or aminoglycosides, minocycline, betalacatams	—
Ochrobactrum anthropi	(39,40,42,51,61, 133,134)	Environment, water sources, human GI tract	CRI, endocarditis, peritonitis, bacteremia	TMP/SMZ, ciprofloxacin, imipenem, aminoglycosides	+/−
Pediococcus pentosaceus	(77)	GI tract (used in food processing industry)	CRI, bacteremia	Penicillin + beta-lactamase inhibitors, aminoglycosides, (cave: vancomycin resistance!)	?
Pseudomonas spp. (*nonaeruginosa*)	(12,21)	Water sources, plants, animal sources, general and hospital environment, oral flora	CRI, UTI, wound infection, septic arthritis	Imipenem, ceftazidime, piperacillin, ciprofloxacin, polymyxin, aminoglycosides	+
Ralstonia (*Pseudomonas*) *pickettii*	(29)	Water sources, (wet) hospital equipment and solutions	CRI, bacteremia, meningitis, UTI, RTI	Imipenem, ceftazidime, piperacillin, tobramycin	+

Organism	Refs	Source	Infection	Antibiotics[a]	
Roseomonas gilardii	(30,31)		CRI, bacteremia	Ciprofloxacin	
Rothia (*Stomatococcus*) spp.	(72,106)	Oral flora/upper respiratory tract, dental caries, and plaque	CRI, bacteremia, oral cavity infection, endocarditis	Penicillin, erythromycin, aminoglycosides, TMP/SMZ, vancomycin, cephalosporins, ciprofloxacin, tetracycline	-/+
Sphingomonas (*Pseudomonas*) *paucimobilis*	(12,21, 32–35)	Water sources, plants, air, hospital equipment	CRI, peritonitis, UTI, meningitis, empyema, wound infection, spleric abscess, bacteremia	Ceftazidime, piperacilline, imipenem, TMP/SMZ	+
Stenotrophomonas maltophilia	(12,33,36–38,146)	Water sources, plants, animal sources, natural & hospital environment	CRI, pneumonia, UTI, endocarditis, wound infection, corneal ulcers	Ceftazidime, TMP/SMZ, (imipenem-resistant)	+
Tsukamurella spp.	(112–114)	Environment	CRI, pneumonia, meningitis	TMP/SMZ, imipenem, 3. gen. cephalosporins, amikacin, ciprofloxacin	+

GI = gastrointestinal tract, CRI = catheter-related infection, UTI = urinary tract infection, TMP/SMZ = trimethoprim-sulfamethoxazole, CNS = central nervous system, CSF = cerebrospinal fluid, RTI = respiratory tract infection catheter removal (based on case reports): + necessary, +\- probably necessary, -\+ possibly necessary, -probably not necessary, ? unclear.
[a] Antibiotics successfully employed or in vitro susceptible.

case of CRI due to *M. neoaurum* was reported from the United States (120). The immunocompetent patient recovered solely by removal of the Hickman catheter. Since the infection seemed to be polymicrobial in retrospect, the pathogenetic role of the mycobacterium remains unclear. CRI with *M. neoaurum* in a child with ALL cleared after removal of the catheter alone (121).

Other mycobacteria, such as *M. aurum* (122), *M. septicum* sp. nov. (123), and *M. smegmatis* (124), have also been isolated from blood from immunocompromised patients with indwelling devices. All patients recovered after removal of the catheter and antibiotic therapy for several weeks according to susceptibility testing.

Polymicrobial Infections

Clusters of nosocomial infections focusing on a single organism, either because it is an unusual pathogen or because it appears in a large cluster, are easily identified and frequently reported. Ponce de Leon et al. (125) were the first to report a cluster of epidemiologically related polymicrobial bloodstream infections related to indwelling catheters, involving two or more common organisms such as *S. epidermidis*, *S. aureus*, *Pseudomonas* spp., *Enterobacter* spp., and *C. albicans*. Bacteremia due to several different organisms (in place of a single causative pathogen) may be a first hint to consider CRI. In another study, polymicrobial bacteremia was shown to be especially frequent in neutropenic patients; 34% (29/86) of all bacteremic episodes versus 3% (1/30) in nonneutropenic patients (126). Intravascular catheters were the most common source of bacteremia in these cases, but the higher incidence of polymicrobial bacteremia was also assumed to be due to the repeated occurrence of cutaneous and mucosal lesions in these patients. Among ICU patients, the incidence of true polymicrobial bacteremia was 8.4%, with Enterobacteriaceae being the most common pathogen (127). The prognosis of patients with polymicrobial bacteremia was not any worse than for those with monomicrobial bloodstream infections. Mortality was even significantly lower than in a cohort of patients with bacteremia due to a single organism. Since intravascular devices were the most common source (42.8%), the authors recommended removing these devices, even though they did not compare the outcome in patients with or without catheters left in place. In 1999, Martino et al. reported 45 episodes of catheter-related infections due to various species of nonfermenting gram-negative bacteria in 115 patients with hematological malignancies and solid tumors (128). Twenty-eight percent of all CRI were polymicrobial, and *Acinetobacter* spp. and *Pseudomonas* spp. were the most prevalent organisms isolated.

CONCLUSIONS

The review of the different case reports and case series illustrates that saprophytic and environmental organisms can realize their potential for causing CRI. So-called avirulent or saprophytic organisms from the patient's own skin flora or from the environment that are present on the hands of health care workers inserting or handling the catheter may cause CRI, especially in the immunocompromised host. Therefore, the catalog of miscellaneous pathogens summarized in Table 4 may only represent the tip of the iceberg. Bacteremia due to uncommon pathogens is frequently reported, but information is seldom given as to whether the infection might have been catheter-related, even though intravascular devices seem to be the main source of bacteremia due to these organisms. The rapid development of medical technology leading to the use of new indwelling medical devices in patients increasingly at high risk for any nosocomial infection will furthermore increase the incidence of these newcomers among the pathogens causing CRI. Under such circumstances, *Peptostreptococcus anaerobius* (127), *Propionibacterium* spp. (127), and probably others, including other anaerobe bacteria (129), might already now be added to the list of pathogens causing CRI. Mortality and the rate of complications such as endocarditis or septic phlebitis seem to be low in cases with CRI due to these organisms. Still, a therapeutic dilemma could occur, since some of these pathogens express intrinsic resistance against standard antibiotics used in the empirical treatment of CRI, such as glycopeptides. At present, no general advice regarding whether the device should be removed, or if and which antibiotic is needed can be given.

Despite their rising importance, infections due to miscellaneous pathogens are likely to stay underreported, since the organisms can be easily misidentified in the laboratory. The lack of prolonged incubation times, specific atmospheric conditions, special media, and complete databases of automated microbiological identification systems are factors contributing to this diagnostic problem. All efforts should be made to identify unusual organisms isolated from blood cultures or catheter tips of patients with assumed CRI to the species level, in order to broaden our knowledge of the spectrum of infections caused by these pathogens, which at present are often regarded as contaminants.

REFERENCES

1. Tebbs SE, Elliott TS. Modification of central venous catheter polymers to prevent in vitro microbial colonisation. Eur J Clin Microbiol Infect Dis 1994; 13:111–117.
2. Dunne WM Jr, Tillman J, Murray JC. Recovery of a strain of *Agrobacterium radiobacter* with a mucoid phenotype from an immunocompromised child with bacteremia. J Clin Microbiol 1993; 31:2541–2543.
3. Hsueh PR, Teng LJ, Yang PC, Chen YC, Ho SW, Luh KT. Recurrent catheter-related infection caused by a single clone of *Mycobacterium chelonae* with two colonial morphotypes. J Clin Microbiol 1998; 36:1422–1424.
4. Soriano F, Ponte C, Galiano MJ. Adherence of *Corynebacterium urealyticum*

(CDC group D2) and *Corynebacterium jeikeium* to intravascular and urinary catheters. Eur J Clin Microbiol Infect Dis 1993; 12:453–456.

5. Ronveaux O, Jans B, Suetens C, Carsauw H. Epidemiology of nosocomial bloodstream infections in Belgium, 1992-1996. Eur J Clin Microbiol Infect Dis 1998; 17:695–700.

6. Richards MJ, Edwards JR, Culver DH, Gaynes RP. Nosocomial infections in medical intensive care units in the United States. National Nosocomial Infections Surveillance System. Crit Care Med 1999; 27:887–892.

7. Richards MJ, Edwards JR, Culver DH, Gaynes RP. Nosocomial infections in pediatric intensive care units in the United States. National Nosocomial Infections Surveillance System. Pediatrics 1999; 103:e39.

8. Kiehn TE, Armstrong D. Changes in the spectrum of organisms causing bacteremia and fungemia in immunocompromised patients due to venous access devices. Eur J Clin Microbiol Infect Dis 1990; 9:869–872.

9. Castagnola E, Conte M, Venzano P, Garaventa A, Viscoli C, Barretta MA, Pescetto L, Tasso L, Nantron M, Milanaccio C, Giacchino R. Broviac catheter-related bacteraemias due to unusual pathogens in children with cancer: case reports with literature review. J Infect 1997;34215–218.

10. Smith TL, Pullen GT, Crouse V, Rosenberg J, Jarvis WR. Bloodstream infections in pediatric oncology outpatients: a new healthcare systems challenge. Infect Control Hosp Epidemiol 2002; 23:239–243.

11. Pedro-Botet MM, Modol JM, Valles X, Romeu J, Sopena N, Gimenez ML, Tor J, Clotet B, Sabria M. Changes in bloodstream infections in HIV-positive patients in a university hospital in Spain (1995–1997). Int J Infect Dis 2002; 6:17–22.

12. Elting LS, Bodey GP. Septicemia due to *Xanthomonas* species and non-aeruginosa *Pseudomonas* species: increasing incidence of catheter-related infections. Medicine (Baltimore) 1990; 69:296–306.

13. Panlilio AL, Beck-Sague CM, Siegel JD, Anderson RL, Yetts SY, Clark NC, Duer PN, Thomassen KA, Vess RW, Hill BC. Infections and pseudoinfections due to povidone-iodine solution contaminated with *Pseudomonas cepacia*. Clin Infect Dis 1992; 14:1078–1083.

14. Pegues DA, Carson LA, Anderson RL, Norgard MJ, Argent TA, Jarvis WR, Woernle CH. Outbreak of *Pseudomonas cepacia* bacteremia in oncology patients. Clin Infect Dis 1993; 16:407–411.

15. Castagnola E, Tasso L, Conte M, Nantron M, Barretta A, Giacchino R. Central venous catheter-related infection due to *Comamonas acidovorans* in a child with non-Hodgkin's lymphoma. Clin Infect Dis 1994; 19:559–560.

16. Ender PT, Dooley DP, Moore RH. Vascular catheter-related *Comamonas acidovorans* bacteremia managed with preservation of the catheter. Pediatr Infect Dis J 1996; 15:918–920.

17. Le Moal G, Paccalin M, Breux JP, Roblot F, Roblot P, Becq-Giraudon B. Central venous catheter-related infection due to *Comamonas testosteroni* in a woman with breast cancer. Scand J Infect Dis 2001; 33:627–628.

18. Austin B, Goodfellow M. *Pseudomonas mesophilica*, a new species of pink bacteria isolated from leaf surfaces. Inter J System Bacteriol 1979; 29:373–378.

19. Poirier A, Lapointe R, Claveau S, Joly JR. Bacteremia caused by *Pseudomonas mesophilica*. CMAJ 1-9-1988; 139:411–412.

20. Kaye KM, Macone A, Kazanjian PH. Catheter infection caused by

Methylobacterium in immunocompromised hosts: report of three cases and review of the literature. Clin Infect Dis 1992; 14:1010–1014.

21. Anaissie E, Fainstein V, Miller P, Kassamali H, Pitlik S, Bodey GP, Rolston K. *Pseudomonas putida.* Newly recognized pathogen in patients with cancer. Am J Med 1987; 82:1191–1194.

22. Arduino S, Villar H, Veron MT, Koziner B, Dictar M. CDC group IV c-2 as a cause of catheter-related sepsis in an immunocompromised patient. Clin Infect Dis 1993; 17:512–513.

23. Kostman JR, Solomon F, Fekete T. Infections with *Chryseomonas luteola* (CDC group Ve-1) and *Flavimonas oryzihabitans* (CDC group Ve-2) in neurosurgical patients. Rev Infect Dis 1991; 13:233–236.

24. Lucas KG, Kiehn TE, Sobeck KA, Armstrong D, Brown AE. Sepsis caused by *Flavimonas oryzihabitans.* Medicine (Baltimore) 1994; 73:209–214.

25. Pien FD. Group VE-2 (*Chromobacterium typhiflavum*) bacteremia. J Clin Microbiol 1977; 6:435–436.

26. Conlu A, Rothman J, Staszewski H, Schoch PE, Domenico P, Quadri SM, Cunha BA. *Flavimonas oryzihabitans* (CDC group Ve-2) bacteraemia associated with Hickman catheters. J Hosp Infect 1992; 20:293–299.

27. Marin M, Garcia De Viedma D, Martin-Rabadan P, Rodriguez-Creixems M, Bouza E. Infection of hickman catheter by *Pseudomonas* (formerly *Flavimonas*) *oryzihabitans* traced to a synthetic bath sponge. J Clin Microbiol 2000; 38:4577–4579.

28. Dan M, Gutman R, Biro A. Peritonitis caused by *Pseudomonas putrefaciens* in patients undergoing continuous ambulatory peritoneal dialysis. Clin Infect Dis 1992; 14:359–360.

29. Raveh D, Simhon A, Gimmon Z, Sacks T, Shapiro M. Infections caused by *Pseudomonas pickettii* in association with permanent indwelling intravenous devices: four cases and a review. Clin Infect Dis 1993; 17:877 880.

30. Alcala L, Vasallo FJ, Cercenado E, Garcia-Garrote F, Rodriguez-Creixems F, Bouza E. Catheter-related bacteremia due to *Roseomonas gilardii* sp. nov. J Clin Microbiol 1997; 35:2712.

31. Marin ME, Marco DP, Dibar E, Fernandez CL, Greco G, Flores Y, Ascione A. Catheter-related bacteremia caused by *Roseomonas gilardii* in an immunocompromised patient. Int J Infect Dis 2001; 5, 170–171.

32. Hsueh PR, Teng LJ, Yang PC, Chen YC, Pan HJ, Ho SW, Luh KT. Nosocomial infections caused by *Sphingomonas paucimobilis*: clinical features and microbiological characteristics. Clin Infect Dis 1998; 26:676–681.

33. Martino R, Martinez C, Pericas R, Salazar R, Sola C, Brunet S, Sureda A, Domingo-Albos A. Bacteremia due to glucose non-fermenting gram-negative bacilli in patients with hematological neoplasias and solid tumors. Eur J Clin Microbiol Infect Dis 1996; 15:610–615.

34. Salazar R, Martino R, Sureda A, Brunet S, Subira M, Domingo-Albos A. Catheter-related bacteremia due to *Pseudomonas paucimobilis* in neutropenic cancer patients: report of two cases. Clin Infect Dis 1995; 20:1573–1574.

35. Decker CF, Hawkins RE, Simon GL. Infections with *Pseudomonas paucimobilis.* Clin Infect Dis 1992; 14:783 784.

36. Herrero Romero M, Gomez Gomez MJ, Pachon Diaz J, Cisneros Herreros JM. Bacteriemias por *Stenotrophomonas maltophilia*: epidemiologica, caracteristicas clinicas y factores pronosticos. Rev Clin Esp 2000; 200:315–317.

37. Friedman ND, Korman TM, Fairely CK, Franklin JC, Spelman DW. Bacteremia due to *Stenotrophomonas maltophilia*: an analysis of 45 episodes. J Infect 2002; 45:47–53.

38. Ratnalingham RA, Peckham D, Denton M, Kerr K, Conway S. *Stenotrophomonas maltophilia* bacteremia in two patients with cystic fibrosis associated with totally implantable venous access devices. J Infect 2002; 44:53–55.

39. Kern WV, Oethinger M, Kaufhold A, Rozdzinski E, Marre R. *Ochrobactrum anthropi* bacteremia: report of four cases and short review. Infection 1993; 21:306–310.

40. Cieslak TJ, Robb ML, Drabick CJ, Fischer GW. Catheter-associated sepsis caused by *Ochrobactrum anthropi*: report of a case and review of related nonfermentative bacteria. Clin Infect Dis 1992; 14:902–907.

41. Cieslak TJ, Raszka WV. Catheter-associated sepsis due to *Alcaligenes xylosoxidans* in a child with AIDS. Clin Infect Dis 1993; 16:592–593.

42. Gransden WR, Eykyn SJ. Seven cases of bacteremia due to *Ochrobactrum anthropi*. Clin Infect Dis 1992; 15:1068–1069.

43. Gröschel D, Cody LD, Tieman C. Nosocomial infections with *Achromobacter xylosoxidans* in cancer patients [abstract]. Program and abstracts of the 19th ICAAC. Washington DC: American Society for Microbiology, 1979:1458–1459.

44. Legrand C, Anaissie E. Bacteremia due to *Achromobacter xylosoxidans* in patients with cancer. Clin Infect Dis 1992; 14:479–484.

45. Manfredi R, Nanetti A, Ferri M, Chiodo F. Bacteremia and respiratory involvement by *Alcaligenes xylosoxidans* in patients infected with the human immunodeficiency virus. Eur J Clin Microbiol Infect Dis 1997; 16:933–938.

46. Knippschild M, Schmid EN, Uppenkamp M, Konig E, Meusers P, Brittinger G, Hoffkes HG. Infection by *Alcaligenes xylosoxidans* subsp. *xylosoxidans* in neutropenic patients. Oncology 1996; 53:258–262.

47. Hernandez JA, Martino R, Pericas R, Sureda A, Brunet S, Domingo-Albos A. *Achromobacter xylosoxidans* bacteremia in patients with hematologic malignancies. Haematologica 1998; 83:284–285.

48. Kay SE, Clark RA, White KL, Peel MM. Recurrent *Achromobacter piechaudii* bacteremia in a patient with hematological malignancy. J Clin Microbiol 2001; 39:808–810.

49. Duggan JM, Goldstein SJ, Chenoweth CE, Kauffman1 CA, Bradley SF. *Achromobacter xylosoxidans* bacteremia: report of four cases and review of the literature. Clin Infect Dis 1996; 23:569–576.

50. Edmond MB, Riddler SA, Baxter CM, Wicklund BM, Pasculle AW. *Agrobacterium radiobacter*: a recently recognized opportunistic pathogen. Clin Infect Dis 1993; 16:388–391.

51. Alnor D, Frimodt-Moller N, Espersen F, Frederiksen W. Infections with the unusual human pathogens Agrobacterium species and *Ochrobactrum anthropi*. Clin Infect Dis 1994; 18:914–920.

52. Hulse M, Johnson S, Ferrieri P. Agrobacterium infections in humans: experience at one hospital and review. Clin Infect Dis 1993; 16:112–117.

53. Maki DG. Nosocomial bacteremia. An epidemiologic overview. Am J Med 1981; 70:719–732.

54. Stamm WE, Colella JJ, Anderson RL, Dixon RE. Indwelling arterial catheters as a source of nosocomial bacteremia. An outbreak caused by *Flavobacterium* Species. N Engl J Med 1975; 292:1099–1102.

55. Nulens E, Bussels B, Bols A, Gordts B, Van Landuyt HW. Recurrent bacteremia by *Chryseobacterium indologenes* in an oncology patient with a totally implanted intravascular device. Clin Microbiol Infect 2001; 7:391–393.

56. Hsueh PR, Teng LJ, Ho SW, Hsieh WC, Luh KT. Clinical and micro-biological characteristics of *Flavobacterium indologenes* infections associated with indwelling devices. J Clin Microbiol 1996; 34:1908–1913.

57. Hsueh PR, Teng LJ, Yang PC, Ho SW, Hsieh WC, Luh KT. Increasing incidence of nosocomial *Chryseobacterium indologenes* infections in Taiwan. Eur J Clin Microbiol Infect Dis 1997; 16:568–574.

58. Sader HS, Jones RN, Pfaller MA. Relapse of catheter-related *Flavobacterium meningosepticum* bacteremia demonstrated by DNA macrorestriction analysis. Clin Infect Dis 1995; 21:997–1000.

59. Kish MA, Buggy BP, Forbes BA. Bacteremia caused by *Achromobacter* species in an immunocompromised host. J Clin Microbiol 1984; 19:947–948.

60. Yu WL, Lin CW, Wang DY. Clinical and microbiologic characteristics of *Ochrobactrum anthropi* bacteremia. J Formos Med Assoc 1998; 97:106–112.

61. Gill MV, Ly H, Mueenuddin M, Schoch PE, Cunha BA. Intravenous line infection due to *Ochrobactrum anthropi* (CDC Group Vd) in a normal host. Heart Lung 1997; 26:335–336.

62. Rello J, Coll P, Net A, Prats G. Infection of pulmonary artery catheters. Epidemiologic characteristics and multivariate analysis of risk factors. Chest 1993; 103:132–136.

63. Siddiqui MN, Ahmed I, Farooqi BJ, Ahmed M. Myonecrosis due to *Aeromonas hydrophila* following insertion of an intravenous cannula: case report and review. Clin Infect Dis 1992; 14:619–620.

64. Papasian CJ, Downs NJ, Talley RL, Romberger DJ, Hodges GR. *Bordetella bronchiseptica* bronchitis. J Clin Microbiol 1987; 25:575–577.

65. Qureshi MN, Lederman J, Neibart E, Bottone EJ. *Bordetella bronchiseptica* recurrent bacteraemia in the setting of a patient with AIDS and indwelling Broviac catheter. Int J STD AIDS 1992; 3:291–293.

66. Hsueh PR, Teng LJ, Yang PC, Ho SW, Luh KT. Indwelling device-related bacteremia caused by serum-susceptible *Campylobacter coli*. J Clin Microbiol 1997; 35:2178–2180.

67. Wong GW, Oppenheimer SJ, Vaudry W. CSF shunt infection by unencapsulated *Haemophilus influenzae*. Clin Infect Dis 1993; 17:519–520.

68. Goutzmanis JJ, Gonis G, Gilbert GL. *Kingella kingae* infection in children: ten cases and a review of the literature. Pediatr Infect Dis J 1991; 10:677–683.

69. Buchman AL, Pickett MJ, Mann L, Ament ME. Central venous catheter infection caused by *Moraxella osloensis* in a patient receiving home parenteral nutrition. Diagn Microbiol Infect Dis 1993; 17:163–166.

70. Patterson JE, Sweeney AH, Simms M, Carley N, Mangi R, Sabetta J, Lyons RW. An analysis of 110 serious enterococcal infections. Epidemiology, antibiotic susceptibility, and outcome. Medicine (Baltimore) 1995; 74:191–200.

71. Ruoff KL, de la ML, Murtagh MJ, Spargo JD, Ferraro MJ. Species identities

of enterococci isolated from clinical specimens. J Clin Microbiol 1990; 28:435–437.

72. Van Goethem GF, Louwagie BM, Simoens MJ, Vandeven JM, Verhaegen JL, Boogaerts MA. *Enterococcus casseliflavus* septicaemia in a patient with acute myeloid leukaemia. Eur J Clin Microbiol Infect Dis 1994; 13:519–520.

73. Peces R, Gago E, Tejada F, Laures AS, Alvarez-Grande J. Relapsing bacteraemia due to *Micrococcus luteus* in a haemodialysis patient with a Perm-Cath catheter. Nephrol Dial Transplant 1997; 12:2428–2429.

74. von Eiff C, Kuhn N, Herrmann M, Weber S, Peters G. *Micrococcus luteus* as a cause of recurrent bacteremia. Pediatr Infect Dis J 1996; 15:711–713.

75. Basaglia G, Carretto E, Barbarini D, Moras L, Scalone S, Marone P, De Paoli P. Catheter-related bacteremia due to *Kocuria kristinae* in a patient with ovarian cancer. J Clin Microbiol 2002; 40:311–313.

76. Atkins JT, Tillman J, Tan TQ, Demmler GJ. *Pediococcus pentosaceus* catheter-associated infection in an infant with gastroschisis. Pediatr Infect Dis J 1994; 13:75–76.

77. Ascher DP, Zbick C, White C, Fischer GW. Infections due to *Stomatococcus mucilaginosus*: 10 cases and review. Rev Infect Dis 1991; 13:1048–1052.

78. Dealler S, Malnick H, Cammish D. Intravenous line infection caused by Corynebacterium CDC group ANF-1. J Hosp Infect 1993; 23:319–320.

79. Kerr KG, Anson JJ, Patmore R, Smith G. Intravenous line infections (letter). J Hosp Infect, 1993, 73–75.

80. Oteo J, Aracil B, Ignacio AJ, Luis Gomez-Garces J. Bacteriemias significativas por *Corynebacterium amycolatum*: un patógeno emergente. Enferm Infecc Microbiol Clin 2001; 19:103–106.

81. Moore C, Norton R. *Corynebacterium aquaticum* septicaemia in a neutropenic patient. J Clin Pathol 1995; 48:971–972.

82. Vasseur E, Broc V, Cocheton JJ. Septicemia due to *Corynebacterium aquaticum* in an HIV-seropositive patient with an implantable chamber catheter. Presse Med 1998; 27:1476–1477.

83. Riebel W, Frantz N, Adelstein D, Spagnuolo PJ. Corynebacterium JK: a cause of nosocomial device-related infection. Rev Infect Dis 1986; 8:42–49.

84. Fish DN, Danziger LH. Neglected pathogens: bacterial infections in persons with human immunodeficiency virus infection. A review of the literature (1). Pharmacotherapy 1993; 13:415–439.

85. Wang CC, Mattson D, Wald A. *Corynebacterium jeikeium* bacteremia in bone marrow transplant patients with Hickman catheters. Bone Marrow Transplant 2001; 27:445–449.

86. Cavendish J, Cole JB, Ohl CA. Polymicrobial central venous catheter sepsis involving a multiantibiotic-resistant strain of *Corynebacterium minutissimum*. Clin Infect Dis 1994; 19:204–205.

87. Rupp ME, Stiles KG, Tarantolo S, Goering RV. Central venous catheter-related *Corynebacterium minutissimum* bacteremia. Infect Control Hosp Epidemiol 1998; 19:786–789.

88. Tumbarello M, Tacconelli E, Del Forno A, Caponera S, Cauda R. *Corynebacterium striatum* bacteremia in a patient with AIDS. Clin Infect Dis 1994; 18:1007–1008.

89. Wood CA, Pepe R. Bacteremia in a patient with non-urinary-tract infection due to *Corynebacterium urealyticum*. Clin Infect Dis 1994; 19:367–368.
90. Bizette GA, Kemmerly SA, Cole JT, Bradford HB Jr, Peltier BH. Sepsis due to coryneform group A-4 in an immunocompromised host. Clin Infect Dis 1995; 21:1334–1336.
91. Campbell PB, Palladino S, Flexman JP. Catheter-related septicemia caused by a vancomycin-resistant Coryneform CDC group A-5. Pathology 1994; 26:56–58.
92. Grove DI, Der-Haroutian V, Ratcliff RM. Aureobacterium masquerading as *'Corynebacterium aquaticum'* infection: case report and review of the literature. J Med Microbiol 1999; 48:965–970.
93. Lau SK, Woo PC, Woo GK, Yuen KY. Catheter-related Microbacterium bacteremia identified by 16S rRNA gene sequencing. J Clin Microbiol 2002; 40:2681–2685.
94. McCaughey C, Damani NN. Central venous line infection caused by Brevibacterium epidermidis. J Infect 1991; 23:211 212.
95. Tuazon CU, Murray HW, Levy C, Solny MN, Curtin JA, Sheagren JN. Serious infections from Bacillus sp. JAMA 1979; 241:1137–1140.
96. Sliman R, Rehm S, Shlaes DM. Serious infections caused by *Bacillus* species. Medicine (Baltimore) 1987; 66:218–223.
97. Richard V, Van der AP, Snoeck R, Daneau D, Meunier F. Nosocomial bacteremia caused by *Bacillus* species. Eur J Clin Microbiol Infect Dis 1988; 7:783–785.
98. Cotton DJ, Gill VJ, Marshall DJ, Gress J, Thaler M, Pizzo PA. Clinical features and therapeutic interventions in 17 cases of Bacillus bacteremia in an immunosuppressed patient population. J Clin Microbiol 1987; 25:672–674.
99. Weber DJ, Saviteer SM, Rutala WA, Thomann CA. In vitro susceptibility of *Bacillus* spp. to selected antimicrobial agents. Antimicrob Agents Chemother 1988; 32:642–645.
100. Carretto E, Barbarini D, Marzani FC, Fumagalli P, Monzillo V, Marone P, Emmi V. Catheter-related bacteremia due to *Lactobacillus rhamnosus* in a single- lung transplant recipient. Scand J Infect Dis 2001; 33:780–782.
101. Katner HP, Joiner TA. *Listeria monocytogenes* sepsis from an infected indwelling i.v. catheter in a patient with AIDS. South Med J 1989; 82:94–95.
102. Dominguez EA, Patil AA, Johnson WM. Ventriculoperitoneal shunt infection due to *Listeria monocytogenes*. Clin Infect Dis 1994; 19:223–224.
103. Schafer FJ, Wing EJ, Norden CW. Infectious endocarditis caused by *Rothia dentocariosa*. Ann Intern Med 1979; 91:747–748.
104. Dzierzanowska D, Miksza-Zytkiewicz R, Czerniawska M, Linda H, Borowski J. Sensitivity of *Rothia dentocariosa*. J Antimicrob Chemother 1978; 4:469–471.
105. Isaacson JH, Grenko RT. *Rothia dentocariosa* endocarditis complicated by brain abscess. Am J Med 1988; 84:352–354.
106. Nivar-Aristy RA, Krajewski LP, Washington JA. Infection of an arteriovenous fistula with *Rothia dentocariosa*. Diagn Microbiol Infect Dis 1991; 14:167–169.
107. Buchman AL, McNeil MM, Brown JM, Lasker BA, Ament ME. Central

venous catheter sepsis caused by unusual *Gordona* (*Rhodococcus*) species: identification with a digoxigenin-labeled rDNA probe. Clin Infect Dis 1992; 15:694–697.

108. Pham AS, De I, Rolston KV, Tarrand JJ, Han XY. Catheter-related becteremia caused by the nocardioform actinomycete *Gordonia terrae*. Clin Infect Dis 2003; 36:524–527.

109. Rubin J, Kirchner K, Walsh D, Green M, Bower J. *Fungal peritonitis* during continuous ambulatory peritoneal dialysis: a report of 17 cases. Am J Kidney Dis 1987; 10:361–368.

110. Miron D, Dennehy PH, Josephson SL, Forman EN. Catheter-associated bacteremia with *Nocardia nova* with secondary pulmonary involvement. Pediatr Infect Dis J 1994; 13:416–417.

111. Lee AC, Yuen KY, Lau YL. Catheter-associated nocardiosis. Pediatr Infect Dis J 1994; 13:1023–1024.

112. Shapiro CL, Haft RF, Gantz NM, Doern GV, Christenson JC, O'Brien R, Overall JC, Brown BA, Wallace RJ Jr, *Tsukamurella paurometabolum*: a novel pathogen causing catheter-related bacteremia in patients with cancer. Clin Infect Dis 1992; 14:200–203.

113. Lai KK. A cancer patient with central venous catheter-related sepsis caused by *Tsukamurella paurometabolum* (*Gordona aurantiaca*). Clin Infect Dis 1993; 17:285–287.

114. Maertens J, Wattiau P, Verhaegen J, Boogaerts M, Verbist L, Wauters G. Catheter-related bacteremia due to *Tsukamurella pulmonis*. Clin Microbiol Infect 1998; 4:51–53.

115. Gaviria JM, Garcia PJ, Garrido SM, Corey L, Boeckh M. Nontuberculous mycobacterial infections in hematopoietic stem cell transplant recipients: characteristics of respiratory and catheter- related infections. Biol Blood Marrow Transplant 2000; 6:361–369.

116. Raad II, Vartivarian S, Khan A, Bodey GP. Catheter-related infections caused by the *Mycobacterium fortuitum* complex: 15 cases and review. Rev Infect Dis 1991; 13:1120–1125.

117. Schelonka RL, Ascher DP, McMahon DP, Drehner DM, Kuskie MR. Catheter-related sepsis caused by *Mycobacterium avium* complex. Pediatr Infect Dis J 1994; 13:236–238.

118. Davison MB, McCormack JG, Blacklock ZM, Dawson DJ, Tilse MH, Crimmins FB. Bacteremia caused by *Mycobacterium neoaurum*. J Clin Microbiol 1988; 26:762–764.

119. Holland DJ, Chen SC, Chew WW, Gilbert GL. *Mycobacterium neoaurum* infection of a Hickman catheter in an immunosuppressed patient. Clin Infect Dis 1994; 18:1002–1003.

120. George SL, Schlesinger LS. *Mycobacterium neoaurum*—an unusual cause of infection of vascular catheters: case report and review. Clin Infect Dis 1999; 28:682–683.

121. Woo PC, Tsoi HW, Leung KW, Lum PN, Leung AS, Ma CH, Kam KM, Yuen KY. Identification of *Mycobacterium neoaurum* isolated from a neutropenic patient with catheter-related bacteremia by 16S rRNA sequencing. J Clin Microbiol 2000; 38:3515–3517.

122. Esteban J, Fernandez-Roblas R, Roman A, Molleja A, Jimenez MS, Soriano F. Catheter-related bacteremia due to *Mycobacterium aurum* in an immunocompromised host. Clin Infect Dis 1998; 26:496–497.

123. Schinsky MF, McNeil MM, Whitney AM, Steigerwalt AG, Lasker BA, Floyd MM, Hogg GG, Brenner DJ, Brown JM. *Mycobacterium septicum* sp. nov., a new rapidly growing species associated with catheter-related bacteraemia. Int J Syst Evol Microbiol 2000; 50 Pt 2:575–581.

124. Skiest DJ, Levi ME. Catheter-related bacteremia due to *Mycobacterium smegmatis*. South Med J 1998; 91:36–37.

125. Ponce dl, Critchley S, Wenzel RP. Polymicrobial bloodstream infections related to prolonged vascular catheterization. Crit Care Med 1984; 12:856–859.

126. D'Antonio D, Pizzigallo E, Iacone A, Dell'Isola M, Fioritoni G, Betti S, Piergallini A, Di Gianfilippo R, Olioso P, Torlontano G. Occurrence of bacteremia in hematologic patients. Eur J Epidemiol 1992; 8:687–692.

127. Rello J, Quintana E, Mirelis B, Gurgui M, Net A, Prats G. Polymicrobial bacteremia in critically ill patients. Intensive Care Med 1993; 19:22–25.

128. Martino R, Gomez L, Pericas R, Salazar R, Sola C, Sierra J, Garau J. Bacteraemia caused by non-glucose-fermenting gram-negative bacilli and *Aeromonas* species in patients with haematological malignancies and solid tumours. Eur J Clin Microbiol Infect Dis 2000; 19:320–323.

129. Haug JB, Harthug S, Kalager T, Digranes A, Solberg CO. Bloodstream infections at a Norwegian university hospital 1994; 19:246–256.

130. Yu WL, Wang DY, Lin CW, Tsou MF. Endemic *burkholderia cepacia* bacteraemia: clinical features and antimicrobial susceptibilities of isolates. Scand J Infect Dis 1999; 31:293–298.

131. Kaitwatcharachai C, Silpapojakul K, Jitsurong S, Kalnauwakul S. An outbreak of *Burkholderia cepacia* bacteremia in hemodialysis patients: an epidemiologic and molecular study. Am J Kidney Dis 2000; 36:199–204.

132. Ramos JM, Domine M, Ponte MC, Soriano F. Bacteremia caused by *Alcaligenes (Achromobacter) xylosoxidans*. Description of 3 cases and review of the literature. Enferm Infecc Microbiol Clin 1996; 14:436–440.

133. Saavedra J, Garrido C, Folgueira D, Torres MJ, Ramos JT. *Ochrobactrum anthropi* bacteremia associated with a catheter in an immunocompromised child and review of the pediatric literature. Pediatr Infect Dis J 1999; 18:658–660.

134. Stiakaki E, Galanakis E, Samonis G, Christidou A, Maraka S, Tselentis Y, Kalmanti M. *Ochrobactrum anthropi* bacteremia in pediatric oncology patients. Pediatr Infect Dis J 2002; 21:72–74.

135. Yu WL, Wang DY, Lin CW. *Agrobacterium radiobacter* bacteremia in a patient with chronic obstructive pulmonary disease. J Formos Med Assoc 1997; 96:664–666.

136. Dube MP, Sattler FR. Catheter-related bacteremia due to *Mycobacterium avium* complex. Clin Infect Dis 1996; 23:405–406.

137. Suara R, Whitlock J, Spearman P. *Mycobacteria fortuitum* central venous catheter-related bacteremia in an infant with renal sarcoma. Pediatr Hematol Oncol 2001; 18:363–365.

138. Linde HJ, Hahn J, Holler E, Reischl U, Lehn N. Septicemia Due to *Acinetobacter junii*. J Clin Microbiol 2002; 40:2696–2697.
139. Ku SC, Hsueh PR, Yang PC, Luh KT. Clinical and microbiological characteristics of bacteremia caused by *Acinetobacter lwoffii*. Eur J Clin Microbiol Infect Dis 2000; 19:501–505.
140. Hammerberg O, Bialkowska-Hobrzanska H, Gopaul D. Isolation of *Agrobacterium radiobacter* from a central venous catheter. Eur J Clin Microbiol Infect Dis 1991; 10:450–452.
141. Roilides E, Mueller BU, Letterio JJ, Butler K, Pizzo PA. *Agrobacterium radiobacter* bacteremia in a child with human immunodeficiency virus infection. Pediatr Infect Dis J 1991; 10:337–338.
142. Potvliege C, Vanhuynegem L, Hansen W. Catheter infection caused by an unusual pathogen. *Agrobacterium radiobacter*. J Clin Microbiol 1989; 27:2120–2122.
143. Lu DC, Chang SC, Chen YC, Luh KT, Lee CY, Hsieh WC. *Burkholderia cepacia* bacteremia: a retrospective analysis of 70 episodes. J Formos Med Assoc 1997; 96:972–978.
144. Lu PL, Hsueh PR, Hung CC, Chang SC, Luh KT, Lee CY. Bacteremia due to *Campylobacter* species: high rate of resistance to macrolide and quinolone antibiotics. J Formos Med Assoc 2000; 99:612–617.
145. Maertens J, Delforge M, Vandenberghe P, Boogaerts M, Verhaegen J. Catheter-related bacteremia due to *Ewingella americana*. Clin Microbiol Infect 2001; 7:103–104.
146. Ladhani S, Gransden W. Septicaemia due to glucose non-fermenting, gram-negative bacilli other than *Pseudomonas aeruginosa* in children. Acta Paediatr 2002; 91:303–306.

11

Central-Venous Catheters

Harald Seifert

Institute for Medical Microbiology, Immunology and Hygiene
University of Cologne
Cologne, Germany

Bernd Jansen

Department of Hygiene and Environmental Medicine
Johannes Gutenberg University
Mainz, Germany

Andreas F. Widmer

Division of Infectious Diseases and Infection Control
University of Basel Hospitals and Clinics
Basel, Switzerland

Barry M. Farr

Department of Internal Medicine
University of Virginia Health System
Charlottesville, VA

INTRODUCTION

Intravascular devices are indispensable for administration of fluids and electrolytes, blood products, drugs, and nutritional support. Patients frequently need a central venous catheter (CVC) to administer chemotherapy for malignant diseases and for total parenteral nutrition. In addition, intensive care units (ICU) use these devices for continuous hemodynamic monitoring of their critically ill patients. Most catheters are made of polyurethane, silicon, or rarely Teflon. A more recent development is the antimicrobial coating of catheters that shall prevent microbial colonization and subsequent infection. More than 20 million patients (over 50%) admitted to U.S. hospitals receive infusion therapy each year (1), and a similar figure of 63% was noted in a European multicenter study (2). Complications arising from intravascular access catheters are frequently observed and generally underestimated. Most importantly, they are largely preventable. Complications of intravascular devices have been known for a long time and were first published only two years after the introduction of plastic catheters in 1945 (3).

This chapter focuses on the epidemiology, microbiology, treatment and prevention of infectious complications associated with CVCs.

DEFINITIONS AND TERMINOLOGY

The first *Guidelines for Prevention of Intravascular Catheter-Related Infections* was issued in 1981 by the Centers for Disease Control (CDC) (4), updated in 1995 (5), and in 2002 a state-of-the art guideline was published by O'Grady et al. (6). The definitions used for catheter-related infections in this chapter are based on the current 2002 guideline (6). It is important to recognize the difference between surveillance definitions for primary bloodstream infections (BSI) and clinical definitions for catheter-related infections. While the former include the term *catheter-associated BSI*, which involves less stringent criteria, and are used for surveillance purposes such as the National Nosocomial Infections Surveillance System (NNIS), the latter are based on clinical and microbiologic diagnostic criteria and include the more specific term *catheter-related BSI*.

A *catheter-associated bloodstream infection* (*CABSI*) is defined by the following: 1) the presence of a vascular access device that terminates at or close to the heart or one of the great vessels. An umbilical artery or vein catheter is considered a central line; and 2) a BSI that is considered to be associated with a central line "if the line was in use during the 48-h period before development of the BSI." If the time interval between onset of infection and device use is <48 hr, there must be compelling evidence that the infection is related to the central line.

This surveillance definition includes all BSIs occurring in patients with CVCs in whom there is no evidence of infection at a distant site and is therefore inherently associated with an overestimation of the true incidence of catheter-related infections.

The clinical definitions for *catheter-related infections* (CRI) include 1) *localized catheter colonization* (formerly classified as local CRI), defined as significant growth of >15 colony-forming units (CFU) obtained by semi-quantitative or roll-plate culture or $>10^3$ CFU by quantitative culture from a proximal or distal catheter segment, or from the catheter hub in the absence of accompanying clinical symptoms; 2) *exit-site infection*, defined as erythema, tenderness, induration, or purulence within 2 cm of the skin at the exit site of the catheter in the absence of a positive blood culture; 3) *tunnel infection*, defined as tenderness, induration, or purulence >2 cm from the catheter insertion site and along the subcutaneous tract along a tunneled catheter in the absence of a positive blood culture; 4) *pocket infection* defined as purulent fluid in the subcutaneous pocket of a totally implanted intravascular catheter with or without necrosis of the overlying skin in the absence of a positive blood culture; and 5) microbiologically documented *catheter-related bloodstream infection (CRBSI)*. The diagnosis of CRBSI requires microbiologically proven bacteremia or fungemia in a patient with an intravascular catheter, clinical manifestations of infection (i.e., fever, chills or hypotension), and no apparent source for the BSI except the catheter. In addition, one of the following should also be present: isolation of the same microorganism (i.e., identical species and antibiogram) from a semiquantitative [>15 CFU from catheter tip or subcutaneous segment (7)] or quantitative [>10^3 CFU/catheter segment after sonication (8)] culture of a catheter segment and from the blood (preferably drawn from a peripheral vein); two simultaneously obtained quantitative blood cultures drawn through the catheter and by venipuncture with a >5:1 ratio (catheter vs. peripheral); and differential time period to positivity of >2 hr of CVC-drawn vs. peripherally obtained blood culture as determined by an automated blood culture system (9,10).

The microbiological methods applied for the diagnosis of different features of catheter-related infections are described in detail in Chapter 3. In the absence of laboratory confirmation, defervescence after removal of an implicated catheter from a patient with BSI may be considered *indirect* evidence of CRBSI.

SIGNS AND SYMPTOMS OF CENTRAL VENOUS CATHETER-RELATED BLOODSTREAM INFECTION

In contrast to peripheral catheters, central venous CRBSI rarely presents with the classical signs of local infection such as redness, induration, pain, and purulent discharge. In a study of neutropenic patients with CRBSI, Seifert and colleagues observed local signs of infection in only 22% of cases and mild inflammation predominated whereas purulent discharge was not observed (10). Clinical sepsis with no obvious source of the infection is the most frequent clinical clue to the diagnosis of CRBSI. The differential diagnosis in a patient with fever and a CVC must therefore always include CRBSI even if careful inspection does not reveal any clinical evidence of exit-site infection.

Catheter-related bloodstream infection is rarely complicated by septic thrombophlebitis (Fig. 1) which manifests as a large inflamed area around the site of insertion, distension of superficial veins, and prominent venous collaterals. Continuously positive blood cultures after catheter removal and despite adequate antimicrobial treatment may herald the presence of suppurative

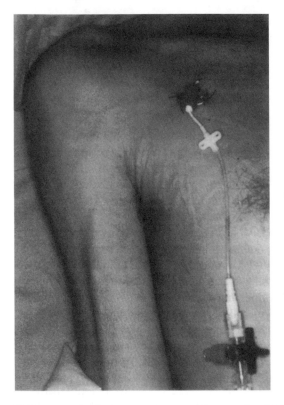

Figure 1 *Staphylococcus aureus* catheter-related bloodstream infection. Erythema, distension of superficial veins, and appearance of prominent venous collaterals as clinical evidence of septic thrombophlebitis. (Photograph taken by T. Bregenzer, M.D.)

thrombophlebitis, and if the large veins are involved local clinical signs are usually absent.

EPIDEMIOLOGY

Nosocomial BSI is the third most common type of nosocomial infection and a leading cause of death in critically ill patients (11). Nosocomial BSIs account for an estimated $6000 increase in hospital costs per infection (12) or $40,000 per survivor in an ICU (13), an extra week of hospital stay, and a case-fatality of more than 20% (13,14). The attributable mortality for bloodstream infections in surgical ICUs has been estimated to be 35% (13,15). For the subgroup of CRBSIs, the attributable mortality was 25%, the excess length of ICU stay was 6.5 days and the attributable costs almost $30,000 (16). The majority of hospital-acquired BSIs are associated with the use of a CVC (11). A recent European prevalence study on nosocomial infections underlined the importance of devices as risk factors for nosocomial infections (17). In the

European study on nosocomial infections in intensive care units (EPIC) involving 10,038 patients, the presence of a central venous line was a statistically significant risk factor (OR 4.6, CI_{95} 3.1–6.8) for BSI (18). ICU patients with a CVC have a fivefold risk of developing a BSI compared to ICU patients without a CVC (18). The risk of CRBSI increases over time if expressed as number of infections per catheter (19–21), but remains remarkably stable if measured as incidence density (infections per 1000 catheter days) (22). To adjust for this potential confounder, the CDC recommends reporting nosocomial device-associated infections as number of infections per 1000 device-days (6).

Central venous catheters have gained widespread use in hospitals, especially in ICUs. Approximately 3 million CVCs are inserted annually in the United States (6), and 200,000 in the United Kingdom (23). Catheter-related infections and in particular CRBSI belong to the most frequently observed complications of intravascular catheterization and represent 10–20% of all nosocomial infections. Of all intravascular catheters, CVCs are responsible for 80–90% of CRBSI (24). In the United States approximately 850,000 CRIs and more than 50,000 CRBSIs occur annually (1,25). The rate of nosocomial BSI associated with a CVC varies considerably with hospital size, department, and type of catheter, and is also influenced by patient characteristics such as age, severity of illness, presence of burn trauma as well as by other hospital-related factors including the skills of the personnel responsible for catheter insertion and maintenance. Not surprisingly, large teaching institutions of >500 beds report higher rates of BSIs than do smaller nonteaching hospitals with <200 beds (11). According to the latest report from the NNIS system, CABSI rates ranged from 2.9 infections per 1000 catheter days in cardiothoracic ICUs to 5.9 in medical ICUs to as high as 11.3 in neonatal ICUs (26).

The attributable mortality of CRBSIs ranges from 14% to 28% (1,12, 13,27). Thus, in the United States, an estimated 7000–14,000 deaths annually may be attributable to CRBSIs. More recent studies showed conflicting results: while the French ICU-bacteremia study group found an attributable mortality of 20% in critically ill patients with primary or catheter-related bacteremia and a median ICU excess length of ICU stay of 9.5 days (28), Rello and colleagues did not observe any difference in mortality among ICU patients with CRBSI and those without; however, the hospital stay in the former group was increased by 19.6 days (29). One of the reasons that may explain these differences could be related to the etiologic microorganisms involved: while in the French study only 23% of cases were due to coagulase-negative staphylococci (CoNS), 63% of cases in the study reported by Rello et al. were caused by CoNS.

Of interest, recent data clearly demonstrate that the incidence of CRBSIs is decreasing (26). Application of guidelines, improving technology with new catheters, and better understanding of the pathogenesis may have contributed to the success of infection control (30).

PATIENTS AT INCREASED RISK FOR NOSOCOMIAL CATHETER-RELATED INFECTION

Burn Patients

After a serious burn trauma, the burned skin area is initially almost free of microorganisms. Therefore, a catheter can be introduced immediately after the trauma through a burned skin area and left in place for 2–3 days, if intravascular access sites are limited. Because burned skin becomes rapidly colonized by multiple, frequently Gram-negative bacteria after this time period, these patients are at high risk to acquire CRI and CRBSI (31,32). A prospective study by Franceschi and colleagues demonstrated that the risk for CRI correlated inversely with the distance of the catheter insertion site from the burned wound (33). Therefore, a catheter should be placed as far distant as possible from the burned skin, 2–3 days after the accident. *Pseudomonas aeruginosa* is the most frequently isolated microorganism from catheters in burned patients (33–35).

In the future, the use of coated catheters may be an option for this patient population (36). The International Society for Burn Injuries (ISBI) and the WHO still recommend to change intravascular catheters every 72 hr (37). For pediatric patients, this interval was extended to 7 days (38). In the authors' opinion, this recommendation may no longer be appropriate if the insertion site is remote from the burned skin area or/and a coated catheter is used.

HIV-Infected Patients

AIDS patients are considered to be at higher risk to develop CRI or CRBSI than non-AIDS patients. Raviglione and colleagues reviewed 46 AIDS patients with Hickman catheters: CRI and CRBSI occurred in 23% and 10%, respectively (39). In another study, the catheter was the source of infection in 73% of bacteremic episodes in HIV-positive patients (40). *Staphylococcus aureus* is one of the most frequent microorganisms isolated from catheters of AIDS patients (39,41), probably because of the high proportion of *S. aureus* nasal carriers in this group (55%) and the hosts' inability to control the infection/colonization locally (42). Infection-free survival of CVC was significantly prolonged with tunneled catheters compared to percutaneously placed central catheters ($p < 0.05$) (43). Therefore, a tunneled or a totally implanted catheter is recommended in AIDS patients with diseases requiring life-long IV treatment such as cytomegalovirus infection.

Total Parenteral Nutrition

Total parenteral nutrition (TPN) differs in many ways from other modes of intravascular therapy: 1) catheters used for TPN are needed much longer than other catheters; 2) TPN solutions support the growth of microorganisms, especially Gram-negative bacteria and *Candida* spp. (44–46); 3) the underlying disease of the patient often increases the risk of acquiring nosocomial infections; and 4) frequently remote infections are present that expose the catheter to hematogenous seeding. The incidence of CRBSI in patients receiving TPN ranges from 0% to 14%, on average 3% to 5% (47–49). Common microorganisms encountered are CoNS, *S. aureus, Candida* spp., *Serratia* spp., and *Enterobacter* spp. (50,51). *Malassezia furfur* is a rare but serious infection strongly associated with TPN in young children (52). In such cases of suspected CRBSI, the clinician should advise the microbiology laboratory about the patient being on TPN. *M. furfur* requires specific supplements to grow in standard media (52–54). Catheter-related blood-stream infection caused by *Candida* spp. has been a particular problem in patients on TPN. These patients often receive multiple antibiotics for other infections, a factor that is independently associated with an increased risk for *Candida* infection (55).

Catheter care is a crucial factor in TPN. Ryan and colleagues (56) related CRIs to violation of the infusion delivery system. Snydman et al. estimated the risk of developing CRI six times higher for catheters that were exposed to violations of the catheter care guidelines than those that were not (51).

The optimal catheter type for short-term (<1 month) TPN is probably the single-lumen catheter without stopcocks (51,57). If a triple-lumen catheter is used, the distal port should be avoided for TPN solutions, to minimize the risk of contamination if guidewire exchange should become necessary. Howard and colleagues reported that patients prefer a totally implantable, subcutaneous infusion port for long-term TPN (>3 months) rather than regular central-venous lines (58).

Needleless and protected-needle intravascular access systems have been recommended for use with intravenous lines to reduce the risk of needlestick injuries in health-care workers. However, these devices have higher rates of CRBSI than regular devices (risk ratio 14.9, $p < 0.05$), specifically for patients with TPN. These devices bear critical reevaluation for its use (59). They may protect the health-care worker, but at the same time they put the patient at increased risk for CRBSI.

A difficult clinical task is to decide when to remove a TPN catheter for suspected sepsis. Quantitative cultures are appropriate, if a long-term catheter is in place. For short-term central-venous lines, exchange to a new site or by guidewire is frequently recommended (60); however, in one study, over 90% of the catheters removed for suspected sepsis were not the source of that sepsis (47,60). Bonadimani and colleagues reported successful management of suspected CVC-related sepsis in patients with TPN by guidewire replacement of catheters even in cases with documented catheter colonization (50). Semiquantitative cultures of the blood taken through the catheter may help in deciding when to keep the line or to change it (negative predictive value 100%, positive predictive value 60%) (61). There is no consensus on this issue, but guidewire exchange seems to be a reasonable approach in the early management of septic episodes of patients on TPN.

Antimicrobial agents should be given sequentially through the different ports to expose all inner lumens to high concentrations of the antimicrobial agent (62).

MICROBIOLOGY

The spectrum of microorganisms causing CRIs largely depends on the type of hospital care (e.g., intensive care vs. care on a regular ward), patients' underlying condition such as bone marrow transplant patients or patients undergoing hemodialysis, the type of catheter, and many other variables (1,63–66). The distribution of pathogens also varies by hospital size and affiliation, e.g., teaching vs. nonteaching institution (Table 1). A shift toward Gram-positive bacteria and fungi was observed over the last two decades in nosocomial BSI (26,67) as well as in CRBSI (11,26,28,29). Coagulase-negative staphylococci, *S. aureus*, enterococci, and *Candida* spp. have emerged as the most frequent pathogens associated with intravascular catheters in the last decade (11,28,29,68). At the University of Iowa Hospitals and Clinics, Iowa, USA, BSI increased linearly from 6.7 to 18.4 per 1000 discharges (0.83 to 1.72 episodes per 1000 patient-days) from 1980 to 1992 ($r = 0.87$).

Table 1 Microbiology of Short-Term Central-Venous Catheters

Short-term CVCs used in	Most frequently isolated pathogens		Other typical pathogens
General ward	Gram-positive bacteria	>60%	MRSA accounts for 5–30% of all *S. aureus*
Intensive care unit	Gram-negative bacteria	30–40%	CoNS and *S. aureus* ≈30% MRSA accounts for 10–50% of all *S. aureus*
Immunocompromised host	Coagulase-negative staphylococci (CoNS)	>50%	*S. aureus* including MRSA ≈10% Gram-negative bacilli <10% Rare, but associated with high mortality: *P. aeruginosa*, *Candida* spp.
Total parenteral nutrition	*Staphylococcus aureus*	>30%	CoNS ≈20% *Candida* spp. ≈10%

The relative frequency is an overall estimation; the range is very broad. The spectrum of microorganisms causing CRIs largely depends on the type of hospital care, underlying condition, and many other variables (see details in chapters on CoNS, *S. aureus*, Gram-negative bacilli, and fungi).
Source: Refs. 11, 26, 28, 29, and 74.

Increases in infection rates were due to Gram-positive cocci ($r = 0.96$) and yeasts ($r = 0.95$) and essentially explained by infections caused by CoNS, *S. aureus*, enterococci, and *Candida* species, respectively (15).

For CoNS, methicillin resistance is present in approximately 50% of European and 80% of U.S. strains (68). The increase in *S. aureus* partly relates to the increase in methicillin-resistant *S. aureus* (MRSA) that adds to the number of methicillin-susceptible *S. aureus* (MSSA) (11). The rate of infections with methicillin-resistant *S. aureus* (MRSA) depends on the prevalence of this pathogen within an institution. Between 10% and 60% of *S. aureus* strains are methicillin-resistant in the United States, with rates being higher in ICUs than in general wards (26). The prevalence of MRSA in Europe increases from north (0–5%) to south (30–60%) (18,69) and differs from institution to institution even within a city. In 2002, a German study (70) reported that up to 20% of all nosocomial *S. aureus* infections in ICUs are now caused by MRSA, despite the fact that Germany had belonged to the low-prevalence countries for decades. Therefore, knowledge about the frequency and resistance pattern of the key pathogens is crucial for setting guidelines for empirical treatment of suspected CRBSI. Such information should be regularly updated based on the information of the local resistance patterns. Detailed information about the importance of individual pathogens is discussed elsewhere in this book.

MICROBIOLOGICAL METHODS FOR THE DIAGNOSIS OF CENTRAL-VENOUS CATHETER-RELATED INFECTIONS

The sensitivity and specificity of microbiological methods for diagnosis of CRI and CRBSI depend on the method used in the routine microbiology laboratory. Siegman-Igra and Farr calculated a pooled estimate of the sensitivity, specificity, and cost of the different microbiological methods (71). If the catheter has been removed, sensitivity and specificity were best for quantitative catheter segment cultures (94% and 92%, respectively). However, as there is no gold standard for the diagnosis of CRI, the results of this meta-analysis must be interpreted with caution. Microbiological methods requiring removal of the catheter and in situ methods are recommended for short-term CVCs. Removal of the catheter is both a diagnostic procedure and an appropriate strategy to eliminate this potential source of infection if a febrile episode of unknown source is observed in a patient with an intravascular catheter in place. Diagnostic methods using the catheter tip are most accurate for such cases with either using the roll-plate technique (7) or sonication (8). However, reinsertion of a new catheter or even guidewire replacement might put the patient at risk, e.g., in patients with severe thrombocytopenia. A method with the catheter left in place is more suitable for the diagnosis of CRI in such patients (10,72,73). Examples are quantitative blood cultures taken through the catheter and a peripheral vein, or targeted skin cultures if the patient is on total parenteral nutrition (10,72,74). Many studies indicated higher sensitivity for sonication than for the roll-plate technique (75,76). However, Widmer and Frei recently challenged these results (77). The roll-plate technique possibly excels sonication if the catheter tip is in place <10 days, whereas sonication is probably more appropriate for tips that were in place >10 days. The different microbiological methods are discussed in detail in Chapter 3. For long-term catheters, time to positivity with an automated blood culture system may be the optimal diagnostic technique (9,10,78). However, blood cultures must arrive at the microbiology laboratory within hours after taking the blood including nights and weekends to correctly identify the different growth rates resulting in different times to positivity of samples obtained through the catheter and by peripheral venipuncture (9,10).

CATHETER MATERIALS

Catheter Composition

Most catheters used in the United States are made of polyurethane, polyvinyl chloride (PVC), polyethylene, or silicone. As for peripheral catheters, silicone catheters are associated with a lower risk of infection than PVC catheters (79). Therefore, PVC catheters are rarely used today. A hydrophilic surface was achieved by introducing hydroxyethylmethacrylate into polyurethane catheters. These hydrophilic surfaces reduced the in vitro adhesion of *Staphylococcus epidermidis* compared to hydrophobic polyurethane catheters (80). However, lacking randomized controlled clinical trials, definite conclusions about the contribution of catheter material to CVC-related infection cannot be drawn.

Surface-Modified Catheters and Cuffs

Microorganisms can adhere to any implanted device. Once adhered and embedded in a biofilm, they become in vivo resistant to most antimicrobial agents even if standard susceptibility testing reveals high sensitivity (81). The mode of growth, the influence of bacterial products such as exopolysaccharides from CoNS, and the different susceptibility of planktonic vs. adherent microorganisms partly explain why microorganisms may become resistant in the presence of a foreign body (81–83). In animal models, several investigators succeeded to reduce bacterial adherence by coating the catheters with antimicrobials or antiseptics (84,85). Colonization of the skin at the insertion site is a well-recognized risk factor for the development of CRI and CRBSI (72). In addition, bacteria on the exit sites of percutaneous catheters can migrate rapidly from the entry site into the dermal tunnel along the external catheter surface, perhaps suspended in a fluid film and propelled by capillary action (86). Therefore research was started on cuffs hindering bacteria to move along the catheter from the surface to the intradermal part of the catheter. In addition, polymers with antiadherence properties were developed, followed by impregnated catheters.

Cuffs

A cuff acts as a tissue-interface barrier. A commercially available example is a biodegradable collagen cuff impregnated with silver ions (VitaCuff™) attached to a catheter just prior to insertion. Multiple prospective, randomized clinical trials have shown the use of cuffs to lower the risk of CRI and CRBSI more than threefold compared to noncuffed catheters (19,20,87). However, their efficacy wanes after 2 weeks of catheterization (87), and more recent studies (88,89) could not demonstrate an influence of the cuff on the incidence of CRBSI. The cuff does not prevent intraluminal transmission of pathogens from contaminated hubs or infusates because the cuff is on the outside of the catheter. The importance of the hub as source of infection increases with the length of catheter dwelling time. Therefore, the protection provided by the cuff wanes over time due to loss of silver ions and increasing importance of the intraluminal pathway. Today, cuffs are rarely used.

Antimicrobially Coated Catheters

The advantages and shortcomings of antimicrobial catheters to prevent CRI and CRBSI are discussed in detail in Chapter 5.

In animal studies, catheters coated with an antiseptic, antimicrobial agent (84,90) or even with nonsteroidal anti-inflammatory agents (91) reduced the bacterial colonization of the catheter. Chlorhexidine-coated catheters decreased biofilm formation and bacterial adherence on catheters (90). Benzalkonium chloride also lowers the degree of bacterial colonization in vitro (80). In elegant animal studies performed by Sherertz et al., coating of catheters with dicloxacillin, clindamycin, and fusidic acid decreased the risk of infection compared with uncoated control catheters ($p < 0.05$) (85).

Most Swan–Ganz pulmonary artery catheters used in the United States are heparin-bonded to maintain patency and coated with benzalkonium chloride which also provides short-term, but broad-spectrum antimicrobial activity (92). In a study by Kamal et al., CVCs pretreated with a cationic surfactant and the antibiotic cefazolin lowered the rate of CRI from 14% to 8% in a surgical ICU ($p < 0.004$) (93); however, the catheter must be coated immediately before use which is time-consuming and needs special training.

The two most extensively studied antimicrobial catheters to date which are also in clinical use as CVCs in the United States and elsewhere are catheters containing chlorhexidine and silver sulfadiazine (CHSS) (Arrowgard Blue™ and Arrowgard Plus™, Arrow International, USA) and a catheter containing minocycline and rifampin (MR) (Cook Spectrum™, Cook Critical Care, USA). Most of the clinical studies on antimicrobial catheters so far have dealt with these two catheter types, the majority of them with the

CHSS catheter and have revealed a trend toward lowering the incidence of CRBSI. In a meta-analysis by Veenstra et al. (94) it was shown that the use of the CHSS catheter in short-term catheterization reduced the risk for CRBSI approximately by one-half. With the MR catheter, two important studies have shown a benefit in reducing the incidence of CRBSI (36,95). A clinical study with 234 patients, randomized to receive a triple-lumen catheter pre-coated with rifampin–minocycline or without precoating, showed that none of the patients with a precoated catheter had CRBSI compared to seven in the control group ($p = 0.01$) (36). Significantly less infectious complications were observed with the MR-coated catheter directly than with the CHSS catheter (95). The better performance of the MR catheter might have resulted from the fact that in contrast to the CHSS catheter, the MR catheter is coated on both the internal and the external surface (96), and a longer-lasting surface activity of the antibiotic MR combination in comparison to CHSS has been observed (96a). However, the second generation of CHSS catheters also contains an external and internal coating, and a higher concentration of chlorhexidine (Arrowgard Blue Plus™). Clinical studies with this new catheter are needed before a superiority of the MR catheter over CHSS catheters can be assumed.

The cost-effectiveness of such impregnated catheters has been deduced for both types of catheters (97,98). In the current U.S. guideline on the prevention of intravascular CRI (6), the use of an antimicrobial or antiseptic-impregnated catheter is emphasized in adults "whose catheter is expected to remain in place more than 5 days if, after implementing a comprehensive strategy to reduce rates of CRBSI, the CRBSI rate remains above the goal set by the individual institution based on benchmark rates." A similar recommendation is given in the British guideline (99), whereas the use of antimicrobial catheters is an unresolved issue in the current German guideline (100).

The emergence of pathogens resistant to minocycline and/or rifampin is a cause of concern that is discussed in detail in Chapter 5.

THERAPY OF INFECTIONS

Suspected Catheter-Related Infection or Catheter-Related Bloodstream Infection

Clinicians are often faced with an acute febrile episode with an unknown source of infection rather than a known catheter-related infectious complication. Removal of the catheter is recommended if little risks associated with a new insertion, such as bleeding or pneumothorax, is anticipated for the patient. In >70% of such episodes, fever has been traced down to a different source, and the catheter has thus been unnecessarily replaced (56,60). In addition, CRIs due to CoNS can be successfully treated with antibiotics without removal of the device (101). Therefore a British guideline recommends obtaining culture results from exit-site swabs and blood cultures drawn from the CVC and a separate peripheral venipuncture before catheter removal is considered (102). However, this procedure requires quantitative blood cultures, a test rarely available routinely in the clinical microbiology laboratory. In addition, failure to remove the catheter puts the patient at high risk for sustained bacteremia, septic thrombosis, and endocarditis (103–105). Serious complications have been reported after an episode of CRBSI with *S. aureus* or fungi: 25% of patients with *S. aureus* CRBSI develop complications and 68% of patients with fungal CRBSI have persistent fungemia (104,106,107). The crude mortality is reported to be 16% for *S. aureus* and 52% for fungal CRBSI (104,106). Given the possibility of severe complications, it is wise to replace a short-term CVC if clinically possible. Hematology–oncology units may follow a less strict policy because CoNS are the most common pathogens and allow antimicrobial treatment with the catheter left in situ with very little risk for the patient. In these patients, blood culture results with determination of the differential time to positivity (DTP, see above) may help identify the catheter as the source of infection, and may thus guide clinical management with regard to catheter removal or antibiotic lock therapy (10). It must be kept in mind, however, that recurrent bacteremia occurs in 20% even with CoNS if the catheter is not removed (101). In summary, removal of the catheter should always be attempted for short-term CVCs unless a high risk is associated with the exchange, and CRI or CRBSI is less likely. Guidewire exchange is not recommended if there is purulence at the insertion site, or CRI or CRBSI is highly probable.

The empirical antimicrobial regimen for CRBSI depends on the resistance pattern of the most frequent pathogens of the institution. In institutions with a high prevalence of MRSA (e.g., >10%), a combination of a glycopeptide such as vancomycin in combination with an aminoglycoside or a quinolone is appropriate against the bacterial pathogens likely to be encountered with an infected catheter.

Treatment of Established Infections

Antimicrobial treatment depends on the microorganism(s) isolated from the catheter tip or with other culture techniques. In most instances, removal of the device and antimicrobial treatment for 7–14 days is appropriate for short-term central-venous lines. Persistent bacteremia may indicate septic thrombosis and should prompt immediate diagnostic procedures. Removal of short-term catheters is often useful for both diagnosis and therapy. For long-dwelling catheters, removal is often more difficult and more expensive, but is still indicated in certain situations. Initial severity of illness and the microbial etiology help to determine whether the long-term catheter must be removed. For mild to moderate cases, an attempt to treat and salvage the catheter is often chosen; for such therapy a combination of 2 weeks of parenteral therapy combined with antibiotic lock therapy (see below) has been recommended for patients with no evidence of complications such as endocarditis that would indicate the use of a longer duration of parenteral therapy (108). If the infection is due to fungi, the probability of salvage is significantly lower and death significantly higher if the catheter is left in place (109,110). So salvage has not been recommended for fungal infections (108). *Staphylococcus aureus* has been associated with significantly worse outcomes in some (111) but not all studies. For example, in one study of hemodialysis catheter-related bloodstream infections, all of the 12 patients with *S. aureus* CRBSI were cured and their catheters salvaged using parenteral and antibiotic lock therapy (112). In another study of hemodialysis catheter-related *S. aureus* BSI, none of the 50 patients died of the infection (113). Such data suggest that initial severity of illness may be used to determine whether catheter salvage should be attempted with this pathogen. A small study suggested that after a brief period of parenteral therapy antibiotic lock therapy was as effective as antibiotic lock therapy plus continued parenteral therapy for curing CRBSI and salvaging the infected catheter (114). More studies are needed to confirm the safety and efficacy of this approach, which the authors suggest could significantly lower antimicrobial pressure in the hospital setting. Another recent article showed that the concentration of heparin used for combination with an antimicrobial in antibiotic-lock therapy was important because lower heparin concentrations (e.g., <1000 U/mL) were associated with precipitation whereas higher heparin concentrations (e.g., 3500–10,000 U/mL) were not (115). A proposal for the clinical approach to patients presenting with suspected CRBSI is given in Fig. 2.

Coagulase-Negative Staphylococci

Coagulase-negative staphylococci are the most frequently involved pathogens in CRBSI. Most infections with long-term catheters can be treated without removal of the device (62,74). This also appears to be true for short-term CVCs. However, Raad et al., investigating 70 cases of CRBSI caused by CoNS, observed recurrent bacteremia in 20% of patients when the catheter was not removed (101), whereas 80% were successfully treated keeping the catheter in place. In addition, mortality was not influenced by treatment with or without catheter removal ($p > 0.1$). Therefore, the only risk with this kind of management is recurrent bacteremia without serious complications that would make catheter removal mandatory.

A glycopeptide such as vancomycin or teicoplanin is the treatment of choice because most CoNS are methicillin-resistant (68). However, an antistaphylococcal penicillin such as flucloxacillin should be used, if antimicrobial susceptibility testing reveals susceptibility. Coagulase-negative staphylococci adhere to plastic surfaces and become embedded in a biofilm layer that provides a measure of protection from antibacterial agents (116). Failure of glycopeptide antibiotics to cure device-related infection is not due to poor penetration of drugs into biofilm but likely due to a diminished antimicrobial effect on the bacteria in the biofilm environment (117).

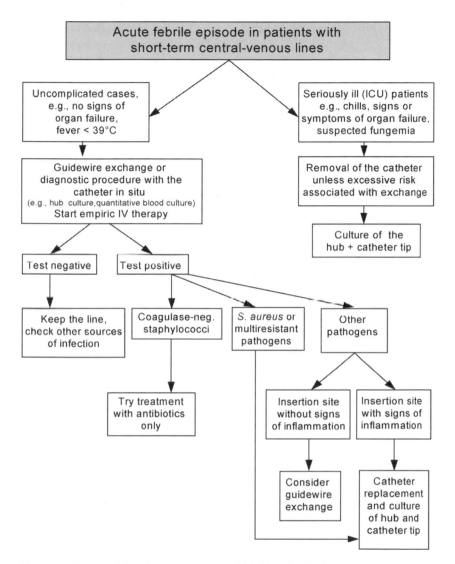

Figure 2 Proposal for the management of febrile episodes in patients with suspected catheter-related infection of catheter-related bloodstream infection.

Rifampin is highly efficacious against adherent CoNS, and antibiotic combinations with rifampin are much more effective against orthopedic implant-related infections than those without rifampin (81,82). However, little data are available for infections involving intravascular catheters. Minocycline and rifampin have been used to cover the plastic surface of the catheter (coated catheters) resulting in a significant reduction of CRBSI episodes (36). Antimicrobial treatment should last 5–7 days if the catheter is removed. If the catheter is not removed, treatment should be extended to ≥14 days. However, the optimal duration of treatment is not well established.

Alternatively, the antibiotic lock technique for long-term catheters probably kills even adherent CoNS by its high intraluminal concentration that is well above peak levels in blood.

Staphylococcus aureus

S. aureus CRBSI frequently ends in septic complications. Twenty-five percent of patients experiencing an episode of *S. aureus* CRBSI develop complications, and one in seven will die (106). Raad and Sabbagh recommended 10 days of antibiotic therapy for uncomplicated cases (105), but this duration has been questioned by others (118). Uncomplicated cases were defined as those who became afebrile within ≤3 days of therapy *and* have negative blood cultures documented. Fourteen days of antimicrobial therapy appear to suffice for uncomplicated cases and have been recommended by the recent Infectious Diseases Society of America (IDSA) guidelines for the management of intravascular CRI (1,108). Complicated cases, e.g., those with septic metastasis, require antimicrobial treatment of 4–6 weeks (119).

A recent study found that 16 (23%) of 69 patients with *S. aureus* CRBSI developed endocarditis detected by transesophageal echocardiography (TEE); the same study found that transthoracic echocardiography (TTE) detected only 27% of those considered to have endocarditis (120). A recent guideline, therefore, suggested that TEE be performed when available and not contraindicated to exclude endocarditis before deciding to give just 14 days of parenteral therapy (108). Another study that did not use TEE on patients with uncomplicated *S. aureus* BSI found that none of 62 patients treated for 10–14 days relapsed or developed endocarditis, however. The authors concluded that clinical criteria were sufficient to detect complications such as endocarditis and that subclinical endocarditis may be cured by 10–14 days of high-dose parenteral therapy (121).

Vancomycin has been the drug of choice for serious MRSA infection, but the outcome of MRSA infections has generally been worse than for MSSA infection even when adjusted for severity of underlying illness (122,123). Part of this worse outcome likely relates to an increased frequency of initially receiving a drug inactive against the infection, but another part may be due to suboptimal results with vancomycin therapy as compared with beta-lactam therapy for MSSA infections. Recent studies have suggested that linezolid may also provide better results than vancomycin, at least when used to treat MRSA pneumonia (124).

Gram-Negative Rods

Gram-negative rods can be treated with a short course of appropriate antibiotics, unless there is evidence for *P. aeruginosa* CRBSI. *P. aeruginosa* BSIs have a higher mortality than those with other bacteria (125), and treatment should include an antipseudomonal β-lactam and an aminoglycoside, preferably tobramycin (126). A promising alternative against *P. aeruginosa* CRBSI is the combination of high-dose ciprofloxacin and piperacillin–tazobactam (127). However, only limited clinical data are available as for meropenem which may be another option.

There are no randomized clinical trials to determine the optimal duration of therapy. Uncomplicated cases respond to a 7–10-day course of appropriate antibiotics, if the catheter is removed (6).

Candida spp. and Moulds

Candida spp. are isolated from episodes of CRBSI in up to 20% (26,28). In cancer patients, overall mortality after an episode of fungal CRBSI may exceed 50% (55). In patients not having received prior fluconazole as a prophylactic or therapeutic agent, fluconazole is appropriate for *Candida* CRBSI pending definite species identification and/or susceptibility testing. Fluconazole remains the therapy of choice for *C. albicans* as well as for most other nonalbicans *Candida* spp. *Candida* spp. less susceptible or resistant to fluconazole such as *C. glabrata* and *C. krusei* have emerged as more frequent causes of infection in recent years, mainly after a previous course of fluconazole for prophylaxis or treatment in immunocompromised patients (128). However, these pathogens were recently observed also without previous exposure to fluconazole (129). Therefore the microbiology laboratory should always identify yeasts to species level to guide appropriate treatment. If a patient had been receiving fluconazole prophylaxis or if *C. glabrata* and *C. krusei* have been identified, caspofungin may be administered pending susceptibility results. This agent is only available for intravenous therapy. Voriconazole, approved for treatment of aspergillus infection, is a reasonable alternative and is available for parenteral and oral therapy. Both agents are very expensive and should only be considered if the pretest probability is high for a nonalbicans *Candida* spp.

Bloodstream infections involving *Candida* spp. always require a change of catheter, because higher mortality and prolonged fungemia have been observed if the catheter remains in place (104,130,131). For molds, amphotericin B, voriconazole, or caspofungin is the preferred agent: amphotericin, if not applied in a liposomal formulation, is the least expensive drug, but also the drug with the most frequent and serious side effects.

Antibiotic Lock

As mentioned above, bacteria adhere to surfaces of catheters rendering them resistant to usual concentration of antibiotics. Therefore several groups studied the impact of antimicrobial agents that are given into the lumen of the catheter for treatment of low-grade CRIs and CRBSIs. A vancomycin "lock" has been most frequently used in combination with systemic therapy (108). A promising, but not well-documented, new option is the antibiotic lock with ethanol (132). A more detailed discussion of antibiotic lock therapy is included in Chapter 4.

PREVENTION STRATEGIES

An overview of the different strategies to prevent CRI and CRBSI is given in Chapter 5 "Prevention and Control of Catheter-Related Infections." The most important preventive measures applied specifically for short-term CVCs are summarized below.

Surveillance for Catheter-Associated Bloodstream Infection and Catheter-Related Bloodstream Infection

Catheter-related bloodstream infections are largely preventable and are therefore part of most surveillance systems for infection control. Patients, hospitals, resources, and equipment differ from hospital to hospital and from country to country. Therefore, guidelines and recommendations must be adjusted to the local setting. Simple surveillance data can help to optimize resources for prevention. The surveillance definition (6) of CABSI facilitates simple surveillance on a local level and data are expressed as number of BSIs per 1000 catheter days. The minimum data required are therefore the total number of CVC days and the number of BSIs. The number of patient-days may be a surrogate, if CVC days are unavailable. Surveillance should focus on high-risk areas such as ICUs, if resources are limited.

Recently, a German report by Zuschneid et al. (133) on infection rates in ICUs participating in the German system for surveillance of nosocomial infections (KISS) showed a decrease in primary BSIs from 2.1 to 1.5 per 1000 CVC days, corresponding to an overall relative reduction of 28.6% during a 2-year observational period among a total of 84 ICUs. Although specific reasons for this reduction are difficult to determine, besides new research findings, improved guidelines, intensified education of medical personnel, and introduction of specific prevention measures, it has been assumed that a modification of behavior under surveillance is at least partially responsible for the decrease in infection rates (Hawthorne effect).

Optimal Site of Insertion

Central venous catheters can be inserted from a peripheral vein [e.g., midline catheters, peripherally inserted central catheters (PICC)] or directly into a large vein (subclavian, jugular, axilla, femoral access). The jugular access is associated with a statistically significant increased risk of infection compared to subclavian vein insertion (21,134–137). These studies report an average colonization rate of CVCs inserted into the jugular vein of 27% compared to 4% in CVCs inserted into the subclavian vein ($p < 0.05$). The differences may be due to increased colonization by respiratory pathogens at the internal jugular insertion site (138), the difficulty of fixation, the mechanical stress caused by head movements, and insufficient adherence of catheter dressings. This long-term complication must be weighed against the noninfectious risks at the time of insertion such as pneumothorax and severe bleeding by inadvertent puncture of the subclavian artery. The subclavian catheter is easier to keep dry and clean; both factors are associated with a lower risk of infection. For patients undergoing elective surgery such as coronary bypass surgery, the jugular access is probably the better choice because short-time catheterization is anticipated (<3–7 days), and acute complication rates during insertion are of concern. For prolonged catheterization, infectious complications probably outweigh those associated with insertion. Therefore, the subclavian access may be preferable for medical ICU patients who require prolonged catheterization. The femoral access is another option, but associated with higher rates of complications; therefore, tunneling of such catheters is an option (139). Noninfectious risks should also be considered when choosing the femoral access. In a randomized clinical trial, deep vein thrombosis occurred in 25% after femoral catheterization compared to 0% in the jugular/subclavian group (140).

Barrier Precautions

Full barrier precautions including the use of mask, cap, sterile gloves, gown, and large sterile drape have been shown to significantly reduce the risk of CRI and CRBSI (66,135). Strict asepsis at the time of insertion is a crucial step for effective infection control. It is unknown if mask and cap are mandatory, but they might provide an additional level of safety. The environment where the catheter is inserted does not play a major role: two randomized studies could not demonstrate a difference in the infection rate between the study group (insertion in the operating theater) and the control group (insertion in wards) (66,135).

Disinfection of the Skin

Cutaneous antisepsis of the insertion site is regarded as one of the most important measures for preventing CRI and CRBSI (6). However, the optimal disinfectant to use for catheter insertion sites is still a matter of debate. The use of highly concentrated acetone for defatting the catheter insertion site is unwarranted (141). In 1981, Maki and Band demonstrated that an ointment containing polymyxin, neomycin, and bacitracin reduced the rate of CRI from 6.5% to 2.2% (142); however, three *Candida* infections including one case of candidemia occurred in this treatment arm. In addition, topical ointments do not have to be sterile under the pharmacopeia's requirement, and a large outbreak of fungal infections was caused by a contaminated topical ointment (143). Maki et al. prospectively tested three different disinfectants, alcohol, povidone-iodine, and chlorhexidine, to evaluate their efficacy in reducing CRI and CRBSI (144). Alcohol and povidone-iodine had clearly higher associated rates of CRI and CRBSI than chlorhexidine, 7.1% and 9.3% vs. 2.3%, respectively ($p < 0.02$); however, the differences were only seen in CRBSI due to CoNS, and only by pooling of the data. Daily application of povidone-iodine did not reduce colonization of central-venous lines in another large study (137). A hand-washing system using chlorhexidine at the University of Iowa reduced the rate of nosocomial infections significantly compared to one using alcohol (145), supporting the preference for chlorhexidine. However, in a randomized clinical trial addressing the effectiveness of alcohol vs. chlorhexidine for surgical scrub, alcohol was significantly more efficacious than chlorhexidine (146). Alcoholic preparations are most suitable because of their rapid action (within 30 sec), broad spectrum, and minimal side-effects. However, there is no residual effect after evaporation of the alcohol. Therefore, chlorhexidine or povidone-iodine might be added to extend the antimicrobial effect (remanent effect). Unfortunately, there are no commercially available preparations of alcoholic chlorhexidine approved for use at intravenous catheter insertion sites in the United States. Disinfectants without alcohol need 3–5 min for microbial killing, a waiting time frequently not respected in a busy hospital.

Catheter Dressings

In the early 1980s, transparent dressings were frequently used to allow convenient visual inspection of the insertion site without prior removal of the dressing. Furthermore, only weekly changes were considered to be necessary, saving nursing time and dressing supply. A well-designed randomized, prospective study showed a higher risk for CRI with the transparent dressing than with gauze (RR 2.6) (147). Other studies that included mainly patients on total parenteral nutrition did not confirm these results (148–151). However, moisture under the dressing increased the risk for CRI (RR > 3), a factor that was more frequently seen in the transparent dressing group (148). A meta-analysis found that transparent dressings led to a threefold increased risk for CRBSI compared with gauze dressings (152). Four independent studies demonstrated higher bacterial counts under transparent dressings than under gauze (21,147,152,153). Other studies, however, found no significant differences (148,149,154). Today, the new highly permeable transparent dressings are not associated with higher rates of CRI or CRBSI (64), even if they are still associated with higher levels of microbial colonization. A replacement of the dressing is necessary if it is has become damp, loosened, or soiled (6). Especially for short-term CVCs (including hemodialysis and pulmonary artery catheters), gauze dressings should be replaced every 2 days and transparent dressings at least every 7 days, whereas dressings used on implanted or tunneled CVC sites should be replaced no more than once a week. However, daily inspection of the insertion site is crucial to detect early local signs of CRI.

Routine Exchange of Central-Venous Catheters

The recent literature supports the idea of *not* routinely changing CVCs (Fig. 2) (34,155–157). No recommendations for a routine exchange are given by the current U.S. guideline for prevention of intravascular device-related infections (6); however, catheters inserted in emergency situations should be replaced as soon as possible, e.g., within 24–48 hr.

The risk for CRI or CRBSI increases linearly with the duration the catheter remains in place (21,157). Noninfectious complications are more frequent with routine change than with a policy to keep the line as long as clinically indicated (156). However, a policy including routine changes always lets physicians reconsider the indication for continuous central-venous access. This regular check will not work with a policy of keeping the line as long as clinically indicated. Therefore, it is important to train the staff to strictly limit the time of catheterization because each additional day of catheterization puts the patient at increased risk for CRI and CRBSI (158).

Guidewire Exchange vs. New Puncture

Guidewire exchange is the preferred method to change a pulmonary artery catheter to a CVC or to replace a malfunctioning catheter (6). The risk of infection after guidewire exchange is not yet established. One large randomized clinical trial showed an increased risk (155), whereas other studies did not support this finding (22,159–161). For patients on total parenteral nutrition, Bonadimani and colleagues reported successful catheter guidewire replacement for suspected CVC-related sepsis even in cases with documented catheter colonization (50). Other authors do not support guidewire exchange for febrile patients with suspected CRI or CRBSI (1,60). The current U.S. guideline for prevention of intravascular device-related infections (6) allows for guidewire exchange for suspected CRI only in the absence of local signs of infection such as inflammation and purulent discharge. Another exchange to a new site becomes necessary, if the culture result of the removed catheter indicates significant catheter colonization. Therefore, the clinician must weigh the risks for complications associated with the procedure against the risks of recurrent infection.

Intravenous Therapy Teams

Prospective studies demonstrated a significantly higher incidence rate of phlebitis among catheters inserted and maintained by floor staff than among those devices inserted and/or maintained by a specifically appointed IV therapy team (162,163). In addition, these catheter teams have also been shown to be highly cost-effective (48,163). A randomized controlled trial has been performed with peripheral catheters only (163). The rate of phlebitis was 1% in the staff-inserted group and 0.2% in the team-inserted group. However, as mentioned above, catheter material and catheter care have changed over time, and findings from older studies may not necessarily apply for today's conditions. As pointed out by Puntis and colleagues, staff training is a key factor in reducing catheter-related infections (158). It is conceivable that professional teams are less likely to inadvertently contaminate the catheter than nurses on the ward without specific training. However, most CVCs are inserted in ICUs where all health-care workers should have appropriate training in catheter care.

Antimicrobial Prophylaxis

Several studies indicated that systemic antimicrobial prophylaxis at the time of insertion of long-term catheters reduced the risk for CRBSI (164–167). However, two randomized trials failed to show a benefit from antimicrobial prophylaxis (168,169). Recently, a systematic review of the prophylactic use of antibiotics prior to the insertion of tunneled long-term CVCs revealed that the prophylactic use of vancomycin/teicoplanin decreased the number of Gram-positive infections (170). This issue remains controversial for long-term catheters, but it is currently not recommended for short-term CVCs. Some data indicate that prophylaxis may be warranted in neonates weighing <1000 g or in patients undergoing bone marrow transplantation (171). However, increased prophylactic use of glycopeptides may be associated with the emergence of vancomycin-resistant enterococci.

SUMMARY

Diagnosis of CRI and CRBSI remains difficult. Clinical signs of infection are frequently absent making the laboratory diagnosis very important. However, the optimal microbiological method to confirm a clinical diagnosis of CRI or CRBSI is still controversial. Removal of the catheter, quantitative culture of the catheter segment, and empirical antimicrobial treatment are recommended for episodes of suspected BSI related to short-term catheters. As an exception, most episodes due to CoNS can be treated with antimicrobial agents without catheter removal. Many different approaches are necessary for the prevention of these serious nosocomial infections. In the future, commercially available, coated catheters may help to further reduce the incidence of CRI and CRBSI; however, despite numerous studies their role still remains to be defined. The current CDC guideline as well as other national guidelines for the prevention of intravascular catheter-related infections may help to adapt the current science to hospital practice (6). However, much remains to be learned about the pathogenesis, prevention, and treatment of CRI and CRBSI.

REFERENCES

1. Maki DG. Pathogenesis, prevention, and management of infections due to intravascular devices used for infusion therapy. In: Bisno AL, Waldvogel FA,

eds. Infections Associated with Indwelling Medical Devices. Washington, D.C.: American Society for Microbiology, 1994:155–212.

2. Nyström B, Larsen SO, Dankert J, Daschner F, Greco D, Grönroos P, Jepsen OB, Lystad A, Meers PD, Rotter M. Bacteraemia in surgical patients with intravenous devices: a European multicentre incidence study. The European Working Party on Control of Hospital Infections. J Hosp Infect 1983; 4:338–349.

3. Neuhof H, Seley GP. Acute suppurative phlebitis complicated by septicemia. Surgery 1947; 21:831–842.

4. Centers for Disease Control Working Group. Guidelines for prevention of intravenous therapy-related infections. Infect Control 1981; 3:62–79.

5. Pearson ML. Guideline for prevention of intravascular device-related infections. Hospital Infection Control Practices Advisory Committee. Infect Control Hosp Epidemiol 1996; 17:438–473.

6. O'Grady NP, Alexander M, Dellinger EP, Gerberding JL, Heard SO, Maki DG, Masur H, McCormick RD, Mermel LA, Pearson ML, Raad II, Randolph A, Weinstein RA. Guidelines for the prevention of intravascular catheter-related infections. The Hospital Infection Control Practices Advisory Committee, Center for Disease Control and Prevention. Pediatrics 2002; 110:e51.

7. Maki DG, Weise CE, Sarafin HW. A semiquantitative culture method for identifying intravenous-catheter-related infection. N Engl J Med 1977; 296:1305–1309.

8. Sherertz RJ, Raad II, Belani A, Koo LC, Rand KH, Pickett DL, Straub SA, Fauerbach LL. Three-year experience with sonicated vascular catheter cultures in a clinical microbiology laboratory. J Clin Microbiol 1990; 28:76–82.

9. Blot F, Nitenberg G, Chachaty E, Raynard B, Germann N, Antoun S, Laplanche A, Brun-Buisson C, Tancrede C. Diagnosis of catheter-related bacteraemia: a prospective comparison of the time to positivity of hub-blood versus peripheral-blood cultures. Lancet 1999; 354:1071–1077.

10. Seifert H, Cornely O, Seggewiss K, Decker M, Stefanik D, Wisplinghoff H, Fatkenheuer G. Bloodstream infection in neutropenic cancer patients related to short-term nontunnelled catheters determined by quantitative blood cultures, differential time to positivity, and molecular epidemiological typing with pulsed-field gel electrophoresis. J Clin Microbiol 2003; 41:118–123.

11. Richards MJ, Edwards JR, Culver DH, Gaynes RP. Nosocomial infections in medical intensive care units in the United States. National Nosocomial Infections Surveillance System [see comments]. Crit Care Med 1999; 27:887–892.

12. Arnow PM, Quimosing EM, Beach M. Consequences of intravascular catheter sepsis. Clin Infect Dis 1993; 16:778–784.

13. Pittet D, Tarara D, Wenzel RP. Nosocomial bloodstream infection in critically ill patients. Excess length of stay, extra costs, and attributable mortality. JAMA 1994; 271:1598–1601.

14. Maki DG. Nosocomial bacteremia. An epidemiologic overview. Am J Med 1981; 70:719–732.

15. Pittet D, Wenzel RP. Nosocomial bloodstream infections. Secular trends in rates, mortality, and contribution to total hospital deaths. Arch Intern Med 1995; 155:1177–1184.

16. Pittet D, Hulliger S, Auckenthaler R. Intravascular device-related infections in critically ill patients. J Chemother 1995; 7(suppl 3):55–66.
17. Ruden H, Gastmeier P, Daschner FD, Schumacher M. Nosocomial and community-acquired infections in Germany. Summary of the results of the First National Prevalence Study (NIDEP). Infection 1997; 25:199–202.
18. Vincent JL, Bihari DJ, Suter PM, Bruining HA, White J, Nicolas-Chanoin MH, Wolff M, Spencer RC, Hemmer M. The prevalence of nosocomial infection in intensive care units in Europe. Results of the European Prevalence of Infection in Intensive Care (EPIC) Study. EPIC International Advisory Committee. JAMA 1995; 274:639–644.
19. Flowers RH, Schwenzer KJ, Kopel RF, Fisch MJ, Tucker SI, Farr BM. Efficacy of an attachable subcutaneous cuff for the prevention of intravascular catheter-related infection. A randomized, controlled trial [see comments]. JAMA 1989; 261:878–883.
20. Maki DG, Cobb L, Garman JK, Shapiro JM, Ringer M, Helgerson RB. An attachable silver-impregnated cuff for prevention of infection with central venous catheters: a prospective randomized multicenter trial. Am J Med 1988; 85:307–314.
21. Richet H, Hubert B, Nitemberg G, Andremont A, Buu-Hoi A, Ourbak P, Galicier C, Veron M, Boisivon A, Bouvier AM, Ricome JC, Wolff MA, Pean Y, Berardi-Grassias L, Bourdaiu JL, Hautefort B, Laaban JP, Tillant D. Prospective multicenter study of vascular-catheter-related complications and risk factors for positive central-catheter cultures in intensive care unit patients. J Clin Microbiol 1990; 28:2520–2525.
22. Eyer S, Brummitt C, Crossley K, Siegel R, Cerra F. Catheter-related sepsis: prospective, randomized study of three methods of long-term catheter maintenance. Crit Care Med 1990; 18:1073–1079.
23. Elliott TSJ, Faroqui MH, Tebbs SE, Armstrong RF, Hanson GC. An audit programme for central venous catheter-associated infections. J Hosp Infect 1995; 30:181–191.
24. Jarvis WR, Edwards JR, Culver DH, Hughes JM, Horan T, Emori TG, Banerjee S, Tolson J, Henderson T, Gaynes RP, et al. Nosocomial infection rates in adult and pediatric intensive care units in the United States. National Nosocomial Infections Surveillance System. Am J Med 1991; 91:185S–191S.
25. Norwood S, Ruby A, Civetta J, Cortes V. Catheter-related infections and associated septicemia. Chest 1991; 99:968–975.
26. National Nosocomial Infections Surveillance (NNIS) System Report, Data Summary from January 1992–June 2001, issued August 2001. Am J Infect Control 2001; 29:404–421.
27. Smith RL, Meixler SM, Simberkoff MS. Excess mortality in critically ill patients with nosocomial bloodstream infections. Chest 1991; 100:164–167.
28. Renaud B, Brun-Buisson C. ICU-Bacteremia Study Group. Outcomes of primary and catheter-related bacteremia. A cohort and case-control study in critically ill patients. Am J Respir Crit Care Med 2001; 163:1584–1590.
29. Rello J, Ochagavia A, Sabanes E, Roque M, Mariscal D, Reynaga E, Valles J. Evaluation of outcome of intravenous catheter-related infections in critically ill patients. Am J Respir Crit Care Med 2000; 162:1027–1030.

30. Eggimann P, Harbarth S, Constantin MN, Touveneau S, Chevrolet JC, Pittet D. Impact of a prevention strategy targeted at vascular-access care on incidence of infections acquired in intensive care. Lancet 2000; 355(9218):1864–1868.

31. Maki DG, Jarrett F, Sarafin HW. A semiquantitative culture method for identification of catheter-related infection in the burn patient. J Surg Res 1977; 22:513–520.

32. Pruitt BA Jr, Stein JM, Foley FD, Moncrief JA, O'Neill JA Jr. Intravenous therapy in burn patients. Suppurative thrombophlebitis and other life-threatening complications. Arch Surg 1970; 100:399–404.

33. Franceschi D, Gerding RL, Phillips G, Fratianne RB. Risk factors associated with intravascular catheter infections in burned patients: a prospective, randomized study. J Trauma 1989; 29:811–816.

34. Gregory JA, Schiller WR. Subclavian catheter changes every third day in high risk patients. Am Surg 1985; 51:534–536.

35. Husain MT, Karim QN, Tajuri S. Analysis of infection in a burn ward. Burns 1989; 15:299–302.

36. Raad I, Darouiche R, Dupuis J, Abi-Said D, Gabrielli A, Hachem R, Wall M, Harris R, Jones J, Buzaid A, Robertson C, Shenaq S, Curling P, Burke T, Ericsson C. Central venous catheters coated with minocycline and rifampin for the prevention of catheter-related colonization and bloodstream infections. A randomized, double-blind trial. The Texas Medical Center Catheter Study Group. Ann Intern Med 1997; 127:267–274.

37. Latarjet J. A simple guide to burn treatment. International Society for Burn Injuries in collaboration with the World Health Organization. Burns 1995; 21:221–225.

38. Sheridan RL, Weber JM, Peterson HF, Tompkins RG. Central venous catheter sepsis with weekly catheter change in paediatric burn patients: an analysis of 221 catheters. Burns 1995; 21:127–129.

39. Raviglione MC, Battan R, Pablos-Mendez A, Aceves-Casillas P, Mullen MP, Taranta A. Infections associated with Hickman catheters in patients with the acquired immunodeficiency virus. Am J Med 1989; 86:780–786.

40. Jacobson MA, Gellermann H, Chambers H. *Staphylococcus aureus* bacteremia and recurrent staphylococcal infection in patients with acquired immunodeficiency syndrome and AIDS-related complex. Am J Med 1988; 85:172–176.

41. Buchman AL, Guss W, Ament ME. *Staphylococcus aureus* Hickman catheter infections. Am J Med 1991; 91:103–104.

42. Raviglione MC, Mariuz P, Pablos-Mendez A, Battan R, Ottuso P, Taranta A. High *Staphylococcus aureus* nasal carriage rate in patients with acquired immunodeficiency syndrome or AIDS-related complex. Am J Infect Control 1990; 18:64–69.

43. Stanley HD, Charlebois E, Harb G, Jacobson MA. Central venous catheter infections in AIDS patients receiving treatment for cytomegalovirus disease. J Acquir Immune Defic Syndr 1994; 7:272–278.

44. D'Angio R, Quercia RA, Treiber NK, McLaughlin JC, Klimek JJ. The growth of microorganisms in total parenteral nutrition admixtures. JPEN J Parenter Enteral Nutr 1987; 11:394–397.

45. Gilbert M, Gallagher SC, Eads M, Elmore MF. Microbial growth patterns in

a total parenteral nutrition formulation containing lipid emulsion. JPEN J Parenter Enteral Nutr 1986; 10:494–497.

46. Goldmann DA, Martin WT, Worthington JW. Growth of bacteria and fungi in total parenteral nutrition solutions. Am J Surg 1973; 126:314–318.

47. Armstrong CW, Mayhall CG, Miller KB, Newsome HH Jr, Sugerman HJ, Dalton HP, Hall GO, Hunsberger S. Clinical predictors of infection of central venous catheters used for total parenteral nutrition. Infect Control Hosp Epidemiol 1990; 11:71–78.

48. Faubion WC, Wesley JR, Khalidi N, Silva J. Total parenteral nutrition catheter sepsis: impact of the team approach. JPEN J Parenter Enteral Nutr 1986; 10:642–645.

49. McCarthy MC, Shives JK, Robison RJ, Broadie TA. Prospective evaluation of single and triple lumen catheters in total parenteral nutrition. JPEN J Parenter Enteral Nutr 1987; 11:259–262.

50. Bonadimani B, Sperti C, Stevanin A, Cappellazzo F, Militello C, Petrin P, Pedrazzoli S. Central venous catheter guidewire replacement according to the Seldinger technique: usefulness in the management of patients on total parenteral nutrition. JPEN J Parenter Enteral Nutr 1987; 11:267–270.

51. Snydman DR, Murray SA, Kornfeld SJ, Majka JA, Ellis CA. Total parenteral nutrition-related infections. Prospective epidemiologic study using semi-quantitative methods. Am J Med 1982; 73:695–699.

52. Dankner WM, Spector SA, Fierer J, Davis CE. *Malassezia* fungemia in neonates and adults: complication of hyperalimentation. Rev Infect Dis 1987; 9:743–753.

53. Garcia CR, Johnston BL, Corvi G, Walker LJ, George WL. Intravenous catheter-associated *Malassezia furfur* fungemia. Am J Med 1987; 83:790–792.

54. Halpin TC, Dahms BB. Complications associated with intravenous lipids in infants and children. Acta Chir Scand 1983; 517(suppl):169–177.

55. Wey SB, Mori M, Pfaller MA, Woolson RF, Wenzel RP. Risk factors for hospital-acquired candidemia. A matched case-control study. Arch Intern Med 1989; 149:2349–2353.

56. Ryan JA Jr, Abel RM, Abbott WM, Hopkins CC, Chesney TM, Colley R, Phillips K, Fischer JE. Catheter complications in total parenteral nutrition. A prospective study of 200 consecutive patients. N Engl J Med 1974; 290:757–761.

57. Yeung C, May J, Hughes R. Infection rate for single lumen v triple lumen subclavian catheters. Infect Control Hosp Epidemiol 1988; 9:154–158.

58. Howard L, Claunch C, McDowell R, Timchalk M. Five years of experience in patients receiving home nutrition support with the implanted reservoir: a comparison with the external catheter. JPEN J Parenter Enteral Nutr 1989; 13:478–483.

59. Danzig LE, Short LJ, Collins K, Mahoney M, Sepe S, Bland L, Jarvis WR. Bloodstream infections associated with a needleless intravenous infusion system in patients receiving home infusion therapy. JAMA 1995; 273:1862–1864.

60. Pettigrew RA, Lang SD, Haydock DA, Parry BR, Bremner DA, Hill GL. Catheter-related sepsis in patients on intravenous nutrition: a prospective study of quantitative catheter cultures and guidewire changes for suspected sepsis. Br J Surg 1985; 72:52–55.

61. Vanhuynegem L, Parmentier P, Potvliege C. In situ bacteriologic diagnosis of total parenteral nutrition catheter infection. Surgery 1988; 103:174–177.

62. Benoit JL, Carandang G, Sitrin M, Arnow PM. Intraluminal antibiotic treatment of central venous catheter infections in patients receiving parenteral nutrition at home. Clin Infect Dis 1995; 21:1286–1288.

63. Garrison RN, Wilson MA. Intravenous and central catheter infections. Surg Clin North Am 1994; 74:557–570.

64. Maki DG, Stolz SS, Wheeler S, Mermel LA. A prospective, randomized trial of gauze and two polyurethane dressings for site care of pulmonary artery catheters: implications for catheter management. Crit Care Med 1994; 22:1729–1737.

65. Mermel LA, Maki DG. Infectious complications of Swan–Ganz pulmonary artery catheters. Pathogenesis, epidemiology, prevention, and management. Am J Respir Crit Care Med 1994; 149:1020–1036.

66. Raad II, Hohn DC, Gilbreath BJ, Suleiman N, Hill LA, Bruso PA, Marts K, Mansfield PF, Bodey GP. Prevention of central venous catheter-related infections by using maximal sterile barrier precautions during insertion. Infect Control Hosp Epidemiol 1994; 15:231–238.

67. Wisplinghoff H, Bischoff T, Tallent SM, Seifert H, Wenzel RP, Edmond MB. Nosocomial bloodstream infections in United States hospitals: analysis of 24,000 cases from a prospective nationwide surveillance study. Clin Infect Dis 2004. In press.

68. Rupp ME, Archer GL. Coagulase-negative staphylococci: pathogens associated with medical progress. Clin Infect Dis 1994; 19:231–243.

69. Voss A, Milatovic D, Wallrauch Schwarz C, Rosdahl VT, Braveny I. Methicillin-resistant *Staphylococcus aureus* in Europe. Eur J Clin Microbiol Infect Dis 1994; 13:50–55.

70. Meyer E, Jonas D, Schwab F, Rueden H, Gastmeier P, Daschner FD. Design of a surveillance system of antibiotic use and bacterial resistance in German intensive care units (SARI). Infection 2003; 31:208–215.

71. Siegman-Igra Y, Anglim AM, Shapiro DE, Adal KA, Strain BA, Farr BM. Diagnosis of vascular catheter-related bloodstream infection: a meta-analysis. J Clin Microbiol 1997; 35:928–936.

72. Raad II, Baba M, Bodey GP. Diagnosis of catheter-related infections: the role of surveillance and targeted quantitative skin cultures. Clin Infect Dis 1995; 20:593–597.

73. Cercenado E, Ena J, Rodriguez-Creixems M, Romero I, Bouza E. A conservative procedure for the diagnosis of catheter-related infections. Arch Intern Med 1990; 150:1417–1420.

74. Groeger Js, Lucas AB, Thaler HT, Friedlander-Klar H, Brown AE, Kiehn TE, Armstrong D. Infectious morbidity associated with long term use of venous access devices in patients with cancer. Ann Intern Med 1993; 119:1168–1174.

75. Raad II, Sabbagh MF, Rand KH, Sherertz RJ. Quantitative tip culture methods and the diagnosis of central venous catheter-related infections. Diagn Microbiol Infect Dis 1992; 15:13 20.

76. Sherertz RJ, Heard SO, Raad II. Diagnosis of triple-lumen catheter infection: comparison of roll plate, sonication, and flushing methodologies. J Clin Microbiol 1997; 35:641–646.

77. Widmer AF, Frei R. Diagnosis of Central-Venous Catheter-Related Infection: Comparison of the Roll-Plate and Sonication Technique in 1000 Catheters. Interscience Conference on Antimicrobial Agents and Chemotherapy 2003, Chicago, IL, 2003 [K-2036].

78. Raad I, Hanna HA, Alakech B, Chatzinikolaou I, Johnson MM, Tarrand J. Differential time to positivity: a useful method for diagnosing catheter-related bloodstream infections. Ann Intern Med 2004; 140:18–25.

79. Mitchell A, Atkins S, Royle GT, Kettlewell MG. Reduced catheter sepsis and prolonged catheter life using a tunnelled silicone rubber catheter for total parenteral nutrition. Br J Surg 1982; 69:420–422.

80. Tebbs SE, Elliott TS. Modification of central venous catheter polymers to prevent in vitro microbial colonisation. Eur J Clin Microbiol Infect Dis 1994; 13:111–117.

81. Widmer AF, Frei R, Rajacic Z, Zimmerli W. Correlation between in vivo and in vitro efficacy of antimicrobial agents against foreign body infections. J Infect Dis 1990; 162:96–102.

82. Widmer AF, Gaechter A, Ochsner PE, Zimmerli W. Antimicrobial treatment of orthopedic implant-related infections with rifampin combinations. Clin Infect Dis 1992; 14:1251–1253.

83. Zimmerli W, Frei R, Widmer AF, Rajacic Z. Microbiological tests to predict treatment outcome in experimental device-related infections due to *Staphylococcus aureus*. J Antimicrob Chemother 1994; 33:959–967.

84. Sherertz RJ, Carruth WA, Hampton AA, Byron MP, Solomon DD. Efficacy of antibiotic-coated catheters in preventing subcutaneous *Staphylococcus aureus* infection in rabbits. J Infect Dis 1993; 167:98–106.

85. Sherertz RJ, Forman DM, Solomon DD. Efficacy of dicloxacillin-coated polyurethane catheters in preventing subcutaneous *Staphylococcus aureus* infection in mice. Antimicrob Agents Chemother 1989; 33:1174–1178.

86. Cooper GL, Schiller AL, Hopkins CC. Possible role of capillary action in pathogenesis of experimental catheter-associated dermal tunnel infections. J Clin Microbiol 1988; 26:8–12.

87. Groeger Js, Lucas AB, Coit D, LaQuaglia M, Brown AE, Turnbull A, Exelby P. A prospective, randomized evaluation of the effect of silver impregnated subcutaneous cuffs for preventing tunneled chronic venous access catheter infections in cancer patients. Ann Surg 1993; 218:206–210.

88. Dahlberg PJ, Agger WA, Singer JR, Yutuc WR, Newcomer KL, Schaper A, Rooney BL. Subclavian hemodialysis catheter infections: a prospective, randomized trial of an attachable silver-impregnated cuff for prevention of catheter-related infections. Infect Control Hosp Epidemiol 1995; 16:506–511.

89. Smith HO, DeVictoria CL, Garfinkel D, Anderson P, Goldberg GL, Soeiro R, Elia G, Runowicz CD. A prospective randomized comparison of an attached silver-impregnated cuff to prevent central venous catheter-associated infection. Gynecol Oncol 1995; 58:92–100.

90. Greenfeld JI, Sampath L, Popilskis SJ, Brunnert SR, Stylianos S, Modak S. Decreased bacterial adherence and biofilm formation on chlorhexidine and silver sulfadiazine-impregnated central venous catheters implanted in swine. Crit Care Med 1995; 23:894–900.

91. Farber BF, Wolff AG. The use of nonsteroidal anti-inflammatory drugs to prevent adherence of *Staphylococcus epidermis* to medical polymers. J Infect Dis 1992; 166:861–865.

92. Mermel LA, Stolz SM, Maki DG. Surface antimicrobial activity of heparin-bonded and antiseptic-impregnated vascular catheters. J Infect Dis 1993; 167: 920–924.

93. Kamal GD, Pfaller MA, Rempe LE, Jebson PJ. Reduced intravascular catheter infection by antibiotic bonding. A prospective, randomized, controlled trial. JAMA 1991; 265:2364–2368.

94. Veenstra DL, Saint S, Saha S, Lumley T, Sullivan SD. Efficacy of antiseptic-impregnated central venous catheters in preventing catheter-related bloodstream infection: a meta-analysis. JAMA 1999; 281:261–267.

95. Darouiche RO, Raad II, Heard SO, Thornby JI, Wenker OC, Gabrielli A, Berg J, Khardori N, Hanna H, Hachem R, Harris RL, Mayhall G. A comparison of two antimicrobial-impregnated central venous catheters. Catheter Study Group. N Engl J Med 1999; 340:1–8.

96. Raad I, Darouiche R, Hachem R, Mansouri M, Bodey GP. The broad-spectrum activity and efficacy of catheters coated with minocycline and rifampin. J Infect Dis 1996; 173:418–424.

96a. Crnich CJ, Maki DG. The promise of novel technology for the prevention of intravascular device-related bloodstream infection: I. Pathogenesis and short-term devices. Clin Infect Dis 2002; 34:1232–1242.

97. Maki DG, Stolz SM, Wheeler S, Mermel LA. Prevention of central venous catheter-related bloodstream infection by use of an antiseptic-impregnated catheter. A randomized, controlled trial. Ann Intern Med 1997; 127:257–266.

98. Veenstra DL, Saint S, Sullivan SD. Cost-effectiveness of antiseptic-impregnated central venous catheters for the prevention of catheter-related bloodstream infection. JAMA 1999; 282:554–560.

99. Pratt RJ, Pellowe C, Loveday HP, Robinson N, Smith GW, Barrett S, Davey P, Harper P, Loveday C, McDougall C, Mulhall A, Privett S, Smales C, Taylor L, Weller B, Wilcox M, Department of Health (England). The epic project: developing national evidence-based guidelines for preventing health-care associated infections. Phase I: Guidelines for preventing hospital-acquired infections. Department of Health (England). J Hosp Infect 2001; 47(suppl):S3–S82.

100. Trautmann M, Jansen B, Frey P, Hummler H, Rasche M, Scheringer I, Schwalbe B. Prävention Gefäßkatheter-assoziierter Infektionen. Bundesgesundheitsbl Gesundheitsforsch Gesundheitsschutz 2002; 45:907–924.

101. Raad I, Davis S, Khan A, Tarrand J, Elting L, Bodey GP. Impact of central venous catheter removal on the recurrence of catheter-related coagulase-negative staphylococcal bacteremia. Infect Control Hosp Epidemiol 1992; 13: 215–221.

102. Elliott TS, Faroqui MH, Armstrong RF, Hanson GC. Guidelines for good practice in central venous catheterization. Hospital Infection Society and the Research Unit of the Royal College of Physicians. J Hosp Infect 1994; 28: 163–176.

103. Burgert SJ, Classen DC, Burke JP, Blatter DD. Candidal brain abscess asso-

ciated with vascular invasion: a devastating complication of vascular catheter-related candidemia. Clin Infect Dis 1995; 21:202–205.

104. Lecciones JA, Lee JW, Navarro EE, Witebsky FG, Marshall D, Steinberg SM, Pizzo PA, Walsh TJ. Vascular catheter-associated fungemia in patients with cancer: analysis of 155 episodes. Clin Infect Dis 1992; 14:875–883.

105. Raad II, Sabbagh MF. Optimal duration of therapy for catheter-related *Staphylococcus aureus* bacteremia: a study of 55 cases and review. Clin Infect Dis 1992; 14:75–82.

106. Jernigan JA, Farr BM. Short-course therapy of catheter-related *Staphylococcus aureus* bacteremia: a meta-analysis. Ann Intern Med 1993; 119:304–311.

107. Malanoski GJ, Samore MH, Pefanis A, Karchmer AW. *Staphylococcus aureus* catheter-associated bacteremia. Minimal effective therapy and unusual infectious complications associated with arterial sheath catheters. Arch Intern Med 1995; 55:1161–1166.

108. Mermel LA, Farr BM, Sherertz RJ, Raad II, O'Grady N, Harris JS, Craven DE. Infectious Diseases Society of America; American College of Critical Care Medicine; Society for Healthcare Epidemiology of America. Guidelines for the management of intravascular catheter-related infections. Clin Infect Dis 2001; 32:1249–1272.

109. Raad I, Hanna H, Boktour M, Girgawy E, Danawi H, Mardani M, Kontoyiannis D, Darouiche R, Hachem R, Bodey GP. Management of central venous catheters in patients with cancer and candidemia. Clin Infect Dis 2004; 38:1119–1127.

110. Kibbler CC, Seaton S, Barnes RA, Gransden WR, Holliman RE, Johnson EM, Perry JD, Sullivan DJ, Wilson JA. Management and outcome of bloodstream infections due to *Candida* species in England and Wales. J Hosp Infect 2003; 54:18–24.

111. Fowler VG, Sanders LL, Sexton DJ. Outcome of *Staphylococcus aureus* bacteremia according to compliance with recommendations of infectious diseases specialist: experience with 244 patients. Clin Infect Dis 1998; 27:478–486.

112. Capdevila JA, Segarra A, Planes AM, Gasser I, Gavalda J, Pahissa A. Long term follow-up of patients with catheter related sepsis (CRS) treated without catheter removal [Abstract J3]. Programs and Abstracts of the 35th Interscience Conference of Antimicrobial Agents and Chemotherapy. San Francisco.

113. Peacock SJ, Curtis N, Berendt AR, Bowler IC, Winearls CG, Maxwell P. Outcome following haemodialysis catheter-related *Staphylococcus aureus* bacteremia. J Hosp Infect 1999; 41:223–228.

114. Viale P, Pagani L, Petrosillo N, Signorini L, Colombini P, Macri G, Cristini F, Gattuso G, Carosi G. Italian Hospital and HIV Infection Group. Antibiotic lock-technique for the treatment of catheter-related bloodstream infections. J Chemother 2003; 15:152–156.

115. Droste JC, Jeraj HA, MacDonald A, Farrington K. Stability and in vitro efficacy of antibiotic-heparin lock solutions potentially useful for treatment of central venous catheter-related sepsis. J Antimicrob Chemother 2003; 51:849–855.

116. Farber BF, Kaplan H, Clogston AG. *Staphylococcus epidermidis* extracted slime inhibits the antimicrobial action of glycopeptide antibiotics. J Infect Dis 1990; 161:37–40.

117. Darouiche RO, Dhir A, Miller AJ, Landon GC, Raad II, Musher DM. Vancomycin penetration into biofilm covering infected prostheses and effect on bacteria. J Infect Dis 1994; 170:720–723.

118. Widmer AF, Pittet D. Optimal duration of therapy for catheter-related *Staphylococcus aureus* bacteremia. Clin Infect Dis 1992; 14:1259–1260.

119. Raad I, Narro J, Khan A, Tarrand J, Vartivarian S, Bodey GP. Serious complications of vascular catheter-related *Staphylococcus aureus* bacteremia in cancer patients. Eur J Clin Microbiol Infect Dis 1992; 11:675–682.

120. Fowler VG Jr, Sanders LL, Kong LK, McClelland RS, Gottlieb GS, Li J, Ryan T, Sexton DJ, Roussakis G, Harrell LJ, Corey GR. Infective endocarditis due to *Staphylococcus aureus*: 59 prospectively identified cases with follow-up. Clin Infect Dis 1999; 28:106–114.

121. Pigrau C, Rodriguez D, Planes AM, Almirante B, Larrosa N, Ribera E, Gavalda J, Pahissa A. Management of catheter-related *Staphylococcus aureus* bacteremia: when may sonographic study be unnecessary? Eur J Clin Microbiol Infect Dis 2003; 22:713–719.

122. Cosgrove SE, Sakoulas G, Perencevich EN, Schwaber MJ, Karchmer AW, Carmeli Y. Comparison of mortality associated with methicillin-resistant and methicillin-susceptible *Staphylococcus aureus* bacteremia: a meta-analysis. Clin Infect Dis 2003; 36:53–59.

123. Blot SI, Vandewoude KH, Hoste EA, Colardyn FA. Outcome and attributable mortality in critically ill patients with bacteremia involving methicillin-susceptible and methicillin-resistant *Staphylococcus aureus*. Arch Intern Med 2002; 162:2229–2235.

124. Kollef MH, Rello J, Cammarata SK, Croos-Dabrera RV, Wunderink RG. Clinical cure and survival in Gram-positive ventilator-associated pneumonia: retrospective analysis of two double-blind studies comparing linezolid with vancomycin. Intensive Care Med 2004; 30:388–394.

125. Hilf M, Yu VL, Sharp J. Antibiotic therapy for *Pseudomonas aeruginosa* bacteremia: outcome correlation in a prospective study of 200 patients. Am J Med 1989; 87:540–547.

126. Chamot E, Boffi El Amari E, Rohner P, Van Delden C. Effectiveness of combination antimicrobial therapy for *Pseudomonas aeruginosa* bacteremia. Antimicrob Agents Chemother 2003; 47:2756–2764.

127. Hyatt JM, Nix DE, Stratton CW, Schentag JJ. In vitro pharmacodynamics of piperacillin, piperacillin–tazobactam, and ciprofloxacin alone and in combination against *Staphylococcus aureus*, *Klebsiella pneumoniae*, *Enterobacter cloacae*, and *Pseudomonas aeruginosa*. Antimicrob Agents Chemother 1995; 39:1711–1716.

128. Pfaller MA, Diekema DJ. International Fungal Surveillance Participant Group. Twelve years of fluconazole in clinical practice: global trends in species distribution and fluconazole susceptibility of bloodstream isolates of *Candida*. Clin Microbiol Infect 2004; 10(suppl 1):11–23.

129. Iwen PC, Kelly DM, Reed EC, Hinrichs SH. Invasive infection due to *Candida krusei* in immunocompromised patients not treated with fluconazole. Clin Infect Dis 1995; 20:342–347.

130. Rex JH, Bennett JE, Sugar AM, Pappas PG, Serody J, Edwards JE, Washburn RG. Intravascular catheter exchange and duration of candidemia.

NIAID Mycoses Study Group and the Candidemia Study Group. Clin Infect Dis 1995; 21:994–996.

131. Nucci M, Colombo AL, Silveira F, Richtmann R, Salomao R, Branchini ML, Spector N. Risk factors for death in patients with candidemia. Infect Control Hosp Epidemiol 1998; 19:846–850.

132. Dannenberg C, Bierbach U, Rothe A, Beer J, Korholz D. Ethanol-lock technique in the treatment of bloodstream infections in pediatric oncology patients with Broviac catheter. J Pediatr Hematol Oncol 2003; 25:616–621.

133. Zuschneid I, Schwab F, Geffers C, Ruden H, Gastmeier P. Reducing central venous catheter-associated primary bloodstream infections in intensive care units is possible: data from the German nosocomial infection surveillance system. Infect Control Hosp Epidemiol 2003; 24:501–505.

134. Gil RT, Kruse JA, Thill-Baharozian MC, Carlson RW. Triple- vs single-lumen central venous catheters. A prospective study in a critically ill population. Arch Intern Med 1989; 149:1139–1143.

135. Mermel LA, McCormick RD, Springman SR, Maki DG. The pathogenesis and epidemiology of catheter-related infection with pulmonary artery Swan–Ganz catheters: a prospective study utilizing molecular subtyping. Am J Med 1991; 91(suppl 3B):197S–205S.

136. Pinilla JC, Ross DF, Martin T, Crump H. Study of the incidence of intra-vascular catheter infection and associated bacteremia in critically ill patients. Crit Care Med 1983; 11:21–25.

137. Prager RL, Silva J Jr. Colonization of central venous catheters. South Med J 1984; 77:458–461.

138. Michel L, McMichan JC, Bachy JL. Microbial colonization of indwelling central venous catheters: statistical evaluation of potential contaminating factors. Am J Surg 1979; 137:745–748.

139. Timsit JF, Bruneel F, Cheval C, Mamzer MF, Garrouste-Orgeas M, Wolff M, Misset B, Chevret S, Regnier B, Carlet J. Use of tunneled femoral catheters to prevent catheter-related infection. A randomized, controlled trial. Ann Intern Med 1999; 130:729–735.

140. Trottier SJ, Veremakis C, Brien JO, Auer AI. Femoral deep vein thrombosis associated with central venous catheterization: results from a prospective, randomized trial. Crit Care Med 1995; 23:52–59.

141. Maki DG, McCormack KN. Defatting catheter insertion sites in total parenteral nutrition is of no value as an infection control measure. Controlled clinical trial. Am J Med 1987; 83:833–840.

142. Maki DG, Band JD. A comparative study of polyantibiotic and iodophor ointments in prevention of vascular catheter-related infection. Am J Med 1981; 70:739–744.

143. Orth B, Frei R, Itin PH, Rinaldi MG, Speck B, Gratwohl A, Widmer AF. Outbreak of invasive mycoses caused by *Paecilomyces lilacinus* from a contaminated skin lotion. Ann Intern Med 1996; 125:799–806.

144. Maki DG, Ringer M, Alvarado CJ. Prospective randomised trial of povidone-iodine, alcohol, and chlorhexidine for prevention of infection associated with central venous and arterial catheters. Lancet 1991; 338:339–343.

145. Doebbeling BN, Stanley GL, Sheetz CT, Pfaller MA, Houston AK, Annis L, Li N, Wenzel RP. Comparative efficacy of alternative hand-washing agents in

reducing nosocomial infections in intensive care units. N Engl J Med 1992; 327:88–93.

146. Widmer AF, Perschmann M, Gasser TC, Frei R. Alcohol vs chlorhexidine-gluconate for preoperative hand scrub: a randomized cross-over clinical trial [abstr]. Interscience Conference on Antimicrobial Agents and Chemotherapy, Orlando, Florida, 1994.

147. Conly JM, Grieves K, Peters B. A prospective, randomized study comparing transparent and dry gauze dressings for central venous catheters. J Infect Dis 1989; 159:310–319.

148. Maki DG, Ringer M. Evaluation of dressing regimens for prevention of infection with peripheral intravenous catheters. Gauze, a transparent polyure-thane dressing, and an iodophor-transparent dressing. JAMA 1987; 258:2396–2403.

149. Ricard P, Martin R, Marcoux JA. Protection of indwelling vascular catheters: incidence of bacterial contamination and catheter-related sepsis. Crit Care Med 1985; 13:541–543.

150. Young GP, Alexeyeff M, Russell DM, Thomas RJ. Catheter sepsis during parenteral nutrition: the safety of long-term OpSite dressings. JPEN J Parenter Enteral Nutr 1988; 12:365–370.

151. Vazquez RM, Jarrard MM. Care of the central venous catheterization site: the use of a transparent polyurethane film. JPEN J Parenter Enteral Nutr 1984; 8:181–186.

152. Hoffmann KK, Weber DJ, Samsa GP, Rutala WA. Transparent polyurethane film as an intravenous catheter dressing. JAMA 1992; 267:2072–2076.

153. Moro ML, Vigano EF, Cozzi Lepri A. Risk factors for central venous catheter-related infections in surgical and intensive care units. The Central Venous Catheter-Related Infections Study Group. Infect Control Hosp Epidemiol 1994; 5:253–264.

154. Hoffmann KK, Western SA, Kaiser DL, Wenzel RP, Groschel DH. Bacterial colonization and phlebitis-associated risk with transparent polyurethane film for peripheral intravenous site dressings. Am J Infect Control 1988; 16:101–106.

155. Bregenzer T, Conen D, Sakmann P, Widmer AF. Is routine replacement of peripheral intravenous catheters necessary? Arch Intern Med 1998; 158:151–156.

156. Cobb DK, High KP, Sawyer RG, Sable CA, Adams RB, Lindley DA, Pruett TL, Schwenzer KJ, Farr BM. A controlled trial of scheduled replacement of central venous and pulmonary-artery catheters. N Engl J Med 1992; 327:1062–1068.

157. Widmer AF, Nettleman M, Flint K, Wenzel RP. The clinical impact of culturing central venous catheters. A prospective study. Arch Intern Med 1992; 152:1299–1302.

158. Puntis JW, Holden CE, Smallman S, Finkel Y, George RH, Booth IW. Staff training: a key factor in reducing intravascular catheter sepsis. Arch Dis Child 1991; 66:335–337.

159. Armstrong CW, Mayhall CG, Miller KB, Newsome HH, Sugerman HJ, Dalton HP, Hall GO, Hunsberger S. Clinical predictors of infection on central venous catheters used for total parenteral nutrition. Infect Control Hosp Epidemiol 1991; 12:407–411.

160. Michel LA, Bradpiece HA, Randour P, Pouthier R. Safety of central venous

catheter change over guidewire for suspected catheter-related sepsis. A prospective randomized trial. Int Surg 1988; 73:180–186.

161. Snyder RH, Archer FJ, Endy T, Allen TW, Condon B, Kaiser J, Whatmore D, Harrington G, McDermott CJ. Catheter infection. A comparison of two catheter maintenance techniques. Ann Surg 1988; 208:651–653.

162. Hershey CO, Tomford JW, McLaren CE, Porter DK, Cohen DI. The natural history of intravenous catheter-associated phlebitis. Arch Intern Med 1984; 144:1373–1375.

163. Tomford JW, Hershey CO, McLaren CE, Porter DK, Cohen DI. Intravenous therapy team and peripheral venous catheter-associated complications: a prospective controlled study. Arch Intern Med 1984; 44:1191–1194.

164. Bock SN, Lee RE, Fisher B, Rubin JT, Schwartzentruber DJ, Wei JP, Callender DP, Yang JC, Lotze MT, Pizzo PA, et al. A prospective randomized trial evaluating prophylactic antibiotics to prevent triple-lumen catheter-related sepsis in patients treated with immunotherapy. J Clin Oncol 1990; 8:161–169.

165. Lim SH, Smith MP, Machin SJ, Goldstone AH. Teicoplanin and prophylaxis of Hickman catheter insertions. Eur J Surg Suppl 1992; 567:39–42.

166. Lim SH, Smith MP, Salooja N, Machin SJ, Goldstone AH. A prospective randomized study of prophylactic teicoplanin to prevent early Hickman catheter-related sepsis in patients receiving intensive chemotherapy for haematological malignancies. J Antimicrob Chemother 1991; 28:109–116.

167. Lim SH, Smith MP, Machin SJ, Goldstone AH. A prospective randomized study of prophylactic teicoplanin to prevent early Hickman catheter-related sepsis in patients receiving intensive chemotherapy for haematological malignancies. Eur J Haematol 1993; 51:10–13.

168. McKee R, Dunsmuir R, Shitby M, Garden OJ. Does antibiotic prophylaxis at the time of catheter insertion reduce the incidence of catheter-related sepis in intravenous nutrition. J Hosp Infect 1985; 6:419–425.

169. Ranson MR, Oppenheim BA, Jackson A, Kamthan AG, Scarffe JH. Double-blind placebo controlled study of vancomycin prophylaxis for central venous catheter insertion in cancer patients. J Hosp Infect 1990; 15:95–102.

170. van de Wetering MD, van Woensel JB. Prophylactic antibiotics for preventing early central venous catheter gram positive infections in oncology patients. Cochrane Database Syst Rev, 2003, (2):CD003295.

171. Vassilomanolakis M, Plataniotis G, Koumakis G, Hajichristou H, Skouteri H, Dova H, Efremidis AP. Central venous catheter-related infections after bone marrow transplantation in patients with malignancies: a prospective study with short-course vancomycin prophylaxis. Bone Marrow Transplant 1995; 15:77–80.

12

Peripheral Venous Catheters

C. Glen Mayhall

University of Texas Medical Branch at Galveston
Galveston, Texas, U.S.A.

INTRODUCTION

Intravascular cannulae are among the most commonly used devices in the delivery of modern healthcare. It has been estimated that 150 million intravascular devices are purchased by hospitals and clinics each year in the United States (1). The overwhelming majority of these cannulae are peripheral venous catheters (PVC) and needles. Approximately 25 million patients per year in the United States receive infusion therapy through peripheral intravenous cannulae (2). Phlebitis or inflammation at the site of vessel cannulation commonly occurs, ranging from 15 to 70% in adults (2–6), and 10 to 13% in children (7,8). However, the great majority of instances of phlebitis are aseptic (not related to infection), and the phenomenon appears most closely related to the physicochemical characteristics of the materials from which catheters are constructed and the type of infusate administered through the catheters (2–8). Few PVCs removed from patients with phlebitis are found to be colonized on semiquantitative culture (2,4,7,9–12).

Because inflammation at the catheter site raises the suspicion of infection, because infection cannot be ruled out without removal and culture of the catheter, and because there is a statistically significant relationship between phlebitis and catheter-related infection (2), aseptic phlebitis will be discussed as well as catheter-related colonization and infection.

PATHOGENESIS OF PERIPHERAL VENOUS CATHETER-RELATED PHLEBITIS, COLONIZATION, AND INFECTION

Phlebitis

The pathogenesis of phlebitis is related to the effects of various physical and chemical factors on the cannulated blood vessel.

Physical Factors

Physical factors related to the development of aseptic phlebitis include cannula composition, cannula length, cannula bore, distortion of the cannula tip, anatomical location of the cannula tip, trauma at venipuncture, rate of flow of infusate, duration of cannulation, and manipulation of the cannula in situ (2,5–8,10,11,13–19). The effect of catheter composition is related to both the direct irritant effect of the material used (polyvinyl chloride and polyethylene are more irritating than Teflon and polyurethane) and stiffness of the catheter (the relatively stiffer Teflon cannula is more irritating than the more flexible silicone catheter) (6,11,13,14).

While certain plastics are less likely than others to cause phlebitis, the surface characteristics and etching of the catheter surface during the manufacturing process are probably more important than the type of plastic (6,15). Longer cannulas are more often associated with thrombophlebitis than shorter catheters, perhaps due to the greater difficulty of insertion of longer catheters, resulting in more trauma (16). Large bore catheters are more often associated with phlebitis than small bore catheters, probably due to the decreased blood flow around large bore catheters, particularly when they are inserted into small veins (6). Distortion or damage to the catheter tip has been shown to be significantly related to phlebitis (Fig. 1) (5). Cannulae inserted in the dorsum of the hand, the wrist, the lower extremities, or over the joints without joint immobilization have been associated with phlebitis (2,6), but studies attempting to relate location of cannula insertion in the upper extremity to phlebitis have yielded inconsistent results (13). Trauma at the time of insertion has been associated with phlebitis. Thus, phlebitis may be more likely to occur when cannulae are inserted as a sheath around the venipuncture needle than when cannulae are inserted through a needle (17). The rate of flow of infusates may be important with slower infusion rates, particularly with more irritant solutions, leading to more irritation of the vein (18). The duration of cannulation is an established risk factor for development of phlebitis in both adults and children (2,6–8,16–18). However, the duration of cannulation is less important in children, and catheters may be left in place up to 144 hours without much risk of phlebitis (8). Manipulation of the cannula in situ by more frequent dressing changes (daily versus every other day) has been found to be significantly related to the development of phlebitis (10).

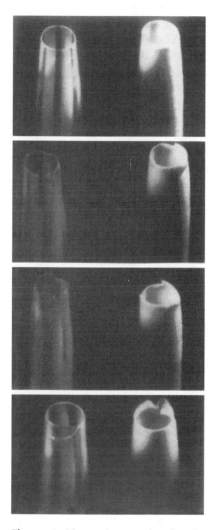

Figure 1 Photomicrographs showing damage to the tips of Vialon and Teflon catheters. The Vialon catheter is shown on the left and the Teflon catheter on the right of each panel. The top two panels show damage gradings of 0 and 1 and the lower two panels show damage gradings of 2 and 3.

Chemical Factors

Several chemical factors predispose to the development of phlebitis, including pH and osmolarity of the infusate, inherent irritating properties of certain infusates, and particulate matter in the infusate.

Low pH of infusates is associated with phlebitis (6,13,17,19–22). Thus, glucose solutions have a pH of 3.4 to 5 to prevent caramelization during autoclaving, and it has been shown that neutralization of the acidic pH of glucose solutions results in reduced rates of phlebitis (19–21). Solutions with high osmolarity (greater than 600 mOsm/L) are also associated with phlebitis (23). Certain chemicals in infusates are inherently irritating to venous endothelium, including benzodiazepines, barbiturates, and other anesthetic agents, and cephalosporin antibiotics (13). Other antibiotics that may cause phlebitis when given intravenously are vancomycin, metronidazole, erythromycin, and amphotericin B. Particulate matter (extraneous, mobile, undissolved substances), including rubber, chemicals, glass, cellulose fibers, and fungi, may be present in parenteral solutions (13). Particulates may irritate the venous endothelium and cause inflammation. That particulates may induce phlebitis is supported by two randomized controlled studies of in-line filtration of parenteral fluids, which showed either that in-line filtration prolonged the phlebitis-free survival of infusions (24) or reduced the per-day incidence of phlebitis with a significant reduction on day three (p < 0.001) (25). However, not all studies of in-line filtration have demonstrated a protective effect against phlebitis (26).

Plastic Catheters Versus Steel Needles

Steel needles have frequently been used as the cannula of first choice for short-term infusions due to the belief that they present a lower risk of phlebitis and infection. In the only randomized clinical trial of steel needles versus a plastic (Teflon) catheter by Tully and colleagues, there was no significant difference between the two types of cannula with respect to colonization/infection (27). However, phlebitis was significantly more likely to occur with Teflon catheters and infiltration significantly more likely to occur with steel needles. In a study of the complications of steel needles used for infusion therapy in patients with hematological malignancy, Band and Maki noted higher rates of aseptic phlebitis with steel needles than Tully and colleagues (33.8 versus 8.8%) and higher rates of catheter-related infection (5.4 versus 1.5%) and catheter-related bacteremia (2.1 versus 0%) (28). Thus, steel needles may pose a higher risk of infectious and noninfectious complications in patients with underlying malignancies.

Catheter-Related Colonization and Infection

Microbial Adherence

Microorganisms may cause cannula-related infection by migrating into the subcutaneous catheter tract, by entering the lumen of the cannula after catheter hub contamination, or by colonizing (seeding) the cannula hematogenously with microorganisms from some other site in the body. However, one of the most important factors determining whether a microorganism can cause catheter colonization or catheter-related infection is its ability to adhere to catheter surfaces.

The degree of adherence of microorganisms to catheters is determined by the materials from which catheters are manufactured, physical characteristics of catheter surfaces, deposition of host proteins on catheter surfaces, and certain characteristics of microorganisms that allow them to attach to surfaces, including elaboration of an extracellular polysaccharide substance known as glycocalyx or slime. Using scanning electron microscopy, Locci and colleagues demonstrated irregularities on the internal and external surfaces of unused intravenous catheters (29). These authors suggested that such defects might provide sites of attachment for bacteria that came into contact with catheter surfaces. Ashkenazi and coworkers showed by scanning electron microscopy that bacteria adhered initially to irregularities on the inner and outer surfaces of the catheters (30). Other undefined characteristics of various catheter materials appear to play a role in binding of microorganisms to these surfaces as well. Thus, bacteria adhered least to siliconized steel needles and Teflon catheters and most to polyethylene and polyvinyl chloride catheters (30,31).

Host proteins, including fibronectin, fibrinogen, and laminin, are deposited onto the surface of catheters after their insertion. Bacteria, particularly *Staphylococcus aureus* and coagulase-negative staphylococci, adhere to these proteins (32,33). *Staphylococcus aureus* binds most strongly to fibronectin and fibrinogen and coagulase-negative staphylococci most strongly to fibronectin

The surface characteristic of bacteria most important in binding to a catheter surface is hydrophobicity (30). Thus, hydrophobic bacteria such as *S. aureus* and *Serratia marcescens* bind better to catheter surfaces than do less hydrophobic species like *Escherichia coli*.

Some strains of bacteria, particularly strains of coagulase-negative staphylococci, produce an extracellular glycocalyx composed of either polysaccharide or glycoprotein that is purported to provide a mechanism for adherence to surfaces (34). While slime may protect microorganisms from host phagocytic cells and antimicrobial agents, initial attachment does not appear to be mediated by slime (32). However, slime has an adverse effect on the host response, which appears to be mediated by interference with induction of normal T-cell proliferation and a direct lytic effect on some of these cells (35). Slime also interferes with the antimicrobial activity of vancomycin and teicoplanin (36). When slime was added to wells containing vancomycin and an inoculum of *Staphylococcus epidermidis*, the minimum inhibitory concentration (MIC) was increased fourfold when compared with wells containing the same concentration of antibiotic and inoculum, but without slime. Slime also reversed the synergistic effect of vancomycin with gentamicin against *S. epidermidis*. Addition of slime had no effect on the MICs of cefazolin, clindamycin, rifampin, and LY146032.

Colonization of the Subcutaneous Catheter Tract

The most important pathogenetic mechanism by which microorganisms cause catheter colonization and catheter-related infection is migration of microorganisms from the skin surface around the point at which the catheter penetrates the skin into the subcutaneous catheter tract (Fig. 2). Maki and Mermel list 10 categories of evidence that support this pathogenetic mechanism as the most important mechanism (37), and some of this evidence will be discussed below.

There are several studies demonstrating that microorganisms recovered from skin at the catheter site are the etiologic agents of catheter colonization and catheter-related infections. These studies show a correlation between a

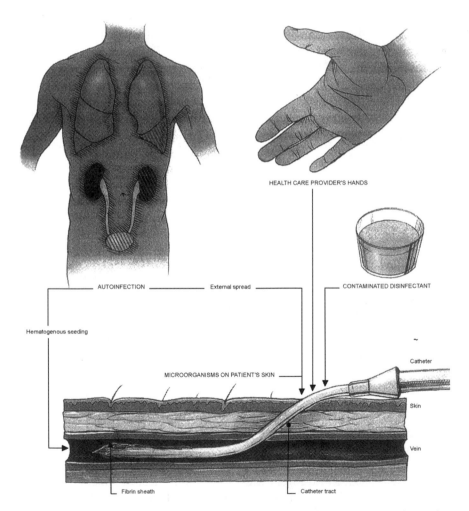

Figure 2 Sources of peripheral venous catheter infection. Microorganisms that contaminate the skin at the catheter insertion site may migrate into the subcutaneous catheter tract, multiply to high concentrations, and eventually colonize the fibrin sheath present on the intravascular portion of the catheter.

high density of microorganisms on the skin at the catheter site and the occurrence of catheter colonization or catheter-related infection (38–40), and in two of these studies, the species recovered from the skin was usually the causative agent of the catheter colonization or catheter-related infection (38,39). While the latter studies assessed only central venous catheters used for total parenteral nutrition, there is no reason to believe that the mechanism of colonization/infection would be different for PVCs.

Patients with burns have a higher density of microorganisms on the surface of the burn wound than is found on normal skin, and these patients have a higher incidence of catheter-related infections than do patients without burns (41–43). In addition, cutaneous colonization at the catheter insertion site at the time of catheter removal was a risk factor for catheter-related infection (relative risk = 6.16), and the incidence of catheter-related infection correlated inversely with the distance of the catheter insertion site from the burn wound (43).

Further support for the skin as a source of microorganisms that cause catheter-related infections is provided by reports of outbreaks of catheter-related infections associated with application of contaminated antiseptics to the skin prior to insertion of intravascular devices (44–46).

As a corollary to the above observations, the more effective removal of microorganisms from the skin around the site at which the catheter is inserted results in a lower catheter-related infection rate. Thus, Maki and associates observed that preparation of the skin with chlorhexidine prior to catheter insertion was associated with a significantly lower rate of catheter-related infection and bacteremia than when povidone-iodine or 70% alcohol were used for skin preparation (47).

Additional evidence for migration of microorganisms from the skin surface into the subcutaneous catheter tract as the most important pathogenetic mechanism for development of catheter-related infections are the observations that microorganisms are found mainly on the external surfaces of colonized catheters when they are examined microscopically on removal and that the presence of microorganisms on the external surfaces of catheters is related to the occurrence of catheter-related bacteremia. Thus, on removal, Cooper and Hopkins cultured intravascular catheters semiquantitatively and then Gram-stained them (48). The direct catheter Gram-stain technique was 100% sensitive and 96.9% specific for catheter colonization as defined by semiquantitative culture. Microorganisms were observed on the external surface of all 41 catheters with a positive semiquantitative culture, but on the internal (lumenal) surface of only four catheters. That the external surface of the catheter is the source for microorganisms that cause catheter-related bacteremia is shown by the observation that a positive semiquantitative catheter culture is highly correlated with the occurrence of bacteremia (48–50).

Finally, when bovine collagen cuffs impregnated with silver ions are placed subcutaneously at the catheter insertion site at the time of catheter insertion, the rate of catheter-related infection is significantly decreased. Thus, Maki and coworkers observed a decrease in infection rates of from 28.9% with control noncuffed catheters to 9.1% with cuffed catheters ($p = 0.002$) (51). Likewise, Flowers and associates noted a reduction in the rate of catheter colonization of from 34.5% with noncuffed control catheters to 7.7% with cuffed catheters ($p = 0.02$) (50). The marked reduction in catheter colonization or catheter-related infection by blocking the entrance to the subcutaneous catheter tract with a silver impregnated bovine collagen cuff provides strong evidence that migration of microorganisms from the skin surface into the catheter tract is the most important pathogenetic mechanism for development of catheter-related infections.

Hub Contamination

The data for hub contamination as a mechanism for development of catheter colonization or catheter-related infection for short-term catheters is less convincing than that for migration of microorganisms into the subcutaneous catheter tract. Contamination of the hub may be the most important mechanism for colonization and catheter-related infection involving long-term catheters (>30 days) (52), but the evidence for hub contamination as an important mechanism in short-term catheters (<30 days) is much less convincing. First, there is no validated standardized technique for culturing catheter hubs, and the meaning of positive qualitative cultures is unclear. Second, in some of the studies, when isolates of the same species were recovered from both hub and catheter tip, they were considered to be the same strain if they had the same antibiogram. The development of molecular typing has shown that antibiograms may be nonspecific markers for determining when two isolates are from the same clone. Third, most of the studies implicating contamination of the hub as the pathogenetic mechanism for development of catheter colonization and catheter-related infection are flawed by using historic controls (53), by failing to explain why the majority of catheters with contaminated hubs also have positive semiquantitative catheter (external surface) cultures (54), and combining short-term and long-term catheters in the same study (55). The most convincing data supporting hub contamination as an important mechanism for catheter-related infection is that published by deCicco and colleagues (56).

After migrating down the subcutaneous catheter tract or, less commonly, down the lumenal surface of the catheter, microorganisms may reach and adhere to the fibrin sheath that forms around the intravascular portion of all catheters as early as 24 hours after their insertion (57). Multiplication in the fibrin sheath may lead to shedding of microorganisms into the bloodstream, giving rise to catheter-related bacteremia. Thrombus formation at the catheter tip may perpetuate the multiplication of microorganisms (42,58). If multiplication takes place to the extent that microorganisms invade the venous wall or an intraluminal abscess develops, the patient has a life-threatening infection termed septic or suppurative thrombophlebitis (42).

Hematogenous Seeding

Another mechanism by which catheter-related infection develops is hematogenous seeding (53,54). Microorganisms that enter the bloodstream from another source may adhere to the fibrin sheath surrounding the intravascular portion of the catheter. Catheter-related infection develops much less commonly by hematogenous seeding than by migration of microorganisms down the external or internal surfaces of catheters. Likewise, contaminated infusion fluids are uncommonly the source of microorganisms that cause catheter-related infection (2,12,28).

CLINICAL MANIFESTATIONS

Phlebitis

The presence of fever is not necessary for the diagnosis of aseptic phlebitis. Phlebitis is diagnosed by the presence of local signs of inflammation without evidence of infection, i.e., without the presence of purulent drainage from the catheter insertion site. The local signs of phlebitis include erythema, palpable venous cord, tenderness, pain, increased warmth, induration, swelling, and lymphangitis (2–4,9,12,59).

Catheter-Related Infection

Catheter-related infection may also be manifested by the same local signs of inflammation observed to occur with aseptic phlebitis, as noted in the Introduction. Patients with catheter-related infection may have fever, and in some cases, a purulent discharge may be noted at the site of catheter insertion (10,60).

Septic thrombophlebitis may occur in any patient with an intravenous catheter, but burn patients are at a particularly high risk of this complication (42). Septic thrombophlebitis may complicate both central and peripheral venous cannulation (42,61). Most patients with septic thrombophlebitis have fever and signs of sepsis, and 72 to 100% have bacteremia (42,61). Baker and associates reported on a series of cases of septic thrombophlebitis in a population of patients with intravenous catheters and persons who abused drugs in the community (61). Local signs of septic thrombophlebitis included local pain in 83% of patients, swelling in 37%, erythema and edema in 62%, abscess in 43%, a palpable cord in 20%, lymphadenopathy in 13%, and spontaneous drainage of pus in 9% (61). Local signs of septic thrombophlebitis in burn patients may occur in less than 50% of cases (42). It must also be kept in mind that signs and symptoms of septic thrombophlebitis may not appear for days after the intravenous cannula is removed (62). The most common systemic complication of septic thrombophlebitis is septic embolism, usually to the lungs (61).

ETIOLOGY OF INFECTIONS ASSOCIATED WITH PERIPHERAL VENOUS CATHETERS

Catheter Colonization and Catheter-Site Infections

Catheter colonization (>15 cfu on semiquantitative culture without local signs of infection) and catheter-related site infection (purulent drainage from the point at which the catheter penetrates the skin) may occur and be limited to the catheter tract or may also give rise to bacteremia.

Adults

There is no national database that compiles data on the etiology of colonization or catheter-related infection for PVCs. The only data available are from published studies from individual institutions. Maki and Ringer observed that for Teflon catheters, 4.7% were colonized with coagulase-negative staphylococci, 0.2% with *S. aureus*, and none with Gram-negative bacilli or yeasts. For polyurethane catheters, 6.7% were colonized by coagulase-negative staphylococci, none by *S. aureus* or Gram-negative bacilli, and 0.2% by yeasts (2). In a second study, Maki and Ringer found that 4.9% of 2088 PVCs were colonized by coagulase-negative staphylococci, 0.1% by *S. aureus*, and none by Gram-negative bacilli or yeasts (12). The most common microorganism colonizing PVCs in the series of Righter and coworkers was *S. epidermidis*. *S. aureus* accounted for only two of 59 isolates and Gram-negative bacilli for two of 59 isolates (4). Of 42 colonized PVCs, Bregenzer and associates found that 36 of 42 (87.5%) catheter isolates were coagulase-negative staphylococci, two of 42 (4.8%) were *Proteus mirabilis*, one of 42 (2.4%) was *S. aureus*, one of 42 (2.4%) was a viridans species of *Streptococcus*, one of 42 (2.4%) was *Corynebacterium xerosis*, and one of 42 (2.4%) was a mixture of coagulase-negative staphylococci and enterococci (63).

Children

In a study of 50 PVCs in neonates, Wilkins and colleagues found 13 cannulae (26%) to be positive on semiquantitative culture. Of 22 isolates from these catheters, 19 were *S. epidermidis*, one was *Staphylococcus haemolyticus*, one was *Staphylococcus warneri*, and one was *S. aureus* (62). In their study of intravenous catheters in neonates, Cronin and colleagues recovered 43 isolates at a colony count of ≥15 cfu on semiquantitative culture of 631 PVCs (64). Thirty-four of 43 (79%) were coagulase-negative staphylococci. Only one (2.3%) was *S. aureus*; the remaining isolates were *Enterococcus* (five or 11.6%), *E. coli* (two or 4.7%), and *Candida parapsilosis* (one or 2.3%).

In a study of children with a mean age of 4.9 ± 5 years, Shimandle and coworkers observed that 92 of 348 (26%) PVCs were colonized (65). Ninety-two of 107 (86%) isolates from colonized peripheral venous catheters were coagulase-negative staphylococci. Eight of 107 (7.5%) isolates were other low-virulence skin or environmental bacteria, five of 107 (4.7%) were *Candida* species, one of 107 (0.9%) was *S. aureus*, and one of 107 (0.9%) was *Klebsiella pneumoniae*.

In older children from general medical wards in a childrens' hospital, Garland and associates found 12 of 115 (10.4%) PVCs to be colonized (66). Eleven of the 12 (91.6%) were colonized by *S. epidermidis* and one (8.4%) was colonized by an alpha hemolytic *Streptococcus*. In a later study of critically ill children, Garland and associates found 54 (11.8%) of 459 PVCs to be colonized (8). Coagulase-negative staphylococci were recovered from 51 of 54 (94.4%) catheters. *Enterococcus faecalis* and β-hemolytic *Streptococcus* were each recovered from two catheters and yeasts were recovered from four catheters.

It would appear, from the limited data available, that the overwhelming majority of catheter colonizations and local catheter-related infections of PVCs in both adults and children are caused by Gram-positive cocci. Most of the Gram-positive coccal isolates are coagulase-negative staphylococci. There are rare isolates of *S. aureus*, Gram-negative bacilli, and yeasts.

Catheter-Related Bacteremia

Catheter-related bacteremia uncommonly complicates the use of PVCs in adults or children.

Adults

No cases of bacteremia were identified in either of the two studies of PVCs by Maki and Ringer (2,12), and Righter and coworkers and Bregenzer and associates observed no cases of bacteremia in their series (4,63). The best data on the etiology of catheter-related bacteremias that complicate the use of PVCs in adults is from a multicenter study in Australia (67). Collignon and his coworkers found that *S. aureus* was most often the cause of bacteremia associated with PVCs. Gram-positive cocci were the cause in 181 of 240 (75.4%) episodes and *S. aureus* was the cause in 149 of 240 (62.1%) of the episodes. Gram-negative bacilli accounted for 55 of 240 (22.9%) episodes and fungi for only four of 240 (1.7%) episodes.

Children

There are also few data on the cause of catheter-related bacteremias in children. The seven bacteremias in neonates in the study of Cronin and colleagues were all caused by coagulase-negative staphylococci, and *Entero-coccus* was also isolated from the blood of one of these patients (64). Systemic *Candida* infections in neonates may also be associated with the use of PVCs (68). In their study on the complications of PVCs in critically ill children,

Garland and associates observed a single case of catheter-related bacteremia caused by Group A, B-hemolytic *Streptococcus* (8).

Patients with Human Immunodeficiency Virus (HIV) Infection

Unpublished data from a cohort study of HIV-infected patients at five Veterans Affairs Hospitals revealed that *S. aureus* (41%) was the most common cause of peripheral intravenous catheter-related bacteremia in this population (Gaynes, R, Hospital Infections Program, Centers for Disease Control and Prevention (CDC) personal communication, 1995). Fifteen of the 55 cases (27.3%) of peripheral venous catheter-related bacteremia had coagulase-negative staphylococci isolated from blood, followed by *K. pneumoniae* (7.3%), *Pseudomonas aeurginosa* (7.3%), *E. coli* (3.6%), *Candida albicans* (3.6%), and other microorganisms (12.7%). The etiologies of catheter-related colonization and infection are shown in Table 1.

Catheter-Related Septic Thrombophlebitis

As with catheter-related infection and catheter-related bacteremia, the most common causes of septic thrombophlebitis are Gram-positive cocci (42,61,69). *S. aureus* is by far the most frequently isolated Gram-positive coccus (42,61,69). Gram-negative bacilli make up approximately 20% of isolates (61,69). Yeasts do not appear to be a common cause of septic thrombophlebitis except in burn patients (42,61,69).

Gram-positive cocci cause most of the cases of catheter-related infection, catheter-related bacteremia, and catheter-related septic thrombophlebitis. In adults, most cases of catheter colonization and catheter site infection are caused by coagulase-negative staphylococci, while *S. aureus* is the most common cause of catheter-related bacteremia and septic thrombophlebitis. On the other hand, coagulase-negative staphylococci are the most common cause of both catheter site infection and catheter-related bacteremia in children.

EPIDEMIOLOGY OF PERIPHERAL VENOUS CATHETER-RELATED PHLEBITIS AND COLONIZATION/INFECTION

Rates of Catheter-Related Phlebitis and Colonization/Infection

Phlebitis

Adults: Rates of aseptic phlebitis range from 2.3 to 51.9% (2,4,5,10–12,16,27,28,63,70,71). The high variability of rates cannot be accounted for by

Table 1 Etiologies of Peripheral Venous Catheter-Related Infections

Authors (Reference)	Microorganisms	Number of isolates	Percentage of total isolates
Adults			
Maki and Ringer (2)	Coagulase-negative	59	96.7
(Catheter isolates	staphylococci		
≥15 cfu)	*Staphylococcus aureus*	1	1.6
	Yeast	1	1.6
Righter et al. (4)	*S. epidermidis*	26	44.1
(Catheter isolates	*Streptococcus* species	13	22.0
≥15 cfu)	*Neisseria* species	4	6.8
	Yeast	4	6.8
	Micrococcus species	3	5.1
	Diptheroids	3	5.1
	S. aureus	2	3.4
	Bacillus species	2	3.4
	Serratia marcescens	1	1.7
	Acinetobacter species	1	1.7
Maki and Ringer (12)	Coagulase-negative	103	98.1
(Catheter isolates	staphylococci		
≥15 cfu)	*S. aureus*	2	1.9
Collignon (67)	*S. aureus*	149	62.1
(Blood isolates)	Coagulase-negative	26	10.8
	staphylococci		
	Streptococcus species	3	1.3
	Enterococcus species	2	0.8
	Corynebacterium species	1	0.4
	Escherichia coli	3	1.3
	Klebsiella species	15	6.3
	Enterobacter species	12	5.0
	Serratia species	4	1.7
	Other Enterobacteriaceae	5	2.1
	Pseudomonas species	7	2.9
	Other Gram-negative	9	3.8
	microorganisms		
	Candida albicans	4	1.7
Bregenzer et al. (63)	*S. epidermidis*	36	85.7
(Catheter isolates	*Proteus mirabilis*	2	4.8
≥15 cfu)	*S. aureus*	1	2.4
	Viridans streptococci	1	2.4
	Corynebacterium xerosis	1	2.4
	S. epidermidis and enterococci	1	2.4
Gaynes (Personal	*S. aureus*	21	38.2
Communication)	Coagulase-negative	15	27.3
(Blood isolates,	staphylococci		
HIV-positive	*K. pneumoniae*	4	7.3
patients)	*P. aeruginosa*	4	7.3

Table 1 Continued

Authors (Reference)	Microorganisms	Number of isolates	Percentage of total isolates
	E. coli	2	3.6
	C. albicans	2	3.6
	Other microorganisms	7	12.7
Children			
Wilkins et al. (62)	S. epidermidis	19	86.4
(Catheter isolates	S. aureus	1	4.5
≥15 cfu)	S. haemolyticus	1	4.5
	S. warneri	1	4.5
Cronin et al. (64)	Coagulase-negative	34	79.1
(Catheter isolates	staphylococci[a]		
≥15 cfu)	S. aureus	1	2.3
	Enterococcus[a]	5	11.6
	E. coli	2	4.7
	C. parapsilosis	1	2.3
Shimandle et al. (65)	Coagulase-negative	92	86
(Catheter isolates	staphylococci		
≥15 cfu)	Other skin and	8	7.5
	environmental bacteria		
	Candida species	5	4.7
	S. aureus	1	0.9
	K. pneumoniae	1	0.9
Garland et al. (66)	S. epidermidis	11	91.7
(Catheter isolates	Streptococcus species	1	8.3
≥15 cfu)			
Garland et al. (8)	Coagulase-negative	78	86.7
(Catheter isolates	staphylococci		
≥15 cfu)[b]	S. pyogenes	2	2.2
	E. faecalis	2	2.2
	Yeasts	4	4.3
	C. parapsilosis	3	3.3
	Malassezia furfur	1	1.1

[a] Some of these catheter isolates may have caused bacteremia.
[b] Catheters cultured by both semiquantitative and quantitative techniques.

differences in definitions of phlebitis or by differences in materials from which the catheters are constructed. In the overwhelming majority of published reports, the rates of phlebitis range from 16.7 to 51.9% (2,4,5,10–12,16,28,63,70). It is of interest that the most carefully performed study found the lowest rate of phlebitis (2.3%) (71).

Children: Only three studies in children report rates of aseptic phlebitis (7,8,65). The reported rates range from 1.1 to 13%. It is unclear why children have lower rates of phlebitis than adults. The differences in rates between children and adults cannot be accounted for by differences in definitions of phlebitis or differences in the materials from which catheters were manufactured.

Catheter Site Colonization/Infection

Adults: Local catheter-related colonization/infection in PVCs has been reported to occur at a much lower rate than aseptic phlebitis. In seven studies in which the semiquantitative catheter culture technique of Maki and coworkers (9) was used to culture peripheral intravenous cannulae on removal, the colonization/infection rates ranged from 1.4 to 6.9% (2,4,10,12,27,28,63). Differences in colonization/infection rates could not be accounted for by differences in catheter materials or time in situ. However, the study that yielded a cannula colonization/infection rate of 5.4% for steel needles was carried out in a population of patients with hematological malignancies (28).

Children: In four studies of PVCs in children in which catheters were cultured by the technique of Maki and coworkers (9) on removal, rates of catheter colonization/infection ranged from 10.4 to 26% (7,8,65,66). In two studies in neonates in which catheters were cultured by the technique of Maki and coworkers (9), rates were 26 and 13%, respectively (62,64). The differences between the rates in children and adults could not be accounted for by differences in culture techniques, catheter materials, or time in situ.

Rates of Catheter-Related Bacteremia

Adults: In six of nine studies of PVCs, no cases of catheter-related bacteremia were identified (2,4,10,12,27,63). In the other three studies, catheter-related bacteremia occurred at a rate of 0.08 to 1.9% (28,70,71). In the multicenter study by Collignon and coworkers from Australia, peripheral intravenous catheter-related bacteremia occurred at a rate of between 0 and 1.28 cases per 1000 catheters purchased; this translated to a rate of 0.1% (67). In the unpublished cohort study of HIV-infected patients at five Veterans Affairs Hospitals, there were 66 PVC-related bloodstream infections (BSI) for a rate of 1.5 bloodstream infections per 1000 catheter-days (Gaynes, R, Hospital Infections Program, CDC, personal communication, 1995). Fifty-five of these patients had only PVCs (i.e., did not have a central line as well) for a rate of 1.2 BSI per 1000 catheter-days.

Children: Peripheral venous catheter-related bacteremia rates are also very low in children. In four published studies, there were no cases of bacteremia (7,62,65,66), and in one report, the bacteremia rate was 0.15% (8).

Taken together, these data indicate that both adult and pediatric patients with PVCs are at a very low risk for catheter-related bacteremia.

Rates of Catheter-Related Septic Thrombophlebitis

No cohort studies of septic thrombophlebitis that complicate the use of PVCs have been published, and therefore, rates for this complication are unknown. However, since bacteremia is a prominent manifestation of septic thrombophlebitis and the rate of peripheral intravenous cannula-related bacteremia is very low, the rate of septic thrombophlebitis complicating the insertion of PVCs would also be expected to be very low.

Risk Factors for Phlebitis and Catheter-Site Colonization and Infection

Phlebitis

Adults: Risk factors for phlebitis have been identified in three prospective studies of PVCs using similar definitions for phlebitis and multivariable analysis of the data (2,5,71). All three studies identified duration of cannulation as a risk factor. Risk factors identified by two of the three studies included infusion of antibiotics and use of Teflon rather than polyurethane catheters (2,5). All three studies identified one risk factor related to female gender, i.e., female sex (2), cesarean section (5), and hospitalization in an obstetrics and gynecology hospital (71). Other risk factors included cannula tip damage (5), having a high-risk diagnosis (cancer, immunodeficiency diseases), catheter order (higher rates of phlebitis for catheters inserted after the first catheter), and an interaction of length and order (length of catheterization increased the risk of phlebitis only for first catheters) (71). In a second analysis, Maki and Ringer identified risk factors for severe phlebitis, defined as a phlebitis score higher than the 77th percentile of all phlebitis scores (2). In addition to duration, female sex, infusion of antibiotics, and use of Teflon rather than polyurethane catheters the discrete proportional hazards model for severe phlebitis identified having had phlebitis with a previous catheter, having catheter-related infection, insertion of catheters in the spring months rather than in the winter, insertion of a catheter in the forearm rather than the hand or wrist, insertion of a catheter in the emergency room or operating room rather than the ward and insertion on the ward rather than in an intensive care unit as risk factors.

Children: Only one prospective study using a standard definition of phlebitis and multivariable techniques for analysis of data has been published in the pediatric literature (7). Using multiple linear regression, Nelson and Garland identified parenteral nutrition, infusion of nafcillin and aminoglycosides, and older age (those who developed phlebitis had a mean age of about six years while those without phlebitis had a mean age of about four years) as independent risk factors for phlebitis in children.

Catheter-Site Colonization and Infection

Adults: Five prospective studies of peripheral catheter colonization/ local catheter-related infection have been published (12,28,72–74). In only two of these studies were catheters (steel needles) cultured semiquantitatively on removal (12,28). In one of these publications, Band and Maki assessed risk factors for colonization/local infection of steel needles in patients with hematological malignancy (28). Using only univariate statistical analytical techniques, they identified local inflammation and needle placements exceeding 72 hours as risk factors. In the only study using semiquantitative cultures of catheters and multivariable statistical analysis, Maki and Ringer found colonization of the catheter site, colonization of the hub, moisture or blood beneath the dressing, and longer duration of catheter placement (3.8 ± 1.8 days versus 2.7 ± 1.6 days) to be risk factors for local catheter-related infection (12). They identified systemic antimicrobial therapy as protective (relative risk 0.47, 95% confidence interval 0.31–0.73).

Ena and associates carried out a cross-sectional study of phlebitis and catheter-related infection in a university-affiliated hospital in Madrid, Spain (72). Catheters were not cultured, and local catheter-related infection was diagnosed by local signs of inflammation and/or fever not attributable to other causes. Of 353 intravascular catheters, 273 (77.3%) were peripheral intravenous catheters. Risk factors identified by logistical regression analysis were infection at any other body site, inappropriate catheter care (defined as any deviation from Centers for Disease Control and Prevention guidelines for catheter care), and inappropriate length of catheter use (not defined). A hospital stay of longer than 14 days had a borderline relationship with catheter-related infection. The data on risk factors from this study have to be interpreted with caution, because catheters were not cultured, and because 22.7% of the catheters were not PVCs.

Nelson and colleagues carried out a prospective study of 100 PVCs to examine the impact of improperly dressed insertion sites on inflammation at these sites (73). On removal of catheters, the sites were scored for signs of inflammation using a score of zero to five for each of the signs, including tenderness, erythema, exudate, edema, and vein occlusion. Catheters were not cultured. They considered that the presence of two or more of these signs was indicative of infection, tissue damage, or irritation. Data were analyzed only by univariate analysis. They observed that 68 catheters were improperly dressed, due either to use of nonsterile materials or improperly applied sterile dressings. Forty-nine of 68 (72%) improperly dressed PVCs had signs of inflammation while only five of 32 (16%) of the properly dressed sites had signs of inflammation. This study is difficult to interpret, because catheters were not cultured and data were analyzed only by univariate statistics.

Hirschmann and coworkers performed a multicenter study in three Austrian hospitals to assess the effect of different types of hand hygiene on the occurrence of signs of inflammation at insertion sites (74). They recorded the presence of erythema, swelling, pain, pus at the insertion site, and fever of unknown origin and defined "infectious" complications as the presence of one or more of these signs. Catheters were not cultured. The authors also collected data on other variables, and data were analyzed by logistical regression. They observed that use of nonsterile disposable latex gloves or hand disinfection with alcohol were significantly protective against infection compared to no hand treatment or washing with nonmedicated soap. Insertion in the operating room compared to insertion in the ward or outpatient department was also significantly protective. Female gender and a duration of insertion ≥49 hours were risk factors for infectious complications. As in the latter two studies, interpretation of the findings in this study must be viewed with caution due to the absence of catheter cultures.

Children: Only one prospective study has been published in the pediatric literature that used a standard culture technique to identify colonized catheters or local catheter-related infection and multivariable analysis of the data to identify risk factors for local catheter-related colonization or infection. Shimandle and coworkers defined catheter colonization as growth of ≥15 cfu of bacteria or fungi and high-level colonization as growth of ≥ 200 cfu (65). Univariate analysis revealed significant associations between catheter colonization and the site of catheter insertion (antecubital fossa), days of catheter placement, and a protective effect of antibiotic administration.

On multivariable analysis, only days of catheter placement were significantly associated with catheter colonization. When the authors evaluated high-level colonization by multivariable analysis, catheter colonization was significantly increased by site of insertion and increased duration of catheter placement. Antibiotic use for up to three days was significantly protective.

Garland and associates conducted a prospective study of complications of PVCs in critically ill children and analyzed their data using multivariable techniques, but cultured catheters with unvalidated modifications of a semiquantitative culture technique (9) and a quantitative culture technique (75). They found infusion of diazepam, infusion of lipids, catheter duration greater than 144 hours, and age equal to or less than one year to be independent risk factors for catheter colonization (8).

Cronin and coworkers performed a prospective study and assessed risk factors for colonization of multiple types of catheters, but stratified their analysis by catheter type (64). Using only univariate analytical techniques, they identified duration of catheterization (longer than three days), absence of antibiotic therapy in the four days prior to catheter removal, use of the catheter for infusion of hyperalimentation solution, and low birthweight (less than 1500 grams) as risk factors for PVC colonization.

In a prospective study in which only 40% of the catheters were cultured and data were analyzed only by univariate techniques, Garland and associates were unable to find a significant relationship between catheter colonization and age, gender, race, conditions of catheter placement (elective versus emergency situation, site, catheter size, number of catheters), local complications including extravasation and phlebitis, and duration of catheterization (66). There was a borderline relationship between absence of antibiotic infusion through the catheter and catheter colonization. All of the studies noted a protective effect or borderline protective effect of antibiotic therapy, and three of the studies found an increased duration of catheter placement to be a risk factor. Otherwise, there was little agreement between these studies with respect to risk factors for catheter colonization, and the data should be interpreted cautiously because of differences in study populations and deficiencies in study design and data analysis.

Risk Factors for Peripheral Venous Catheter-Related Bacteremia

No studies have been published that assess risk factors for peripheral venous catheter-related bacteremia. Except for patients with HIV infection, bacteremias associated with PVCs are so uncommon that huge numbers of patients would have to be enrolled in a multicenter study. Given the low morbidity and mortality attributed to such bacteremias, it is unlikely that such a study will ever be done.

However, in patients with HIV infection, peripheral venous catheter-related bacteremias appear to be more common. Lambotte and associates studied a potential relationship between PVCs and nosocomial bacteremia in patients with HIV infection (76). They did a retrospective case-control study. Cases were patients who developed bacteremia ≥72 hours after admission and controls were patients without bacteremia matched to cases by length of stay equal to or greater than time to bacteremia in the case patient. Only a univariate analysis was done. Patients with a known source of bacteremia were not selected as controls. Cases were significantly more likely to have had a PVC inserted in the 48 hours before the first positive blood culture than were controls. This finding could be viewed with greater confidence if the data had been analyzed with a multivariable statistical technique.

DIAGNOSIS OF CATHETER COLONIZATION, LOCAL CATHETER-RELATED INFECTION, AND CATHETER-RELATED BACTEREMIA

Clinical Manifestations

Although local signs of inflammation (palpable cord, erythema, tenderness, swelling) may be associated with positive catheter cultures (see "Catheters" under "Application of Microbiological Techniques" Section) (9,40), it is clear that local signs of inflammation occur most often with negative catheter cultures (aseptic phlebitis) (2,4,10). The only local sign that is diagnostic of local catheter-related infection is drainage of purulent fluid from the site at which the catheter penetrates the skin (10,60,75). Thus, in the absence of purulent drainage, local signs of inflammation alone are an indication to remove the catheter and submit it for appropriate culture (see "Catheters" under "Application of Microbiological Techniques" Section), but without purulent drainage, local signs of inflammation alone are not diagnostic of catheter-related infection. On the other hand, the absence of signs of inflammation at the catheter site does not rule out catheter colonization/ catheter-related infection, i.e., does not predict that catheter cultures will be negative (4,9,10,77).

Septic thrombophlebitis should be considered in patients who have fever and a positive blood culture without an obvious source and who have a PVC in place or who have had a PVC recently removed (42,61). Local signs of infection may occur in less than half of these patients (42,78). When local signs of inflammation are present, they may include pain, swelling, erythema, palpable cord, lymphadenopathy, purulent drainage, and local abscess (61).

Septic thrombophlebitis should be considered in the absence of local signs at presently or recently cannulated venous sites in patients with persistent fever and bacteremia with no identifiable source. This may be particularly important in burn patients (42,78). All currently and recently cannulated veins should be examined for signs of inflammation and purulent drainage. An attempt should be made to express purulent fluid from previously cannulated sites. In patients with continuing fever and bacteremia with no identifiable source and negative findings on examination of current and previously cannulated venous sites, it may be necessary to surgically explore these sites, starting in the area of the vein where the tip of the previous cannula was likely to have been positioned (42,78). For patients with ongoing fever and bacteremia with an unknown source who have an intravascular catheter(s) in place, the catheter(s) should be removed and submitted for appropriate cultures (see "Catheters" under "Application of Microbiological Techniques" Section). Any purulent drainage should be cultured and a Gram-stained smear examined microscopically.

Application of Microbiological Techniques for Diagnosis of Catheter Colonization and Catheter-Related Infections

Cultures

The three types of specimens that may be cultured to establish the diagnosis of catheter colonization/catheter-related infection are purulent drainage from a site of venous cannulation, the cannula, and the patient's blood.

Purulent Drainage from the Catheter Site: When local catheter-related infection is suspected, the cannulated site should be carefully assessed for the presence of purulent drainage and any purulent fluid sampled carefully with a sterile swab to avoid contamination from skin around the cannula site. The swab should be promptly submitted for culture.

Catheters: Culture of a catheter in broth has a high sensitivity but low specificity, because even a single bacterial cell from the surrounding skin that contaminates the catheter on removal will give rise to a positive broth culture after overnight incubation. Thus, a negative broth culture indicates that the catheter is not colonized or that there is no local cannula-related infection, but a positive culture in broth is difficult to interpret.

To improve on the diagnostic accuracy of catheter cultures, Maki and coworkers developed a semiquantitative culture technique in which catheter segments were rolled across the surface of an agar plate using a flamed forceps (9). They found that cultures yielding ≥15 cfu were significantly associated with local inflammation and septicemia. Maki and coworkers considered that a positive catheter culture (≥15 cfu) indicated catheter-related infection. However, since Maki and coworkers' description of this culture technique, it has become clear that many catheters removed from inflamed sites are culture-negative (2,4,10,12) and that catheters that yield >15 cfu on semiquantitative culture may be from sites with no signs of local inflammation (7,8). Thus, a positive semiquantitative catheter culture is currently considered to represent catheter colonization rather than catheter-related infection. However, because catheter colonization is considered to be a precursor of catheter-related infection, and because colonized catheters may give rise to bacteremia (77), catheter colonization is considered an adverse event.

Collignon and colleagues reevaluated the semiquantitative catheter culture technique of Maki and coworkers (9) nearly a decade later and found that the technique was still a useful indicator of central venous catheter-related bacteremia (49). However, they noted that a threshold of ≥5 cfu improved the sensitivity of the technique with no change in specificity. Since these authors cultured only the tips of central venous catheters, it is unclear how their observations might apply to PVCs.

Because the semiquantitative catheter culture technique cultures only the outside of the catheter, has a low positive predictive value, and ≥1000 cfu can be quantitated per catheter segment, quantitative culture techniques were developed to overcome these deficiencies in the semiquantitative culture technique (75,77,79). Catheters were immersed in broth and the lumina were flushed with broth followed by quantitative culture of the broth (79), or catheters were sonicated in broth followed by quantitative culture of the broth (75,77). The sensitivity, specificity, positive, and negative predictive values for the quantitative broth sonication technique were 93, 95, 76, and 99%, respectively (77). However, only the study by Cleri and associates clearly included PVCs and they considered $> 10^3$ cfu as the threshold for infection, because counts of $\geq 10^3$ cfu were associated with bacteremia (79). Since 111 of 149 catheters in this study were PVCs, it would appear that this diagnostic technique could be applied to PVCs. In the reports of the quantitative sonication technique, either the types of catheters studied were not reported (75) or only central venous catheters were included (77).

Thus, it is unclear whether the broth sonication technique can be applied to PVCs.

Another quantitative culture technique that has been used to diagnose catheter-related infection is quantitative culture of blood samples obtained simultaneously from the intravascular cannula and from a peripheral vein (40,80–82). When the concentration of microorganisms in blood obtained from the catheter exceeds the concentration of microorganisms in peripheral venous blood by ≥ fourfold (82), ≥ sevenfold (81), or ≥ tenfold (40), catheter-related infection is diagnosed. None of the studies have included PVCs. This culture technique is particularly useful for central venous catheters, because it permits catheter-related infection to be ruled out without removing the catheter. This is important for central venous catheters, because they are more expensive to insert than PVCs and because insertion may be associated with serious complications. Given the relatively low cost and risk for insertion of PVCs, it is likely that simply removing a suspect PVC and inserting a new one at another site would be more cost-effective than differential quantitative blood cultures.

Microscopic Examination of Stained Catheter Segments

In 1985, Cooper and Hopkins reported on a technique that involved direct Gram staining of catheter segments immediately after removal (48). They cultured the catheter segments by the semiquantitative technique of Maki and coworkers (9) prior to Gram staining and compared the semiquantitative culture results with the results of microscopic examination of Gram-stained catheter segments. Sensitivity of the Gram stain technique was 100%, specificity was 96.9%, the positive predictive value was 83.9%, and the negative predictive value was 100%. All bacteremias were associated with catheters considered positive by the Gram stain technique. Unfortunately, only eight (2.4%) of the catheters were PVCs, making conclusions about application of this technique to PVCs tenuous.

Zufferey and coworkers developed a technique for microscopical examination of catheters stained directly by acridine orange (83). These authors also cultured the catheters using the semiquantitative method of Maki and coworkers (9) prior to staining them with acridine orange. Compared to the semiquantitative cultures, the direct acridine orange-staining technique had a sensitivity of 84%, a specificity of 100%, a positive predictive value of 86%, and a negative predictive value of 99%. The overall agreement with semiquantitative culture was 98%. Four hundred ninety-eight of the 710 (70%) catheters studied were PVCs. Thus, it would appear that this technique could be applied to PVCs.

Coutlée and colleagues (84) also compared direct staining of catheter segments with Gram stain and acridine orange with the semiquantitative culture method (9). These investigators found a lower sensitivity, specificity, positive predictive value, and negative predictive value for direct Gram staining and direct acridine orange staining than did Cooper and Hopkins (48) and Zufferey and coworkers (83), respectively. Except for fungal infections, Coutlée and colleagues did not consider either of these direct staining techniques very useful for diagnosis of catheter-related infections. However, unlike the studies of Cooper and Hopkins and Zufferey and coworkers, the study of Coutlée and colleagues was retrospective and included only 99 catheters. Twenty-three percent of the catheters in the latter study were PVCs. While microscopical examination of directly stained catheters may be laborious, it would appear that such techniques provide valid data for diagnosing or excluding catheter-related infection. Since only eight PVCs were studied by Cooper and Hopkins (48), more data are needed on the application of the direct Gram-staining technique to PVCs.

Definitions of Catheter Colonization, Local Catheter-Related Infection, and Catheter-Related Bacteremia

1. Catheter Colonization. Recovery of ≥ 15 cfu from the catheter on semiquantitative culture (9), or $> 10^3$ cfu from the catheter using the quantitative culture technique of Cleri and associates (79) in the absence of purulent drainage from the point at which the catheter penetrates the skin.
2. Local Catheter-Related Infection. Purulent drainage from the point at which the catheter penetrates the skin.
3. Septic Thrombophlebitis. Presence of purulent fluid in the lumen of a vein or histopathological evidence of invasion of the venous wall by microorganisms on venous wall biopsy.
4. Catheter-Related Bacteremia. Same species of microorganism recovered from blood cultures and either culture of purulent drainage from the point at which the catheter penetrates the skin or from a positive semiquantitative (9) or quantitative (79) culture of the catheter and no other identifiable source for the bacteremia. (For coagulase-negative staphylococci, there must be at least two positive blood cultures and the isolates from blood must have the same antibiogram as the isolate from the catheter).

SPECIAL TYPES OF PERIPHERAL VENOUS CATHETERS

Heparin Lock Cannulae

Heparin lock cannulae were developed by Stern and colleagues to permit intermittent dosing of intravenous antibiotics in patients with cystic fibrosis and complicating pulmonary infections (85). Since that time, heparin locks have been used extensively, but few studies have been published on the infectious complications encountered with use of these devices.

Adults

The only study of heparin lock cannulae in adults was published by Ferguson and associates in 1976 (86). They noted a phlebitis rate of 12%. Cultures were performed on 119 heparin lock needles on removal. Qualitative cultures were taken by first flushing the heparin lock with brain heart infusion broth and then removing the needle tip and placing it in the same type of broth. Fifty-three percent of cannulae associated with phlebitis had a positive flush culture versus 1% positive flush cultures in cannulae not related to phlebitis ($p = 2.3 \times 10^{-8}$). On the other hand, positive needle tip cultures were not significantly related to phlebitis ($p > 0.50$). None of the patients with heparin locks developed bacteremia. Microorganisms isolated from heparin lock flush cultures and needle tip cultures included *S. epidermidis*, *Micrococcus* species, and aerobic diphtheroids.

Risk factors for a positive flush culture included duration of usage (>96 hours), number of different drugs infused or injected through the heparin lock, and the number of manipulations of the device. The only risk factor for a positive needle tip culture was the number of manipulations. Only two episodes of phlebitis (injection of medication into infiltrated heparin-lock needles) occurred prior to 96 hours of heparin lock needle dwell time. The authors dismissed the microorganisms recovered from needle tip cultures as contaminants picked up on needle removal. If it is assumed that only a positive flush culture is indicative of cannula-related infection, then the infection rate is 0% up to 96 hours and 21% after 96 hours.

The only report in the literature on bacteremia associated with the use of heparin lock needles is a letter to the editor by Agger and Maki (87). They described two cases of bacteremia in two patients with leukemia and heparin locks in place. They stated that needle-related septicemia may occur more frequently in patients with cancer and other immunocompromising conditions.

Children

Taylor and coworkers have published the only study on heparin locks in children (88). They randomized 39 newborn infants in an intermediate care nursery to receive parenteral medications by a heparin lock catheter or by an intravenous line kept patent by a continuous low infusion rate. None of the patients in the study developed thrombophlebitis, local catheter-related infection, or bacteremia. The only significant difference in the two groups was that patients with the continuous infusion had more episodes of subcutaneous infiltration.

Midline Catheters

Midline catheters are three- to eight-inch PVCs made of silicone or polyurethane and inserted into larger peripheral veins in the vicinity of the antecubital fossa with the tip lying distal to the central veins (89). There are four published studies that assess the risk of infection associated with the use of midline catheters (89–92). All are prospective observational studies. Harwood and colleagues studied 41 catheters in 27 children and young adults with cystic fibrosis (90). They observed no phlebitis and no infections, but neither condition was defined by the authors.

Mermel and associates studied 251 midline catheters in 238 patients (89). Infections were well-defined and both catheter hubs and catheter segments were cultured on removal. They were able to obtain 140 catheters for culture. The rate of phlebitis was 15.7% or 18.3 per 1000 catheter-days. Catheter colonization occurred at a rate of 4.2% or 5 per 1000 catheter-days and bacteremia at a rate of 0.7% or 0.8 per 1000 catheters-days. Significant growth was noted from 3% of the hubs and 0.7% of infusate specimens. Microorganisms recovered from colonized catheters included coagulase-negative staphylococci, *K. pneumoniae*, and *S. aureus*. The one case of bacteremia was caused by *S. aureus*.

Although the number of catheter colonizations was small, Mermel and associates used Poisson regression to show that catheter colonization occurred at a significantly higher rate in catheters in place for less than eight days compared to those in place for eight to 14 days. They interpreted this to mean that midline catheters do not need to be changed on a regular basis if the patient has no unexplained fever or purulent drainage at the insertion site.

Williams and associates studied an ultrafine polyurethane midline catheter (external diameter of 0.8 mm [22G] used for peripheral parenteral nutrition in 45 adult patients (91). Seven of the 45 (15.6%) patients developed clinical signs of peripheral vein thrombophlebitis (PVT). Six of these seven catheters were positive on culture. The culture technique and criteria for a positive culture were not described. The cumulative daily risk for the occurrence of PVT was 0.016 episodes per day. None of the patients developed sepsis.

Lesser and coworkers studied the use of a small number of midline catheters in low-birthweight infants and compared the performance of midline catheters with PCVs (92). Catheters were not cultured on removal. Nine midline catheters were compared with 23 PVCs. The mean dwell time for midline catheters was 9.0 ± 1.4 days and for PVCs it was 3.1 ± 0.5 days (p < 0.05). There were no suspected or confirmed episodes of sepsis associated with either type of catheter.

Of the published studies, only the study of Mermel and associates has an adequate number of patients/catheters to define rates of phlebitis, catheter colonization, and catheter-related bacteremia (89). More studies of midline catheters are needed with adequate power and multivariable analytical techniques to establish the rates of complications and risk factors for colonization/infection of midline catheters.

Peripherally Inserted Central Venous Catheters (PICCs)

Insertion of catheters into central veins by way of a peripheral vein rather than a subclavian or jugular vein was first introduced by Bottino and colleagues for administration of chemotherapeutic agents and blood products to patients with malignant neoplasms (93). These catheters are silicone elastomer (Silastic) catheters inserted through large veins in the antecubital fossa.

In normal hosts, rates of phlebitis have ranged from 2.2 to 11.5% (94–97). Local catheter site infections have been assessed in only two studies. Giuffrida and associates noted a 0.4% cumulative incidence of suppurative thrombophlebitis in their patients with PICCs (98), and Pauley and coworkers observed a cumulative incidence of catheter colonization of 5% using a semiquantitative culture technique (99). Rates of catheter-related bacteremia have been reported in four studies and range from 2.2 to 0.6% (94,96) or 0.48 and 0.9 infections per 1000 catheter-days (95–97). Rates of local catheter-related infection are similar to those for short PVCs. Catheter-related bacteremia rates for PICCs are about the same as those associated with short PVCs and are much lower than those for centrally inserted central venous catheters.

Raad and colleagues found higher rates of catheter-related infections for PICCs inserted into cancer patients (100). Local catheter-related colonization and infection occurred at a rate of 12.3% and the PICC-related bacteremia rate was 3.9%. Strahilevitz and colleagues did a study of PICCs inserted into 40 patients with acute myeloid leukemia (101). All catheters were inserted by interventional radiologists. Insertion site infections were defined as sites with a purulent discharge that yielded growth on culture. There were 1.4 insertion site infections per 1000 catheter-days and 4.68 bloodstream infections per 1000 catheter-days. Although it would appear that catheter-associated infection rates may be higher in cancer patients, more studies are needed to determine whether use of PICCs in these patients is associated with higher infection rates.

Using semiquantitative catheter cultures (9) and univariate analytical techniques, Paz-Fumagalli and coworkers studied 38 PICCs in patients with spinal cord injury (102). All catheters were inserted by interventional radiologists. These authors observed a catheter insertion site colonization/infection rate of 2.1 per 1000 catheter-days and no bacteremias. The cumulative incidence of phlebitis was reduced from 16.5% for short PVCs to 2.4% for PICCs.

Skiest and colleagues carried out a prospective observational cohort study on patients with HIV infection/AIDS (103). The mean CD_4 cell count was 35 cells/μL (range 0–323 cells/μL). The catheters were inserted by a nurse trained in PICC placement or by an interventional radiologist. Catheters were not cultured. Catheter insertion sites were observed for signs of inflammation. The rate of phlebitis was 0.6 per 1000 catheter-days, and the rate of bacteremia was 0.8 per 1000 catheter-days. It would appear that the rates of catheter-associated infections including bacteremias in HIV/AIDS patients are similar to those in patients without HIV infection.

Two studies in children have been published. Infections related to the use of PICCs were defined as catheter-associated sepsis or catheter sepsis.

Results of catheter cultures and blood cultures were not analyzed separately. Thiagarajan and associates studied 441 PICC insertions in patients with a mean age of 3.4 years (104). Nine of 441 (2%) PICCs had catheter-associated sepsis (positive blood or catheter tip culture). Microorganisms cultured from blood or catheter tip included coagulase-negative staphylococci, enterococci, *E. coli*, and *Candida* species.

Foo and colleagues studied both PICCs and tunneled central venous lines (TCVLs) in very low birthweight infants (105). Catheters were not cultured. Catheter-related infections were defined as a positive blood culture in the presence of a catheter and treated by the NICU team with antibiotics. TCVLs had an incidence rate of infection of 19.9 infections per 1000 catheter-days and PICCs had a rate of 18.9 infections per 1000 catheter-days. Infections were caused by coagulase-negative staphylococci, enterococci, *Klebsiella oxytoca*, *Enterobacter cloacae*, and *C. albicans*.

In patients without cancer, most catheter-related infections were caused by coagulase-negative staphylococci, but other microorganisms isolated included *S. aureus*, streptococci, *Candida* species, and Gram-negative bacilli (94,95,97,99). Raad and colleagues also found that the latter microorganisms were commonly isolated from blood in cancer patients whose PICCs were complicated by bacteremia, but also isolated *S. marcescens*, *Mycobacterium cheloni*, *E. faecalis*, and *Acinetobacter anitratus* (100). In leukemia patients with PICCs, Strahilevitz and colleagues also recovered *E. coli*, *K. pneumoniae*, *E. cloacae*, *Citrobacter freundii*, *Capnocytophaga* sp., and *Clostridium perfringens* from blood cultures (101).

The data on risk factors for PICC colonization/infection are scant. The only attempt to elucidate risk factors for infections that complicate the use of PICCs was in the study published by Raad and colleagues (100). In a univariate analysis, these investigators identified therapy for acute lymphocytic or acute myelocytic leukemia as the only factor significantly associated with PICC-related infections. Treatment with corticosteroids, neutropenia, thrombocytopenia, renal insufficiency, and bone marrow transplantation were not identified as risk factors for catheter-related infection in patients with PICCs. There was no difference in catheter colonization rates between those patients who received antibiotics and those who did not. Raad and colleagues also noted that site inflammation with negative catheter cultures occurred in 40 of 154 (26%) PICCs, but in only five of 188 (2.7%) subclavian central venous catheters.

Peripherally Implantable Venous Access Devices

Through the decade of the '90s, the peripherally implantable venous access device (arm port) has been introduced and now substantial data have accumulated on the techniques for insertion, and on the longevity and complications associated with use of these devices (106–111). These devices are usually inserted by interventional radiologists.

The device has a port chamber with a titanium body and a silicone rubber septum (Fig. 3). The catheter attached to the chamber is made of radiopaque soft polyurethane, has a 6 Fr outer diameter, and is 76 cm in length (Pharmacia Deltec, St. Paul, MN, USA) (109). The device may be inserted into the upper arm or forearm (109,111) (Fig. 4). The imaging techniques used for insertion include venography, fluoroscopy, and ultrasonography.

After insertion of the catheter into the brachial, basilic, or cephalic vein, a subcutaneous pocket is created for the P.A.S. port chamber in the arm. After connecting the catheter to the chamber and suturing the chamber into the pocket, the incision is closed (106–108,111).

With the exception of one study (106), catheters have not been cultured for suspected catheter-associated infections. Signs of local inflammation in skin and soft tissues over the device have been recorded. Purulent drainage and purulent fluid in port pockets and blood have been cultured. Infections that occurred within 30 days after insertion were considered early infections and those that occurred after 30 days were considered late infections (107,108). Early infections were considered to be procedurally related and late infections were considered to be due to breaks in technique during use or due to immunosuppression in the patients (107,108).

The incidence rates of infectious complications associated with use of these devices have been consistently low in published studies. Published incidence rates range from 0.29 infections per 1000 device-days to 0.8 infections per 1000 device-days (7,8,10–13).

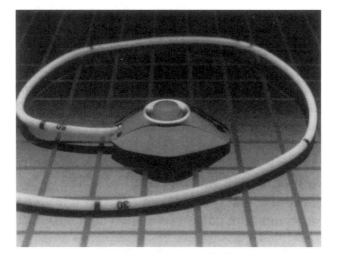

Figure 3   P.A.S. port device with catheter attached. The chamber is made of titanium, the septum of silicone rubber, and the catheter of radiopaque polyurethane.

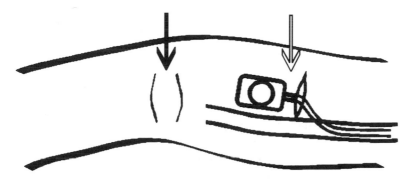

Figure 4   The typical position of the port in the upper extremity is shown in this line drawing. The black arrow shows the antecubital fossa and the open arrow shows the relationship of the catheter venous entry site to the port location.

In one study, no infections were observed in 105 implanted devices (109). The mean times that the devices were indwelling ranged from 87.7 days to 258.3 days (8–12).

In two studies, the authors also studied the complications of P.A.S. ports in patients with HIV infection (108,110). In this population, the incidence rates of infections complicating use of these devices was somewhat higher than rates in non-HIV patients with a range of 0.69 infections per 1000 device-days to 1.1 infections per 1000 device-days. However, the rates in both non-HIV and HIV infected patients were quite low.

The causative microorganisms of infections that complicate the use of these devices were similar to those that have been isolated from infections that complicated the use of other types of intravascular devices. *Staphylococcus aureus* has been recovered most frequently (107,110,111,113). Other isolates have included coagulase-negative staphylococci, *Enterococcus* species, *Propionibacterium acnes*, *P. aeruginosa*, *A. antitratus*, *E. cloacae*, *Serratia liquefaciens*, and *C. albicans* (107,110,111,113).

The advantages of arm ports over chest ports are that they are smaller and more concealed and tend to be much less of an undesirable external sign of severe disease to patients (112). Since they can be inserted by interventional radiologists in the radiology suite, same-day service is feasible and insertion in radiology is less expensive than insertion in the operating room. Further, pneumothorax and damage to vessels and nerves can be avoided (108,112). Another complication that can be avoided is catheter fracture between the clavicle and first rib (111). Finally, these devices can be used in patients with HIV infection with a low risk of device-associated infection (108,110).

The disadvantages of arm ports include the smaller diaphragm, which is more difficult to access, requiring finer needles, and the finer needles, smaller nipple, and longer catheter result in a higher resistance to infusion. Thus, the arm ports are less suited for rapid or massive effusions such as in the treatment

of leukemia or administration of large volumes of parenteral nutrition fluids
(113).

E. Peripheral Parenteral Nutrition

Although peripherally inserted central venous catheters are now being used to
administer parenteral nutrition fluids [peripheral parenteral nutrition (PPN)],
there are few published data on rates of infection that complicate this type of
therapy. In a study of only nine patients receiving parenteral nutrition by
PICCs, Stokes and Hill observed no infections and no thrombophlebitis
(114). Nordenström and associates prospectively studied 142 surgical patients
receiving PPN and recorded the incidence and severity of infusion phlebitis,
but did not assess the incidence, etiology, or risk factors for infections that
complicate the administration of parenteral nutrition fluids by this route
(115). They noted an overall incidence of phlebitis of 18%, but showed that
the incidence of phlebitis was significantly lower when a compounded mixture
of fluids was administered compared to infusion of fluids from separate
bottles.

Alhimyary and coworkers studied 135 PICC lines inserted into 126 non-
intensive care unit patients for PPN (116). They compared the outcomes in the
latter patients with 105 patients with 135 triple lumen central subclavian
venous catheters with one port designated exclusively for the administration
of TPN. Two catheter-related infections developed in the subclavian line
group and in none of the patients with a PICC line. One patient in the
subclavian catheter group developed a pneumothorax at the time of catheter
placement. Three patients in the PICC group developed phlebitis. This is the
largest study to date on the infectious complications of PPN. The results
suggest that the risk of catheter-related infections is low when PICCs are used
for infusion of parenteral nutrition fluids.

Two of the latter studies show that delivery of parenteral nutrition fluids
by PICCs is very effective in meeting the nutritional needs of patients
(114,115). However, prospective, randomized controlled trials and prospective cohort studies analyzed using multivariable techniques are needed to
better define the rates of complicating infections, etiologies of these infections,
and risk factors for infections associated with delivery of parenteral nutrition
fluids by this route.

PREVENTION OF PHLEBITIS AND PERIPHERAL VENOUS
CATHETER-RELATED INFECTIONS

Phlebitis

Catheter Materials

In three prospective controlled studies (two randomized), the rate of aseptic
phlebitis for polyurethane catheters versus Teflon catheters was lower, by 27

to 46% (2,5,11). Thus, it would appear that, when all other factors are equal, use of polyurethane catheters would provide the lowest risk of phlebitis.

Rotation of Catheter Sites

Previous recommendations that PVCs be rotated to a new site every 48 to 72 hours were based on an increase in risk of catheter-related infections when these devices remained in situ for longer than 48 to 72 hours. However, catheter-related infection rates for PVCs are currently so low that recommendations for rotation of sites in adults are now based on reducing the incidence of phlebitis (12,71,117). New recommendations from the Centers for Disease Control and Prevention (CDC) call for replacement of short peripheral venous catheters at least every 72–96 hours (117). Phlebitis is less of a problem in pediatric patients, and it does not appear necessary to rotate PVC sites in children (7,8,65,117).

Vein Selected for Cannulation

For midline catheters and PICC lines, insertion into the basilic vein may be associated with significantly less thrombophlebitis and extravasation than insertion into the cephalic vein (118).

Buffering Acidic Solutions

As noted in the "Chemical Factors" Section, acidic solutions are associated with aseptic phlebitis. Several studies have shown that buffering acidic solutions substantially reduces the occurrence of phlebitis (17,21,119).

Avoiding Use of Solutions with High Osmolarity

As noted in the "Chemical Factors" Section, solutions with an osmolarity greater than 600 mOsm/L are associated with a significant increase in phlebitis. This was noted to be particularly associated with infusion of amino acids and solutions with a high potassium content infused into small veins (23). It has been recommended that osmolarity be maintained below 600 mOsm/L, that very high concentrations of potassium be avoided, that infusions of such fluids not be administered by small veins, and that catheter insertion sites be rotated daily (23).

Use of Transdermal Glyceryl Trinitrate

It has been postulated that irritation of the endothelium of veins by insertion of cannulae causes venoconstriction and that this contributes to phlebitis. However, this mechanism of the pathogenesis of thrombophlebitis has recently been challenged by a study published by Everitt (120). He performed a study on the changes in caliber of veins caused by insertion of a fine-bore polyurethane catheter and infusion of a hypertonic, acidic nutritional emulsion. He used ultrasound to measure vein caliber. Vein caliber was measured at the point of catheter insertion and at the position of the catheter tip. Mean vein diameter was slightly greater at the point of venipuncture (not statistically significant) and at the position of the catheter tip, where mean vein diameter was statistically significantly increased. Mean vein diameter was greater at both points on day seven, and on the final day of catheters that were removed for complications, the mean diameter at both points was significantly greater. This study strongly suggests that venoconstriction is not the pathogenetic mechanism for thrombophlebitis.

In the past, based on the belief that venoconstriction caused thrombophlebitis, it was postulated that application of an agent close to the insertion site that would keep the vein dilated might reduce the incidence of phlebitis (121). Two randomized clinical trials in which glyceryl trinitrate, a vasodilator, was applied near the cannula insertion site showed a significant reduction in phlebitis compared to placebo (121,122). O'Brien and coworkers studied the cost-effectiveness of transdermal glyceryl trinitrate prophylaxis using a Markov process and concluded that such prophylaxis would be cost-effective for cannulae that remained in place for more than 50 hours (123). The only side effect noted with transdermal glyceryl trinitrate was headache easily managed with simple analgesics (122). While transdermal glyceryl trinitrate appears promising for prophylaxis of infusion phlebitis, it is unclear what its mechanism of action is, given the study of Everitt (120). More studies on the mechanism of action, efficacy, safety, and cost-effectiveness of glyceryl trinitrate are needed before recommending that such prophylaxis be widely adopted.

Inline Filtration of Infusion Fluids

It has been postulated that particulate contamination of infusion fluids is an important cause of infusion phlebitis (24–26). However, randomized controlled clinical trials of inline filters have yielded conflicting results (24–26,124). Given that inline filters have not been shown to be efficacious in the prevention of infusion phlebitis or infections associated with intravenous infusions, that certain drugs given in low doses may suffer a loss in potency as a result of filtration (125), and that inline filters add to the cost of infusion therapy, their routine use in infusion therapy cannot be recommended. Filters may be required for infusion of certain drugs, and filters should be used in accordance with pharmaceutical manufacturers' recommendations.

Catheter-Related Colonization and Infection

Detailed recommendations for the prevention of PVC-related infections are provided in Table 2. Some of the most important aspects of prevention of infections that complicate the use of PVCs are discussed in more detail below.

Catheter Selection

Microorganisms adhere more avidly to polyethylene and polyvinyl chloride, and catheters constructed from these materials are associated with a higher

Table 2   Recommendations for the Prevention of Peripheral Venous Catheter-Related Infections

Recommendation	Category[a]
I. Health care worker education and training	
A. Educate health care workers regarding the indications for intravascular catheter use, proper procedures for the insertion and maintenance of intravascular catheters, and appropriate infection-control measures to prevent intravascular catheter-related infections.	IA
B. Periodically assess knowledge of and adherence to guidelines for all persons who insert and manage intravascular catheters.	IA
C. Ensure appropriate nursing staff levels in ICUs to minimize the incidence of catheter-related bloodstream infections (CRBSIs).	IB
II. Surveillance	
A. Monitor the catheter sites visually or by palpation through the intact dressing on a regular basis, depending on the clinical situation of individual patients. If patients have tenderness at the insertion site, fever without obvious source, or other manifestations suggesting local or bloodstream infection (BSI), the dressing should be removed to allow thorough examination of the site.	IB
B. Encourage patients to report to their health care provider any changes in their catheter site or any new discomfort.	II
C. Record the operator, date, and time of catheter insertion and removal, and dressing changes on a standardized form.	II
D. Do not routinely culture catheter tips.	IA
III. Hand hygiene	
A. Observe proper hand hygiene procedures, either by washing hands with conventional antiseptic-containing soap and water or with waterless alcohol-based gels or foams. Observe hand hygiene before and after palpating catheter insertion sites, as well as before and after inserting, replacing, accessing, repairing, or dressing an intravascular catheter. Palpation of the insertion site should not be performed after the application of antiseptic, unless aseptic technique is maintained.	IA
B. Use of gloves does not obviate the need for hand hygiene.	IA
IV. Aseptic technique during catheter insertion and care	
A. Maintain aseptic technique for the insertion and care of intravascular catheters.	IA

Table 2   Continued

Recommendation	Category[a]
B. Wear clean or sterile gloves when inserting an intravascular catheter as required by the Occupational Safety and Health Administration Bloodborne Pathogens Standard.	IC
Wearing clean gloves rather than sterile gloves is acceptable for the insertion of peripheral intravascular catheters if the access site is not touched after the application of skin antiseptics. Sterile gloves should be worn for the insertion of arterial and central venous catheters.	IA
C. Wear clean or sterile gloves when changing the dressing on intravascular catheters.	IC
V. Catheter insertion	
Do not routinely use arterial or venous cutdown procedures as a method to insert catheters.	IA
VI. Catheter site care	
A. Cutaneous antisepsis	
1. Disinfect clean skin with an appropriate antiseptic before catheter insertion and during dressing changes. Although a 2% chlorhexidine-based preparation is preferred, tincture of iodine, an iodophor, or 70% alcohol can be used.	IA
2. No recommendation can be made for the use of chlorhexidine in infants aged <2 months.	Unresolved issue
3. Allow the antiseptic to remain on the insertion site and to air dry before catheter insertion. Allow povidone-iodine to remain on the skin for at least two minutes, or longer if it is not yet dry before insertion.	IB
4. Do not apply organic solvents (e.g., acetone and ether) to the skin before insertion of catheters or during dressing changes.	IA
VII. Catheter-site dressing regimens	
A. Use either sterile gauze or sterile, transparent, semipermeable dressing to cover the catheter site.	IA
B. Tunneled CVC sites that are well-healed might not require dressings.	II
C. If the patient is diaphoretic, or if the site is bleeding or oozing, a gauze dressing is preferable to a transparent, semipermeable dressing.	II
D. Replace catheter-site dressing if the dressing becomes damp, loosened, or visibly soiled.	IB
E. Change dressings at least weekly for adult and adolescent patients, depending on the circumstances of the individual patient.	II

Table 2 Continued

Recommendation	Category[a]
F. Do not use topical antibiotic ointment or creams on insertion sites (except when using dialysis catheters) because of their potential to promote fungal infections and antimicrobial resistance.	IA
G. Do not submerge the catheter under water. Showering should be permitted if precautions can be taken to reduce the likelihood of introducing organisms into the catheter (e.g., if the catheter and connecting device are protected with an impermeable cover during the shower).	II
VIII. Selection and replacement of intravascular catheters	
A. Select the catheter, insertion technique, and insertion site with the lowest risk for complications (infectious and noninfectious) for the anticipated type and duration of IV therapy.	IA
B. Promptly remove any intravascular catheter that is no longer essential.	IA
C. Do not routinely replace central venous or arterial catheters solely for the purposes of reducing the incidence of infection.	IB
D. Replace peripheral venous catheters at least every 72–96 hours in adults to prevent phlebitis (128). Leave peripheral venous catheters in place in children until IV therapy is completed, unless complications (e.g., phlebitis and infiltration) occur.	IB
E. When adherence to aseptic technique cannot be ensured (i.e., when catheters are inserted during a medical emergency), replace all catheters as soon as possible and after no longer than 48 hours.	II
F. Use clinical judgment to determine when to replace a catheter that could be a source of infection (e.g., do not routinely replace catheters in patients whose only indication of infection is fever). Do not routinely replace venous catheters in patients who are bacteremic or fungemic if the source of infection is unlikely to be the catheter.	II
G. Replace any short-term CVC if purulence is observed at the insertion site, which indicates infection.	IB
H. Replace all CVCs if the patient is hemodynamically unstable and CRBSI is suspected.	II
I. Do not use guidewire techniques to replace catheters in patients suspected of having catheter-related infection.	IB
IX. Replacement of administration sets[b], needleless systems, and parenteral fluids	
A. Administration sets	
1. Replace administration sets, including secondary sets and add-on devices, no more frequently than	IA

Table 2 Continued

Recommendation	Category[a]
at 72-hour intervals, unless catheter-related infection is suspected or documented.	
2. Replace tubing used to administer blood, blood products, or lipid emulsions (those combined with amino acids and glucose in a 3-in-1 admixture or infused separately) within 24 hours of initiating the infusion.	IB
If the solution contains only dextrose and amino acids, the administration set does not need to be replaced more frequently than every 72 hours.	II
3. Replace tubing used to administer propofol infusions every six or 12 hours, depending on its use, per the manufacturer's recommendation.	IA
B. Needleless intravascular devices	
1. Change the needleless components at least as frequently as the administration set.	II
2. Change caps no more frequently than every 72 hours or according to manufacturers' recommendations.	II
3. Ensure that all components of the system are compatible to minimize leaks and breaks in the system.	II
4. Minimize contamination risk by wiping the access port with an appropriate antiseptic and accessing the port only with sterile devices.	IB
C. Parenteral fluids	
1. Complete the infusion of lipid-containing solutions (e.g., 3-in-1 solutions) within 24 hours of hanging the solution.	IB
2. Complete the infusion of lipid emulsions alone within 12 hours of hanging the emulsion. If volume considerations require more time, the infusion should be completed within 24 hours.	IB
3. Complete infusions of blood or other blood products within four hours of hanging the blood.	II
4. No recommendation can be made for the hang time of other parenteral fluids.	Unresolved issue
X. IV-injection ports	
A. Clean injection ports with 70% alcohol or an iodophor before accessing the system.	IA
B. Cap all stopcocks when not in use.	IB
XI. Preparation and quality control of IV admixtures	
A. Admix all routine parenteral fluids in the pharmacy in a laminar-flow hood using aseptic technique.	IB

Table 2 Continued

Recommendation	Category[a]
B. Do not use any container of parenteral fluid that has visible turbidity, leaks, cracks, or particulate matter, or if the manufacturer's expiration date has passed.	IB
C. Use single-dose vials for parenteral additives or medications when possible.	II
D. Do not combine the leftover content of single-use vials for later use.	IA
E. If multidose vials are used	
1. Refrigerate multidose vials after they are opened if recommended by the manufacturer.	II
2. Cleanse the access diaphragm of multidose vials with 70% alcohol before inserting a device into the vial.	IA
3. Use a sterile device to access a multidose vial and avoid touch contamination of the device before penetrating the access diaphragm.	IA
4. Discard multidose vial if sterility is compromised.	IA
XII. Inline filters	
Do not use filters routinely for infection-control purposes.	IA
XIII. IV-therapy personnel	
Designate trained personnel for the insertion and maintenance of intravascular catheters.	IA
XIV. Prophylactic antimicrobials	
Do not administer intranasal or systemic antimicrobial prophylaxis routinely before insertion or during use of an intravascular catheter to prevent catheter colonization or BSI.	IA

Peripheral Venous Catheters, Including Midline Catheters, in Adult and Pediatric Patients	
I. Selection of peripheral catheter	
A. Select catheters on the basis of the intended purpose and duration of use, known complications (e.g., phlebitis and infiltration), and experience of individual catheter operators.	IB
B. Avoid the use of steel needles for the administration of fluids and medication that might cause tissue necrosis if extravasation occurs.	IA
C. Use a midline catheter or PICC when the duration of IV therapy will likely exceed six days.	IB
II. Selection of peripheral-catheter insertion site	
A. In adults, use an upper- instead of a lower-extremity site for catheter insertion. Replace a catheter inserted in a lower-extremity site to an upper-extremity site as soon as possible.	IA
B. In pediatric patients, the hand, the dorsum of the foot, or the scalp can be used as the catheter insertion site.	II

Table 2 Continued

Recommendation	Category[a]
C. Replacement of catheter	
1. Evaluate the catheter insertion site daily, by palpation through the dressing to discern tenderness and by inspection if a transparent dressing is in use. Gauze and opaque dressings should not be removed if the patient has no clinical signs of infection. If the patient has local tenderness or other signs of possible CRBSI, an opaque dressing should be removed and the site inspected visually.	II
2. Remove peripheral venous catheters if the patient develops signs of phlebitis (e.g., warmth, tenderness, erythema, and palpable venous cord), infection, or a malfunctioning catheter.	IB
3. In adults, replace short, peripheral venous catheters at least every 72–96 hours to reduce the risk for phlebitis. If sites for venous access are limited and no evidence of phlebitis or infection is present, peripheral venous catheters can be left in place for longer periods, although the patient and the insertion sites should be closely monitored.	IB
4. Do not routinely replace midline catheters to reduce the risk for infection.	IB
5. In pediatric patients, leave peripheral venous catheters in place until IV therapy is completed, unless a complication (e.g., phlebitis and infiltration) occurs.	IB
III. Catheter and catheter-site care	
A. Do not routinely apply prophylactic topical antimicrobial or antiseptic ointment or cream to the insertion site of peripheral venous catheters.	IA

[a] As in previous guidelines issued by CDC and HICPAC, each recommendation is categorized on the basis of existing scientific data, theoretical rationale, applicability, and economic impact. The CDC/HICPAC system for categorizing recommendations is as follows:

Category IA.	Strongly recommended for implementation and strongly supported by well-designed experimental, clinical, or epidemiological studies.
Category IB.	Strongly recommended for implementation and supported by some experimental, clinical, or epidemiological studies, and a strong theoretical rationale.
Category IC.	Required by state or federal regulations, rules, or standards.
Category II.	Suggested for implementation and supported by suggestive clinical or epidemiological studies or a theoretical rationale.
Unresolved Issue.	Represents an unresolved issue for which evidence is insufficient or no consensus regarding efficacy exists.

[b] Administration sets include the area from the spike of tubing entering the fluid container to the hub of the vascular access device. However, a short extension tube might be connected to the catheter and might be considered a portion of the catheter to facilitate aseptic technique when changing administration sets. (Modified from Ref. 117.)

rate of catheter colonization than are catheters made from Teflon and polyurethane (2,30,31). Thus, it would appear that use of polyurethane catheters in adults would provide the lowest rates of aseptic phlebitis (as noted in "Adults" under "Risk Factors for Phlebitis and Catheter-Site Colonization" Section) and catheter colonization (2,5,11). Data are insufficient on which catheters are most appropriate for use in children.

Catheter Insertion

Site of Insertion: For many years, it has been taught that in adults, PVCs should not be inserted into veins in the lower extremity, because PVCs in the lower extremity are at a higher risk of infection than those inserted into the upper extremity. It would appear that concern for a higher risk of infection for PVCs inserted into the lower extremity is based on anecdotal reports published 42–44 years ago (126–128). There are no prospective observational cohort studies or randomized clinical trials to support a higher risk of infection for PVCs inserted into the lower extremity. As will be noted in Table 2, the CDC's new guidelines on prevention of intravascular device-related infections still recommend the upper extremity as the preferred site for insertion of PVCs in adults.

Antiseptic Preparation of the Site: Short peripheral venous catheters should be inserted using aseptic no-touch technique after application of an antiseptic to the skin overlying the vein to be cannulated. There are few published data on which to base selection of an antiseptic for preparation of the skin prior to insertion of the catheter. It would appear that tincture of iodine is more effective than an iodophor for skin preparation prior to venipuncture to obtain blood for culture (129), but this does not necessarily translate to greater effectiveness than an iodophor for skin preparation prior to cannulation of a vein. The only randomized controlled trial of antiseptics used for skin preparation prior to insertion of an intravascular catheter was published by Maki and colleagues (47). However, this was a study of central venous and arterial catheters, and it may not be possible to extrapolate these findings to PVCs. The authors showed that 2% aqueous chlorhexidine gluconate was significantly more effective than 70% isopropyl alcohol and 10% povidone-iodine solution in preventing catheter-related infection and catheter-related bacteremias. In the absence of studies on antisepsis for the insertion of PVCs in adults, it is reasonable to conclude that 2% aqueous chlorhexidine gluconate may be the antiseptic of choice, pending publication of randomized clinical trials on antiseptics for preparation of PVC insertion sites.

Garland and associates carried out a prospective, nonrandomized study of successive cohorts of neonates. During the first six months, 10% povidone-iodine was used for skin preparation at PVC insertion sites, followed by use of 0.5% chlorhexidine gluconate in 70% isopropyl alcohol for the next six months (130). The rate of catheter colonization was 9.3% with povidone-iodine and 4.7% with 0.5% chlorhexidine gluconate in 70% isopropyl alcohol (p = 0.01). Using logistical regression, the authors showed that 0.5% chlorhexidine gluconate in 70% isopropyl alcohol was significantly better than 10% povidone-iodine and that heavy skin colonization before catheter insertion was a risk factor for catheter colonization.

There are no published data on the efficacy of procedures for insertion of midline catheters or PICCs. For insertion of midline catheters, Mermel and coworkers cleansed the insertion site with povidone-iodine, followed by 70% ethyl alcohol and then povidone-iodine again. The insertion site was draped with large, sterile sheet drapes, and the operator wore a mask and sterile gloves (89).

The procedure for insertion of PICCs varies from center to center. The site has usually been prepped with povidone-iodine (95,100), and masks may be worn (95,98). All reports mentioned that the operator wore sterile gloves (95,96,98,100).

Device Securement

There are few published data on how intravascular catheters should be secured. In a randomized controlled trial, Yamamoto and colleagues studied the efficacy of a new device designed to anchor PICCs and other central venous catheters (131). Eighty-five patients were randomized to receive a new device to anchor their PICC, and 85 were randomized to have their PICC secured with a suture. The new device (StatLock® [Venetec International, San Diego, CA]) is sutureless and has an adhesive on the back side, which is applied to the skin. Catheter-related bloodstream infections were diagnosed using CDC definitions. The patients randomized to the sutureless, adhesive-backed device had significantly fewer systemic infections than the patients whose PICC was secured with a suture. Although it is unknown how the sutureless, adhesive-backed securement device reduces catheter-related systemic infections, it is postulated that a suture at the insertion site promotes bacterial colonization of the site (131).

Application of Topical Antimicrobial Ointments to the Insertion Site

Application of an antimicrobial ointment to the site where the catheter penetrates the skin is based on the most important pathogenetic mechanism for catheter site colonization and infection. Thus, theoretically, it would be expected that a topical antimicrobial agent applied at the entrance to the subcutaneous catheter tract might block the migration of microorganisms into the tract and reduce the risk of colonization and infection. However, this approach to prevention of infection has generally been disappointing. Moran and coworkers conducted the first randomized controlled trial of topical antibiotic prophylaxis 37 years ago (132). They observed a significant protective effect of a topical preparation containing neomycin, polymyxin, and bacitracin applied to venous cutdown sites. Two randomized controlled trials of percutaneously inserted catheters by Norden (133) and Zinner and associates (134) in the 1960s using a topical preparation of polymyxin B, neomycin and bacitracin yielded equivocal results. Colonization/infection rates with pathogens were the same for the topical antibiotic and placebo groups, but colonization/infection with pathogens developed more slowly in the antibiotic group (133), or catheters in the antibiotic group were colonized with fewer pathogens (134). In both studies, yeasts were recovered only from catheters to which the topical antibiotics had been applied.

In a randomized clinical trial, Maki and Band compared the prophylactic effects of polymyxin, neomycin, bacitracin (PNB) ointment, and an iodophor ointment with no ointment (135). These authors observed a significant (but what they interpreted as a marginal effect) reduction in catheter-related infections in the PNB group compared to the group who received no ointment. The iodophor ointment did not provide a significant protective effect compared to the group without ointment, and neither PNB nor the iodophor ointment reduced the incidence of catheter-related bacteremia. The maximum protective effect of PNB was seen with catheters that remained in place for more than four days. Three of four *Candida* infections, including one septicemia, occurred in the PNB group.

Topical antimicrobial agents applied to catheter insertion sites appear to provide only marginal protection against bacteria and may increase the risk of infections due to yeasts. If topical antimicrobial agents have any role in the prevention of PVC colonization or catheter-related infection, it may be for catheters that remain in place for more than four days.

Catheter Site Dressings

The catheter insertion site should be covered with a sterile dressing after catheter placement. The dressings applied usually consist of sterile gauze covered with adhesive tape or a polyurethane film. Gauze and tape dressings act as a partial barrier to contamination and permit escape of moisture so that the catheter site remains dry. However, gauze and tape dressings are not impermeable to external moisture and require removal for inspection of the catheter insertion site. On the other hand, polyurethane film dressings are impermeable to moisture from external sources and permit patients to shower without removing the dressing or risking contamination of the site, and they allow for inspection of the catheter site without removing the dressing because they are transparent. A potential disadvantage of polyurethane film dressings is that, due to their impermeability, they may trap moisture under the dressing at the catheter insertion site and provide a moist occluded environment conducive to multiplication of microorganisms.

Two controlled trials, one randomized (136) and one nonrandomized (137), from the mid 1980s showed a significantly increased rate of catheter colonization for PVCs covered with a polyurethane dressing when compared to gauze dressings. In neither study did catheter colonization correlate with phlebitis, and Craven and colleagues observed no difference in the incidence of bacteremia between patients with gauze dressings and those with polyurethane dressings (136). In a meta-analysis that included seven studies, Hoffmann and associates found a significant increase in catheter colonization for PVCs dressed with polyurethane film when compared with those dressed with gauze, but there was no difference in the incidence of bacteremia related to the type of dressing used (138).

Other studies have shown no difference in catheter colonization between polyurethane film and gauze dressings. Hoffmann and coworkers performed a randomized controlled trial of polyurethane film versus gauze dressings applied to PVC sites (139). They randomized 300 patients to the polyurethane group and 298 to the gauze group. No differences in catheter colonization or catheter-related bacteremia were observed. In the largest randomized clinical trial of dressings applied to PVC sites published to date, Maki and Ringer randomized 2088 patients to one of four groups: **(a)** sterile gauze replaced every other day, **(b)** gauze left in place for the duration of catheterization, **(c)** polyurethane film left on for the lifetime of the catheter, and **(d)** an iodophor-transparent dressing also left on for the lifetime of the catheter (12). There was no difference in rates of catheter colonization between the dressing groups. None of these catheters were associated with bacteremia. This very large, well-designed, and well-executed controlled trial offers convincing evidence that polyurethane film dressings are as safe as gauze and tape dressings and that none of these dressings need to be routinely replaced during the lifetime of the catheter. This will likely hold true for the future with the introduction of new polyurethane films that are more permeable to moisture and that reduce the accumulation of moisture under the dressing (140).

Maintenance of the Catheter and Infusion System

Given the findings of Maki and Ringer noted above and the absence of data to support routine dressing changes as an infection control measure for PVCs, it would appear that such routine changes need not be done. In accordance with the CDC Guidelines on Intravascular Device-Related Infections Prevention (117), the catheter site should be assessed on a regular basis by visually inspecting or palpating the catheter insertion site for tenderness through the intact dressing. The site should be visually inspected if the patient develops tenderness at the insertion site, fever without an obvious source, or symptoms of local or bloodstream infection. The dressing should be replaced if it becomes damp, loosened, or visibly soiled. In the most recent CDC guidelines, it is recommended that dressings be changed at least weekly for adult and adolescent patients, depending on the circumstances of the individual patient (117). It may be necessary to change dressings more frequently in diaphoretic patients.

PVCs should be removed and inserted at a new site every 72 to 96 hours, not to prevent catheter colonization or catheter-related infection, but to reduce the incidence of phlebitis (117). Since intravenous administration sets may be left in place at least 72 hours (117,141–143), it may be convenient to change the catheter and administration set at the same time.

Specialized Intravenous Therapy Personnel

Two nonrandomized studies using historical controls have shown that when specially trained personnel were used to maintain central venous catheter sites, there was a substantially lower rate of catheter-related infections than when catheter sites were maintained by personnel without special training (144,145). One nonrandomized controlled trial using an intravenous therapy team versus residents and ward nurses to insert and care for PVCs has been published (3). There was a significantly reduced rate of phlebitis and the rates of cellulitis and septic thrombophlebitis were reduced tenfold for catheters inserted and maintained by the intravenous therapy team. However, before intravenous therapy teams can be recommended for prevention of catheter-related infections, randomized controlled clinical trials that assess both the efficacy and cost of such programs must be carried out.

REFERENCES

1. Maki DG, Mermel LA. Infections due to infusion therapy. In: Bennett JV, Brachman PS, eds. Hospital Infections. 4th ed. Philadelphia: Lippincott-Raven, 1998:689.
2. Maki DG, Ringer M. Risk factors for infusion-related phlebitis with small peripheral venous catheters. A randomized controlled trial. Ann Intern Med 1991; 114:845–854.
3. Tomford JW, Hershey CO, McLaren CE, Porter DK, Cohen DI. Intravenous therapy team and peripheral venous catheter-associated complications. Arch Intern Med 1984; 144:1191–1194.
4. Righter J, Bishop LA, Hill B. Infection and peripheral venous catheterization. Diagn Microbiol Infect Dis 1983; 1:89–93.
5. Gaukroger PD, Roberts JG, Manners TA. Infusion thrombophlebitis: a prospective comparison of 645 Vialon and Teflon cannulae in anaesthetic and postoperative use. Anaesth Intens Care 1988; 16:265–271.
6. Turnidge J. Hazards of peripheral intravenous lines. Med J Aust 1984; 141: 37–40.
7. Nelson DB, Garland JS. The natural history of Teflon catheter-associated phlebitis in children. AJDC 1987; 141:1090–1092.
8. Garland JS, Dunne WM Jr, Havens P, Hintermayer M, Bozzette MA, Wincek J, Bromberger T, Scavers M. Peripheral intravenous catheter complications in critically ill children: a prospective study. Pediatrics 1992; 89:1145–1150.
9. Maki DG, Weise CE, Sarafin HW. A semiquantitative culture method for identifying intravenous-catheter-related infection. N Engl J Med 1977; 296:1305–1309.
10. Gantz NM, Presswood GM, Goldberg R, Doern G. Effects of dressing type and change interval on intravenous therapy complication rates. Diagn Microbiol Infect Dis 1984; 2:325–332.

11. McKee JM, Shell JA, Warren TA, Campbell VP. Complications of intravenous therapy: a randomized prospective study-Vialon vs. Teflon. J Intraven Nurs 1989; 12:288–295.

12. Maki DG, Ringer M. Evaluation of dressing regimens for prevention of infection with peripheral intravenous catheters. Gauze, a transparent polyurethane dressing, and an iodophor-transparent dressing. JAMA 1987; 258:2396–2403.

13. Lewis GBH, Hecker JF. Infusion thrombophlebitis. Br J Anaesth 1985; 57:220–233.

14. Madan M, Alexander DJ, McMahon MJ. Influence of catheter type on occurrence of thrombophlebitis during peripheral intravenous nutrition. Lancet 1992; 339:101–103.

15. Bair JN, Peterson RV. Surface characteristics of plastic intravenous catheters. Am J Hosp Pharm 1979; 36:1707–1711.

16. Collin J, Collin C, Constable FL, Johnston IDA. Infusion thrombophlebitis and infection with various cannulas. Lancet 1975; ii:150–152.

17. Eremin O, Marshall V. Complications of intravenous therapy: reduction by buffering of intravenous fluid preparation. Med J Aust 1977; 2:528–531.

18. Ross SA. Infusion phlebitis. Selected factors. Nurs Res 1972; 21:313–318.

19. Hessov I, Bojsen-Møller M. Experimental infusion thrombophlebitis. Importance of the pH of glucose solutions. Europ J Intens Care Med 1976; 2:97–101.

20. Tse RL, Lee MW. pH of infusion fluids: a predisposing factor in thrombophlebitis. JAMA 1971; 215:642.

21. Fonkalsrud EW, Pederson BM, Murphy J, Beckerman JH. Reduction of infusion thrombophlebitis with buffered glucose solutions. Surgery 1968; 63:280–284.

22. Elfving G, Saikku K. Effect of pH on the incidence of infusion thrombophlebitis. Lancet 1966;i:953.

23. Gazitua R, Wilson K, Bistrian BR, Blackburn GL. Factors determining peripheral vein tolerance to amino acid infusions. Arch Surg 1979; 114:897–900.

24. Allcutt DA, Lort D, McCollum CN. Final inline filtration for intravenous infusions: a prospective hospital study. Br J Surg 1983; 70:111–113.

25. Falchuk KH, Peterson L, McNeil BJ. Microparticulate-induced phlebitis. Its prevention by in-line filtration. N Engl J Med 1985; 312:78–82.

26. Maddox RR, John JF Jr, Brown LL, Smith CE. Effect of inline filtration on postinfusion phlebitis. Clin Pharm 1983; 2:58–61.

27. Tully JL, Friedland GH, Baldini LM, Goldmann DA. Complications of intravenous therapy with steel needles and Teflon catheters. Am J Med 1981; 70:702–706.

28. Band JD, Maki DG. Steel needles used for intravenous therapy. Morbidity in patients with hematologic malignancy. Arch Intern Med 1980; 140:31–34.

29. Locci R, Peters G, Pulverer G. Microbial colonization of prosthetic devices. I. Microtopographical characteristics of intravenous catheters as detected by scanning electron microscopy. Zbl Bakt Hyg, I Abt Orig B 1981; 173:285–292.

30. Ashkenazi S, Weiss E, Drucker MM. Bacterial adherence to intravenous catheters and needles and its influence by cannula type and bacterial surface hydrophobicity. J Lab Clin Med 1986; 107:136–140.

31. Sheth NK, Franson TR, Rose HD, Buckmire FLA, Cooper JA, Sohnle PG.

Colonization of bacteria on polyvinyl chloride and Teflon intravascular catheters in hospitalized patients. J Clin Microbiol 1983; 18:1061–1063.

32. Herrmann M, Vaudaux PE, Pittet D, Auckenthaler R, Lew PD, Schumacher-Perdreau F, Peters G, Waldvogel FA. Fibronectin, fibrinogen, and laminin act as mediators of adherence of clinical staphylococcal isolates to foreign material. J Infect Dis 1988; 158:693–701.

33. Vaudaux P, Suzuki R, Waldvogel FA, Morgenthaler JJ, Nydegger UE. Foreign body infection: role of fibronectin as a ligand for the adherence of *Staphylococcus aureus*. J Infect Dis 1984; 150:546–553.

34. Peters G, Locci R, Pulverer G. Microbial colonization of prosthetic devices. II. Scanning electron microscopy of naturally infected intravenous catheters. Zbl Bakt Hyg, I Abt Orig B 1981; 173:293–299.

35. Gray ED, Peters G, Verstegen M, Regelmann WE. Effect of extracellular slime substance from *Staphylococcus epidermidis* on the human cellular immune response. Lancet 1984; i:365–367.

36. Farber BF, Kaplan MH, Clogston AG. *Staphylococcus epidermidis* extracted slime inhibits the antimicrobial action of glycopeptide antibiotics. J Infect Dis 1990; 161:37 40.

37. Maki DG, Mermel LA. Infections due to infusion therapy. In: Bennett JV, Brachman PS, eds. Hospital Infections. 4th ed. Philadelphia: Lippincott-Raven, 1998:697–699.

38. Bjornson HS, Colley R, Bower RH, Duty VP, Schwartz-Fulton JT, Fischer JE. Association between microorganism growth at the catheter insertion site and colonization of the catheter in patients receiving total parenteral nutrition. Surgery 1982; 92:720–727.

39. Snydman DR, Gorbea HF, Pober BR, Majka JA, Murray SA, Perry LK. Predictive value of surveillance skin cultures in total-parenteral-nutrition-related infection. Lancet 1982; ii:1385–1388.

40. Armstrong CW, Mayhall CG, Miller KB, Newsome HH Jr, Sugerman HJ, Dalton HP, Hall GO, Hunsberger S. Clinical predictors of infection of central venous catheters used for total parenteral nutrition. Infect Control Hosp Epidemiol 1990; 11:71–78.

41. Maki DG, Jarrett F, Sarafin HW. A semiquantitative culture method for identification of catheter-related infection in the burn patient. J Surg Res 1977; 22:513–520.

42. Pruitt BA Jr, McManus WF, Kim SH, Treat RC. Diagnosis and treatment of cannula-related intravenous sepsis in burn patients. Ann Surg 1980; 191:546–554.

43. Franceschi D, Gerding RL, Phillips G, Fratianne RB. Risk factors associated with intravascular catheter infections in burned patients: a prospective, randomized study. J Trauma 1989; 29:811–815.

44. Dixon RE, Kaslow RA, Mackel DC, Fulkerson CC, Mallison GF. Aqueous quaternary ammonium antiseptics and disinfectants. Use and misuse. JAMA 1976; 236:2415–2417.

45. Frank MJ, Schaffner W. Contaminated aqueous benzalkonium chloride. An unnecessary hospital infection hazard. JAMA 1976; 236:2418–2419.

46. Kahan A, Philippon A, Paul G, Weber S, Richard C, Hazebroucq G, Degeorges M. Nosocomial infections by chlorhexidine solution contaminated with *Pseudomonas pickettii* (biovar VA-1). J Infect 1983; 7:256–263.

47. Maki DG, Ringer M, Alvarado CJ. Prospective randomised trial of povidone-iodine, alcohol, and chlorhexidine for prevention of infection associated with central venous and arterial catheters. Lancet 1991; 338:339–343.

48. Cooper GL, Hopkins CC. Rapid diagnosis of intravascular catheter-associated infection by direct gram staining of catheter segments. N Engl J Med 1985; 312:1142–1147.

49. Collignon PJ, Soni N, Pearson IY, Woods WP, Munro R, Sorrell TC. Is semiquantitative culture of central vein catheter tips useful in the diagnosis of catheter-associated bacteremia? J Clin Microbiol 1986; 24:532–535.

50. Flowers RH III, Schwenzer KJ, Kopel RF, Fisch MJ, Tucker SI, Farr BM. Efficacy of an attachable subcutaneous cuff for the prevention of intravascular catheter-related infection. A randomized, controlled trial. JAMA 1989; 261:878–883.

51. Maki DG, Cobb L, Garman JK, Shapiro JM, Ringer M, Helgerson RB. An attachable silver-impregnated cuff for prevention of infection with central venous catheters: a prospective randomized multicenter trial. Am J Med 1988; 85:307–314.

52. Raad I, Costerton W, Sabharwal U, Sacilowski M, Anaissie E, Bodey GP. Ultrastructural analysis of indwelling vascular catheters: a quantitative relationship between luminal colonization and duration of placement. J Infect Dis 1993; 168:400–407.

53. Sitges-Serra A, Liñares J, Pérez JL, Jaurrieta E, Lorente L. A randomized trial on the effect of tubing changes on hub contamination and catheter sepsis during parenteral nutrition. J Parenter Enter Nutr 1985; 9:322–325.

54. Liñares J, Sitges-Serra A, Garau J, Pérez JL, Martín R. Pathogenesis of catheter sepsis: a prospective study with quantitative and semiquantitative cultures of catheter hub and segments. J Clin Microbiol 1985; 21:357–360.

55. Salzman MB, Isenberg HD, Shapiro JF, Lipsitz PJ, Rubin LG. A prospective study of the catheter hub as the portal of entry for microorganisms causing catheter-related sepsis in neonates. J Infect Dis 1993; 167:487–490.

56. deCicco M, Panarello G, Chiaradia V, Fracasso A, Veronesi A, Testa V, Santini G, Tesio F. Source and route of microbial colonisation of parenteral nutrition catheters. Lancet 1989; ii:1258–1261.

57. Hoshal VL Jr, Ause RG, Hoskins PA. Fibrin sleeve formation on indwelling subclavian central venous catheters. Arch Surg 1971; 102:353–358.

58. Stillman RM, Soliman F, Garcia L, Sawyer PN. Etiology of catheter-associated sepsis. Correlation with thrombogenicity. Arch Surg 1977; 112:1497–1499.

59. Hershey CO, Tomford JW, McLaren CE, Porter DK, Cohen DI. The natural history of intravenous catheter-associated phlebitis. Arch Intern Med 1984; 144:1373–1375.

60. Hampton AA, Sherertz RJ. Vascular-access infections in hospitalized patients. Surg Clin North Am 1988; 68:57–71.

61. Baker CC, Petersen SR, Sheldon GF. Septic phlebitis: a neglected disease. Am J Surg 1979; 138:97–103.

62. Wilkins EGL, Manning D, Roberts C, Davidson DC. Quantitative bacteriology of peripheral venous cannulae in neonates. J Hosp Infect 1985; 6:209–217.

63. Bregenzer T, Conen D, Sakmann P, Widmer AF. Is routine replacement of peripheral intravenous catheters necessary? Arch Intern Med 1998; 158:151–156.

64. Cronin WA, Germanson TP, Donowitz LG. Intravascular catheter colonization and related bloodstream infection in critically ill neonates. Infect Control Hosp Epidemiol 1990; 11:301–308.

65. Shimandle RB, Johnson D, Baker M, Stotland N, Karrison T, Arnow PM. Safety of peripheral intravenous catheters in children. Infect Control Hosp Epidemiol 1999; 20:736–740.

66. Garland JS, Nelson DB, Cheah T, Hennes HH, Johnson TM. Infections complications during peripheral intravenous therapy with Teflon catheters: a prospective study. Pediatr Infect Dis J 1987; 6:918–921.

67. Collignon PJ. Intravascular catheter associated sepsis: a common problem. Med J Aust 1994; 161:374–378.

68. Leibovitz E, Iuster-Reicher A, Amitai M, Mogilner B. Systemic candidal infections associated with use of peripheral venous catheters in neonates: a 9-year experience. Clin Infect Dis 1992; 14:485–491.

69. Fry DE, Fry RV, Borzotta AP. Nosocomial blood-borne infection secondary to intravascular devices. Am J Surg 1994; 167:268–272.

70. Collins RN, Braun PA, Zinner SH, Kass EH. Risk of local and systemic infection with polyethylene intravenous catheters. A prospective study of 213 catheterizations. N Engl J Med 1968; 279:340–343.

71. Tager IB, Ginsberg MB, Ellis SE, Walsh NE, Dupont I, Simchen E, Faich GA, The Rhode Island Nosocomial Infection Consortium. An epidemiologic study of the risks associated with peripheral intravenous catheters. Am J Epidemiol 1983; 118:839–851.

72. Ena J, Cercenado E, Martinez D, Bouza E. Cross-sectional epidemiology of phlebitis and catheter-related infections. Infect Control Hosp Epidemiol 1992; 13:15–20.

73. Nelson RRS, Tebbs SE, Richards N, Elliott TSJ. An audit of peripheral catheter care in a teaching hospital. J Hosp Infect 1996; 32:65–69.

74. Hirschmann H, Fux L, Podusel J, Schindler K, Kundi M, Rotter M, Wewalka G. The influence of hand hygiene prior to insertion of peripheral venous catheters on the frequency of complications. J Hosp Infect 2001; 49:199–203.

75. Sherertz RJ, Raad II, Belani A, Koo LC, Rand KH, Pickett DL, Straub SA, Fauerbach LL. Three-year experience with sonicated vascular catheter cultures in a clinical microbiology laboratory. J Clin Microbiol 1990; 28:76–82.

76. Lambotte O, Lucet J-C, Fleury L, Joly-Guillou M-L, Bouvet E. Nosocomial bacteremia in HIV patients: the role of peripheral venous catheters. Infect Control Hosp Epidemiol 2000; 21:330–333.

77. Raad II, Sabbagh MF, Rand KH, Sherertz RJ. Quantitative tip culture methods and the diagnosis of central venous catheter-related infections. Diag Microbiol Infect Dis 1992; 15:13–20.

78. O'Neill JA Jr, Pruitt BA Jr, Foley FD, Moncrief JA. Suppurative thrombophlebitis-a lethal complication of intravenous therapy. J Trauma 1968; 8:256–267.

79. Cleri DJ, Corrado ML, Seligman SJ. Quantitative culture of intravenous catheters and other intravascular inserts. J Infect Dis 1980; 141:781–786.

80. Wing EJ, Norden CW, Shadduck RK, Winkelstein A. Use of quantitative bacteriologic techniques to diagnose catheter-related sepsis. Arch Intern Med 1979; 139:482–483.

81. Fan ST, Teoh-Chan CH, Lau KF. Evaluation of central venous catheter sepsis by differential quantitative blood culture. Eur J Clin Microbiol Infect Dis 1989; 8:142–144.

82. Capdevila JA, Planes AM, Palomar M, Gasser I, Almirante B, Pahissa A, Crespo E, Martínez-Vásquez JM. Value of differential quantitative blood cultures in the diagnosis of catheter-related sepsis. Eur J Clin Microbiol Infect Dis 1992; 11:403–407.

83. Zufferey J, Rime B, Francioli P, Bille J. Simple method for rapid diagnosis of catheter-associated infection by direct acridine orange staining of catheter tips. J Clin Microbiol 1988; 26:175–177.

84. Coutlée F, Lemieux C, Paradis J. Value of direct catheter staining in the diagnosis of intravascular-catheter-related infection. J Clin Microbiol 1988; 26:1088–1090.

85. Stern RC, Pittman S, Doershuk CF, Matthews LW. Use of a "heparin lock" in the intermittent administration of intravenous drugs. A technical advance in intravenous therapy. Clin Pediatr 1972; 11:521–523.

86. Ferguson RL, Rosett W, Hodges GR, Barnes WG. Complications with heparin-lock needles. A prospective evaluation. Ann Intern Med 1976; 85:583–586.

87. Agger WA, Maki DG. Septicemia from heparin-lock needles. Ann Intern Med 1977; 86:657.

88. Taylor J, Shannon R, Kilbride HW. Heparin lock intravenous line. Use in newborn infants. A controlled trial. Clin Pediatr 1989; 28:237–240.

89. Mermel LA, Parenteau S, Tow SM. The risk of midline catheterization in hospitalized patients. A prospective study. Ann Intern Med 1995; 123:841–844.

90. Harwood IR, Greene LM, Kozakowski-Koch JA, Rasor JS. New peripherally inserted midline catheter: a better alternative for intravenous antibiotic therapy in patients with cystic fibrosis. Pediatr Pulmonol 1992; 12:233–239.

91. Williams N, Wales S, Irving MH. Prolonged peripheral parenteral nutrition with an ultrafine cannula and low-osmolality feed. Brit J Surg 1996; 83:114–116.

92. Lesser E, Chhabra R, Brion LP, Suresh BR. Use of midline catheters in low birth weight infants. J Perinatol 1996; 16:205–207.

93. Bottino J, McCredie KB, Groschel DHM, Lawson M. Long-term intravenous therapy with peripherally inserted silicone elastomer central venous catheters in patients with malignant diseases. Cancer 1979; 43:1937–1943.

94. Lam S, Scannell R, Roessler D, Smith MA. Peripherally inserted central catheters in an acute-care hospital. Arch Intern Med 1994; 154:1833–1837.

95. Abi-Nader JA. Peripherally inserted central venous catheters in critical care patients. Heart Lung 1993; 22:428–434.

96. Loughran SC, Borzatta M. Peripherally inserted central catheters: a report of 2506 catheter days. J Parenter Enter Nutr 1995; 19:133–136.

97. Duerksen DR, Papineau N, Siemens J, Yaffe C. Peripherally inserted central catheters for parenteral nutrition: a comparison with centrally inserted catheters. J Parenter Enter Nutr 1999; 23:85–89.

98. Giuffrida DJ, Bryan-Brown CW, Lumb PD, Kwun K, Rhoades HM. Central vs peripheral venous catheters in critically ill patients. Chest 1986; 90:806–809.

99. Pauley SY, Vallande NC, Riley EN, Jenner NM, Gulbinas DG. Catheter-related colonization associated with percutaneous inserted central catheters. J Intraven Nurs 1993; 16:50–54.

100. Raad I, Davis S, Becker M, Hohn D, Houston D, Umphrey J, Bodey GP. Low infection rate and long durability of nontunneled silastic catheters. A safe and cost-effective alternative for long-term venous access. Arch Intern Med 1993; 153:1791–1796.

101. Strahilevitz J, Lossos IS, Verstandig A, Sasson T, Kori Y, Gillis S. Vascular access via peripherally inserted central venous catheters (PICCs): experience in 40 patients with acute myeloid leukemia at a single institute. Leukemia Lymphoma 2001; 40:365–371.

102. Paz-Fumagalli R, Miller YA, Russell BA, Crain MR, Beres RA, Mewissen MW. Impact of peripherally inserted central catheters on phlebitic complications of peripheral intravenous therapy in spinal cord injury patients. J Spinal Cord Med 1997; 20:341–344.

103. Skiest DJ, Abbott M, Keiser P. Peripherally inserted central catheters in patients with AIDS are associated with a low infection rate. Clin Infect Dis 2000; 30:949–952.

104. Thiagarajan RR, Ramamoorthy C, Gettmann T, Bratton SL. Survey of the use of peripherally inserted central venous catheters in children. Pediatrics 1997; 99:1–4.

105. Foo R, Fujii A, Harris J-A, LaMorte W, Moulton S. Complications in tunneled CVL versus PICC lines in very low birth weight infants. J Perinatol 2001; 21:525–530.

106. Brant-Zawadzki M, Anthony M, Mercer EC. Implantation of P.A.S. Port venous access device in the forearm under fluoroscopic guidance. Am J Radiol 1993; 160:1127–1128.

107. Kaufman JA, Salamipour H, Geller SC, Rivitz SM, Waltman AC. Long-term outcomes of radiologically placed arm ports. Radiology 1996; 201:725–730.

108. Hills JR, Cardella JF, Cardella K, Waybill PN. Experience with 100 consecutive central venous access arm ports placed by interventional radiologists. J Vasc Interv Radiol 1997; 8:983–989.

109. Hata Y, Morita S, Morita Y, Awatani T, Takasaki M, Horimi T, Ozawa Z. Peripheral insertion of a central venous access device under fluoroscopic guidance using a peripherally accessed system (PAS) port in the forearm. Cardiovasc Intervent Radiol 1998; 21:230–233.

110. Whigham CJ, Goodman CJ, Fisher RG, Greenbaum MC, Thornby JI, Thomas JW. Infectious complications of 393 peripherally implantable venous access devices in HIV-positive and HIV-negative patients. J Vasc Interv Radiol 1999; 10:71–77.

111. Bodner LJ, Nosher JL, Patel KM, Siegel RL, Biswal R, Gribbin CE, Tokarz R. Peripheral venous access ports: outcomes analysis in 109 patients. Cardiovasc Intervent Radiol 2000; 23:187–193.

112. Carey PC, Mann DV, Pearce SZ, Windsor ACJ, Pullyblank AM, Guillou PJ, Monson JRT. Long-term circulatory access via a peripheral implantable port. Br J Surg 1993; 80:600–601.

113. Lundberg G, Wahlberg L, Rickberg A, Olofsson P. PAS-port: a new

implantable vascular access device for arm placement: Experiences from the first two years. Eur J Surg 1995; 161:323–326.

114. Stokes MA, Hill GL. Peripheral parenteral nutrition: a preliminary report on its efficacy and safety. J Parenter Enter Nutr 1993; 17:145–147.

115. Nordenström J, Jeppsson B, Lovén L, Larsson J. Peripheral parenteral nutrition: effect of a standardized compounded mixture on infusion phlebitis. Br J Surg 1991; 78:1391–1394.

116. Alhimyary A, Fernandez C, Picard M, Tierno K, Pignatone N, Chan HS, Malt R, Souba W. Safety and efficacy of total parenteral nutrition delivered via a peripherally inserted central venous catheter. Nutr Clin Prac 1996; 11:199–203.

117. Centers for Disease Control and Prevention Guidelines for the prevention of intravascular catheter-related infections. MMWR 2002; 51(No. RR-10):13–16.

118. Everitt NJ, McMahon MJ. Influence of fine-bore catheter length on infusion thrombophlebitis in peripheral intravenous nutrition: a randomised controlled trial. Ann R Coll Surg Engl 1997; 79:221–224.

119. Fonkalsrud EW, Carpenter K, Masuda JY, Beckerman JH. Prophylaxis against postinfusion phlebitis. Surg Gynecol Obstet 1971; 133:253–256.

120. Everitt NJ. Effect of prolonged infusion on vein calibre: a prospective study. Ann R Coll Surg Engl 1999; 81:109–112.

121. Khawaja HT, Campbell MJ, Weaver PC. Effect of transdermal glyceryl trinitrate on the survival of peripheral intravenous infusions: a double-blind prospective clinical study. Br J Surg 1988; 75:1212–1215.

122. Wright A, Hecker JF, Lewis GBH. Use of transdermal glyceryl trinitrate to reduce failure of intravenous infusion due to phlebitis and extravasation. Lancet 1985; ii:1148–1150.

123. O'Brien BJ, Buxton MJ, Khawaja HT. An economic evaluation of trans-dermal glyceryl trinitrate in the prevention of intravenous infusion failure. J Clin Epidemiol 1990; 43:757–763.

124. Rusho WJ, Bair JN. Effect of filtration on complications of postoperative intravenous therapy. Am J Hosp Pharm 1979; 36:1355–1356.

125. Butler LD, Munson JM, DeLuca PP. Effect of inline filtration on the potency of low-dose drugs. Am J Hosp Pharm 1980; 37:935–941.

126. Bansmer G, Keith D, Tesluk H. Complications following use of indwelling catheters of inferior vena cava. JAMA 1958; 167:1606–1611.

127. McNair TJ, Dudley HAF. The local complications of intravenous therapy. Lancet 1959; ii:365–368.

128. Crane C. Venous interruption for septic thrombophlebitis. N Engl J Med 1960; 262:947–951.

129. Strand CL, Wajsbort RR, Sturmann K. Effect of iodophor vs iodine tincture skin preparation on blood culture contamination rate. JAMA 1993; 269:1004–1006.

130. Garland JS, Buck RK, Maloney P, Durkin DM, Toth-Lloyd S, Duffy M, Szocik P, McAuliffe TL, Goldmann D. Comparison of 10% povidone-iodine and 0.5% chlorhexidine gluconate for the prevention of peripheral intra-venous catheter colonization in neonates: a prospective trial. Pediatr Infect Dis J 1995; 14:510–516.

131. Yamamoto AJ, Solomon JA, Soulen MC, Tang J, Parkinson K, Lin R,

Schears GJ. Sutureless securement device reduces complications of peripherally inserted central venous catheters. J Vasc Interv Radiol 2002; 13:77–81.

132. Moran JM, Atwood RP, Rowe MI. A clinical and bacteriologic study of infections associated with venous cutdowns. N Engl J Med 1965; 272:554–560.

133. Norden CW. Application of antibiotic ointment to the site of venous catheterization-a controlled trial. J Infect Dis 1969; 120:611–615.

134. Zinner SH, Denny-Brown BC, Braun P, Burke JP, Toala P, Kass EH. Risk of infection with intravenous indwelling catheters: effect of application of antibiotic ointment. J Infect Dis 1969; 120:616–619.

135. Maki DG, Band JD. A comparative study of polyantibiotic and iodophor ointments in prevention of vascular catheter-related infection. Am J Med 1981; 70:739–744.

136. Craven DE, Lichtenberg DA, Kunches LM, McDonough AT, Gonzalez MI, Heeren TC, McCabe WR. A randomized study comparing a transparent polyurethane dressing to a dry gauze dressing for peripheral intravenous catheter sizes. Infect Control 1985; 6:361–366.

137. Kelsey MC, Gosling M. A comparison of the morbidity associated with occlusive and non-occlusive dressings applied to peripheral intravenous devices. J Hosp Infect 1984; 5:313–321.

138. Hoffmann KK, Weber DJ, Samsa GP, Rutala WA. Transparent polyurethane film as an intravenous catheter dressing. A meta-analysis of the infection risks. JAMA 1992; 267:2072–2076.

139. Hoffmann KK, Western SA, Kaiser DI, Wenzel RP, Groschel DHM. Bacterial colonization and phlebitis–associated risk with transparent polyurethane film for peripheral intravenous site dressings. Am J Infect Control 1988; 16:101–106.

140. Maki DG, Stolz S, Wheeler S. A prospective, randomized, three-way clinical comparison of a novel, highly permeable, polyurethane dressing with 206 Swan-Ganz pulmonary artery catheters: OpSite IV3000 vs Tegaderm vs gauze and tape. I. Cutaneous colonization under the dressing, catheter-related infection. In: Maki DG, ed. Improving Catheter Site Care. London: Royal Society of Medicine, 1991:61–66.

141. Josephson A, Gombert ME, Sierra MF, Karanfil LV, Tansino GF. The relationship between intravenous fluid contamination and the frequency of tubing replacement. Infect Control 1985; 6:367–370.

142. Snydman DR, Donnelly-Reidy M, Perry LK, Martin WJ. Intravenous tubing containing burettes can be safely changed at 72 hour intervals. Infect Control 1987; 8:113–116.

143. Maki DG, Botticelli JT, LeRoy ML, Thielke TS. Prospective study of replacing administration sets for intravenous therapy at 48- vs 72-hour intervals. JAMA 1987; 258:1777 1781.

144. Nelson DB, Kien CL, Mohr B, Frank S, Davis SD. Dressing changes by specialized personnel reduce infection rates in patients receiving central venous parenteral nutrition. J Parenter Enter Nutr 1986; 10:220–222.

145. Faubion WC, Wesley JR, Khalidi N, Silva J. Total parenteral nutrition catheter sepsis: impact of the team approach. J Parenter Enter Nutr 1986; 10:642–645.

13

Infectious Complications of PA Pulmonary Artery Catheters, Cordis Introducers, and Peripheral Arterial Catheters

Leonard A. Mermel

Brown Medicine School and Rhode Island Hospital
Providence, Rhode Island, U.S.A.

Dennis G. Maki

University of Wisconsin Hospital and Clinics
Madison, Wisconsin, U.S.A.

PA PULMONARY ARTERY CATHETERS

Introduction

Balloon-tipped pulmonary artery (PA) catheters have come into widespread use since their inception in the early 1970s (1). On average, 16.1% of patients in U.S. intensive care units (ICUs) have PA catheters at some time during their ICU stay (range <0.1% to 40.5% for patients in neonatal and surgical ICUs, respectively (2)). More than one million PA catheters are sold in the United States each year and the annual cost associated with their use exceeds $2 billion per year (3). Nevertheless, controversy surrounds the utility and safety of this device. An uncontrolled, observational study suggested that PA catheter use was associated with increased mortality and cost (4). This finding prompted a consensus conference, which suggested that based on the available literature, use of PA catheters improves outcomes in many clinical scenarios; however, uncertainty remains in its use for many conditions. The complex and unique features of the PA catheter present challenges to the user of this device unlike any other catheter used in caring for critically ill patients (5). Not surprisingly, the consensus panel suggested that clinician knowledge about PA catheter use and complications needs to be improved upon (6). More recently, a meta-analysis of randomized, controlled trials revealed that PA catheter-guided strategies to care for patients led to a significant reduction in morbidity (7).

In this chapter, we review the incidence and pathogenesis of PA catheter-related infections, risk factors associated with their occurrence, and recommendations for the treatment and prevention of such infections.

Features of the Catheter

PA catheters are among the most complex intravascular devices used in clinical medicine, consisting of a polyvinyl chloride or polyurethane catheter, which is placed through a percutaneous, indwelling Teflon introducer into a central great vein, through the right side of the heart, and into the pulmonary artery (Fig. 1). Most PA catheters are inserted into the subclavian or internal jugular vein and, far less frequently, into a femoral vein. One of the catheter lumens is used to inflate a balloon on the catheter tip. This allows the catheter to float in the bloodstream and occlude a small pulmonary artery for measurement of a wedged PA or left-atrial pressure. Two additional lumina of the catheter are attached to transducers, permitting continuous pressure monitoring within the pulmonary artery (PA lumen) and the cannulated central vein (CVP lumen) and measurement of the PA occlusive (wedge) pressure when the balloon is inflated. A protective plastic sleeve is usually attached to the end of the introducer covering the extravascular portion of the catheter, allowing the PA catheter to be advanced or pulled back without incurring touch contamination. Pressurized bags of heparin-containing flush solution are attached to the PA and CVP lumens and each is connected to a chamber dome, which interfaces with an electromechanical transducer and a continuous-flow device.

Incidence of Infection

Many prospective studies have addressed the incidence of PA catheter-related infection (8–36). Cultures of introducers, in addition to PA catheter segments, were systematically performed in several large studies (28,30,32,36,37). In two of these studies (30,37), cultures of all potential sources of infection were done and molecular subtyping techniques were used to reliably determine concordance among the isolates. Table 1 summarizes the results of 16 prospective studies in which cultures of at least 75 PA catheters were tested, and rates of catheter-related bloodstream infections were reported. In those prospective studies using semiquantitative (20,23–25,27–32,37) or quantitative catheter

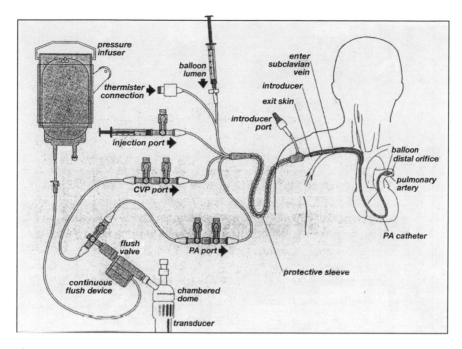

Figure 1 Schematic of a Swan-Ganz catheter placed through a Teflon introducer sheath, with an external protective plastic sleeve over the extravascular portion of the pulmonary artery (PA) catheter. Note: Some PA catheters do not have the injection port depicted. (From Ref. 5.)

culture methods (26,35,36), 2.3 to 47.3% of PA catheters or introducers were colonized (weighted mean 17.0% [95% CI 16.4–17.5%] and median 14.2% incidence of catheter colonization, respectively). From these studies, the incidence of catheter-related bloodstream infection ranged from 0 to 5.3%. The weighted mean and median incidence of catheter-related bloodstream infection was 1.6 [95% CI 1.5–1.6%] and 0.8%, respectively. The incidence of PA catheter-related bloodstream infection is substantially lower than that reported for other types of short-term, noncuffed central venous catheters used in the same patient population (39). Many of the prospective studies of PA catheters may have underestimated the true incidence of PA catheter-related bloodstream infection since routine cultures of introducers, hubs, and infusate were not done.

Microbial Profile

Coagulase-negative staphylococci, predominantly *Staphylococcus epidermidis*, are the most common pathogens associated with PA catheter infection. Of the episodes of PA catheter colonization and bloodstream infection

Table 1 Incidence of Swan-Ganz Pulmonary Artery Catheter-Related Infection

Study	Catheter (n)	Where most catheters inserted	Catheterization (mean days)	Catheter culture method	Catheter colonized (%)	Catheter-related bloodstream infection (%)	(Per 1000 catheter-days)
Elliot et al. (9)	116	ICU	4	Broth	63.7	1.7	3.9
Michel et al. (19)	153	OR	4	Broth	19.0	0	0
Kaye et al. (20)	133	ICU	NR	SQ	9.8	2.3	NR
Groeger et al. (21)	76	ICU	3	NR[a]	26.3	3.9	13.2
Richard et al. (22)	109	OR	2	SQ	8.3	0	0
Parsa et al. (23)	90	ICU	NR	SQ	NR	1.1	NR
Damen et al. (24)	794	OR	1	SQ	2.3	0	0
Damen and Van Der Twell (25)	123	OR	1	SQ	10.6	0	0
Heard et al. (26)	87	ICU	NR	QS	18.0	5.3	NR
Fisher et al. (27)	169	NR	4	SQ	14.2	2.3	8.4
Eyer et al. (28)	156	ICU	6	SQ[a]	5.9	4.6	6.9
Horowitz et al. (29)	158	ICU	3	SQ	29.1	2.5	8.0
Mermel et al. (30)	297	OR	3	SQ[a]	21.9	0.7	2.3
Bach et al. (31)	159	OR	2	SQ	5.0	0	0
Bull et al. (32)	241	OR	2	SQ[a]	47.3	0.8	NR
Maki et al. (37)	442	OR	3	SQ[a]	21.7	1.1	3.6
Cohen et al. (38)	166	ICU	4	SQ	16.9	4.8	NR
Blot et al. (36)	79	ICU	3	QV	8.9	0	0
Kac et al. (35)	164	OR	6	QV	11.6	0.6	0.9

Abbreviations: Broth = qualitatively, by immersion in liquid medium; SQ = semiquantitative roll plate; QS = quantitative by sonication; QV = quantitative by vortex method; ICU = intensive care unit; OR = operating room; NR = not reported.

[a] Introducer sheaths and the catheters were cultured. Hubs and infusate from each lumen of the introducer sheath and PA catheter were cultured, and molecular subtyping was done to confirm true device-related bloodstream infection.

(From Ref. 5.)

reported in the literature, 56 and 37%, respectively, were due to coagulase-negative staphylococci; 19 and 11%, respectively, were due to enteric gram-negative bacilli; 7 and 16%, respectively, were due to *Candida*; and 5 and 26%, respectively, were due to *Staphylococcus aureus*. *Candida* and *S. aureus* each account for a higher percentage of PA catheter-related bloodstream infections than catheter colonization, reflecting their greater pathogenicity (Fig. 2).

Risk Factors

Multivariate analysis has been used to identify independent risk factors exclusively for PA catheter-associated infection (25,30,33,35). Use of these catheters in patients under one year of age and for three or more days in children, placement with lesser barrier precautions [relative risk (RR) 2.1], placement in internal jugular rather than subclavian vein (RR 4.3), heavy cutaneous colonization of the insertion site (RR 5.5), and catheterization longer than three (RR 3.8), four [odds ratio (OR) 9.8], or five days (OR 14.4), have each been found to be independent predictors of an increased risk of catheter colonization. Antibiotic use is associated with reduced risk (OR 0.23). In combined studies of central venous and PA catheters using multivariate analysis (40–43), the following risk factors were associated with catheter-related infection: bacteremia or candidemia originating from another site of infec-

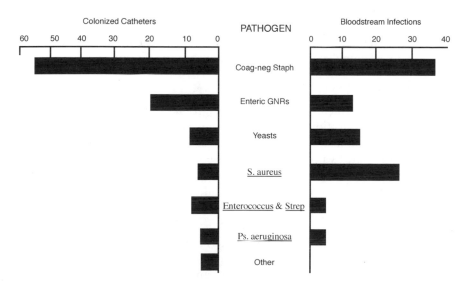

Figure 2 Microbial profile of Swan-Ganz catherer-related infection—local (catheter colonization) and bloodstream infection based on pooled data from 14 prospective studies providing complete microbiological data on all infected catheters. (From Ref. 5.)

tion; heavy colonization of the insertion site or hub; catheterization exceeding four or seven days; difficult catheter insertion; second catheterization; internal jugular vein cannulation; use of polyurethane transparent dressing; patients in a coronary care unit or on the surgery service. Based on this information, physicians should rigorously assess the need for PA catheters each day with the intent of removing the device as soon as it is no longer absolutely necessary for care of a patient. The catheter should be inserted with full barrier precautions, ideally in the subclavian rather than the internal jugular site.

Colonization of the Insertion Site

A number of prospective studies of PA and central venous catheters have found heavy colonization of the insertion site to be an independent risk factor of catheter-related infection (30,40,42–45). Therefore, prevention of PA catheter-related infection requires interventions that lead to the greatest reduction in microbial colonization of the insertion site.

Site of Insertion

Insertion of a PA catheter in an internal jugular vein rather than a subclavian vein is independently associated with a significantly increased risk of infection (30). This may be due to heavier cutaneous colonization (46), greater potential for contamination by respiratory secretions (47), and greater difficulty maintaining a catheter dressing on an internal jugular vein insertion site. Thus, placement of central venous and PA catheters in a subclavian vein rather than an internal jugular vein is preferable in patients who are not at increased risk of mechanical complications such as bleeding, or pneumothorax.

Skill of the Inserter

The experience of the inserter has not been found to be a risk factor for PA catheter-related infection, but few studies have adequately examined this risk factor (33,48). Difficult catheter insertion requiring three or more punctures has been associated with a 15-fold increase in the risk of central venous and PA catheter infection (40). After three unsuccessful attempts, we believe that another, more experienced individual should try to insert the catheter.

Barrier Precautions

Use of maximal barrier precautions—sterile gloves, a long-sleeved surgical gown, a surgical mask and hat, and a large sterile sheet drape—in contrast to using only sterile gloves, a surgical mask, and a small fenestrated drape—is associated with a twofold reduction in the risk of PA catheter-related colonization (30). In another prospective study, wearing a sterile gown, in addition to a mask, hat, and gloves, and applying a cutaneous antiseptic for five minutes, led to a threefold reduction in PA catheter colonization compared to catheters inserted by clinicians not wearing a gown and spending less time preparing the insertion site (32). Maximal barrier precautions during central venous catheter insertion has been shown to reduce the incidence of catheter-related bloodstream infection fivefold (49,50). Based on these findings, maximal barrier precautions should be the standard of care during insertion of all central venous catheters, including PA catheters.

Guide Wires

In one prospective study including PA catheters, patients were randomized to one of three groups: catheter exchange every seven days over a guide wire; catheter removal and insertion of a new catheter every seven days; or no routine catheter change (28). There was no significant difference in the incidence of catheter-related bloodstream infection or colonization among the three groups. A more recent prospective, randomized trial of central venous and PA catheters found nearly a twofold increase in the incidence of catheter-related bloodstream infection with catheters placed at an old site over a guide wire (51); however, guide wire exchange reduced the risk of mechanical complications. We believe that PA catheters should not be routinely replaced over a guide wire, but that if it is considered necessary to do so because of limited sites for access, the inserter should done a new set of sterile gloves after removing the old catheter and insert the new one over a guide wire, and cultures of the old catheter should always be done.

Duration of Catheterization

Most prospective studies of PA catheters using univariate analysis have shown that the risk of infection increases with the duration of catheterization (8,19,20,26,30,34,40,52,53), but not all investigations have found such an association (9,14,16,28,54). Three studies using multivariate analysis found a strong association between prolonged catheterization and an increased risk of PA catheter colonization (25,30,33). The actuarial risk of PA catheter-related bloodstream infection is low during the first four days, but rises sharply thereafter (9,20,30,37) (Fig. 3). As noted above, studies using multivariate analysis have shown that the risk of catheter colonization rises sharply beyond three days (RR or OR for three, four, and five days of catheterization = 3.8, 9.8, and 14.4, respectively). These data suggest that a PA catheter should ideally be removed within three days unless there are extenuating circumstances. In two prospective studies, central venous and PA catheters were randomized to regularly scheduled replacement at three days (51) or seven days (28) versus no routine replacement. In both studies, the incidence of catheter colonization and bloodstream infection was not significantly different in the two populations. In a meta-analysis, routine catheter replacement at set intervals was not associated with a reduced risk of central venous catheter infection (55) and routine PA catheter replacement is not recommended.

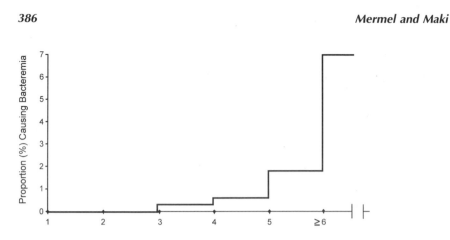

Figure 3 Relationship between the duration of Swan-Ganz catheterization and the actuarial risk of catheter-related bloodstream infection, based on pooled data (988 catheters) from four prospective studies (9,20,30,37). (From Ref. 5.)

Dressings

The importance of the cutaneous microflora in the pathogenesis of vascular catheter-related infection (5) suggests that the dressing applied to the insertion site could have an important effect on the risk of infection. There have been three large prospective, randomized trials of polyurethane dressings compared with gauze dressings used to cover PA catheter insertion sites (22,37,56); none found a significant difference in the incidence of catheter-related infection. The largest trial found no increased risk of catheter colonization or bloodstream infection when two types of polyurethane dressings, changed every five days, were compared to gauze dressing changed every other day (37). These data suggest that polyurethane dressings may be used safely to cover the site of PA catheter insertion. However, if blood is oozing from the insertion site, a gauze dressing should be used until this resolves (56).

Heparin-Bonded Catheters

Heparin is bonded to the external surface of PA catheters in an effort to reduce thrombosis on a catheter surface during the early period after insertion (57). Because the benzalkonium chloride used to bond heparin has intrinsic antimicrobial activity, heparin-bonded PA catheters exhibit surface activity against a wide range of microbial pathogens, including *Candida albicans* (58). An analysis of prospective studies of PA catheter-related infection suggests that heparin bonding with benzalkonium chloride reduces the risk of infection (Table 2). A recent study using electron microscopy found thrombus formation and platelet aggregation on PA catheter balloon tips, but not the catheter shafts, as soon as 24 hours after insertion, despite heparin-bonding of the catheters (59). Thus, the currently marketed heparin-bonded PA catheters in

Table 2 Rates of Catheter-Related Bloodstream Infection Found in Prospective Studies of Heparin-Bonded and Nonheparin-Bonded Pulmonary Artery Catheters

	Heparin-bonded catheters	Nonbonded catheters
Studies (n)	3	3
Total catheters studied (n)	1260	341
Catheter-related bacteremia per 100 catheters		
Mean	1.0	2.8
Range	0–2.3	0–4.6
Per 1000 catheter-days		
Mean	3.6	6.7
Range	0–8.4	0–13.2

(From Ref. 58.)

the United States may well have little impact on thrombus formation at the tip of the catheter. This is important since thrombus formation increases the risk of catheter infection (60). Lastly, these catheters should not be used in patients with heparin-induced thrombocytopenia (61).

Other Risk Factors

Three studies have found an increased risk of PA catheter-related infection in patients with a remote focus of infection during catheterization (14,19,26). Two studies found that administration of total parenteral nutrition through PA catheters did not increase the risk of catheter-related infection (29,30), and in one study, steroid use was associated with PA catheter-related infection (26).

Sources of Infection

There are numerous microbial reservoirs from which pathogens may gain access to a catheterized patient's bloodstream (Fig. 1): skin flora at the insertion site can invade the transcutaneous tract and colonize the introducer and PA catheter extraluminally; microbes colonizing any of the three PA catheter hubs or the introducer hub can enter the catheter lumen during hub manipulation and contaminate the infusate, or the infusate may become contaminated by the manufacturer or during preparation in the hospital prior to use; microbes from the hands of health-care workers can also contaminate the extravascular portion of the PA catheter and gain access when the catheter is advanced through the introducer when repositioned; and the intravascular portion of the introducer or PA catheter may become colonized hematogenously from a distant focus of infection.

Two small studies have demonstrated concordance among isolates from the introducer and PA catheter tip (15,21). Such concordance was demonstrated in all three cases of PA catheter-related bloodstream infection in one of the studies (21). Combining the results of two larger and more recent studies (35,62), there were 31 instances where the PA catheter or introducer had significant catheter colonization. In these studies, there were 17 instances where both the PA and introducer segments had significant growth, 11 instances where only the introducer segment had significant growth, and three instances where only the PA catheter segment had significant growth. Therefore, culturing both the PA catheter and introducer is important to maximize the yield of catheter cultures.

Two studies found occasional low-level contamination of injectate used for cardiac output measurements, usually with coagulase-negative staphylococci (12,16). This was not associated with PA catheter colonization or bloodstream infection.

A number of investigators (15,16,21,26,30,37,63–66) have demonstrated low-level contamination of the extravascular portion of the PA catheter inside the external protective plastic sleeve (mean frequency of contamination, 9%). Concordance with colonized PA catheters, however, was uncommon, and concordance with bloodstream infection was rare (21,64). One randomized trial of these sleeves paradoxically found a slightly higher rate of catheter-related bloodstream infection among patients whose catheters were maintained with a sleeve rather than without one (21). This may have been due to greater manipulation of the catheters with protective sleeves. Another study found no significant difference in colonization of PA catheters protected or unprotected by a sleeve (48); however, the mean duration of catheterization was only one day, and there were no bloodstream infections. In the most recent large, prospective, randomized clinical trial (38), a dramatic reduction in bloodstream infections was associated with the use of protective sleeves in PA catheters left in situ for an average of 3.5 days (10.2 and 0% without and with the protective sleeve, respectively [p < 0.002]). Use of protective sleeves over PA catheters should now be the standard of care.

There are conflicting data regarding the risk of seeding an introducer or PA catheter hematogenously from a distant focus of infection. Hematogenous seeding of PA catheters or introducers was demonstrated in all seven exposed catheters in one study (12) and in seven of nine exposed catheters in another (21). However, most investigators have found hematogenous seeding of introducer or PA catheters to be infrequent (16,17,30,37,55). This variability may reflect differences in the pathogens involved and types of infection seen in these investigations.

Conclusively demonstrating the source of microbes causing PA catheter-related bloodstream infection requires obtaining cultures from all potential sources of infection and utilizing molecular fingerprinting techniques to unequivocally determine concordance among isolates. In a prospective study of 297 PA catheters (30), colonization was found among 58 introducers and 20 PA catheters, and there were two cases of catheter-related bloodstream infection. Seventeen of the 20 colonized PA catheters had concordant growth on the introducer. Using molecular subtyping, 80% of colonized catheters had concordant growth with organisms isolated from the insertion site, 17% with contaminated hubs, and 19% with organisms found on the extravascular portion of the PA catheter within the protective sleeve. Isolates from colonized PA catheters were most likely to show concordance with colonized introducer (71%). Only two of the 38 catheters exposed to bloodstream infection originating from a remote focus of infection became colonized hematogenously. In another study using molecular subtyping of clinical isolates, 5 of 442 PA catheters were associated with bloodstream infection (37).

All seven cases of PA catheter-associated bloodstream infections in which molecular fingerprinting was employed were associated with concordant growth of the introducer, whereas only three had concordant growth of the PA catheter segment itself (30,37). In each case, the introducer had been in place for at least five days. Since most clinicians use an introducer, it is the only point of contact between a catheter segment and skin at the insertion site. Based on this data, microbial pathogens appear to migrate extraluminally along the transcutaneous tract of the introducer, but in only an occasional case do they migrate distally to the PA catheter itself and cause bloodstream infection. Contamination of the introducer with skin flora during insertion may also be responsible for the strong association between introducer colonization and bloodstream infection. Frequent manipulation of the introducer hub also contributes to the association between introducer colonization and PA catheter-related bloodstream infection. Four of the seven bloodstream infections were associated with concordant growth at the insertion site, and an equal number involved concordant growth at the catheter hub. Two of the seven PA catheter-related bloodstream infections involved contaminated infusate; however, infusate specimens were obtained only at the time of catheter removal, and this may underestimate the incidence of infusate contamination and the potential importance of this source of bloodstream infection. The extravascular portion of the PA catheter under the protective sleeve was colonized with concordant growth of organisms in one case of PA catheter-related bloodstream infection. Therefore, despite the advent of this technologic advance, PA catheter colonization underneath the protective sleeve may still occur, with serious consequences. Hematogenous seeding of the PA catheter was demonstrated in only one of the seven cases of PA catheter-related bloodstream infections. Although this supports most of the earlier studies, which did not employ molecular fingerprinting, lower thresholds to collect blood cultures by some clinicians may have led to an underestimation of this association.

In summary, it appears that the insertion site and the catheter hub are equally important sources of the microbes causing most serious PA catheter-related infections. The introducer, rather than the PA catheter itself, is the throughway for most pathogens invading the bloodstream. This likely reflects the fact that the introducer, not the PA catheter, is in direct contact with the skin.

Epidemics

Although there have been at least 28 epidemics of nosocomial sepsis associated with arterial pressure monitoring (67–71), few were traced to hemodynamic monitoring with PA catheters. In one outbreak, five cases of PA catheter-related Enterobacter bacteremia were traced to failure of chemical disinfection involving reusable plastic chamber domes in the monitoring circuit (72). The essential steps in dealing with a nosocomial epidemic of bloodstream infection have been outlined elsewhere (73) and should be followed if this is suspected.

Pathogenesis

After PA catheter insertion, microbial pathogens colonizing the insertion site or hub can quickly migrate toward the catheter tip and into the bloodstream (74,75). In some instances, extensive biofilm can be seen covering the PA catheter surface 24 hours after insertion and, in half of PA catheters, at the time of removal (17). The biofilm consists of a bacterial polysaccharide glycocalyx slime substance, host-derived proteins, and platelets. Bacterial adhesins promote attachment to intravascular catheters (76). Platelets and thrombus can be found on the balloon of PA catheters as soon as 24 hours after catheter insertion (59). Catheter-associated thrombus is associated with an increased risk of infection (60,77,78) since platelets and host-derived proteins—fibronectin, thrombospondin, vitronectin, and Von Willibrand's factor—enhance binding of microbial pathogens, such as *S. aureus*, to the catheter surface (79–82). Once microbes are bound to a catheter, they may be difficult to eradicate for various reasons: the protective nature of the polysaccharide glycocalyx slime substance (83); the inability of neutrophils to kill these adherent bacteria (84); and reduced antibiotic susceptibility of these sessile bacteria, compared to planktonic ones (85).

Types of Infection

The animal model of infective endocarditis involves placing a vascular catheter into the internal jugular vein of a laboratory animal and passing the catheter into the right ventricle, producing a sterile vegetation. Bacteria are then introduced into the bloodstream, which infect the vegetation, producing a syndrome similar to infective endocarditis in humans (86–88). To function properly, PA catheters must be passed through the right atrium and ventricle, leaving patients particularly vulnerable to developing endocarditis. Noninfective endocardial lesions (endocardial hemorrhage, thrombi, valvular thickening, or overt vegetations) are quite common after PA catheterization (9,89–98) and are found in as many as 91% of autopsies (96). These lesions would seem likely to predispose patients to infective endocarditis. Approximately 2% of patients who had undergone PA catheterization shortly before death have autopsy findings consistent with infective endocarditis (89–91,99–104). Most cases of PA catheter-related endocarditis occurred after prolonged catheterization (91,99,104–107), and involved the right atrium or ventricular endocardium or the tricuspid or pulmonic valves, as single or multiple lesions (91,105–107). Pulmonic valve vegetations appear to derive almost exclusively from PA catheters.

Septic thrombophlebitis is an occasional complication of central venous catheter use (108–111). Local signs of venous occlusion may be seen, such as ipsilateral neck, chest wall, or arm swelling, yet the insertion site is often devoid of inflammation. Persistent high-grade bacteremia or fungemia despite removal of an infected PA catheter usually indicates septic thrombophlebitis or infective endocarditis, particularly when it involves staphylococci or *Candida* (108–111). Only a single case of great central vein septic thrombophlebitis associated with PA catheterization has been reported (110). This may reflect the fact that the duration of catheterization is generally shorter with PA catheters than other central venous catheters. Underreporting of this catastrophic form of catheter-related bloodstream infection events is also very likely.

Septic pulmonary emboli and infarction can also be seen in patients with PA catheter-related bloodstream infection, secondary to septic thrombophlebitis (100) or infective endocarditis (89,91,99–102). Rarely, pulmonary artery mycotic aneurysm may complicate PA catheter infection (105) or lung abscess and empyema, deriving from secondary infection of a coexistent pulmonary infarct (112,113).

Diagnosis of Infection

The signs and symptoms of patients with intravascular catheter-related bloodstream infection are indistinguishable from bloodstream infection due to other etiologies. Nevertheless, there are certain clinical findings that significantly increase the likelihood that bloodstream infection is secondary to a central venous or pulmonary artery catheter: bloodstream infection in a nonsurgical patient; bacteremia due to *S. aureus*, coagulase-negative staphylococci, or *Candida*; central venous catheter in situ; and no identifiable localized infection (114).

The utility of obtaining cultures of multiple PA catheter segments is unclear since it increased the yield in one study (115), but not in another one (62). Using a combination of two culture techniques increases the yield (116); culturing multiple PA catheter segments is impractical for routine cultures in the clinical microbiology laboratory. Performing central venous and PA catheter cultures at the bedside using the roll-plate technique also increases the yield of catheter cultures (117). As noted in the section "Sources of Infection", it is important to culture both the PA catheter and introducer since culture of the PA catheter alone has a sensitivity of only 65% and will miss catheter infections involving only the introducer (35,62).

Management of Infection

Guidelines for the management of intravascular catheter-related infections have recently been published (118). Unexplained fever in a patient without severe sepsis—hypotension, mental status changes, or decreased urine output—should prompt the patient's physician to obtain blood cultures. If quantitative blood cultures or differential time to blood culture positivity using continuously monitored automated systems are available, one set of blood cultures can be obtained through the catheter and the other set from a peripheral vein. If quantitative blood cultures are unavailable, two sets of percutaneously drawn blood cultures should be obtained, and consideration should be made for removing the catheter. If an intravascular catheter is still necessary for optimal patient care, a new catheter can be inserted in another site or in the original site over a guide wire. However, the second catheter should be removed if the original one is found to be heavily colonized. Rapid diagnostic tests, such as Gram stain or acridine orange stain of blood obtained through the catheter, may also be used. Gram stain of the insertion site may also be helpful in this setting.

In the case of a septic patient with a PA catheter in place and in whom (a) there is no obvious other source of infection or purulence at the insertion site, (b) bloodstream infection has already been documented with staphylococci or *Candida*, or (c) the catheter has been in situ for more than four days, the catheter should be removed in its entirety, including the introducer and PA catheter. Both should be sent for culture, in addition to obtaining blood cultures. Failure to remove a colonized PA catheter associated with bacteremia or candidemia places the patient at undue risk of developing septic great central vein thrombophlebitis or infective endocarditis. If continued hemodynamic monitoring is necessary, this can be accomplished with insertion of a PA catheter into a new site or by noninvasive means (119). If the original catheter remained in place, but quantitative blood cultures revealed a marked step up in the number of organisms that grew from the catheter-drawn, as compared to the percutaneously-drawn blood cultures (120), or if catheter-drawn blood cultures reveal growth two or more hours before simultaneously obtained percutaneously-drawn blood cultures (121,122), the catheter should also be removed. Lastly, if the insertion site or catheter hub have significant numbers of pathogens found on quantitative culture or Gram stain, consideration should be made for removal of the PA catheter in its entirety.

Removal of a heavily colonized intravascular catheter will often lead to resolution of a patient's fever (123). However, a parenteral course of antibiotics should be considered in the clinical setting of a febrile patient with negative blood cultures in whom the removed PA catheter is heavily colonized, especially by *S. aureus* or *Candida*, and there is no other source of the fever. This is because the catheter was in close proximity to the tricuspid and pulmonic valves, which may be more susceptible to becoming secondarily infected due to catheter-induced endocardial and valvular lesions (90–92,94,124). This recommendation may be especially important if the patient is known to have underlying valvular heart disease, especially a prosthetic valve (125). There are no available data to dictate the appropriate duration of antibiotic therapy in this setting, but a brief five- to seven-day course of antimicrobial therapy is reasonable.

If empirical antimicrobial therapy is used, pending the results of blood and catheter cultures, vancomycin should be considered to cover methicillin-resistant staphylococci in those institutions where there is a high incidence of MRSA and MRSE (118). Addition of an antibiotic effective against nosocomial gram-negative bacilli may be reasonable, based on the clinical setting. Definitive therapy of PA catheter-related bloodstream infection should be based on microbiological identification and susceptibility of the pathogens involved. The appropriate duration of antibiotic therapy for PA catheter-related bloodstream infection should be determined by a number of factors: the presence of underlying valvular heart disease or evidence of an endovascular infection—endocarditis or septic thrombophlebitis; evidence of a distant metastatic infection; or persistent, high-grade bacteremia after catheter withdrawal and initiation of appropriate antimicrobial therapy (118,126). If endocarditis is suspected, transesophageal echocardiography has greater sensitivity than transthoracic echocardiography for detecting vegetations—especially small vegetations, those involving prosthetic valves, or those in the right side of the heart (127–129).

Septic thrombophlebitis of the central great veins should be suspected, in the setting of persistent bacteremia or fungemia without evidence of endocarditis. The diagnosis can often be made by noninvasive techniques, such as ultrasonography (130), computerized tomography (130–132), or magnetic resonance imaging (132). Although venography remains the diagnostic standard (107,108,131), a recent prospective study found that color duplex ultrasonograpy has a sensitivity and specificity of 82% each in the diagnosis of upper extremity thrombosis (133). If bacteremia due to pathogens other than *S. aureus* clears within three days and the patient is without underlying valvular heart disease or clinical evidence of endocarditis, septic thrombophlebitis, or metastatic infection, parenteral antimicrobial therapy should be administered for seven to 14 days (118). However, with uncomplicated catheter-related *S. aureus* bacteremia, 14 days of parenteral antimicrobial therapy may be considered (127,134–140) in selected patients without evidence of infective endocarditis on transesophageal echocardiography after catheter removal (118), although some controversy remains regarding short course therapy for *S. aureus* bloodstream infection (141). All patients with catheter-related candidemia should receive antimicrobial therapy, even if the patient's fever resolves after catheter withdrawal and subsequent blood cultures are negative (142–144). Candidemia that rapidly clears should be treated with intravenous amphotericin B or fluconazole administered over 14 days (142,144–146), or a newer antifungal agent such as caspofungin (147).

Infective endocarditis originating from a colonized PA catheter should be treated similar to endocarditis unrelated to a catheter, with prolonged parenteral bactericidal antimicrobial therapy, using a dosage regimen appropriate for endocarditis (148). However, for patients with right-sided, catheter-related bacterial endocarditis, a corollary may be drawn between these patients and those who have acquired right-sided endocarditis secondary to IV drug use, in whom two weeks of parenteral antibiotic therapy may be effective when there has been rapid resolution of bacteremia and no evidence of septic pulmonary emboli (137,139).

PA catheter-related septic thrombophlebitis of the central great veins can be reliably treated in most instances, without surgical intervention. With bacterial infection, a four-week course of parenteral antimicrobial therapy is recommended (108,110,118,149). Anticoagulation should also be considered unless contraindicated (108,110,118,149). Thrombolytic therapy used in the setting of central great vein septic thrombophlebitis does not appear to improve outcome and is not recommended (150).

All patients with PA catheter-related bloodstream infection should be monitored closely after completing therapy, especially patients with prolonged bloodstream infection, to detect late-appearing metastatic infection or relapse of the original endovascular infection.

Prevention of Infection

Preventive strategies aimed at reducing the risk of intravascular catheter-related infection have been reviewed in detail elsewhere (151–153). The risk of catheter-related infection can be reduced by placement of the catheter in the subclavian vein rather than the internal jugular vein (Table 3). However, the reduced risk of infection at the subclavian insertion site should be weighted against the other risks. Although there is a greater likelihood of arterial puncture with internal jugular insertion (158), there is a higher risk of perforating a great central vein with subclavian insertion (159). Since bleeding secondary to vascular injury may be more easily managed when the catheter has been inserted in the internal jugular vein, the latter insertion site may be preferred for patients with coagulopathy or thrombocytopenia.

To reduce the risk of PA catheter-related infection (30,32,46) and exposure to bloodborne pathogens (160), a long-sleeved, sterile surgical gown, sterile gloves, mask, eye protection, and hat should be worn during catheter insertion, and the site should be covered by a large, sterile sheet drape. These same precautions should be undertaken if the catheter is

Table 3 Catheter-Related Infections: Internal Jugular vs. Subclavian Approach

Colonization		Bloodstream infection		
IJ (%)	SC (%)	IJ (%)	SC (%)	Ref.
19	7	—	—	10
16	37[a]	—	—	154
21	10[a]	—	—	155
28	15[a]	—	—	156
22	10[a]	—	—	157
35	14[a]	—	—	41
		10	3[a]	29
27	4[a]	1	0	30
—	—	7	2	38

Abbreviations: IJ = internal jugular vein; SC = subclavian vein.
[a] $p < 0.05$.
(From Ref. 151.)

exchanged over a guide wire. In the latter setting, after vigorously cleansing the insertion site with a cutaneous antiseptic, inserting the guide wire, removing the catheter, and cleansing the site once again with an antiseptic agent, the operator should reglove and ideally redrape the site, as the original gloves and drapes may have become contaminated from manipulation of the original catheter.

Chlorhexidine-based products, especially alcoholic chlorhexidine, is superior to povidone-iodine or alcohol alone at reducing the risk of intravascular catheter-related infection (151,161).

The efficacy of antibiotic prophylaxis during PA catheter insertion has not been studied in a prospective fashion; however, this practice is unwarranted based on prospective studies with central venous catheters (151,153,162).

Use of an external protective plastic sleeve significantly reduces the risk of PA catheter-related infection by minimizing touch contamination during manipulation of the PA catheter (38). Use of heparin-bonded PA catheters is associated with a reduced risk of catheter-related infection because benzalkonium chloride is used on the catheter surface as a cationic surfactant to bond the anionic heparin to the catheters manufactured in the United States (58). Therefore, heparin-bonded catheters should be used rather than non-heparin-bonded catheters unless there are clinical contraindications, such as heparin-induced thrombocytopenia (163,164).

In a large, prospective trial of 442 PA catheters, there was no difference in the incidence of catheter colonization or catheter-related bloodstream infection between gauze and transparent dressing groups (37). For this reason, either standard sterile gauze and tape or polyurethane transparent dressings are acceptable for use on the insertion site of PA catheters.

Additionally, transparent dressings may be left in place up to five days between dressing changes, without increased risk of PA catheter-related infection (37). Newer, more permeable transparent dressings do not appear to reduce the risk of PA catheter-related infection, compared to standard transparent dressings (37). Oozing of blood from the insertion site increases the risk of catheter-related infection (56) and in such instances, gauze dressing should be used until if and when such bleeding resolves.

There are a number of measures aimed at reducing the risk of in-use contamination of PA catheter infusate and components. The delivery system should be manipulated as little as possible. No one should handle or especially enter the system without appropriate hand hygiene. Entering the monitoring circuit for the purpose of blood drawing should be limited as much as possible.

The number of stopcocks in the system should be minimized. Stopcocks should be wiped with a cutaneous antiseptic, such as using an alcohol pledget, prior to manipulation (165). Closed systems used for measuring the cardiac output by thermal dilution appear to reduce the risk of injectate contamination (166). All calibration devices, heparinized solutions, and other apparatus that come in direct contact with the fluid within the monitoring circuit must be sterile (67). Dextrose-containing solutions should not be used in hemodynamic monitoring infusions (67). Totally disposable transducer assemblies are preferred and should not be reused (67). Reusable transducers should be subjected to high-level chemical disinfection or, preferably, sterilization with ethylene oxide between patients, or when the monitoring circuit (chamber dome and continuous-flow device) is replaced (67). Centralized decontamination provides more consistent quality control; however, in an emergent situation, decontamination of reusable transducers with alcohol pledgets does not appear to increase the risk of catheter-related infection (167,168). The addition of sodium metabisulfite to a heparin-containing flush solution reduced the incidence of left atrial catheter-related infections in one study (169). However, before recommending this preventive strategy, prospective randomized studies must be done to confirm these findings and to provide data regarding the safety of these infusions.

If disposable transducers and chamber domes are used with infusions for hemodynamic monitoring, there is no need to replace the transducer assembly and other components of the delivery system, including flush solutions, more frequently than every four days (170). In a recent prospective trial including arterial, central venous, and PA catheters, the pressure-monitoring infusion systems were not replaced at regular intervals (171). Only four of 1991 cultures of infusion fluid had significant growth, and all occurred within 48 hours of a bag change. Routine replacement of the pressure-monitoring infusion system at 72-hour intervals, as was the standard of care in the institution, would not have prevented this contamination. The new policy also led to a significant cost savings to the institution. Based on this information, it appears that the pressure-monitoring infusion system—including the transducer and associated plastic ware, tubing, and flush solutions—may not need routine replacement.

Although there remains some controversy surrounding the safe duration of PA catheterization, the risk of infection is low if the catheter remains in place for no longer than three to four days (Fig. 3). It behooves the user of this device to assess the need for continued catheterization on a daily basis and to remove the catheter as soon as feasible. If PA catheterization beyond four days is considered necessary, there are three options: the catheter may be left in place, accepting that the risk of infection will begin to rise sharply; a new catheter can be placed in a new site, gaining another four days of very low risk; or, using a guide wire, the catheter can be exchanged with a new one. Cultures of the original catheter should be done, and the new catheter should be removed if colonization is found, especially with more pathogenic organisms such as *S. aureus* or *Candida*.

PERIPHERAL ARTERIAL CATHETERS

Introduction

Peripheral arterial catheters are commonly used to monitor the blood pressure and arterial blood gases (pH, PaO_2, $PaCO_2$) and oxygenation of critically ill or unstable patients. At one institution where two years of observational data were reviewed, 48 and 33% of patients admitted to medical and surgical intensive care units, respectively, had arterial catheterization (172). In a survey of U.S. adult ICUs, 40% of patients have arterial catheters (173).

Features of the Catheter

Peripheral arterial catheters are typically made of Teflon or polyurethane. Arterial catheters are complex medical devices (Fig. 4), similar to PA catheters. Besides the arterial catheter itself, an infusion designated for arterial pressure monitoring also includes an extended length of tubing connected to a chamber that interfaces with an electromechanical transducer. A continuous-flow device is in the line and permits periodic flushes to maintain patency of the system. This device is connected to a pressurized bag of heparin-containing flush solution. The infusion system differs from many others used in clinical practice in that the infusate characteristically runs very slowly, the fluid column interfaces with an electromechanical transducer through the diaphragm of a chamber dome, the system may contain multiple stopcocks, and the chamber dome and transducer are often attached to the patient's arm, potentially vulnerable to contamination by cutaneous microflora.

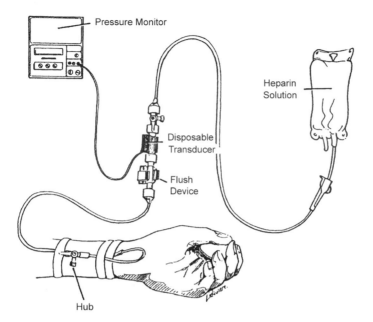

Figure 4 Schematic of a peripheral arterial catheter placed in the radial artery.

During the first decade of widescale use of arterial pressure monitoring in the United States, chamber domes were routinely reused as a cost-saving measure. When it was recognized that failure to reliably decontaminate chamber domes between patients led to many epidemics of gram-negative bacteremia, manufacturers developed disposable chamber domes, which are now widely used. Despite this intervention, the permanent transducers interfacing with disposable chamber domes also became contaminated, leading to infusate contamination and epidemic bloodstream infections. Completely disposable modular systems were then developed, incorporating a continuous-flow device, chamber dome, and electromechanical transducer. Most U.S. hospitals now exclusively use disposable systems. Besides infectious complications, which is the subject of this chapter, it is important to realize that noninfectious complications associated with use of this device are not uncommon (174).

Incidence of Infection

Many prospective studies have addressed the risk of peripheral arterial catheter-related infection (10,20,24,25,28,32,34,54,175–189). However, in only one of these studies were cultures performed of all possible sources of catheter-related infection (185). Table 4 summarizes the 18 studies of at least 75 catheters published after 1980, in which cultures were routinely carried out at the time of catheter withdrawal. In studies using semiquantitative or

Table 4 Incidence of Peripheral Arterial Catheter-Related Infection

Study	Catheters	Catheter culture method	Colonized (%)	Catheter-related bloodstream infection (%)
Pinilla et al. (10)	172	SQ	4.1	0
Kaye et al. (20)	102	NR	13.7	1.0
Shinozaki et al. (177)	170	NR	NR	0.6
Russell et al. (179)	261	NR	NR	1.1
Thomas et al. (178)	68	Q	20.5	NR
Damen et al. (24)	584	SQ	1.2	0
Damen and Van Der Twell (25)	349	SQ	4.3	0
Leroy et al. (183)	164	SQ	22.6	0
Maki and Ringer (185)	489	SQ	3.1	0.8
Eyer et al. (28)	250	SQ	3.6	2.8
Furfaro et al. (186)	340	SQ	2.9	0
Bull et al. (32)	256	SQ	18.0	0.8
Raad et al. (34)	121	SQ	15.5	5.6
Raad et al. (188)	807	SQ	14.7	0
Rijnders et al. (189)	272	QS	15.4	1.5

Abbreviations: SQ = semiquantitative roll-plate method; QV = quantitative by vortex method; QS = quantitative by sonication; NR = not reported.

quantitative catheter culture methods and at least 75 catheters per study, 1.2 to 22.6% of peripheral arterial catheters were colonized (weighted mean and median incidence of colonization is 8.4% [95% CI 8.1–8.6%] and 4.1%, respectively). In these studies, the range of peripheral arterial catheter-related bloodstream infection was 0 to 5.6%. The weighted mean and median incidence of arterial catheter-related bloodstream infection is 0.54% [95% CI 0.50–0.58%] and 0%, respectively. It is not possible to confidently determine the incidence of arterial catheter-related bloodstream infection per 1000 catheter-days since few studies gave information regarding the number of catheter-days. However, a recent large study found an incidence of 1.3% (3.7 per 1000 catheter days) (190).

Microbial Profile

Coagulase-negative staphylococci, predominately *S. epidermidis*, are the most common pathogens responsible for peripheral arterial catheter colonization and bloodstream infection. Fifty-nine percent of arterial catheters are colonized with coagulase-negative staphylococci, 17% with other gram-positive pathogens, 23% with gram-negative bacteria, and 2% with yeast (24,25,54,177,183,184). In these prospective studies, there were only seven catheter-related bloodstream infections —four caused by coagulase-negative staphylococci, two by *Enterococcus*, and one by *Pseudomonas aeruginosa*.

Risk Factors

Two studies used multivariate analysis to determine independent risk factors for catheter-related infection (25,185). Heavy cutaneous colonization of the catheter insertion site (RR 10), age less than one year, prolonged dwell time in children, and insertion in an old site over a guide wire were each independent risk factors for peripheral arterial catheter-related infection. Using univariate analysis, a number of investigators have found other risk factors for peripheral arterial catheter-related infection, as described below.

Insertion Site

Although heavy cutaneous colonization is associated with arterial catheter-related infection (185), there are conflicting data regarding the association of inflammation with arterial catheter colonization. Some investigators (186) have found that inflammation was significantly associated with catheter colonization; others (182,183) have found that inflammation at the catheter insertion site was not predictive of catheter colonization. In one study (184), cultures of the arterial catheter insertion site had a 57 and 100% positive and negative predictive value for catheter infection, respectively. Based on this information, heavy arterial catheter insertion site colonization is associated with infection. The absence of insertion site colonization in a febrile, catheterized patient should suggest arterial catheter infection associated with a colonized catheter hub, contaminated infusate, or another site of infection.

Site of Insertion

Although a number of investigators have compared the incidence of infection associated with radial artery, as compared to femoral artery, insertion (25,54,178,179), only one investigator prospectively randomized catheters to insertion at these two sites (178). Most of the studies were limited by the small number of catheters studied. Combining these investigations, there is a suggestion of an increased risk of infection associated with femoral catheterization—catheter colonization and bloodstream infection 3 and 0.4%, respectively, with radial artery insertion, compared to 7 and 1.3%, respectively, for femoral artery insertion. A confounding variable in these studies is that femoral catheter insertion may be associated with more prolonged dwell time (179). Also, the number of femoral arterial catheters studied is small. Although the largest of these studies did not describe the number of patients who had radial vs. femoral arterial insertion, a significantly increased incidence of catheter colonization in the latter site was noted (25); however, using Kaplan-Meier plots, the risk of infection associated with femoral artery insertion did not increase over time.

Drawing firm conclusions regarding the risk of infection associated with insertion in the femoral vs. the radial artery must await the results of larger prospective, randomized trials. At present, it would appear that decisions regarding which site to use for peripheral arterial catheter insertion should be based on the clinical setting.

Barrier Precautions

In a prospective study of barrier precautions for arterial catheter insertion, investigators using sequential enrollment compared the incidence of catheter-related infection utilizing two different preventive strategies associated with catheter insertion (32). In the first phase, physicians inserting arterial catheters donned hat, mask, and sterile gloves. In the latter half of the study, a surgical gown was also worn by the catheter inserter, and a more prolonged, five-minute skin preparation was done. The incidence of catheter colonization was 23.7% without and 14.7% with full barrier precautions and prolonged skin preparation ($p < 0.001$). It is difficult to determine the efficacy of full barrier precautions from this study since the duration of cutaneous antisepsis also varied. In many of the published studies (Table 4), sterile gloves and drapes were used, but mask, hat, and gown were not worn during arterial catheter insertion. We believe that sterile gloves and drapes are sufficient barrier precautions during insertion of these catheters (see "Prevention of Infection" for further discussion).

Guidewires

A single study prospectively randomized patients (a) to guide wire arterial catheter exchange every seven days, (b) to catheter insertion in a new site every seven days, or (c) to prolonged catheterization without routine guide wire exchange (28). There was no significant difference in the incidence of catheter-related infection in any of these three patient groups; however, the incidence of infection was low and the power of the analysis was very limited based on the small number of patients studied. In a nonrandomized prospective clinical trial (185), the incidence of catheter-related bloodstream infection was 3.7% in patients who had arterial catheters placed in an old site over a guide wire, as compared to 0% in patients whose arterial catheters were inserted in a new site ($p < 0.01$). All six arterial catheter-related bloodstream infections were in the guide wire exchange group. Data from these studies suggest that routine guide wire exchange of peripheral arterial catheters does not reduce the incidence of systemic catheter-related infection, but rather increases the risk.

Duration of Catheterization

A number of investigators found that prolonged catheter insertion was associated with an increased cumulative risk of peripheral arterial catheter-related infection (20,25,32,34,178,183,188,191); however, others did not find this to be the case (28,54,186). Although the cumulative incidence of arterial catheter-related infection increases with time, the risk of infection per day of catheterization (i.e., the incidence density) does not increase with prolonged catheterization (10,183,186). In three prospective trials (177,178,186), the arterial catheter, transducer assembly, and associated plasticware were not routinely changed. The combined incidence of catheter colonization and catheter-related bloodstream infection was 2.9 and 0.2%, respectively—both comparable to median rates for all prospective clinical trials. One group of investigators (170) found that the incidence of transducer fluid contamination was not significantly different when the fluids were randomized to be changed every two days or every four days, yet, the cumulative prevalence of transducer fluid contamination was greater when the fluids were changed every eight days compared with every two days. In another study (177), none of 170 transducer fluid samples were contaminated, despite a policy that allowed the catheters, transducers, and associated plasticware to remain in place without routine changes. More recently, the incidence of transducer fluid contamination was found to be extremely low, despite prolonged arterial and PA catheter dwell times, and routine replacement of the transducer fluid every three days would not have prevented the few cases of contamination that occurred (171). Based on this information, it would appear that routine replacement of peripheral arterial catheters, transducers, and associated plasticware is unnecessary as long as the insertion site is devoid of purulence or fluctuance and the patient does not have unexplained fever or other symptoms of occult infection that may be due to the catheter itself.

Hematogenous Seeding

In prospective studies, only three of 94 arterial catheters exposed to bacteremia or fungemia from a distant focus of infection had concordant growth on the catheter surface when removed (183–186). One episode of rebound bacteremia was observed associated with hematogenous seeding of an arterial catheter (185). Based on this information, it would appear that the risk of hematogenous seeding of arterial catheters is low, similar to the majority of studies of PA catheters. However, return of fever in previously treated bacteremic or fungemic patients should alert the clinician to the possibility of seeding of the catheter, prompting removal of the catheter for culture if no other source of fever is evident.

Dressings

A single study compared the risk of arterial catheter-related bloodstream infection in patients whose catheter insertion site was covered with transparent polyurethane film dressings vs. gauze and tape dressings (56). In this study of 400 arterial catheters, use of transparent dressing replaced every other day increased the risk of catheter-related bloodstream infection more than fivefold. Large, prospective, randomized trials are needed to definitively determine the risk of arterial catheter-associated infection when using transparent vs. gauze and tape dressings. At the present time, we believe that use of gauze and tape dressings on arterial catheter insertion sites may be preferable to transparent polyurethane dressings. One study of multiple catheter types, including arterial catheters, concluded that oozing of blood under dressings increased the risk of infection (56).

Antibiotic Use

Antibiotic use during catheterization has had no impact on the incidence of catheter colonization, including the use of vancomycin (34,183,186). A prospective, randomized trial of central venous catheters also found that prophylactic vancomycin did not reduce the incidence of catheter-related infection (162). Based on these findings and the increased risk of the development of antibiotic resistance with widespread use, antibiotic prophylaxis should not be used for arterial catheter insertion (118).

Cutaneous Antisepsis

In one clinical trial, patients with arterial catheters were prospectively randomized to have the insertion sites cleansed with aqueous chlorhexidine, alcohol, or povidone-iodine (192). The incidence of catheter-related infection was 0.7, 4.3, and 5.6% in each of these groups, respectively. None of the four arterial catheter-related bloodstream infections occurred in the group randomized to chlorhexidine, and the incidence of catheter-related infection was significantly lower than the chlorhexidine group compared to the alcohol and povidone-iodine groups combined (p = .03). In another study (187), the incidence of arterial catheter colonization was 15/1000 catheter-days versus 32/1000 catheter-days in groups randomized to alcoholic chlorhexidine and benzalkonium chloride combination compared with povidone-iodine (p = 0.05). These data suggest that chlorhexidine-containing preparations are the antiseptic agents of choice for cleaning the skin prior to arterial catheter insertion.

Other Risk Factors

In one prospective trial, patients underwent radial arteriography prior to catheter removal (183). Eight percent of the arterial catheters, mean dwell time of 6.5 days, had radiographically evident thrombus formation. However, the incidence of arterial catheter colonization was 25 and 23% in patients with and without evidence of thrombus, respectively. Despite the fact that a number of microbial pathogens, in particular *S. aureus*, have an avidity for binding to host-derived protein components of thrombus (79–81), the association of thrombus and arterial catheter colonization was not demonstrated in this small study.

The use of an arterial catheter with 120 cm of pressure tubing through which blood was drawn back to clear the line of heparin before sampling has been associated with an increased risk of catheter colonization compared to another arterial pressure-monitoring device, which had a one-way valve that did not allow blood backflow into the tubing (186).

F.   Sources of Infection

Bacteria and fungi may gain access to a catheterized patient's bloodstream from skin at the insertion site, stopcock contamination, contamination of the transducer assembly, contamination of infusate during preparation or during catheter use, or intraluminal contamination secondary to drawing blood into the line during an episode of bacteremia or fungemia. Cultures of all potential sources of arterial catheter-related infection were performed in only one study (185). Three percent and 2.9% of infusate and hub specimens had significant growth, respectively. Of the six episodes of primary catheter-related bloodstream infection, two each were due to colonization of the skin, hub, and infusate, respectively; one case of catheter-related bloodstream infection had an unidentifiable source. All six primary catheter-related bloodstream infections occurred in patients whose arterial catheters were exchanged over a guide wire and in whom the insertion site was cleansed with povidone-iodine or alcohol, as compared to chlorhexidine. Information gathered from this investigation supports the fact that there are myriad potential sources of bloodstream infection in patients with arterial catheters and preventive strategies should be aimed at each of these potential reservoirs.

In one study (184), the incidence of transducer fluid contamination increased significantly when the duration of catheterization was greater than two days. These investigators also found that 8 of 14 insertion site cultures with significant growth were associated with concordant growth on a catheter segment. Catheter colonization only occurred in the presence of microbial growth at the insertion site.

Using arterial catheters with a long stagnant column of infusate, another group of investigators found that 12 of 102 transducer fluid cultures had significant microbial growth; four of these 12 fluid samples were associated with concordant bacteremia (185). Investigators using arterial catheters without the stagnant column observed that 23 of 98 infusate specimens drawn through the arterial catheter stopcock had significant growth (183); however, in only four of the 23 instances of contamination was the arterial catheter tip found to be colonized with concordant growth of bacteria or fungi, and there were no associated bloodstream infections. Interestingly, the incidence of infusate contamination increased during the summer months. In another study (177) of arterial catheters assembled without a stagnant column of infusate, none of the 170 transducer fluids had significant growth sampled, despite prolonged catheterization and no routine change of the catheter, transducer assembly, or related plasticware. However, stopcock contamination increased significantly with the duration of catheterization; 10 and 26% of stopcocks used for four or less days vs. five or more days had significant growth, respectively. In a study of peripheral arterial and PA catheters (170), contamination of transducer fluid collected through a stopcock was not significantly different when the transducers were changed every two days or every four days; however, contamination increased significantly when transducer fluids were changed every 8 days as compared to every two days. The single episode of transducer-related bloodstream infection occurred on the day the transducer fluid was initially contaminated and would have been unaffected by more frequently scheduled replacement of the transducer assembly. In another combined study, infusate contamination was exceedingly rare, 0.1%, despite no routinely scheduled component changes (171). The contamination that occurred would not have been avoided had the institution maintained a policy for changing pressure-monitoring components every 3 days.

In some studies, investigators found that the cumulative rate of microbial colonization increased with the duration of catheterization; however, in those prospective studies performed without routinely changing the catheter, transducer, or associated plasticware (177, 178,186), the combined incidence of arterial catheter-associated bloodstream infection was very low—0.15%, despite prolonged dwell time. Thus, routine replacement of pressure-monitoring components does not appear to be necessary.

Blood conservation devices have been developed to eliminate the loss of discard volume of blood, which occurs when drawing blood through arterial catheters. The incidence of arterial infection using these devices compared with standard arterial catheters has not been studied in any prospective, randomized studies. However, the risk of contamination of the internal components of two such devices has been determined in a small study (193). In this study, 20 devices (three different internal sites cultured per device) from each of two currently marketed products were sampled. Thirty-five percent of the internal components from one manufacturer were colonized compared with 15% of the other (p = 0.1). All instances of colonization involved coagulase-negative staphylococci except for one episode each involving bacillus and diptheroids. Apparently none of these cultures correlated from positive cultures from other sites. Therefore, these products pose a potential risk of infection due to skin organisms. How this risk compares to use of arterial catheters without implementing such blood-conserving measures remains unknown at the present time.

Epidemics

Physicians using arterial catheters must remain vigilant in regard to the risk of epidemic bloodstream infection associated with this device. The insidious nature of epidemic arterial catheter-related bloodstream infection is reflected by the fact that these epidemics last, on average, 11 months before being recognized, compared to three months with epidemics of bacteremia derived from other sources (194). There have been 29 epidemics associated with arterial pressure monitoring published between 1971 and 1996 (67–71;

Table 5). Nearly 75% of these epidemics were due to faulty decontamination of the transducer components. This was often the result of using a dilute quaternary ammonium solution, which fostered contamination by resistant nosocomial gram-negative bacilli. Eleven of the 29 epidemics occurred despite using disposable chamber domes with reusable transducer heads. Nine of the epidemics were associated with carriage of the epidemic strain on the hands of healthcare providers. Contamination of fluids that come in contact with the pressure-monitoring device, such as heparinized saline flush solutions or contaminated disinfectant solutions, contaminated calibration systems, and contaminated ice used to chill syringes, have all been associated with epidemics.

Although manufacturers state that disposable equipment should not be reused, reuse of disposable chamber domes has been associated with epidemic bloodstream infections traced to arterial pressure monitoring. To our knowledge, there have been no large epidemics of arterial catheter-related bloodstream infection traced to contaminated infusions used for pressure monitoring in hospitals exclusively using disposable transducers. However, there are two reports of arterial catheter-related bloodstream infections due to gram-negative bacilli in hospitals using disposable transducers (71,195). In one of these reports (195), two infections with unusual environmental bacteria may have been related to preparation of heparinized saline solutions used for pressure monitoring in a nonsterile environment over a sink. However,

Table 5 Epidemiology of Epidemic Bloodstream Infections Traced to Arterial Pressure Monitoring

Epidemiology[a]	Epidemics (n)
Faulty decontamination of transducer components	18
Reusable transducer heads used with disposable chamber domes	11
Reusable chamber domes	6
Reuse of disposable chamber domes	3
Carriage of epidemic organisms on hands of users	9
Contaminated heparinized saline solutions	3
Use of dextrose-containing fluids instead of saline	3
Contaminated disinfectant solution	3
Contaminated calibration system	2
Contaminated ice used to chill syringes for blood–gas specimens	1
Contaminated uncovered, preassembled pressure-monitoring equipment in operating rooms	1

[a] In many of the outbreaks, more than one source or probable mechanism of contamination was implicated.
(From Ref. 67.)

environmental cultures of this area failed to grow the bacteria found in the blood of these two patients. In one epidemic, cleaning operating rooms with a faulty spray disinfection device led to contamination of uncovered pressure-monitoring equipment and gram-negative bacterial bloodstream infections (71).

Many of the outbreaks associated with arterial pressure monitoring were caused by unusual nosocomial, gram-negative bacilli, such as *Serratia*, nonaeruginosa *Pseudomonas, Burkholderia cepacia*, and *Enterobacter* species, which are able to proliferate in fluids with minimal nutritional support (Table 6). Finding such bacteria in blood cultures of patients with arterial pressure monitoring, or blood cultures growing other unusual gram-negative pathogens such as *Achromobacter, Acinetobacter*, or *Flavobacterium*, should alert the clinician to the possibility of an epidemic deriving from contamination of arterial pressure-monitoring systems. A single bacteremia may reflect a sporadic endemic case. However, two or more bacteremias should prompt an immediate investigation to determine the etiology and, if due

Table 6 Microbial Profile of Epidemic Nosocomial Bloodstream Infections Deriving from Contamination of Arterial Pressure-Monitoring Systems

	Epidemics (n)	
Pathogen	Single pathogen	Multiple-organism outbreaks
Serratia marcescens	6	1
Burkholderia cepacia	4	—
Comamonas acidovorans	—	2
Pseudomonas fluorescens	—	2
Pseudomonas aeruginosa	1	1
Stenotrophomonas maltophilia	1	—
Pseudomonas spp.	—	1
Enterobacter cloacae	2	3
Enterobacter aerogenes	1	—
Enterobacter spp.	—	1
Achromobacter xylosoxidans	1	—
Acinetobacter calcoaceticus	1	—
Acinetobacter spp.	—	1
Klebsiella oxytoca	1	1
Klebsiella pneumoniae	—	1
Citrobacter diversus	—	1
Flavobacterium sp.	2	—
Candida parapsilosis	2	—
Candida spp.	1	—

(From Ref. 67.)

to arterial pressure monitoring, to identify the reservoir and mechanism of introduction of these pathogens into the patients' monitoring systems.

Pathogenesis

The pathogenesis of peripheral arterial catheter-related infection is similar to that of PA catheters. Using electron microscopy, biofilms containing bacteria have been observed on the surface of radial and femoral arterial catheters after one day in situ (196). Thus, microbial pathogens may colonize arterial catheters during or shortly after insertion, although early invasion of the bloodstream appears to be uncommon. The reason for the low incidence of bloodstream infections associated with peripheral arterial catheters may be due in part to the fact that the catheter is made of Teflon or polyurethane. There is less bacterial adherence to Teflon (197) or polyurethane (198) than catheters made of other materials such as polyvinychloride. There is also less avid binding of host-derived proteins, such as fibronectin, to polyurethane catheters, compared to catheters made of other materials (198). The bio-burden of microbes at the radial artery insertion site is also significantly less than insertion sites of central venous catheters, and the radial artery site also is less likely to be colonized with microbes other than coagulase-negative staphylococci (46).

     In conclusion, although microbes are commonly found on arterial catheter segments, the catheter material and host immune response appear to act together to limit their proliferation and bloodstream infection.

Types of Infection

Infective endocarditis associated with arterial pressure monitoring is extremely rare. More commonly reported is localized suppurative infection involving the cannulated artery. In one prospective evaluation of arterial catheters (185), a single case of endarteritis was described involving thrombus formation in the artery that contained *Candida*.

     Infected radial artery pseudoaneurysms associated with arterial pressure monitoring has been reviewed (191,199). In one study (191), 12 radial artery infections occurred over two years (for infected and uninfected cases, the mean duration of catheterization was 5.2 and 2.7 days, respectively [p < 0.001]). Five of the 12 developed infected aneurysms, all treated with excision and antibiotics. Of note, these apparently developed despite early antibiotic therapy. The aneurysms developed early in some patients (five and eight days after catheterization, respectively), but aneurysms developed three, five, and seven weeks after catheterization in three other patients. All infected aneurysms involved *S. aureus*. Excised tissue revealed false aneurysm in each case associated with intraluminal thrombosis and dense inflammatory infiltrate in the fibrous wall. Septic emboli of the involved hand was seen in two patients. In the other study (199), six infected aneurysms occurred at one hospital over six years. The duration of radial artery catheterization was significantly longer in patients who developed infected pseudoaneurysms than in patients who had radial arterial catheters in place without this complication—12.5 vs. 4.3 days, respectively (p < 0.05). Patients with this complication were older than noninfected patients admitted to the same intensive care units—72 vs. 54 years, respectively (p < 0.05). The infected patients also appeared to have had more prolonged stays in the intensive care unit prior to the development of this infection. Most of these patients presented with an expanding or fluctuant pulsatile mass at the radial artery insertion site. Some of these symptoms developed as late as six weeks after the catheter had been removed. Five of the six cases of infected radial artery pseudoaneurysms were caused by *S. aureus*. Four infected pseudoaneurysms secondary to radial artery catheterization previously reported in the literature were also due to *S. aureus* (200–202). Infected pseudoaneurysms, predominantly caused by *S. aureus*, have also been reported in association with femoral arterial pressure monitoring (203). Some of the infections involving the radial artery, as well as those associated with brachial artery catheters, have also been associated with Osler's nodes, Janeway lesions, and splinter hemorrhages in the extremity (191,200–202,204) and, in some cases, surrounding erythema, cellulitis, or, rarely, purulent drainage from the catheter insertion site. In summary, radial artery pseudoaneurysm may develop several weeks after catheter removal and administration of antibiotics. *S. aureus* is the most likely pathogen and therapy should consist of bactericidal antistaphylococcal antibiotics and excision of the infected aneurysm. Limiting the duration of arterial catheterization will reduce the risk of developing this complication.

Diagnosis of Infection

The microbiological methods available for the diagnosis of peripheral arterial catheter-related infection are no different from those available for other intravascular devices; unfortunately, there are no systematic investigations comparing the sensitivity and specificity of different methodologies with arterial catheters.

There is varying data in the literature regarding the sensitivity and specificity of inflammation surrounding the catheter insertion site, aiding in the diagnosis of arterial catheter-related infection (182,183,186,191). Insertion site cultures had positive and negative predictive values of 57 and 100%, respectively, in one study (184) and may be of some value in accessing the febrile patients with arterial catheters.

Management of Infection

General recommendations for treatment of patients with intravascular catheter infections has been published (118). The management of peripheral artery catheter-related infection is similar to that of PA catheters. Finding a pulsatile mass around the insertion site while the catheter is in situ, or after catheter withdrawal, should prompt surgical exploration with Gram stain and cultures, and debridement, possibly en bloc resection, if an infected pseudoaneurysm is found. In this setting, intravenous antibiotic therapy should be initiated to cover resistant staphylococci at those institutions with a high incidence of MRSA, such as vancomycin, pending the results of microbiological sensitivity testing, or initiate nafcillin or oxacillin at those hospitals where there is still a low incidence of MRSA.

Prevention of Infection

As previously noted, guidelines for prevention of intravascular catheter infections have been recently published (151,153).

A recent, prospective study of 272 arterial catheters found no significant difference in arterial catheter colonization or catheter-related infection when patients were randomized to have their catheters inserted using sterile gloves, mask, cap, sterile gown, and sheet versus sterile gloves only (189). Although sterile gloves and drapes are likely to be adequate barrier precautions during arterial catheter insertion, a long-sleeved, sterile surgical gown, mask, and eye protection should also be worn to reduce the risk of exposure to potential bloodborne pathogens.

Similar to PA catheters, chlorhexidine is the cutaneous antiseptic of choice for insertion site preparation (185). Regarding dressings used to cover arterial catheter insertion sites, gauze and tape is preferable if there is oozing of blood from the insertion site.

Two randomized trials have shown that heparin flush reduces risk of thrombosis of arterial catheters (205,206). In a study involving arterial and venous catheters, there was a significantly increased likelihood of catheter colonization with intraluminal or extraluminal thrombus formation (OR 6 (207)). This information, and similar findings with PA and other catheters, suggests that heparin should be used as flush solution to prevent thrombus formation and infection in peripheral arterial catheters.

Based on the available data from prospective studies, routine replacement of the arterial catheter, transducer, chamber dome assembly, and associated plasticware at scheduled intervals appears to be unnecessary. Because of the epidemics associated with faulty decontamination of reusable transducers, disposable, single-use transducer assemblies should be used. Other precautions regarding the monitoring equipment are similar to those discussed in the section on prevention of PA catheter-related infections.

There are no prospective studies of innovative arterial catheter hubs or antiseptic-coated arterial catheters. Because of the low incidence of peripheral arterial catheter-related bloodstream infection, it will be difficult to show an impact of any new strategy unless very large numbers of patients are studied. Any new preventive strategy must be shown to be cost-effective, especially since the incidence of infection is so low at the current time. It is important, however, for clinicians using peripheral arterial catheters to assess the need for continued arterial pressure monitoring on a daily basis and remove the catheter as soon as feasible. It is hoped that future technological advances will permit hemodynamic monitoring of patients noninvasively (119), further reducing their risk of hospital-acquired infection.

REFERENCES

1. Swan HJC, Ganz W, Forrester J, Marcus H, Diamond G, Chonette D. Catheterization of the heart in man with use of a flow-directed balloon-tipped catheter. N Engl J Med 1970; 283:447–451.
2. Jeffrey S, Groeger MD, Kalpalatha K, et al. Descriptive analysis of critical care units in the United States: patient characteristics and intensive care unit utilization. Crit Care Med 1993; 21:279–291.
3. Dalen JE, Bone RC. Is it time to pull the pulmonary artery catheter? JAMA 1996; 276:916–918.
4. Connors AF, Speroff T, Dawson NV, et al. The effectiveness of right heart catheterization in the initial care of critically ill patients. JAMA 1996, 276:889–897.
5. Mermel LA, Maki DG. Infectious complications of PA pulmonary artery catheters. Am J Respir Crit Care Med 1994; 149:1020–1036.
6. Taylor RW, Ahrens T, Viejo A, et al. Pulmonary artery catheter consensus conference: consensus statement. Crit Care Med 1997; 25:910–925.
7. Ivanov R, Allen J, Calvin JE. The incidence of major morbidity in critically ill patients managed with pulmonary artery catheters: a meta-analysis. Crit Care Med 2000; 28:615–619.
8. Applefeld JJ, Caruthers TE, Reno DJ, Civetta JM. Assessment of the sterility of long-term cardiac catheterization using thermodilution PA catheter. Chest 1978; 74:377–380.
9. Elliott CG, Zimmerman GA, Clemmer TP. Complications of pulmonary artery catheterization in the care of critically ill patients. Chest 1979; 76:647–652.
10. Pinilla JC, Ross DF, Martin T, Crump H. Study of the incidence of intra-vascular catheter infection and associated septicemia in critically ill patients. Crit Care Med 1983; 11:21–25.
11. Boyd KD, Thomas SJ, Gold J, Boyd AD. A prospective study of com-plications of pulmonary artery catheterizations in 500 consecutive patients. Chest 1983; 84:245–249.
12. Miller JJ, Venus B, Mathru M. Comparison of the sterility of long-term central venous catheterization using single lumen, triple lumen, and pulmonary artery catheters. Crit Care Med 1984; 12:634–637.
13. Samsoondar W, Freeman JB, Coultish I, Oxley C. Colonization of intra-vascular catheters in the intensive care unit. Am J Surg 1985; 149:730–732.
14. Myers ML, Austin TW, Sibbald WJ. Pulmonary artery catheter infections. A prospective study. Ann Surg 1985; 201:237–241.
15. Senagore A, Waller JD, Bonnell BW, Bursch LR, Scholten DJ. Pulmonary

artery catheterization: a prospective study of internal jugular and subclavian approaches. Crit Care Med 1987; 15:35–37.

16. Hudson-Civetta JA, Civetta JM, Martinez OV, Hoffman TA. Risk and detection of pulmonary artery catheter-related infection in septic surgical patients. Crit Care Med 1987; 15:29–34.

17. Passerini L, Phang PT, Jackson FL, Lam K, Costerton JW, King EG. Biofilms on right heart flow-directed catheters. Chest 1987; 92:440–446.

18. Levy JH, Nagle DM, Curling PE, Waller JL, Kopel M, Tobia V. Contamination reduction during central venous catheterization. Crit Care Med 1988; 16:165–167.

19. Michel L, Marsh HM, McMichan JC, Southorn PA, Brewer NS. Infection of pulmonary artery catheters in critically ill patients. JAMA 1981; 245:1032–1036.

20. Kaye W, Wheaton M, Potter-Bynoe G. Radial and pulmonary artery catheter-related sepsis [abstr]. Crit Care Med 1983; 11:249.

21. Groeger J, Carlon GC, Howland WS. Contamination shields for pulmonary artery catheters [abstr]. Crit Care Med 1983; 11:230.

22. Ricard P, Martin R, Marcoux JA. Protection of indwelling vascular catheters: incidence of bacterial contamination and catheter-related sepsis. Crit Care Med 1985; 13:541–543.

23. Parsa MH, Al-Sawwaf M, Shoemaker WC. Complications of pulmonary artery catheterization. Prob Gen Surg 1985; 2:133–144.

24. Damen J, Verhoef J, Bolton DT, et al. Microbiologic risk of invasive hemodynamic monitoring in patients undergoing open-heart operations. Crit Care Med 1985; 13:548–555.

25. Damen J, Ver Der Twell I. Positive tip cultures and related risk factors associated with intravascular catheterization in pediatric cardiac patients. Crit Care Med 1988; 16:221–228.

26. Heard SO, Davis RF, Sherertz RJ, et al. Influence of sterile protective sleeves on the sterility of pulmonary artery catheters. Crit Care Med 1987; 15:499–502.

27. Fisher MA, Maxwell LP, Teba L. Pulmonary artery catheters: risk factors for infection [abstr]. Program and Abstracts of the Twenty-eighth Interscience Conference on Antimicrobial Agents and Chemotherapy, Los Angeles, CA, October 1988; Washington, DC: American Society for Microbiology, 1988:273.

28. Eyer S, Brummitt C, Crossley K, Siegel R, Cerra F. Catheter-related sepsis: prospective, randomized study of three methods of long-term catheter maintenance. Crit Care Med 1990; 18:1073–1079.

29. Horowitz HW, Dworkin BM, Savino JA, Byrne DW, Pecora NA. Central catheter-related infections: comparison of pulmonary artery catheters and triple lumen catheters for the delivery of hyperalimentation in a critical care setting. J Parenter Enteral Nutr 1990; 14:588–592.

30. Mermel LA, McCormick RD, Springman SR, Maki DG. The pathogenesis and epidemiology of catheter-related infection with pulmonary artery PA catheters. A prospective study using molecular subtyping. Am J Med 1991; 38:197S–205S.

31. Bach A, Stubbig K, Geiss HK. Infectious risk of replacing venous catheters by the guide-wire technique. Zbl Hyg 1992; 193:150–159.

32. Bull DA, Neumayer LA, Hunter GC, et al. Improved sterile technique diminishes the incidence of positive line cultures in cardiovascular patients. J Surg Res 1992; 52:106–110.

33. Rello J, Coll P, Net A, Prats G. Infection of pulmonary artery catheters. Epidemiologic characteristics and multivariate analysis of risk factors. Chest 1993; 103:132–136.

34. Raad I, Umphrey J, Khan A, Truett LJ, Bodey GP. The duration of placement as a predictor of peripheral and pulmonary artery catheter infections. J Hosp Infect 1993; 23:17–26.

35. Kac G, Durain E, Amrein C, et al. Colonization and infection of pulmonary artery catheter in ardiac surgery patients: epidemiology and multivariate analysis of risk factors. Crit Care Med 2001; 29:971–975.

36. Blot F, Chachaty E, Raynard B, et al. Mechanisms and risk factors for infection of pulmonary artery catheters and introducer sheaths in cancer patients admitted to an intensive care unit. J Hops Infect 2001; 48:289–297.

37. Maki DG, Stolz SS, Wheeler S, Mermel LA. A prospective, randomized trial of gauze and two polyurethane dressings for site care of pulmonary artery catheters: implications for catheter management. Crit Care Med 1994; 22:1729–1737.

38. Cohen Y, Fosse JP, Karoubi P, et al. The "hands-off" catheter and the prevention of systemic infections associated with pulmonary artery catheter. A prospective study. Am J Respir Crit Care Med 1998; 157:284–287.

39. Hulliger S, Pittet D. Incidence and morbidity of central venous catheter-related infections in intensive care units. Abstracts of The Infectious Diseases Society of America Annual Meeting, Orlando, FL, October 1994; Washington, DC: Infectious Diseases Society of America, 1994:162 [abstr].

40. Maki DG, Will L. Risk factors for central venous catheter-related infection within the ICU. A prospective study of 345 catheters. Program and Abstracts of the Third International Conference of Nosocomial Infections, August, 1990, Atlanta, GA; Atlanta: Centers for Disease Control, National Foundation for Infectious Diseases, 1990:54 [abstr].

41. Richet H, Hubert B, Nitemberg G, et al. Prospective multicenter study of vascular-catheter-related complications and risk factors for positive central-catheter cultures in intensive care unit patients. J Clin Microbiol 1990; 28: 2520–2525.

42. Moro ML, Vigano EF, Lepri AC. Risk factors for central venous catheter-related infections in surgical and intensive care units. Infect Control Hosp Epidemiol 1994; 15:253–264.

43. Charalambous C, Swoboda SM, Dick J, Perl T, Lipsett PA. Risk factors and clinical impact of central line infections in the surgical intensive care unit. Arch Surg 1998; 133:1241–1246.

44. Conly JM, Grieves K, Peters B. A prospective, randomized study comparing transparent and dry gauze dressings for central venous catheters. J Infect Dis 1989; 159:310–319.

45. Armstrong CW, Mayhall CG, Miller KB, et al. Clinical predictors of infection of central venous catheters used for total parenteral nutrition. Infect Control Hosp Epidemiol 1990; 11:71–78.

46. Maki DG. Marked difference in skin colonization of insertion sites for central

venous, arterial and peripheral IV catheters. The major reason for differing risks of catheter-related infection? Program and Abstracts of the Thirtieth Interscience Conference on Antimicrobial Agents and Chemotherapy, Atlanta GA, October 1990; Washington, DC: American Society for Microbiology, 1990:712 [abstr].

47. Michel L, McMichan JC, Bachy JI. Microbial colonization of indwelling central venous catheters: statistical evaluation of potential contaminating factors. Am J Surg 1979; 137:745–748.

48. Damen J, Bolton D. A prospective analysis of 1400 pulmonary artery catheterizations in patients undergoing cardiac surgery. Acta Anaesthesiol Scand 1986; 30:386–392.

49. Raad II, Hohn DC, Gilbreath J, et al. Prevention of central venous catheter-related infections by using maximal sterile barrier precautions during insertion. Infect Control Hosp Epidemiol 1994; 15:231–238.

50. Maki DG. Yes, Virginia, aseptic technique is very important: maximal barrier precautions during insertion reduce the risk of central venous catheter-related bacteremia. Infect Control Hosp Epidemiol 1994; 15:227–230.

51. Cobb DK, High KP, Sawyer RG, et al. A controlled trial of scheduled replacement of central venous and pulmonary-artery catheters. N Engl J Med 1992; 327:1062–1068.

52. Sise MJ, Hollingsworth P, Brimm JE, Peters RM, Virgilio RW, Shackford SR. Complications of the flow-directed pulmonary-artery catheter: A prospective analysis in 219 patients. Crit Care Med 1981; 9:315–318.

53. Civetta JM, Hudson-Civetta JA, Dion L, Ghows MB, Angood PB, Martinez O. Duration of illness effects catheter related infection and bacteremia. Program and Abstracts of the Twenty-seventh Interscience Conference on Antimicrobial Agents and Chemotherapy, New York, NY, October 1987; Washington, DC: American Society for Microbiology, 1987:1141 [abstr].

54. Singh S, Nelson N, Acosta I, Check FE, Puri VK. Catheter colonization and bacteremia with pulmonary and arterial catheters. Crit Care Med 1982; 10:736–739.

55. Cook D, Randolph A, Kernerman P, et al. Central venous catheter replacement strategies: a systematic review of the literature. Crit Car Med 1997; 25:1417–1424.

56. Maki DG, Will L. Colonization and infection associated with transparent dressings for central venous, arterial, and hickman catheters. Program and Abstracts of the Twenty-fourth Interscience Conference on Antimicrobial Agents and Chemotherapy, Washington, DC, October 1984; Washington, DC: American Society for Microbiology, 1984:933 [abstr].

57. Hoar PF, Wilson RM, Mangano DT, Avery GJ, Szarnicki RJ, Hill JD. Heparin bonding reduces thrombogenicity of pulmonary artery catheters. N Engl J Med 1981; 305:993–995.

58. Mermel LA, Stolz SM, Maki DG. Surface antimicrobial activity of heparin-bonded and antiseptic-impregnated vascular catheters. J Infect Dis 1993; 167:920–924.

59. Hofbauer R, Moser D, Kaye AD, et al. Thrombus formation on the balloon of heparin-bonded pulmonary artery catheters: an ultrastructural scanning electron microscope study. Crit Care Med 2000; 28:727–735.

60. Timsit JF, Farkas JC, Boyer JM, et al. Central vein catheter-related thrombosis in intensive care patients. Incidence, risk factors and relationship with catheter-related sepsis. Chest 1998; 114:207–213.

61. Arepally G, Cines DB. Heparin-induced thrombocytopenia and thrombosis. Clin Rev Allergy Immunol 1998; 16:237–247.

62. Valles J, Rello J, Matas L, et al. Impact of using an indwelling introducer on diagnosis of Swan-Ganz pulmonary artery catheter colonization. Eur J Clin Microbiol Infect Dis 1996; 15:71–75.

63. Johnston WE, Prough DS, Royster RL, et al. Short-term sterility of the pulmonary artery catheter inserted through an external plastic shield. Anesthesiology 1984; 61:461–464.

64. Baele P, Pedemonte O, Zech F, Kestens-Servaye Y. Clinical use and bacteriological studies of catheter contamination sleeves. Intens Care Med 1984; 10:297–300.

65. Murray MJ, Wignes M, McMichan JC. Assessment of sterility of pulmonary artery catheters. Anesth Analg 1986; 65:1218–1221.

66. Kopman EA, Sandza JG. Manipulation of the pulmonary-artery catheter after placement: maintenance of sterility. Anesthesiology 1978; 48:373–374.

67. Mermel LA, Maki DG. Epidemic bloodstream infections from hemodynamic pressure monitoring: signs of the times. Infect Control Hosp Epidemiol 1989; 10:47–53.

68. Hekker TAM, Overhage WV, Schneider AJ. Pressure transducers: an overlooked source of sepsis in the intensive care unit. Intens Care Med 1990; 16: 511–512.

69. Gahrn-Hansen B, Alstrup P, Dessau R, et al. Outbreak of infection with *Achromobacter xylosoxidans* from contaminated intravascular pressure transducers. J Hosp Infect 1988; 12:1–6.

70. Thomas A, Lalitha MK, Jesudason MV, John S. Transducer related *Enterobacter cloacae* sepsis in post-operative cardiothoracic patients. J Hosp Infect 1993; 25:211–215.

71. Rudnick JR, Beck-Sague CM, Anderson RL, et al. Gram-negative bacteremia in open-heart-surgery patients traced to probable tap-water contamination of pressure-monitoring equipment. Infect Control Hosp Epidemiol 1996; 17:281–285.

72. Weinstein RA, Emori TG, Anderson RL, Stamm WE. Pressure transducers as source of bacteremia after open heart surgery. Report of an outbreak and guidelines for prevention. Chest 1976; 69:338–344.

73. Maki DG, Mermel LA. Infections due to infusion therapy. In: Bennett JV, Brachman PS, eds. Hospital Infections; Boston: Little Brown, 1998:689–724.

74. Cooper GL, Schiller AL, Hopkins CC. Possible role of capillary action in pathogenesis of experimental catheter-associated dermal tunnel infections. J Clin Microbiol 1988; 26:8–12.

75. Pittet D, Lew PD, Auckenthaler R, Waldvogel FA. Bacterial spread as a pathogenic factor in catheter-related infections. Program and Abstracts of the Thirtieth Interscience Conference on Antimicrobial Agents and Chemotherapy, Atlanta, GA, October 1990; Washington, DC: American Society for Microbiology, 1990:26 [abstr].

76. Dunne WM. Bacterial adhesion: seen any good biofilms lately? Clin Microbiol Rev 2002; 15:155–166.

77. Stillman RM, Seligman F, Garcia L, Sawyer PN. Etiology of catheter-associated sepsis. Correlation with thrombogenicity? Arch Surg 1977; 112:1496–1499.

78. Raad II, Luna M, Khalil SAM, Costerton JW, Lam C, Bodey GP. The relationship between the thrombotic and infectious complications of central venous catheters. JAMA 1994; 271:1014–1016.

79. Herrmann M, Vaudaux PE, Pittet D, et al. Fibronectin, fibrinogen, laminin act as mediators of adherence of clinical staphylococcal isolates to foreign material. J Infect Dis 1988; 158:693–701.

80. Herrmann M, Suchard SJ, Boxer LA, et al. Thrombospondin binds to *Staphylococcus aureus* and promotes staphylococcal adherence to surfaces. Infect Immunol 1991; 59:279–288.

81. Herrmann M, Lai QJ, Albrecht RM, et al. Adhesion of *Staphylococcus aureus* to surface-bound platelets: role of fibrinogen/fibrin and platelet integrins. J Infect Dis 1993; 167:312–322.

82. Herrmann M, Hartleib J, Kehrel B, et al. Interaction of von Willebrand factor with *Staphylococcus aureus*. J Infect Dis 1997; 176:984–991.

83. Donlan RM, Costerton JW. Biofilms: survival mechanisms of clinically relevant microorganisms. Clin Microbiol Rev 2002; 15:167–193.

84. Zimmerli W, Lew PD, Waldvogel FA. Pathogenesis of foreign body infection. Evidence for a local granulocyte defect. J Clin Invest 1984; 73:1191–1200.

85. Zimmerli W, Frei R, Widmer AF, Rajacic Z. Microbiological tests to predict treatment outcome in experimental device-related infections due to *Staphylococcus aureus*. J Antimicrob Chemother 1994; 33:959–967.

86. Garrison PK, Freedman LR. Experimental endocarditis I Staphylococcal endocarditis in rabbits resulting from placement of a polyethylene catheter in the right side of the heart. Yale J Biol Med 1970; 42:394–410.

87. Durack DT, Beeson PB. Experimental bacterial endocarditis I. Colonization of a sterile vegetation. Br J Exp Pathol 1972; 53:44–49.

88. Tsao MMP, Katz D. Central venous catheter-induced endocarditis: human correlate of the animal experimental model of endocarditis. Rev Infect Dis 1984; 6:783–790.

89. Greene JF Jr, Fitzwater JE, Clemmer TP. Septic endocarditis and indwelling pulmonary artery catheters. JAMA 1975; 233:891–892.

90. Ford SE, Manley PN. Indwelling cardiac catheters. An autopsy study of associated endocardial lesions. Arch Pathol Lab Med 1982; 106:314–317.

91. Rowley KM, Clubb KS, Walker Smith GJ, Cabin HS. Right-sided infective endocarditis as a consequence of flow-directed pulmonary-artery catheterization. A clinicopathological study of 55 autopsied patients. N Engl J Med 1984; 311:1152–1156.

92. Pace NL, Horton W. Indwelling pulmonary artery catheters. JAMA 1975; 233:893–894.

93. Katz JD, Cronau LH, Barash PG, Mandel SD. Pulmonary artery flow-guided catheters in the perioperative period. Indications and complications. JAMA 1977; 237:2832–2834.

94. Lange HW, Galliani CA, Edwards JE. Local complications associated with

indwelling PA catheters: autopsy study of 36 cases. Am J Cardiol 1983; 52:1108–1111.

95. Horst HM, Obeid FN, Vij D, Bivins BA. The risks of pulmonary arterial catheterization. Surg Gynecol Obstet 1984; 159:229–232.

96. Connors AF Jr, Castele RJ, Farhat NZ, Tomashefski JF Jr. Complications of right heart catheterization. A prospective autopsy study. Chest 1985; 88:567–572.

97. Becker RC, Martin RG, Underwood DA. Right-sided endocardial lesions and flow-directed pulmonary artery catheters. Cleve Clin J Med 1987; 54:384–388.

98. Melton JG, Kamal GD. Fatal right-sided nonbacterial endocarditis associated with pulmonary artery catheterization. Intensive Care Med 1989; 15.126–128.

99. Ehrie M, Morgan AP, Moore FD, O'Connor NE. Endocarditis with the indwelling balloon-tipped pulmonary artery catheter in burn patients. J Trauma 1978; 18:664–666.

100. Sasaki TM, Panke TW, Dorethy JF, Lindberg RB, Pruitt BA. The relationship of central venous and pulmonary artery catheter position to acute right-sided endocarditis in severe thermal injury. J Trauma 1979; 19:740–743.

101. Powell DC, Bivins BA, Bell RM, Sachatello CR, Griffen WO Jr. Bacterial endocarditis in the critically ill surgical patient. Arch Surg 1981; 116:311–314.

102. Iqbal SM, Hehir RL, Ehrich DA. Right sided endocarditis following PA catheterization: detection by two-dimensional echocardiography. Ultrasound Med Biol 1982; 8:701–704.

103. Van Der Bel-Kahn J, Fowler NO, Doerger P. Right heart catheter lesions: any significance? Am J Clin Pathol 1984; 82:137 147.

104. Ducatman BS, McMichan JC, Edwards WD. Catheter-induced lesions of the right side of the heart. JAMA 1985; 253:791–795.

105. Roush K, Scala-Barnett DM, Donabedian H, Freimer EH. Rupture of a pulmonary artery mycotic aneurysm associated with *Candida endocarditis*. Am J Med 1988; 84:142–144.

106. Soding PF, Klinck JR, Kong A, Farrington M. Infective endocarditis of the pulmonary valve following pulmonary artery catheterisation. Intensive Care Med 1994; 20:222–224.

107. Bernardin G, Milhaud D, Roger PM, et al. Swan-Ganz catheter-related pulmonary valve infective endocarditis: a case report. Intensive Care Med 1994; 20:142–144.

108. Verghese A, Widrich WC, Arbeit RD. Central venous septic thrombophlebitis—the role of medical therapy. Medicine 1985; 64:394–400.

109. Garcia E, Granier I, Geissler A, Boespflug MD, Magnan PE, Durand-Gasselin J. Intensive Care Med 1997; 23:1002–1004.

110. Kaufman J, Demas C, Stark K, Flancbaum L. Catheter-related septic central venous thrombosis current therapeutic options. West J Med 1986; 145:200–203.

111. Topiel MS, Bryan RT, Kessler CM, Simon GL. Case report: treatment of silastic catheter-induced central vein septic thrombophlebitis. Am J Med Sci 1986; 291:425–428.

112. Shin MS, Ho K-J. Cavitary pulmonary lesions complicating use of flow-directed balloon-tipped catheters in two cases. AJR 1979; 132:650–652.

113. McLoud TC, Putman CE. Radiology of the PA catheter and associated pulmonary complications. Radiology 1975; 116:19–22.

114. Mermel LA, Velez LA, Zilz MA, Maki DG. Epidemiologic and microbiologic features of nosocomial bloodstream infection (NBSI) implicating a vascular catheter source: a case-control study of 85 vascular catheter-related and 101 secondary NBSIs. Program and Abstracts of the Thirty-first Interscience Conference on Antimicrobial Agents and Chemotherapy, Chicago, IL, October 1991; Washington, DC: American Society for Microbiology, 1991:454 [abstr].

115. Rello J, Coll P, Net A, Prats G. Evaluation of different catheters' parts for identification of pulmonary artery catheter colonisation. Scand J Infect Dis 1991; 23:655–656.

116. Sherertz R, Heard S, Raad I. Diagnosis of triple-lumen catheter infection: comparison of roll-plate, sonication and flushing methodologies. J Clin Micro 1997; 35:641–646.

117. Hnatiuk OW, Pike J, Stoltzfus D, Lane W. Value of bedside plating of semiquantitative cultures for diagnosis of central venous catheter-related infections in ICU patients. Chest 1993; 103:896–899.

118. Mermel LA, Farr BM, Sherertz RJ, et al. Guidelines for the management of intravascular catheter-related infections. Clin Infect Dis 2001; 32:1249–12724.

119. McIntyre KM, Vita JA, Lambrew CT, Freman J, Loscalzo J. A noninvasive method of predicting pulmonary-capillary wedge pressure. N Engl J Med 1992; 327:1715–1720.

120. Siegman-Igra Y, Anglim AM, Shapiro D, et al. Diagnosis of vascular catheter-related bloodstream infection: a meta-analysis. J Clin Microbiol 1997; 35:928–936.

121. Blot F, Nitenberg G, Chachaty E, et al. Diagnosis of catheter-related bacteraemia: a prospective comparison of the time to positivity of hub-blood versus peripheral-blood cultures. Lancet 1999; 354:1071–1077.

122. Raad, Hanna HA, Alakech B, Chatzinikolaou I, Johnson MM, Tarrand J. Differential time to positivity: a useful method for diagnosing catheter-related bloodstream infections. Ann Intern Med 2004; 140:18–25.

123. Sattler FR, Foderaro JB, Aber RC. *Staphylococcus epidermidis* bacteremia associated with vascular catheters: an important cause of febrile morbidity in hospitalized patients. Infect Control 1984; 5:279–283.

124. Greene JF Jr, Cummings KC. Aseptic thrombotic endocardial vegetations. A complication of indwelling pulmonary artery catheters. JAMA 1973; 225:1525–1526.

125. Terpenning MS, Buggy BP, Kauffman CA. Hospital-acquired infective endocarditis. Arch Intern Med 1988; 148:1601–1603.

126. Raad II, Sabbagh MF. Optimal duration of therapy for catheter-related *Staphylococcus aureus* bacteremia: a study of 55 cases and review. Clin Infect Dis 1992; 14:75–82.

127. Shapiro SM, Young E, De Guzman S, et al. Transesophageal echocardiography. N Engl J Med 1995; 332:1268–1275.

128. Winslow T, Foster E, Adams JR, Schiller NB. Pulmonary valve endocarditis: improved diagnosis with biplane transesophageal echocardiography. J Am Soc Echocardiogr 1992; 5:206–210.

129. Heidenreich PA, Masoudi F, Maini B, et al. Echocardiography in patients with suspected endocarditis: a cost-effectiveness analysis. Am J Med 1999; 107:198–208.

130. Albertyn LE, Alcock MK. Diagnosis of internal jugular vein thrombosis. Radiology 1987; 162:505–508.
131. Mori H, Fukua T, Isomoto I, Maeda H, Hayashi K. CT diagnosis of catheter-induced septic thrombus of vena cava. J Comp Assist Tomogr 1990; 14:236–238.
132. Braun IF, Haffman JC, Malko JA, Petigrew RI, Danniels W, Davis PC. Jugular venous thrombosis: MR imaging. Radiology 1985; 157:357–360.
133. Baarslag HJ, van Beek EJR, Koopman MMW, Reekers JA. Prospective study of color duplex ultrasonography compared with contrast venography in patients suspected of having deep venous thrombosis of the upper extremities. Ann Intern Med 2002; 136:865–872.
134. Mylotte JM, McDermott C. *Staphylococcus aureus* bacteremia caused by infected intravenous catheters. Am J Infect Control 1987; 15:1–6.
135. Ehni WF, Reller LB. Short-course therapy for catheter-associated *Staphylococcus aureus* bacteremia. Arch Intern Med 1989; 149:533–536.
136. Chambers HF, Miller RT, Newman MD. Right-sided *Staphylococcus aureus* endocarditis in intravenous drug abusers: two-week combination therapy. Ann Intern Med 1988; 109:619–624.
137. Bowler I, Conlon C, Crook D, Peto KT. Optimum duration of therapy for catheter related *Staphylococcus aureus* bacteremia: a cohort study of 75 patients. Program and Abstracts of the Thirty-second Interscience Conference on Antimicrobial Agents and Chemotherapy, Anaheim, CA, October 1992; Washington, DC: American Society for Microbiology, 1992:833 [abstr].
138. Torres-Tortosa M, deCueto M, Vergara A, et al. Prospective evaluation of a two-week course of intravenous antibiotics in intravenous drug addicts with infective endocarditis. Eur J Clin Microbiol Infect Dis 1994; 7:559–564.
139. Malanoski GJ, Samore MH, Pefanis A, Karchmer AW. *Staphylococcus aureus* catheter-associated bacteremia. Minimal effective therapy and unusual infectious complications associated with arterial catheters. Arch Intern Med 1995; 155:1161–1166.
140. Rosen AB, Fowler VG, Corey Gr, et al. Ann Intern Med 1999; 130:810–820.
141. Jernigan JA, Farr BM. Short-course therapy of catheter-related *Staphylococcus aureus* bacteremia: a meta-analysis. Ann Intern Med 1993; 119:304–311.
142. Rose HD. Venous catheter-associated candidemia. Am J Med Sci 1978; 275:265–269.
143. Beutler SM, Young LS, Linquist LB, Montomerie JZ, Edwards JE Jr. Delayed complications of candidemia. Program and Abstracts of the Twenty-second Interscience Conference on Antimicrobial Agents and Chemotherapy, Miami, FL, October 1982; Washington, DC: American Society for Microbiology, 1982:496 [abstr].
144. Leccoines JA, Lee JW, Navarro EE, et al. Vascular catheter-associated fungemia in patients with cancer: analysis of 155 episodes. Clin Infect Dis 1992; 14:875–883.
145. Rex JH, Bennett JE, Sugar AM, et al. A randomized trial comparing fluconazole with amphotericin B for the treatment of candidemia in patients without neutropenia. N Engl J Med 1994; 331:1325–1330.
146. Rex JH, Walsh TJ, Sobel JD, et al. Practice guidelines for the treatment of Candidiasis. Clin Infect Dis 2000; 30:662–678.

147. Mora–Buarte J, Betts R, Rotstein C, Colombo AL, Thompson-Moya L, Smietana J, Lupinacci R, Sable C, Kartsonis N, Perfect J. Comparison of caspofungin and amphotericin B for invasive candidiasis. N Engl J Med 2002; 347:2020–2029.

148. Bayer AS, Scheld WM. Endocarditis and intravascular infections. In: Mandell GL, Douglas RG, Bennett JE, eds. Principles and Practices of Infectious Diseases. 5th ed. New York: Churchill Livingstone, 1995:857–917.

149. Strinden WD, Helgerson RB, Maki DG. *Candida* septic thrombosis of the great veins associated with central catheters. Clinical features and management. Ann Surg 1985; 202:653–658.

150. LaQuaglia MP, Caldwell C, Lucas A, et al. A prospective randomized double-blind trial of bolus urokinase in the treatment of established Hickman catheter sepsis in children. J Pediatr Surg 1994; 29:742–745.

151. Mermel LA. Prevention of intravascular catheter-related infections. Ann Intern Med 2000; 132:391–402.

152. Mermel LA. Correction: catheter-related bloodstream infections. Ann Intern Med 2000; 133:395.

153. O'Grady NP, Alexander M, Patchen Dellinger E, et al. Guidelines for the prevention of intravascular catheter-related infections. MMWR 2002; 51(RR-10):1–29.

154. Prager RL, Silva J. Colonization of central venous catheters. South Med J 1984; 77:458–461.

155. Brun-Buisson C, Abrouk F, Legrand P, Huet Y, Larabi S, Rapin M, Diagnosis of central venous catheter-related sepsis. Critical level of quantitative tip cultures. Arch Intern Med 1987; 147:873–877.

156. Collignon P, Soni N, Pearson I, et al. Sepsis associated with central vein catheters in critically ill patients. Intens Care Med 1988; 14:227–231.

157. Gil RT, Kruse JA, Thili-Baharozian MC, Carlson RW. Triple- vs. single-lumen central venous catheters. A prospective study in a critically ill population. Arch Intern Med 1989; 149:1139–1143.

158. Ruesch S, Walder B, Tramer MR. Complications of central venous catheters: internal jugular versus subclavian access—a systematic review. Crit Care Med 2002; 30:454–460.

159. Robinson JF, Robinson WA, Cohn A, Garg K, Armstrong JD. Perforation of the great vessels during central venous line placement. Arch Intern Med 1995; 155:1225–1228.

160. Centers for Disease Control. Recommendations for prevention of HIV transmission in health-care settings. MMWR 1987; 36:1S–18S.

161. Chaiyakunapruk N, Veenstra DL, Lipsky BA, Saint S. Chlorhexidine compared with povidone-iodine solution for vascular catheter-site care: a meta-analysis. Ann Intern Med 2002; 136:792–801.

162. McKee R, Dunsmuir R, Whitby M, Garden OJ. Does antibiotic prophylaxis at the time of catheter insertion reduce the incidence of catheter-related sepsis in intravenous nutrition? J Hosp Infect 1985; 6:419–425.

163. Laster J, Silver D. Heparin-coated catheters and heparin-induced thrombocytopenia. J Vasc Surg 1988; 7:667–672.

164. Moberg PQ, Geary VM, Sheikh FM. Heparin-induced thrombocytopenia: a

possible complication of heparin-coated pulmonary artery catheters. J Cardiothorac Anesth 1990; 4:226–228.

165. Salzman MB, Isenberg HD, Rubin LG. Use of disinfectants to reduce microbial contamination of hubs of vascular catheters. J Clin Microbiol 1993; 31:475–479.

166. Yonkman CA, Hamory BH. Comparison of three methods of maintaining a sterile injectate system during cardiac output determinations. Am J Infect Control 1984; 12:276–281.

167. Talbot GH, Skros M, Provencher M. 70% alcohol disinfection of transducer heads: experimental trials. Infect Control 1985; 6:237–239.

168. Platt R, Lehr JL, Marion S, et al. Safe and cost-effective cleaning of pressure-monitoring transducers. Infect Control Hosp Epidemiol 1988; 9:409–416.

169. Freeman R, Holden MP, Lyon R, Hjersing N. Addition of sodium metabisulphite to left atrial catheter infusates as a means of preventing bacterial colonisation of the catheter tip. Thorax 1982; 37:142–144.

170. Luskin RL, Weinstein RA, Natan C, Chamberlin WH, Kabsin SA. Extended use of disposable pressure transducers: a bacteriologic evaluation. JAMA 1986; 255:916–920.

171. O'Malley MK, Rhame FS, Cerra FB, McComb RC. Value of routine pressure monitoring system changes after 72 hours of continuous use. Crit Care Med 1994; 22:1424–1430.

172. Frezza EE, Mezghebe H. Indications and complications of arterial catheter use in surgical or medical intensive care units: analysis of 4932 patients. Am Surg 1998; 64:127.

173. Durie M, Beckmann U, Gillies D. Incidents relating to arterial cannulation as identified in 7525 reports submitted to the Australian incident monitoring study (AIMS-ICU). Anaesth Intensive Care 2002; 30:60–65.

174. Brown RB, Colodny SM, Drapkin MS, et al. One-day prevalence study of 118 intensive care units. Infect Control Hosp Epidemiol 1995; 16:438 [abstr].

175. Band JD, Maki DG. Infections caused by arterial catheters used for hemodynamic monitoring. Am J Med 1979; 67:735–741.

176. Maki DG, Hassemer CA. Endemic rate of fluid contamination and related septicemia in arterial pressure monitoring. Am J Med 1981; 70:733–738.

177. Shinozaki T, Deane RS, Mazuzan JE, et al. Bacterial contamination of arterial lines. JAMA 1983; 249:223–225.

178. Thomas F, Burke JP, Parker J, et al. The risk of infection related to radial vs femoral sites for arterial catheterization. Crit Care Med 1983; 11:807–812.

179. Russell JA, Joel M, Hudson RJ, Mangano DT, Schlobohm M. Prospective evaluation of radial and femoral artery catheterization sites in critically ill adults. Crit Care Med 1983; 11:936–939.

180. Thomas F, Orme JF, Clemmer TP, Burke JP, Elliott CG, Gardner RM. A prospective comparison of arterial catheter blood and catheter-tip cultures in critically ill patients. Crit Care Med 1984; 12:860–862.

181. Sommers M, Baas LS, Beiting AM. Nosocomial infections related to four methods of hemodynamic monitoring. Heart Lung 1987; 16:13–19.

182. Ducharme FM, Gauthier M, Lacroix J, Lafleur L. Incidence of infection

related to arterial catheterization in children: a prospective study. Crit Care Med 1988; 16:272–276.

183. Leroy O, Billiau V, Beuscart C, et al. Nosocomial infections associated with long-term radial artery cannulation. Intens Care Med 1989; 15:241–246.

184. Norwood SH, Cormier B, McMahon NG, Moss A, Moore V. Prospective study of catheter-related infection during prolonged arterial catheterization. Crit Care Med 1988; 16:836–839.

185. Maki DG, Ringer M. Prospective study of arterial catheter-related infection: incidence, sources of infection and risk factors. Program and Abstracts of the Twenty-ninth Interscience Conference on Antimicrobial Agents and Chemotherapy, Houston, TX, September 1989; Washington, DC: American Society for Microbiology, 1989:1075 [abstr].

186. Furfaro S, Gauthier M, Lacroix J, Nadeau D, Lafleur L, Mathews S. Arterial catheter-related infections in children: a 1-year cohort analysis. Am J Dis Child 1991; 145:1037–1043.

187. Mimoz O, Pieroni L, Lawrence C, et al. Prospective, randomized trial of two antiseptic solutions for prevention of central venous or arterial catheter colonization and infection in intensive care unit patients. Crit Care Med 1996; 24:1818–1823.

188. Raad I, Abi-Said D, Carrasco CH, Umphrey J, Hill LA. The risk of infection associated with intra-arterial catheters for cancer chemotherapy. Infect Control Hosp Epidemiol 1998; 19:640–642.

189. Rijnders BJA, Van Wijngaerden E, Wilmer A, Peetermans WE. Use of full sterile barrier precautions during insertion of arterial catheters: a randomized trial. Clin Infect Dis 2003; 36:743–748.

190. Safdar N, Maki DG. The incidence and pathogenesis of catheter-related bloodstream infection with arterial catheters [abstr]. Program and Abstracts of the Forty-second Interscience Conference on Antimicrobial Agents and Chemotherapy, San Diego, CA, September 2002; Washington, DC: American Society for Microbiology, 2002:299.

191. Swanson E, Freiberg A, Salter DR. Radial artery infections and aneurysms after catheterization. J Hand Surg 1990; 15A:166–171.

192. Maki DG, Ringer M, Alvarado CJ. Prospective randomized trial of povidone-iodine, alcohol, and chlorhexidine for prevention of infection associated with central venous and arterial catheters. Lancet 1991; 338:339–343.

193. Peruzzi WT, Noskin GA, Moen SG, et al. Microbial contamination of blood conservation devices during routine use in the critical care setting: Results of a prospective, randomized trial. Crit Care Med 1996; 24:1157–1162.

194. Beck-Sague CM, Jarvis WR. Epidemic bloodstream infections associated with pressure transducers: a persistent problem. Infect Control Hosp Epidemiol 1989; 10:54–59.

195. Leggiadro RJ, Luedtke GS, Anderson MS, Storgion SA, Bugnitz MC, Barrett FF. Persistent, unusual gram-negative bacteremia associated with arterial pressure monitoring in a pediatric intensive care unit. Infect Control Hosp Epidemiol 1992; 13:556–558.

196. Passerini L, Lam K, Costerton W, King EG. Biofilms on indwelling vascular catheters. Crit Care Med 1992; 20:665–673.

197. Sheth NK, Franson TR, Rose HD, Buckmire FLA, Cooper JA, Sohne PG.

Colonization of bacteria on polyvinyl chloride and Teflon intravascular catheters in hospitalized patients. J Clin Microbiol 1983; 18:1061–1063.

198. Vaudaux P, Pittet D, Haeberli A, et al. Fibronectin is more active than fibrin or fibrinogen in promoting *Staphylococcus aureus* adherence to inserted intravascular catheters. J Infect Dis 1993; 167:633–641.

199. Falk PS, Scuderi PE, Sheretz RJ, Motsinger SM. Infected radial artery pseudoaneurysms occurring after percutaneous cannulation. Chest 1992; 101:490–495.

200. Fanning WL, Aronson M. Osler node, janeway lesions and splinter hemorrhages. Arch Dermatol 1977; 113:648–649.

201. Cohen A, Reyes R, Kirk M, Fulks RM. Osler's nodes, pseudoaneurysm formation, and sepsis complicating percutaneous radial artery cannulation. Crit Care Med 1984; 12:1078–1079.

202. Arnow PM, Costas CO. Delayed rupture of the radial artery caused by catheter-related sepsis. Rev Infect Dis 1988; 10:1035–1037.

203. Soderstrom CA, Wasserman DH, Ransom KJ, Caplan ES, Cowley RA. Infected false femoral artery aneurysms secondary to monitoring catheters. J Cardiovasc Surg 1983; 24:63–68.

204. Maki DG, McCormick RD, Wirtnen GW. Septic endarteritis due to intraarterial catheters for cancer chemotherapy. I. Clinical features. II. Risk factors. III. Guidelines for prevention. Cancer 1979; 44:1228–1240.

205. Kulkarni H, Elsner C, Ouellet D, Zeldin R. Heparinized saline versus normal salinein maintaining patency of the radial arterial catheter. Can J Surg 1994; 37:37–42.

206. Epperson EL. Efficacy of 0.9% sodium chloride injection with and without heparin for maintaining indwelling intermittent injection sites. Clin Pharm 1984; 3:626–629.

207. Narendran V, Gupta G, Todd DA, John E. Bacterial colonization of indwelling vascular catheters in newborn infants. J Paediatr Chil Health 1996; 32:391–396.

14

Long-Term Central Venous Catheters

Issam Raad and Hend A. Hanna

*Department of Infectious Diseases, M. D. Anderson Cancer Center
Houston, Texas, U.S.A.*

INTRODUCTION

Evaluation of Central Venous Catheters

Long-term venous access devices have revolutionized the medical care of chronically ill patients. Clinicians who treated such patients 30 or 40 years ago can particularly appreciate the impact of these devices. With the use of small peripheral venous catheters, the treatment of cancer patients was once complicated by extravasation of toxic agents and thrombosis of peripheral veins, which often limited intravenous chemotherapy. The introduction of long-term silicone venous devices allowed the safe administration of chemo-therapy drugs, blood products, total parenteral nutrition (TPN), fluids, antibiotics, and other substances over an extended period of time. There is no doubt that such devices helped decrease morbidity and mortality and minimized human suffering.

Types of Central Venous Catheters

Four general types of long-term central venous catheters are available (Fig. 1): tunneled catheters, nontunneled catheters, implantable ports, and peripher-ally inserted central catheters (PICCs).

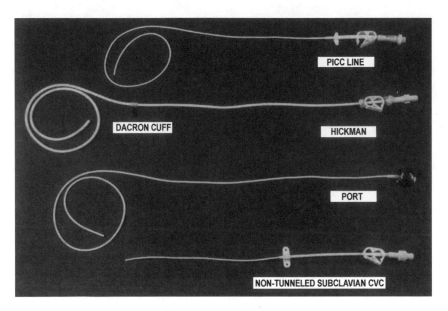

Figure 1 Four types of long-term silicone catheters: PICC line, Hickman (with Dacron cuff), port, and nontunneled subclavian central venous catheters.

Tunneled Catheters

The first tunneled catheter was developed by Broviac in the early 1970s for patients who required long-term TPN (1). Subsequently, Hickman developed another long-term tunneled catheter for patients undergoing bone marrow transplantation (2). In contrast with the thick-walled Hickman and Broviac catheters, Groshong developed a thin-walled catheter characterized by a two-slit valve adjacent to a rounded, closed end that remains closed unless fluids are being infused or blood is being withdrawn. This eliminates the need to clamp the catheter and decreases the risk of intraluminal blood clotting or infusion of air when the catheter is not in use. Tunneled catheters usually exit the body midway between the nipple and the sternum and are tunneled for several inches to the cannulated vein. All tunneled catheters have a Dacron cuff that is located in the proximal subcutaneous segment 5 cm from the exit site. The Dacron cuff becomes enmeshed with fibrous tissue, anchoring the catheter and creating a tissue interface barrier against the migration of skin organisms. Tunneled catheters are available in single-, double-, or triple-lumen cannulae.

Nontunneled Catheters

Nontunneled subclavian silicone catheters have the smallest lumen and external diameter. They can be maintained for extended periods up to

400 days (3). They can be inserted percutaneously in the subclavian vein in outpatient nonsurgical settings. If a nontunneled catheter becomes displaced or a catheter-related infection (CRI) occurs, it can be exchanged over a guide wire.

Implantable Ports

An implantable port consists of a metal or plastic port inserted completely beneath the skin and connected to a catheter tube (4). Ports are usually placed in a subcutaneous pocket of the upper chest wall (central subclavian ports) or in the antecubital area of the arm (peripheral ports). Ports are available as single- or double-lumen catheters with or without the Groshong valve.

Peripherally Inserted Central Catheters

During the last decade, the use of PICCs has gained acceptance as a method for long-term venous access. A PICC is a type of catheter that is inserted peripherally at or above the antecubital space in the cephalic vein, the basilic vein, the medial cephalic vein, or the medial basilic vein and advanced into the central venous system. This catheter is usually inserted percutaneously in an outpatient nonsurgical setting by a trained infusion therapy nurse. It has been shown at our center that these catheters are safe and have a mean duration of placement of 117 days. The PICCs are associated with a low infection rate and low cost (3). Generally, the catheters are composed of silicone elastomers or polyurethane material and may or may not have a Groshong valve. Placement of a PICC requires only local anesthesia and minimal surgery.

EPIDEMIOLOGY OF INFECTIOUS COMPLICATIONS

Uncomplicated, long-term intravenous access contributes significantly to the comfort of patients with a variety of conditions, such as hematologic malignancies, solid tumors, sickle cell anemia, aplastic anemia, endocarditis, burns, Crohn's disease, osteomyelitis, and other cases in which a large vessel is required for safe infusion. Infection remains a significant cause of morbidity for patients with long-term central venous catheters (CVCs). Catheter-related infections can be classified as exit-site infections, tunnel tract infections, port pocket infections, and catheter-related bacteremia or fungemia. Catheter-related bloodstream infections (CRBSIs) and exit-site infections are common to all types of catheters; however, port pocket infections and tunnel infections are specific to implantable devices and tunneled catheters, respectively. Phlebitis is more common with PICCs.

It is difficult to interpret and compare reports of CRIs because of differences in populations, catheter use, length of catheterization, and methods of diagnosing true CRI. Several factors have been reported to correlate with the incidence of infection: type of fluid infused, therapy with interleukin-2, the patient's neutrophil count, and occurrence of catheter thrombosis.

In one study, patients with tunneled catheters that had been placed primarily for TPN experienced a higher rate of infection (22.9%) than patients whose catheters were placed for antibiotic management of infection (12.7%) or patients who received chemotherapy only (4.9%) (5). Patients receiving biologic modifiers such as interleukin-2 have also been shown to have a higher risk for catheter infection caused by staphylococcal organisms (6–8).

In a study conducted by Howell and colleagues of patients with long-term indwelling tunneled CVCs who were followed for a total of 12,410 catheter-days, neutropenia of < 500 neutrophils per mm^3 of blood was the only independent risk factor for catheter-related infection ($P = 0.018$) (9). Catheter infections were significantly more likely to occur during the first week of neutropenia than during the remaining neutropenic days. However, in a study conducted at our center (3), neither neutropenia, bone marrow transplantation, use of high-dose steroids, nor infusion of vesicant chemotherapy agents through the CVC predisposed patients to catheter infection. The only statistically significant risk factor for catheter infection was hematologic malignancy (acute lymphocytic leukemia or acute myelocytic leukemia).

The same was observed by Groeger and colleagues (10) in a study of patients with leukemia who had shorter infection-free periods compared with patients with lymphomas or myeloma ($P = 0.02$), but neutropenia was not evaluated as a risk factor except at the time of catheter insertion. In addition, patients with solid tumors had longer infection-free periods than those who had hematologic diseases ($P = 0.005$) (10). Independent of neutropenia, patients with hematologic malignancies may be at a higher risk of infection because of excessive manipulation of catheters resulting from the high frequency of blood transfusions and blood withdrawals done through the catheter. In a multivariate logistic regression analysis of various risk factors (including neutropenia), blood product transfusions were found to be the only risk factor associated with CRBSI (11).

A recent postmortem study on long-term CVC use conducted at our center demonstrated that 38% of catheterized veins had evidence of mural thrombosis and that vascular mural thrombosis of the catheterized veins was significantly associated with catheter-related septicemia (12). This relationship was independent of other host or catheter variables such as underlying disease, thrombocytopenia, and site and duration of catheterization. It was previously demonstrated at the subclinical microscopic level that the fibrin sheath, which engulfs most indwelling catheters, promotes the adherence of staphylococci and *Candida* spp. Our postmortem study offers evidence that the pathology of mural thrombosis of catheterized veins is associated with clinical catheter-related sepsis. Two other studies evaluating a related question failed to document an association between clotting in the vicinity of the catheter and risk of infection (9,10).

PATHOGENESIS AND MICROBIOLOGY
OF CATHETER-RELATED INFECTION

Adherence Factors

In prospective studies, the most common organisms causing catheter infection have been coagulase-negative staphylococci, *Staphylococcus aureus*, and yeasts. Extensive reviews of cases of long-term CVC sepsis implicated coagulase-negative staphylococci in more than 50% of the infections. Adherence of the bacteria to the catheter surface depends on the interaction of the host, the microbial factors, and the catheter material (13–15).

First, the host considers the catheter a foreign body and reacts by forming a thrombin sleeve around it (16,17). This thrombin layer is rich in fibrin and fibronectin (substances that *S. aureus*, and *Candida* adhere to tightly). Both *S. aureus* and *Candida albicans* are coagulase-producing organisms that benefit from the process of thrombogenesis by adhering tightly to the fibrin-rich layer of the biofilm (18,19). Coagulase-negative staphylococci adhere to fibronectin but not to fibrin (19).

Second, the microbial factors include the production of exopolysaccharides. Microbial organisms, particularly slime-producing coagulase-negative staphylococci, *S. aureus*, and *Candida parapsilosis*, enhance adherence by producing a polysaccharide adhesin, also known as extracellular slime, that constitutes the microbial substance of the biofilm (20–23). The biofilm layer, which is made of microbial and host substances, is conducive not only to the continued adherence of the organisms, but also to their maintenance, because it acts as a barrier that protects embedded organisms from antibiotics, phagocytic neutrophils, macrophages, and antibodies (24–27).

The third factor that plays a role in the adherence process is the catheter material. Several investigators have shown, for example, that *S. aureus* and *Candida* spp. adhere better to polyvinyl chloride catheters than to Teflon catheters (28). Staphylococci preferentially adhere to silicone (29). Several prospective studies in which quantitative catheter cultures were used have shown that the most common organisms causing CRIs are coagulase-negative staphylococci, *S. aureus*, and *Candida* spp. (30–37). *C. albicans* and *C. parapsilosis* account for most of the *Candida* spp. causing CRIs.

Bacterial Colonization

The source of catheter colonization remains a controversial issue. For short-term polyurethane catheters, Maki (38) showed that the skin is the most common source for catheter colonization and catheter-related bacteremia. Sitges-Serra et al. (39–41) have emphasized the hub as the most common source of catheter-related septicemia. To assess the degree of luminal and extraluminal colonization of long-term CVCs, we prospectively studied 359 indwelling silicone CVCs from a cohort of 340 cancer patients. All CVCs were cultured by the roll-plate and sonication quantitative culture techniques. Semiquantitative electron microscopy was done on all CVCs associated with catheter infection and on matched culture-negative controls. External surface colonization, most likely originating from the skin, was predominant in the first 10 days of the catheter placement; luminal colonization, probably originating from the hub, became predominant after 30 days of catheter placement. Luminal colonization increased progressively with duration of catheterization in both premortem and postmortem catheters, supporting the notion that prolonged excessive use of long-term catheters would lead to contaminated hubs and in turn to increased luminal colonization (42). Hence, the hub rather than the insertion site is the major source of long-term catheter colonization.

Port pocket infection, usually caused by Gram-positive cocci, often follows direct inoculation or migration of organisms along the accessing needle into the septum of the port bell. Whereas coagulase-negative staphylococci and *S. aureus* are introduced through the skin and contaminated hubs (38–41), many of the *Candida* infections are thought to seed hematogenously from the gastrointestinal tract and adhere to the fibrin and fibronectin on the surface of the catheter (43). Infusion-related sepsis caused by contaminated infusate is often caused by Gram-negative bacilli such as *Enterobacter*, *Pseudomonas*, *Citrobacter*, and *Serratia* species (13).

COMPARISON OF CATHETERS

Infection Rates

No prospective randomized study in the literature has compared the complications related to the different types of catheters including nontunneled subclavian catheters. The available studies published to date are controversial. Reporting catheter infections according to the percentage of catheters that become infected without considering the duration of catheter use is inappropriate. Many institutions report catheter infection rates as the number of infection episodes per 100 or 1000 patient-days of catheter use. Based on this concept, the incidence of catheter-related infection with both tunneled and nontunneled long-term silicone catheters ranges from 1.0 to 1.9 episodes per 1000 catheter-days. In 13 studies reviewed by Clarke and Raffin (44), 17 studies reviewed by Press et al. (45), and 21 studies reviewed by Decker and Edwards (46), the incidence of long-term CVC infection was found to be in the range of 1.4 per 1000 catheter-days. The review by Howell et al. included 26 studies of 3948 catheters in 3478 adult cancer patients and reported a CVC infection rate of 1.9 per 1000 catheter-days (9).

The study of 108 catheters conducted by Pasqual et al. (47) comparing Groshong and Hickman catheters indicated that there was no significant difference in septic complications resulting from the use of these devices.

Keung et al. (48) conducted a retrospective comparative study of infectious complications associated with 111 long-term CVCs of different types. Using the log rank test and Cox's multivariate analysis, they also found no significant difference in catheter-related infections between Hickman and Groshong catheters or between subcutaneous ports and tunneled catheters. Likewise, Mueller et al. (49), in a prospective randomized trial comparing complications in external tunneled catheters and subcutaneous ports in 100 children and adults, found no significant difference in the incidence of infection between the two types of devices.

Conversely, Gleeson et al. (50) conducted a study on 104 catheters and found that catheter sepsis occurred with 32% of Groshong catheters versus 16.2% of Hickman ports (P = 0.04). Carde and colleagues reported a trial of 100 patients with solid tumors who were randomly assigned to implanted ports or tunneled catheter treatment; the rates of infection were 2% and 11%, respectively (51).

Because of the differences among published studies regarding the rates of infection with different types of catheters, Sariego and colleagues (52) retrospectively reviewed a total of 1422 catheters including 730 single-lumen Hickman catheters, 368 double-lumen Hickman catheters, and 307 single-lumen ports. Overall, 60 catheters were removed, replaced, or both prior to completion of the intended therapy (4%). Reasons for removal were infection in 1% of cases and catheter malfunction in 3%. The percentage of ports removed was significantly greater than the percentage of Hickman catheters removed (P < 0.001). Another study conducted by Mirro and colleagues (53) involving 120 Hickman catheters, 146 Broviac catheters, and 93 implantable ports in children with malignancy showed that, when all causes of catheter failure were considered, such as infection, obstruction, or dislodgment, indwelling ports had a significantly longer duration of use than percutaneous Hickman or Broviac catheters (P = 0.0009). In a prospective observational study conducted on 1630 long-term venous catheters (923 percutaneous catheters and 707 ports), Groeger and colleagues found that the incidence of infection per device per day was 12 times greater with externalized tunneled catheters than with ports (10).

The number of lumens was thought to play a role in catheter-related infections, but in several studies the differences in rates were not statistically significant. One study conducted by Early et al. (54) showed that infection rate was significantly less in the single-lumen catheter than in the double-lumen catheter (one infection per 1210 days versus one infection per 496 days, respectively; P ≤ 0.02); however, this study was retrospective and therefore possibly subject to various types of biases.

We are not aware of a single prospective randomized study where the risk factors for catheter infection (such as underlying diseases, neutropenia, thrombosis, duration of placement, and the various uses of the catheter) were matched among the patients undergoing such comparative evaluation. In the absence of such a study, comparisons are subject to selection bias in this very complicated patient population. However, after reviewing the current literature, one may conclude that ports may be associated with the lowest infection rates. In a large prospective study that included 20,041 nontunneled long-term CVCs, 882 tunneled CVCs, and 2148 ports, the implantable ports were associated with the lowest rate of CRBSI (55).

Durability, Lifestyle, and Cost

Use of the tunneled catheter was thought to be a means of preventing migration of microorganisms from skin along the intercutaneous surface of the catheter. However, analysis of data from The University of Texas M. D. Anderson Cancer Center (3,55) in comparison with published data on tunneled catheters revealed that tunneled cuffed catheters had no distinct advantage over percutaneous nontunneled subclavian silicone catheters. One advantage of percutaneous nontunneled subclavian silicone catheters, such as the Hohn catheters (Davol, Inc., Bard Access System, Salt Lake City, UT), is that they can be inserted in an outpatient setting. These devices can also be removed easily if a catheter-related complication occurs, and they are associated with long durability (mean duration of placement is 149 days), low infection rate (0.073 bloodstream infections per 1000 catheter-days), and significant cost savings when compared to surgically implantable catheters (ports, Hickman, and Broviac) (Table 1) (55). However, percutaneous non-

Table 1 Estimated Insertion Cost (to the Patient) of Catheters at M. D. Anderson Cancer Center

Cost items	Nontunneled		Hickman tunneled CVC	Port
	PICC	Subclavian		
Physician	$116[a]	$374	$953	$953
Clinic	90	90	90	90
Catheter	65	88	95	730
Supplies	149	94	799	799
X-ray	115	115	96	96
Fluoroscopic imaging	—	—	81	81
Coagulation study	47	47	47	47
Anesthesia	—	—	274	274
Operating room	—	—	635	635
Recovery room	—	—	236	236
Hospital room	—	—	—	375
Total	$582	$808	$3,306	$4,316

[a] PICCs are inserted by nurses. The $116 is the nurse's insertion fee.

tunneled subclavian silicone catheters require daily heparin injection and weekly dressing changes, which are disadvantages.

There are several disadvantages to using tunneled catheters. The procedures involved in inserting and removing these devices are more invasive and more costly than some other catheter placement procedures. Daily heparin injections are also required, except for Groshong tunneled CVCs. Because they are external catheters, the patients' body image can be affected, and this serves as a constant reminder of their disease. The daily-to-weekly site care, cost of maintenance (including dressing materials, dressings cost, frequency of flushing, and cap changing), and surgery to insert the device (which necessitates postoperative care for 7 to 10 days) are other disadvantages of tunneled catheter use. However, one advantage of tunneled catheters is that breaks or tears in the device can be repaired easily (56). They can be easily maintained in a home setting and can be removed in an outpatient or inpatient setting (57).

Implantable ports carry less risk of infection and less interference with the patient's body image and lifestyle. In large prospective studies that included ports and other long-term CVCs, the implantable ports were associated with a significantly lower rate of CRBSI when compared with PICCs and tunneled and nontunneled CVCs (55,58). Maintenance is minimal, and there is no visible reminder of the patient's illness. The presence of this device is revealed by only a small bump under the skin, allowing the patient freedom of activity. Implantable ports are preferred in children and patients with active lifestyles, especially those who enjoy water sports. However, disadvantages to the use of implantable catheters are their high cost, the 7- to 10-day postoperative care period after insertion, and the objection of some patients to the needlestick required to access the port. Removal of the port also requires a minor surgical procedure.

The PICCs offer inexpensive outpatient placement that does not require surgery and can usually be performed by a specialized nurse. They are easily removed in an outpatient setting. Their major disadvantages are that daily care is required and that they do affect the patient's body image and activity. Because the catheter is not tunneled and may not be sutured, an occlusive dressing over the exit site is required at all times. In addition, because of their small lumen size, some PICCs are not recommended for blood withdrawal because they tend to collapse when aspirated (59).

The PICC is gaining acceptance as a long-term venous access device (60–65). A review of the literature indicates some detailed description of the complications resulting from the use of this type of catheter. Phlebitis associated with PICCs is reported in 3.8% to 18% of cases (60–62). This phlebitis is mostly aseptic and has been reported to resolve within 24 to 48 hours without the need to remove the catheter (63). Sepsis associated with this type of catheter is low. In a prospective follow-up of 351 PICCs that were inserted for a total of 10,562 catheter-days, 32.8% were removed due to a complication (65). These complications included infection (7.4%, 2.46/1000 catheter-days), phlebitis (6.6%), vein thrombosis (3.4%), PICC occlusion (4%), and mechanical problems (6%). In another prospective observational study of 14,530 PICCs at our institution, we demonstrated that such catheters have a mean duration of placement of 117 days with a CRBSI rate of 0.065/1000 catheter-days (58). This low infection rate was comparable to that of the tunneled and nontunneled subclavian CVCs.

In conclusion, given the high cost of surgically inserted catheters (ports and tunneled devices) and the long durability of nontunneled percutaneous catheters (such as nontunneled subclavian catheters and PICCs), the primary physician should consider the percutaneous nontunneled silicone catheter as the first option when long-term venous access is required in the chronically ill patient. Ports should be considered in children and in patients who have an active life style or are concerned about cosmetic appearance. The role of the externalized tunneled catheter (Hickman or Broviac) devices should be critically reevaluated, given the high cost of their insertion and the lack of significant advantages (infection-free durability) over the PICCs and non-tunneled silicone subclavian catheters.

PREVENTIVE STRATEGIES

Tunneling and Ports

The surgically implantable CVCs represent one of the earliest attempts to prevent the migration of skin organisms along the intercutaneous segment of the catheter. Indeed, the Dacron cuff incorporated into the subcutaneous segment of the tunneled Hickman and Broviac devices does create a tissue interface mechanical barrier against the migration of skin organisms (1,2). The completely implanted subcutaneous ports were developed in the 1980s with the same intention of avoiding the migration of organisms from the skin along the intercutaneous pathway into the bloodstream (4). However, although the bloodstream infection rate of surgically implantable intravascular devices is low, these devices continue to be associated with serious bacteremia and fungemia episodes as well as with tunnel or port site infections (10,66). Given the high cost of inserting and removing such devices, which is in the range of $3000 to $4000 per device, one has to ask the question (3), "Could the same end point of a long durability and low infection rate be achieved by using safe nontunneled silicone catheters?"

Two prospective randomized studies evaluated the effect of catheter tunneling on catheter-related infections (67,68). One study evaluated long-term CVCs (mostly silicone catheters) placed in immunocompromised patients. The risks of catheter-related bacteremia associated with tunneled and nontunneled CVCs were 2% and 5%, respectively. The difference was not significant, most likely due to the relatively small number of patients in each group (107 and 105 patients, respectively). In another study involving short-term polyurethane catheters placed in the internal jugular vein of critically ill patients, tunneled CVCs were associated with a significantly lower rate of catheter-related bacteremia than nontunneled CVCS. Therefore, tunneling of CVCs may decrease the risk of catheter-related bacteremia in the use of short-term polyurethane CVCs. But is the additional cost of tunneling justified in the use of long-term silicone CVCs? Two large prospective observational studies that evaluated long-term silicone CVCs in cancer patients showed that the CRBSI rate associated with a tunneled CVC is comparable to that associated with nontunneled subclavian CVCs and PICCs (55,58).

Maximal Sterile Barriers

At M. D. Anderson Cancer Center, we showed that nontunneled silicone CVCs inserted in the subclavian vein could be maintained for a long period of time (mean duration of stay of 100 days) with a very low infection rate (1.3 per 1000 catheter-days). This is particularly true if these catheters are cared for by a specialized infusion therapy team and are inserted under maximal sterile barrier precautions. We conducted a randomized prospective controlled trial comparing maximal sterile barrier precautions (which involved wearing sterile gloves, a mask, a gown, and a cap and using a large drape) during the insertion of a nontunneled subclavian silicone CVC versus less rigorous procedures (which involved wearing only gloves and using a small drape) as the control (69). The catheter-related sepsis rate was 6.3 times higher in the control group compared to the maximal sterile barrier group ($P = 0.03$). Most (67%) of the catheter-related infections in the control group occurred during the first week postinsertion, whereas all of the infections in the sterile barrier group occurred more than two months following insertion ($P = <0.01$). Cost-benefit analysis of these data showed the use of such precautions as highly cost-effective. Such data are compelling in favor of using maximal sterile barriers during the insertion of nontunneled silicone catheters, particularly in an outpatient nonsurgical setting. What was remarkable about that study, however, was that the catheter-related septicemia rate in the control arm was 0.5 per 1000 catheter-days whereas in the maximal sterile barrier arm the catheter-related septicemia rate was reduced to 0.08 per 1000 catheter-days. The mean duration of stay was 67 to 70 days, and these long-term catheters were followed up to 100 days. Hence, one can conclude that nontunneled silicone catheters (inserted in the subclavian vein or as PICC lines) are associated with a very low infection rate if inserted in an aseptic manner and cared for meticulously (3,55,58,69).

Flushing With Antimicrobials

Because the catheter hub and the catheter lumen could be major sources of colonization, prevention of catheter infection has been attempted through the use of antimicrobial or anticoagulant flush solutions. In several studies, a solution consisting of heparin/vancomycin was used to flush tunneled CVCs and its efficacy was compared to that of heparin alone (70–73). Another prospective randomized study in pediatric patients failed to show any benefit from heparin–vancomycin lock solution over heparin alone in preventing CRBSI (74). Irrespective of its efficacy, there are at least three factors that can potentially limit the use of heparin/vancomycin catheter flush solutions: (a) the incompatibility of heparin and vancomcin (b) the limitation of the activity of vancomycin against Gram-positive bacteria that might lead to superinfection with Gram-negative bacilli and *Candida* spp., and (c) the concern over the development of vancomycin-resistant Gram-positive cocci, given the fact that vancomycin is the drug of choice for the treatment of established infections caused by methicillin-resistant staphylococci and penicillin-resistant enterococci. This concern is particularly heightened during this era of emerging vancomycin-resistant entercocci.

Recently, a flush solution consisting of a new combination of low concentration minocycline and EDTA was developed (75). The latter compound has been shown to have an anticoagulant activity equal to or even stronger than heparin, and this anticoagulant activity is not diminished by the addition of minocycline. Hence, there is no incompatibility between EDTA and minocycline. In contrast, this combination was found to have a broad-spectrum and often synergistic activity against methicillin-resistant staphylococci, Gram-negative bacilli (such as *Escherichia aerogenes* and *Stenotrophomonas maltophilia*), and *C. albicans*. In addition, neither minocycline nor EDTA is used in the treatment of bloodstream infections; hence, the risk of the emergence of organisms resistant to this microbiocidal combination is low and should not result in a therapeutic dilemma. In a rabbit model of vascular catheter-related infection, this combination was found to be highly efficacious in preventing *Staphylococcus epidermidis* bacteremia, catheter-related septic phlebitis, and right-sided endocarditis when compared with heparin (76). This flush solution was also found to prevent the recurrence of catheter and implantable port infections in adult and pediatric cancer patients (75,77).

Antimicrobial Coating of Catheters

In the 1990s, significant progress was made in demonstrating that short-term polyurethane catheters could be coated with various antiseptics and antimicrobial agents, resulting in a significant decrease in catheter-related bacteremia. Kamal and colleagues demonstrated the protective efficacy of bonding short-term CVCs with cefazolin using a cationic bonding surfactant, tridodecyl methylammonium chloride (78). Maki and colleagues coated short-term polyurethane CVCs with silver sulfadiazine/chlorhexidine and demonstrated that such catheters were twofold less likely to become colonized and were at least fourfold less likely to produce bacteremia (79). We coated short-term polyurethane triple-lumen catheters with a combination of minocycline and rifampin and demonstrated that such catheters have broad-spectrum in vitro inhibitory activity against Gram-positive bacteria, Gram-negative bacteria, and *C. albicans* (80). These catheters were also found to be highly efficacious in preventing colonization in a rabbit model and in a multi-center prospective randomized clinical trial (80,81).

In a prospective randomized multicenter clinical trial, short-term polyurethane CVCs impregnated with minocycline and rifampin were 12 times less likely to be associated with CRBSIs and three times less likely to be colonized compared to a first-generation short-term polyurethane CVCs impregnated only externally with chlorhexidine/silver sulfadiazine (82). The catheters impregnated with minocycline and rifampin had the advantage of being coated both on the external surface as well as in the lumen, and the antimicrobial durability of the minocycline/rifampin catheters extended to more than four weeks. The first-generation antiseptic CVCs impregnated with chlorhexidine/silver sulfadiazine only on the external surface did not reduce the risk of CRBSIs in leukemia and lymphoma patients who required catheterization for a mean duration of 20 days. This was attributed to the fact that these first-generation chlorhexidine/silver sulfadiazine antiseptic catheters did not provide any "protection" for the lumen of the CVC (which is of special importance in the pathogenesis of long-term CRBSIs) and had a limited antimicrobial durability of less than two weeks. A second-generation polyurethane CVC impregnated with chlorhexidine and silver sulfadiazine on the external and internal surfaces was shown to retain antimicrobial activity longer than the first generation and may be associated with a better outcome in patients requiring long-term catheterization (83).

Given the luminal protection and the prolonged antimicrobial durabil-ity of CVCs impregnated with minocycline and rifampin, these CVCs were used in the pre-engraftment phase of bone marrow transplant patients and were shown to decrease the risk of staphylococcal bloodstream infections by more than fourfold. However, concerns have been raised through in vitro studies as to the potential development of antibiotic resistance, particularly to rifampin, associated with prolonged use of such antimicrobial catheters. After long-term use of such antimicrobial catheters coated with minocycline and rifampin over a period of 21,888 catheter-days in bone marrow transplant patients between 1997 and 2001, staphylococcal organisms cultured from the blood and catheter tip of bone marrow transplant patients remained highly susceptible, with a MIC_{90} of less than 0.006 µg/mL to both minocycline and rifampin (84). In fact, the breakthrough staphylococcal organisms cultured from the bloodstream and catheter tips of bone marrow transplant patients, after four years of using the antimicrobial catheters impregnated with minocycline and rifampin, were more susceptible to minocycline and rifampin compared to baseline staphylococcal organisms cultured from CRBSIs at the same center prior to the usage of the antimicrobial catheters or to staphylo-coccal organisms cultured from leukemia patients where no antimicrobial catheters were used during the same time period (between 1997 and 2001). Subsequently, a prospective randomized study compared long-term silicone CVCs (nontunneled subclavian silicone catheters and PICCs) impregnated with minocycline/rifampin to uncoated control catheters used in cancer patients. Patients were followed until the catheters were removed or up to three months following insertion. The minocycline/rifampin long-term sili-cone catheters were 13-fold less likely to be associated with CRBSIs than were uncoated catheters (85). Recently, the Centers for Disease Control and Prevention published guidelines on the prevention of intravascular catheter-related infections (86). The use of "an antimicrobial- or antiseptic-impregnated central venous catheter in adults whose catheter is expected to remain in place for more than five days" was strongly recommended (Category 1B) "if, after implementing a comprehensive strategy to reduce rates of catheter-related bloodstream infection, the rate remains above the goal set by the institution based upon benchmark rates and local factors." The comprehensive strategy should include the following three components: educating persons who insert and maintain the catheter's use, use of maxi-mum sterile barrier precautions, and a 2% chlorhexidine skin antiseptic during and every few days after CVC insertion (86). Antimicrobial and antiseptic silicone catheters, which are coated externally and internally and which are associated with a long antimicrobial durability extending beyond four weeks, could play a role in the prevention of infections associated with long-term silicone CVCs used in chronically ill patients.

REFERENCES

1. Broviac JW, Cole JJ, Scribner GH. A silicone rubber atrial catheter for pro-longed parenteral alimentation. Surg Gynecol Obstet 1973; 136–602.
2. Hickman RO, Buckner CD, Clift RA, Sanders JE, Stewart P, Thomas ED. A modified right atrial catheter for access to the venous system in marrow transplant recipients. Surg Gynecol Obstet 1979 *Jun.*; 148(6):871–875.
3. Raad I, Davis S, Becker M, Hohn D, Houston D, Umphrey J, Bodey GP. Low infection rate and long durability of nontunneled silastic catheters: a safe and cost-effective alternative for long-term venous access. Arch Intern Med 1993 *Aug 9*; 153(15):1791–1796.
4. Goodman MS, Wickman R. Venous access devices: an overview. Oncol Nurs Forum 1984; 11:16–23.
5. Fuchs PC, Gustafson ME, King JT, Goodall PT. Assessment of catheter-associated infection risk with the Hickman right atrial catheter. Infect Control 1984 *May*; 5(5):226–230.
6. Syndman DR, Sullivan B, Gill M, Gould JA, Parkinson DR, Atkins DB. Nosocomial sepsis with interleukin-2. Ann Intern Med 1990; 112:102–107.
7. Bock SN, Lee RE, Fisher B, Rubin JT, Schwartzentruber DJ, Wei JP, Callender

DP, Yang JC, Lotze MT, Pizzo PA, et al. A prospective randomized trial evaluating prophylactic antibiotics to prevent triple lumen catheter-related sepsis in patients treated with immunotherapy. J Clin Oncol 1990 *Jan.*; 8(1): 161–169.

8. Murphy PM, Lane HC, Gollin JI, Fauci AS. Marked disparity in incidence of receiving interleukin-2 or interferon-gamma. Ann Intern Med 1988; 108:36–41.

9. Howell PB, Walters PE, Donowitz GR, Farr BM. Risk factors for infection of adult patients with cancer who have tunneled central venous catheters. Cancer 1995; 75(6):1367–1374.

10. Groeger JS, Lucas AB, Thaler HT, Friedlander-Klar H, Brown AE, Kiehn TE, Armstrong D. Infectious morbidity associated with long-term use of venous access devices in patients with cancer. Ann Intern Med 1993 *Dec 15.*; 119(12): 1168–1174.

11. Hanna HA, Raad I. Blood products: a significant risk factor for long-term catheter-related bloodstream infections in cancer patients. Infect Control Hosp Epidemiol 2001; 22:165–166.

12. Raad II, Luna M, Khalil S-AM, Costerton JW, Lam C, Bodey GP. The relationship between the thrombotic and infectious complications of central venous catheters. JAMA 1994; 271(13):1014–1016.

13. Hampton AA, Sherertz RJ. Vascular-access infections in hospitalized patients. Surg Clin North Am 1988; 68:57–71.

14. Elliott TSJ. Intravascular-device infections. J Med Microbiol 1988; 27:161–167.

15. Maki DG. Risk factors for nosocomial infection in intensive care: 'devices vs nature' and goals for the next decade. Arch Intern Med 1989; 149:30–35.

16. Brismar R, Hardstedt C, Jacobson S. Diagnosis of thrombosis by catheter phlebography after prolonged central venous catheterization. Ann Surg 1981; 194:779–783.

17. Ahmed N, Payne RF. Thrombosis after central venous cannulation. Med J Aust 1976; 1:217.

18. Herrmann M, Vaudaux PE, Pittet D, Auckenthaler R, Lew PD, Schumacher-Perdreau F, Peters G, Waldvogel FA. Fibronectin, fibrinogen, and laminin act as mediators of adherence of clinical staphylococcal isolates to foreign material. J Infect Dis 1988 *Oct.*; 158(4):693–701.

19. Vaudaux P, Pittet D, Haeberli A, Huggler E, Nydegger UE, Lew DP, Waldvogel FA. Host factors selectively increase staphylococcal adherence on inserted catheters: a role for fibronectin and fibrinogen or fibrin. J Infect Dis 1989 *Nov.*; 160(5):865–875.

20. Christensen GD, Simpson WA, Bisno AL, Beachey EH. Adherence of slime-producing strains of *Staphylococcus epidermidis* to smooth surfaces. Infect Immun 1982; 37:318–326.

21. Christensen GD, Simpson WA, Younger JJ, Baddour LM, Barrett FF, Melton DM, Beachey EH. Adherence of coagulase-negative staphylococci to plastic tissue culture plates: a quantitative model for the adherence of staphylococci to medical devices. J Clin Microbiol 1985 *Dec.*; 22(6):996–1006.

22. Falcieri E, Vaudaux P, Huggler E, Lew D, Waldvogel F. Role of bacterial exopolymers and host factors on adherence and phagocytosis of *Staphylococcus aureus* in foreign body infection. J Infect Dis 1987; 155:524–531.

23. Costerton JW, Irvin RT, Cheng KJ. The bacterial glycocalyx in nature and disease. Annu Rev Microbiol 1981; 35:299–324.

24. Davenport DS, Massanari RM, Pfaller MA, Bale MJ, Streed SA, Hierbolzer WJ Jr. Usefulness of a test for slime production as a marker for clinically significant infections with coagulase-negative staphylococci. J Infect Dis 1986 *Feb.*; 153(2):332–339.

25. Sheth NK, Franson TR, Sohnle PG. Influence of bacterial adherence to intravascular catheters on in vitro antibiotic susceptibility. Lancet 1985; 2:1266–1268.

26. Farber BF, Kaplan MH, Clogstron AG. *Staphylococcus epidermidis* extracted slime inhibits the antimicrobial action of glycopeptide antibiotics. J Infect Dis 1990; 161:37–40.

27. Costerton JW, Lappin-Scott HM. Behavior of bacteria in biofilms. Am Soc Microbiol News 1989; 55:650–654.

28. Sheth NK, Franson TR, Rose HD, Buckmire FL, Cooper JA, Sohnle PG. Colonization of bacteria on polyvinyl chloride and Teflon intravascular catheter in hospitalized patients. J Clin Microbiol 1983 *Nov.*; 18(5):1061–1063.

29. Sherertz RJ, Carruth WA, Marosok RD, Espeland MA, Johnson RA, Solomon DD. Contribution of vascular catheter material to the pathogenesis of infection: the enhanced risk of silicone in vivo. J Biomed Mater Res 1995; 29:635–645.

30. Collignon PG, Soni N, Pearson IY, Woods WP, Munro R, Sorrell TC. Is semiquantitative culture of central vein catheter tips useful in the diagnosis of catheter-associated bacteremia? J Clin Microbiol 1986; 24:532–535.

31. Moyer MA, Edwards LD, Farley L. Comparative culture methods on 101 intravenous catheters. Arch Intern Med 1983; 143:66–69.

32. Snydman DR, Murray SA, Kornfeld SJ, Majka JA, Ellis CA. Total parenteral nutrition-related infections: prospective epidemiologic study using semiquantitative methods. Am J Med 1982; 73:695–699.

33. Cleri DJ, Corrado ML, Seligman SJ. Quantitative culture of intravenous catheters and other intravascular inserts. J Infect Dis 1980; 141:781–786.

34. Bjornson HS, Colley IR, Bower RH, Duty VP, Schwartz-Fulton JT, Fisher JE. Association between microorganism growth at the catheter insertion site and colonization of the catheter in patients receiving total parenteral nutrition. Surgery 1982; 92:720–726.

35. Brun-Buisson C, Abrouk F, Legrand P, Huet Y, Larabi S, Rapin M. Diagnosis of central venous catheter-related sepsis: critical level of quantitative tip cultures. Arch Intern Med 1987; 147:873–877.

36. Sherertz RJ, Raad II, Balani A, Koo L, Rand K. Three-year experience with sonicated vascular catheter cultures in a clinical microbiology laboratory. J Clin Microbiol 1990; 28:76–82.

37. Raad II, Sabbagh MF, Rand KH, Sherertz RJ. Quantitative tip culture methods and the diagnosis of central venous catheter-related infections. Diagn Microbiol Infect Dis 1991; 15:13–20.

38. Maki DG, Sources of infection with central venous catheters in an ICU: a prospective study. Program and Abstracts of the 28th Interscience Conference on Antimicrobial Agents and Chemotherapy, Los Angeles, 1988:157. Abstract 269.

39. Sitges-Serra A, Puig P, Linares J, Perez JL, Farrero N, Jaurrieta E, Garau J. Hub colonization as the initial step in an outbreak of catheter-related sepsis due

to coagulase negative staphylococci during parenteral nutrition. JPEN 1984 *Nov–Dec.*; 8(6):668–672.

40. Sitges-Serra A, Linares J, Perez JL, Laurrieta E, Lorente L. A randomized trial on the effect of tubing changes on hub contamination and catheter sepsis during parenteral nutrition. JPEN 1985; 9:322–325.

41. Linares J, Sitges-Serra A, Garau J, Perez JL, Martin R. Pathogenesis of catheter sepsis: a prospective study with quantitative and semiquantitative cultures of catheter hub and segments. J Clin Microbiol 1985; 21:357–360.

42. Raad I, Costerton W, Sabbarwal U, Sacilowski M, Anaissie E, Bodey GP. Ultra-structural analysis of indwelling catheters: a quantitative relationship between luminal colonization and duration of placement. J Infect Dis 1993; 168:400–407.

43. Maki DG. Pathogenesis, prevention, and management of infections due to intravascular devices used for infusion therapy. In: Bisno AL, Waldvogel FA, eds. Infections Associated With Indwelling Medical Devices. Washington: American Society for Microbiology, 1989:161–177.

44. Clarke DE, Raffin TA. Infectious complications of indwelling long-term central venous catheters. Chest 1990; 97(4):966–972.

45. Press OW, Ramsey PG, Larson EB, Fefer A, Hickman RO. Hickman catheter infections in patients with malignancies. Medicine 1984; 63(4):189–200.

46. Decker MD, Edwards KM. Central venous catheter infections. Pediatr Clin North Am 1988; 35(3):579–612.

47. Pasquale MD, Campbell JM, Magnant CM. Groshong versus Hickman catheters. Surgery 1992; 174:408–410.

48. Keung Y-K, Watkins K, Chen S-C, Groshen S, Silberman H, Douer D. Comparative study of infectious complications of different types of chronic central venous access devices. Cancer 1994; 73(11):2832–2837.

49. Mueller BU, Skelton J, Callender DPE, Marshall D, Gress J, Longo D, Norton J, Rubin M, Venzon D, Pizzo PA. A prospective randomized trial comparing the infectious complications of the externalized catheters versus a sub-cutaneously implanted device in cancer patients. J Clin Oncol 1992 *Dec.*; 10(12):1943–1948.

50. Gleeson NC, Fiorica JV, Mark JE, Pinelli DM, Hoffman MS, Roberts WS, Cavanagh D. Externalized Groshong catheters and Hickman ports for central venous access in gynecologic oncology patients. Gynecol Oncol 1993 *Dec.*; 51(3): 372–376.

51. Carde P, Cossett-Delaigue MF, LaPlanche A, Chareau I. Classical external indwelling central venous catheter versus totally implanted venous access systems for chemotherapy administration: a randomized trial in 100 patients with solid tumors. Eur J Cancer Clin Oncol 1989; 6:939–944.

52. Sariego J, Bootorabi B, Matsumoto T, Kerstein M. Major long-term compli-cations in 1,422 permanent venous access devices. Am J Surg 1993; 165:249–251.

53. Mirro J Jr, Rao BN, Kumar M, Rafferty M, Hancock M, Austin BA, Fairclough D, Lobe TE. A comparison of placement techniques and complications of externalized catheters and implantable port use in children with cancer. J Pediatr Surg 1990 *Jan.*; 25(1):120–124.

54. Early TF, Gregory RT, Wheeler JR, Snyder SO, Gayle RG. Increased infection rate in double-lumen versus single-lumen Hickman catheters in cancer patients. South Med J 1990; 83(1):34–36.

55. Raad I, Hanna, H, McFadyen S, Marts K, Richardson D, Mansfield P. Non-tunneled Subclavian Central Venous Catheters (NTSC) vs Tunneled central venous Catheters (CVCs) and Ports in Cancer Patients. Proceedings of the 41st Interscience Conference on Antimicrobial Agents and Chemotherapy, Chicago, IL, December 16–19, 2001. Abstract 2049.

56. Anderson MA, Aker SN, Hickman RO. The double-lumen Hickman catheter. Am J Nurs 1982; 82:272–277.

57. Goodman MS, Wickman R. Venous access devices: an overview. Oncol Nurs Forum 1984; 11:16–23.

58. Hanna H, McFadyen S, Marts K, Richardson D, Raad II. Prospective Evaluation of 1.67 Million Catheter-Days of Peripherally Inserted Central Catheters (PICCs) in Cancer Patients: Long Durability and Low Infection Rate. Proceedings of the 41st Interscience Conference on Antimicrobial Agent and Chemotherapy, Chicago, IL, December 16–19, 2001. Abstract 1459.

59. Slater N, Goldfarb IW, Jacob HE, Hill JB, Srodes CH. Experience with long-term outpatient venous access utilizing percutaneously placed silicone elastomer catheters. Cancer 1985; 56:2074–2077.

60. Markel S, Reynen K. Impact on patient care: 2652 PIC catheter days in the alternative setting. J Intravenous Nur 1990; 13(6):347–351.

61. Rutherford C. Insertion and care of multiple lumen peripherally inserted central line catheters. J Intravenous Nurs 1988; 11(1):16–19.

62. Brown JM. Peripherally inserted central catheters: use in homecare. J Intravenous Nurs 1989; 12(3):144–147.

63. Chathas MK. Percutaneous central venous catheters in neonates. JOGNN 1986; 144(11):324–332.

64. Rutherford C. A study of single lumen peripherally inserted central line catheter dwelling time and complications. J Intravenous Nurs 1988; 11(3):169–173.

65. Walshe LJ, Malak SF, Eagan J, Sepkowitz KA. Complication rates among cancer patients with peripherally inserted central catheters. J Clin Oncol 2002; 20(15):3276–3281.

66. Benezra D, Kiehn TE, Gold GWM, Brown AE, Turnbull ADM, Armstrong D. Prospective study of infections in indwelling central venous catheters using quantitative blood cultures. Am J Med 1988; 85:495–498.

67. Andrivet P, Bacquer A, Ngoc C, Ferme C, Letinier JY, Gautier H, Gallet CB, Brun-Buisson C. Lack of clinical benefit from subcutaneous tunnel insertion of central venous catheters in immunocompromised patients. CID 1994 Feb.; 18(2):199–206.

68. Timsit JF, Sebille V, Farkas JC, Misset B, Martin JB, Chevret S, Carlet J. Effect of subcutaneous tunneling on internal jugular catheter-related sepsis in critically ill patients. JAMA 1996 Nov 6; 276(17):1416–1420.

69. Raad II, Hohn DC, Gilbreath BJ, Suleiman N, Hill LA, Bruso PA, Marts K, Mansfield PF, Bodey GP. Prevention of central venous catheter-related infections by using maximal sterile barrier precautions during insertion. Infect Control Hosp Epidemiol 1994 Apr.; 15(4 Pt I):231–238.

70. Schwartz C, Henrickson KJ, Roghmann K, Powell K. Prevention of bacteremia attributed to luminal colonization of tunneled central venous catheters with vancomycin-susceptible organism. J Clin Oncol 1990; 8:1591–1597.

71. Henrickson KJ, Axtell RA, Hoover SM, Kuhn SM, Pritchett J, Kehl SC, Klein JP. Prevention of central venous catheter-related infections and thrombotic events in immunocompromised children by the use of vancomycin/ciprofloxacin/heparin flush solution: a randomized, multicenter, double-blind trial. J Clin Onc 2000; 18:1269–1278.

72. Carratala J, Niubo J, Fernandez-Sevilla A, Juve E, Castellsague X, Berlanga J, Linares J, Gudiol F. Randomized, double-blind trial of an antibiotic-lock technique for prevention of gram-positive central venous catheter-related infection in neutropenic patients with cancer. Antimicrob Agents Chemother 1999; 43:2200–2204.

73. Maki D, Garland J, Alex C, Henrickson K. A randomized trial of a vancomycin–heparin lock solution (VHLS) for prevention of catheter-related bloodstream infection (CRBSI) in a NNICU. 12th Annual Scientific Meeting of the Society for Healthcare Epidemiology of America (SHEA), Salt Lake City, Utah, USA, April 6–9, 2002.

74. Rackoff WR, Weiman M, Jakobowski D, Hirschl R, Stallings V, Bilodeau J, Danz P, Bell L, Lange B. A randomized, controlled trial of the efficacy of a heparin and vancomycin solution in preventing central venous catheter infections in children. J Pediatr 1995; 127:147–151.

75. Raad I, Buzaid A, Rhyne J, Hachem R, Darouiche R, Safar H, Albitar M, Sherertz RJ. Minocycline and ethylenediaminetetraacetate for the prevention of recurrent vascular catheter infections. Clin Infect Dis 1997; 25:149–151.

76. Raad I, Hachem R, Tcholakian RK, Sherertz R. Efficacy of minocycline and EDTA lock solution in preventing catheter-related bacteremia, septic phlebitis, and endocarditis in rabbits. Antimicrob Agents Chemother 2002; 46:327–332.

77. Chatzinikolaou I, Zipf TF, Hanna H, Umphrey J, Roberts WM, Sherertz R, Hachem R, Raad I. Minocycline and Ethylenediaminetetraacetate (M-EDTA) Lock Solution for the Prevention of Implantable Port Infections in Pediatric Cancer Patients. In press, Clinical Infectious Diseases, to be published end of 2002.

78. Kamal GD, Pfaller MA, Rempe LE, Jebson PJR. Reduced intravascular catheter infection by antibiotic bonding. JAMA 1991; 265:2364–2368.

79. Maki DG, Stolz SM, Wheeler S, Mermel LA. Prevention of central venous catheter-related bloodstream infection by use of an antiseptic-impregnated catheter. A randomized, controlled trial. Ann Intern Med 1997; 127:257–266.

80. Raad I, Darouiche R, Hachem R, Mansouri M, Bodey GP. The broad-spectrum activity and efficacy of catheters coated with minocycline and rifampin. J Infect Dis 1996; 173:418–424.

81. Raad I, Darouiche R, Dupuis J, Abi-Said D, Gabrielli A, Hachem R, Wall M, Harris R, Jones J, Buzaid A, Robertson C, Shenaq S, Curling P, Burke T, Ericsson C. Central venous catheters coated with minocycline and rifampin for the prevention of catheter-related colonization and bloodstream infections. A randomized, double-blind trial. The Texas Medical Center Catheter Study Group. Ann Intern Med 1997; 127:267–274.

82. Darouiche RO, Raad II, Heard SO, Thornby JI, Wenker OC, Gabrielli A, Berg J, Khardori N, Hanna H, Hachem R, Harris RL, Mayhall G. A

comparison of two antimicrobial-impregnated central venous catheters. Catheter Study Group. N Engl J Med 1999; 340:1–8.

83. Bassetti S, Hu J, D'Agostino RB Jr, Sherertz RJ. Prolonged antimicrobial activity of a catheter containing chlorhexidine-silver sulfadiazine extends protection against catheter infections in vivo. Antimicrob Agents Chemother 2001; 45:1535–1538.

84. Hanna H, Graviss L, Chaiban G, Dvorak T, Arbuckle R, Estey E, Munsell M, Hachem R, Champlin R, Raad I. Susceptibility patterns of Staphylococcus organisms in leukemia and bone marrow transplant (BMT) services after the use of minocycline/rifampin-impregnated central venous catheters (MR-CVCs) in a cancer hospital. Proceedings of the 42nd Annual Meeting of the Interscience Conference on Antimicrobial Agents and Chemotherapy, San Diego, California, September 27–30, 2002. Abstract #K-74.

85. Hanna H, Benjamin R, Chatzinikolaou I, Richardson D, Marts K, Mansfield P, Raad I. The Role of Long-term Silicone Central Venous Catheters Impregnated with Rifampin and Minocycline (S-CVC-RM) in Preventing Catheter-related Infections: A Prospective Randomized Study. Proceedings of the 38th Conference of the American Society of Clinical Oncology (ASCO), Orlando, Florida, May 18–21, 2002. Abstract #1419.

86. O'Grady NP, Alexander M, Dellinger EP, Gerberding JL, Heard SO, Maki DG, Masur H, McCormick RD, Mermel LA, Pearson ML, Raad II, Randolph A, Weinstein RA. Guidelines for the prevention of intravascular catheter-related infections. Centers for Disease Control and Prevention. Morbidity & Mortality Weekly Report. Recommendations & Reports 51(RR-10):1–29, 2002.

15

Infections Associated with Central Nervous System Implants

Roger Bayston

School of Medicine and Surgical Sciences
University of Nottingham
United Kingdom

GENERAL INTRODUCTION

Implants used in the central nervous system include those for control of cerebrospinal fluid (CSF) pressure, those to measure or monitor it, and devices to deliver long-term intrathecal medication. Other implantable devices such as aneurism clips will not be considered here.

Elevated CSF pressure can arise from cerebral edema due to encephalitis or from imbalance between CSF production and absorption, usually due to obstruction. If it causes secondary anatomical and neurological changes, it is termed hydrocephalus. Treatment of elevated CSF pressure considered to be transient may include the placement of an external ventricular drainage (EVD) system. While these can also be used to control hydrocephalus in the short term, the condition usually requires placement of a permanent shunting device. Removal of excess CSF can also be carried out for short-term pressure control after insertion of a reservoir that allows direct percutaneous ventricular access, although such reservoirs are usually used for administration of drugs such as those used to treat malignancy. Controlled infusion of antispasmodics or analgesics into the spinal theca is used increasingly for either spasticity or otherwise intractable pain. All of these devices are at risk of infection.

HYDROCEPHALUS SHUNTING

Introduction

Hydrocephalus

Hydrocephalus can be caused by any of a variety of conditions that predispose to obstruction of the CSF interventricular pathways (aqueducts) or of the absorptive system, especially the arachnoid villi. These include congenital anomalies, periventricular hemorrhage in babies or subarachnoid hemorrhage in adults, tumors, trauma, meningitis, and idiopathic stenosis of the aqueducts. Currently, most new cases occur in premature infants, but the condition also affects adults. Despite the variety of underlying causes, options for treatment are few. In those cases where the obstruction is within the ventricular system, an attempt can be made endoscopically to fenestrate the floor of the third ventricle, but where this is unsuccessful or where the site of obstruction precludes this approach, shunt placement is the only realistic option.

Hydrocephalus Shunts

The first shunting devices became widely available in the late 1950s, and since then designs have diversified but their function has changed little until recently. They are made mainly of silicone elastomer, sometimes with steel or plastic components (Fig. 1). They consist essentially of a tube placed in the cerebral ventricular system to collect CSF, a second tube to drain the CSF to another body cavity, and a valve to control flow rate and prevent reflux. Some also have inbuilt reservoirs to allow access to ventricular CSF for sampling. In the past decade, more sophisticated devices have been developed, notably those which can have their flow rate adjusted noninvasively using a magnetic programmer that moves a step motor inside the valve. These now often incorporate an antisiphon device. Further developments such as inbuilt pressure-sensing devices can be expected.

Cerebrospinal fluid can be drained to the right cardiac atrium, the pleural cavity, the peritoneal cavity, or to other spaces, but currently in Europe the majority of shunts drain into the peritoneal cavity (ventriculoperitoneal, VP), with about 10–15% draining into the heart (ventriculoatrial, VA) (Fig. 2). Similar shunts can also be used to drain CSF from the lumbar theca to the peritoneal cavity but this route is less commonly used.

Etiology and Pathogenesis of Shunt Infections

Definition of Shunt Infection

In order to avoid confusion when addressing issues of etiology and prevention, shunt infections must be defined. They can be divided into two types, external and internal (1). External shunt infections consist of infection of the extracranial soft tissues surrounding the shunt tubing or valve body, en-

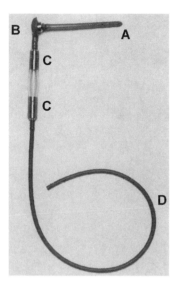

Figure 1 The Holter valve and shunt for control of hydrocephalus. (A) Ventricular catheter; (B) Rickham reservoir for sampling, pressure measurement, etc.; (C) uni directional flow-control valves in a steel housing; (D) distal catheter to right atrium VA shunt or peritoneal cavity (VP shunt). Apart from the valve housings and the base of the reservoir, all parts are silicone.

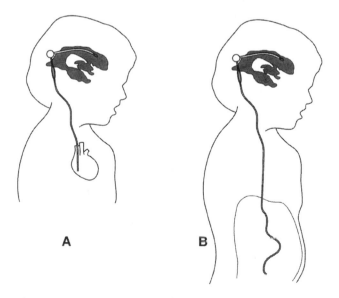

Figure 2 (A) Route of ventriculoatrial shunt for hydrocephalus; (B) route of ventriculoperitoneal shunt.

hanced by the presence of the biomaterial. They usually arise as wound infections soon after surgery. In those with poor skin cover, such as premature neonates or the debilitated elderly, or in those with involuntary head movements, erosion of the healed wound can also occur and the wound become secondarily infected. In most practices, external infections constitute less than 5% of shunt infections. The major infective problem in shunting is internal shunt infection, consisting of colonization of the inner surfaces of the shunt tubing and valve (2).

Costs and Consequences of Shunt Infections

Though the hospital-based costs of shunt infection are recognized as high, with each infection estimated to cost about eight times as much as the original insertion, they are rarely computed. A model for this purpose has been proposed (3). The medical consequences include ventriculitis, abdominal adhesions and abscesses, loculated ventricles (4), sometimes bloodstream infection, and decreased mental acuity (5,6).

Etiology and Causative Organisms

The causative organisms of internal shunt infection are mainly staphylococci, with coagulase-negative staphylococci (CoNS), and particularly *Staphylococcus epidermidis*, predominating (7–11). There are no major differences in causative organisms between VA and VP, with the exception that VP shunt catheters occasionally pierce an abdominal viscus, intestinal bacteria, including anaerobes, are then found. The proportion of CoNS to *S. aureus* varies due to diagnostic criteria and other factors but it is approximately >90% CoNS to <10% *S. aureus*.

The incidence of shunt infection is often cited as about 10% of operations, and the rate generated by a U.K. National Shunt Registry is 11% (12). There is no difference overall in the literature in infection rates between VA and VP shunts (1). However, these figures conceal wide differences (13,14), particularly between age groups. The incidence for adults and older children is about 3–5% in many studies, but in those cases where infants less than 6 months of age are shunted, the incidence is often 10–25% (1,7,9–11). Though various theories have been advanced to explain this high rate, it is probably due to the sequence of life events in these children. Most are born prematurely or with a disability and are first treated in neonatal intensive care facilities. Only later when they have survived and shown evidence of developing hydrocephalus are they shunted, by which time they have received their normal flora from the hospital environment and staff rather than from their parents. One study has supported this, showing both a higher skin bacterial density and a higher number of adhesive staphylococci on the skins of such infants (9).

Soon after shunts became available, infections appeared (15,16), but they were assumed to be either from the operating theatre environment or staff, or else not associated with the shunt surgery but rather caused by

Table 1 Results of Intraoperative Sampling of Incisions During Shunt Insertion

No. of patients sampled	No. positive	No. from patient (range, mean colonies)	No. of unknown origin (range, mean colonies)
100	58	32 1–55, mean 10	26 1–7, mean 2

spontaneous or secondary bacteremias. Results of research have now clarified the position. In summary, the shunt and/or the CSF are contaminated during surgery by organisms from the patient's skin or mucous membranes; hematogenous infection is extremely rare. In one study (17), 58 of 100 incisions were found to contain skin flora at the time of insertion of the shunt, and 32 were found by typing to be indistinguishable from those found on the patient's skin before preparation for surgery (Table 1). In this series, there were 11 shunt infections and 9 of these were due to staphylococci indistinguishable from those in the incision that were derived from the patient. The remaining two were due to bacteria that could not be typed. Contamination of surgical incisions occurs commonly (18). Although the skin surface can be disinfected by agents such as alcoholic chlorhexidine, it is recolonized about 15–20 minutes later by bacteria from the glands and follicles (11,19). The incision is then contaminated from the wound edges (Fig. 3). However, although 32 patients had incisions contaminated with their skin bacteria, only a third of them developed a shunt infection, raising questions about the relative abilities of strains of the bacteria to colonize catheters.

Once in contact with the inner surface of the shunt, staphylococci are able to adhere either to the silicone (2,20) or to the glycoprotein conditioning film,

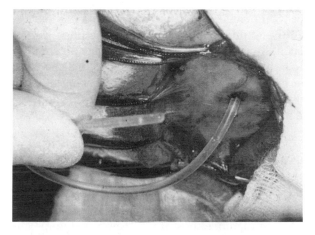

Figure 3 Shunt operation showing opportunities for bacterial access to the ventricles and the shunt system.

derived from the CSF, which is always deposited (21,22). In patients with elevated CSF protein concentrations, this will be deposited more rapidly. There are apparent paradoxes associated with conditioning film, in that CSF protein deposition has been found to reduce bacterial adhesion in some conditions (23) but to enhance it in others (24). Albumen is known to reduce staphylococcal adhesion, whereas other plasma proteins such as fibronectin, laminin, or fibrinogen are known to enhance it. Deposition of a conditioning film is a dynamic process (25), and the glycoproteins predominating will presumably determine the degree of bacterial adherence. Be this as it may, *S. epidermidis* is able to adhere to shunts after insertion (2,20), probably initially by means of vitronectin-binding protein (26). Due to the low concentration of nutrients in the CSF, subsequent proliferation is usually slow, though the low available iron concentrations at least can probably be countered by the presence of catecholamines in the CSF, which have been shown to act as bacterial iron capture agents (27). As proliferation progresses, bacterial stress signals operate to change the phenotype and a biofilm develops. The sequence of events and the biofilm development explain many of the clinical features of shunt infection.

Other Causative Organisms

About 20% of shunt infections are due to other organisms such as coryneforms, propionibacteria, oral streptococci, and occasionally *Candida* spp. and enterobacteria (Table 2) (28–51). In most centers these last two groups constitute less than 3–5% of infections. Again, most appear to be derived from the patient's skin, and *Candida* and enterobacteria or other gram negative bacteria such as *Acinetobacter* spp. are commonly found on the skin of patients who have had courses of broad-spectrum antibiotics and have spent long periods in hospital before shunting. In a review of *Candida* shunt infection (46), the main predisposing factors were found to be recent meningitis or complications of abdominal surgery, each involving long hospital stay and antibiotic treatment. A report of two cases of cryptococcal shunt infection, in apparently immunocompetent patients shunted on the same day by the same surgeon, showed that the two isolates were different on typing and were assumed to be due to preexisting infection (51). In most cases, the causative organisms are capable of adherence to the surfaces of the shunt catheter and of producing biofilms, as is the case with *S. epidermidis*. In some cases of candida infection, pseudohyphae cause shunt obstruction (1).

Shunting of Patients with Postmeningitic Hydrocephalus

Patients with cryptococcal meningitis who develop hydrocephalus will require shunting, and several reports have shown that this is safe after treatment has begun (52,53). Similarly, early shunting is beneficial in tuberculous meningitis complicated by hydrocephalus, and does not carry a risk of either shunt infection or dissemination of tuberculosis (54). However, Lamprecht et al. (55) have reported a high infection rate (due mainly to staphylococci) in patients shunted for tuberculous hydrocephalus.

Table 2 Organisms Other than Staphylococci Reported to Cause Shunt Infections

Organism	Source	Reference
Coryneforms	Kaplan and Weinstein, 1969	28
	Bolton et al., 1975	29
	Moss et al., 1977	30
	O'Regan and Makker, 1979	31
	Bayston, 1989	1
	Hande et al., 1976	32
	Allen and Green, 1986	33
Propionibacteria	Everett et al., 1976	34
	Beeler et al., 1976	35
	Skinner et al., 1978	36
	Brook et al., 1980	37
	Rekate et al., 1980	38
	Lim et al., 1980	39
	Bayston, 1989	1
Listeria spp	Heck et al., 1971	40
	Strife et al., 1976	41
	McLaurin, 1973	42
Peptococcus	Caron et al., 1979	43
Enterobacteria	Denoya et al., 1986	44
Pseudomonas	Basset et al., 1973	45
	Bayston, 1989	1
Candida spp	Sanchez-Portocarro et al., 1994	46
	Bayston, 1989	1
Mixed infections and anaerobes	Brook et al., 1977	47
	Bayston, 1989	1
	Sami et al., 1995	48
	Shinkawa et al., 2001	49
	Park et al., 2000	50

Community-Acquired Meningitis

Meningitis due to *Streptococcus pneumoniae*, *Neisseria meningitidis* or *Hemophilus influenzae* occurs in shunted patients with the same frequency as in the remaining population, and should not be regarded as shunt infection.

Diagnosis and Clinical Features

Symptoms of Shunt Infection and Laboratory Tests

The signs and symptoms of shunt infection differ between VA and VP shunts. In VA shunt infections, the patient may be apparently well, or suffer only minor or vague symptoms, for many years before presenting with illness serious enough to prompt investigation. In the early stages, there may be pyrexia, chills, anorexia, disturbed sleep patterns, and lassitude, though any of these can be intermittent or absent. On investigation, blood culture might yield *S. epidermidis* or a coryneform, and the investigator will be presented with the problem of determining whether this is infection or contamination. A reliable result apart from the documentation of repeatedly positive blood-cultures is the blood hemoglobin level, and those with a VA shunt infection are usually moderately anemic (about 8–10 g/dL). The anemia is refractory to iron therapy. Those patients with VA shunts who have vague symptoms, occasional pyrexias, and anemia should be suspected of having shunt infection. If for any reason the diagnosis is not made within 1–2 years of operation, the persisting discharge of bacteria from the shunt into the bloodstream stimulates production of extremely high concentrations of antibody, leading to immune complex disease. This is manifest by petechial or macular rashes which sometimes become ulcerated, particularly around the ankles; arthropathy with hot, painful joints; and hematuria (1,56). The hematuria indicates immune-complex glomerulonephritis caused by deposition of immune complexes on the glomerular basement membranes and stimulation of cytokine release (1,35,57).

Hypertension and elevated plasma urea and creatinine levels indicate renal failure. At this stage, blood cultures are often negative, presumably because of the high antibody levels. Patients can be referred to inappropriate specialties such as rheumatology, dermatology, hematology, or nephrology, causing further delay in diagnosis (58,59). A simple serological test has been found to be extremely reliable in diagnosing VA shunt infection, even before it becomes symptomatic, and this along with serum C3 and C4 complement titers can confirm the diagnosis of VA shunt infection, with or without immune complex disease (1,60). However, this test is not widely available. When the test was applied to a group of 488 pediatric patients having VA shunts (61), 127 underwent serial serological testing before and up to six months after operation whereas 361 did not. Both groups were followed up conventionally for three years or until a shunt infection was diagnosed. The infection rate was the same (5.5%) in each group, but in the group without serological surveillance there were 10 cases of shunt nephritis, at least one of which was fatal, whereas in the surveillance group there was one case. This patient was diagnosed solely on the basis of serological results as having a shunt infection two weeks postoperatively but she had had an extremely difficult shunt history and the current shunt was working well; a decision was made to treat with antibiotics and observe. She remained clinically well though with intermittently positive blood cultures and rising antibody titers to *S. epidermidis* (>10,240, normal for age ≤160), until she became unwell 17 months later with hematuria. Although the diagnosis in this case was made early, the symptoms presented as late shunt infection. Other than this case, there were no late infections in the surveillance group, but there were 17 in the conventional follow-up group. This and other evidence show that late shunt infection is almost invariably undiagnosed early infection. In view of the ease with which

VA shunt infections can be diagnosed, shunt nephritis should not occur, and from the point of view of infection, VA shunts are as safe as VP shunts.

Ventriculoperitoneal shunt infections usually present as recurrence of the original symptoms of hydrocephalus, because unlike VA infections, they usually result in obstruction of the distal catheter by adhesions or cysts of the greater omentum (62,63). Another major difference is that they usually present within 6–8 months of surgery, probably because of the obstruction. The clinical dilemma consists of differentiating between infective and noninfective obstruction. This can be done on the grounds of clinical history (presenting soon after surgery), presence of erythema along the shunt track, particularly over the torso, and laboratory tests. Blood cultures are almost always negative and are not indicated. The most useful laboratory test is the C-reactive protein (CRP) assay (64,65). Unfortunately, there is no serological test equivalent to that for VA infections. If a patient with a VP shunt has recurrence of symptoms of hydrocephalus within 6–8 months of operation, and if the serum CRP level is raised with no other obvious cause, then shunt infection should be suspected.

When VA or VP shunt infection is suspected on grounds set out earlier, aspiration of ventricular CSF from the shunt reservoir might confirm it. The CSF neutrophil count is not always elevated, but culture is usually positive. A useful guide to the significance of cultures of CoNS is the ability to visualize them on a Gram stain of CSF (66). However, in a significant proportion of cases, the ventricular CSF appears normal and culture-negative in the presence of colonization of the lower catheter. There is a risk of introducing infection by reservoir aspiration, although this is small.

Treatment

Options for Treatment

Early attempts to treat shunt infections with intravenous antibiotics in the same way as other staphylococcal infections were unsuccessful (67,68). This was shown to be due, at least in part, to the poor CSF drug concentrations achieved with intravenous administration. In fact, most antimicrobials commonly used intravenously fail to penetrate the blood/CSF barrier in the absence of inflammation, and the ventriculitis usually associated with shunt infection is not accompanied by a vigorous inflammatory response. This is true of all beta-lactams, which are at an added disadvantage due to the effective excretion pathway from the CSF space (69). A study by Faillace and Tan (70) has shown that, despite satisfactory serum levels, CSF concentrations of gentamicin and vancomycin after intravenous administration were too low to measure in patients without meningeal inflammation. Only a limited range of drugs overcomes this obstacle, these being chloramphenicol, rifampicin, and trimethoprim. Chloramphenicol has been disappointing in this context (71). Nau et al. (72) have reported that rifampicin gives therapeutic CSF levels without meningeal inflammation. Cotrimoxazole has been used with limited success for treatment of *S. epidermidis* VP shunt infections (73). It was later realized that another important factor was the biofilm-mode growth of the bacteria inside the shunt (2,9). Organisms in a biofilm are slow-growing and relatively insusceptible to antimicrobials (74,75). Though attempts to treat shunt infections nonsurgically continued to be made, a study by Shurtleff et al. (68) indicated that antibiotics without surgery had a poor outcome. James et al. (76) later showed conclusively, with a small but well-designed study, that the outcome was considerably better if the infected shunt was removed as part of the treatment. Based on this and other studies, shunt removal as part of the treatment of shunt infection is now accepted. However, even with shunt removal, treatment with intravenous antibiotics, usually dictated by susceptibility results, often still requires a long course with extraventricular drainage (EVD) to control CSF pressure until re-shunting can be undertaken. Insertion of a new shunt is usually delayed until the ventricular CSF can be shown to be "clear." While the absence of microorganisms is an obvious requirement, a normal CSF white blood cell (WBC) count has also been deemed necessary in some practices. The delay to reshunting in a patient who is clinically free from infection can lead to secondary infection from the EVD, and consumes healthcare resources. Whereas this has to be balanced against the catastrophe of recurrence of infection in the new shunt, the significance of a persistently abnormal CSF WBC count in such circumstances is open to question. White blood cells in the CSF are not always neutrophils. Macrophages containing myelin-derived lipid (77) can be mistaken for neutrophils, but these can be found in patients on EVD where CSF pressure control is sometimes less than optimal. Eosinophils are also to be found in the CSF of some patients treated with intraventricular vancomycin (78). A Giemsa stain in cases of persistently abnormal CSF WBC count can be helpful.

Gentamicin has been used to treat CoNS shunt infections but the results have been generally disappointing (1). Rifampicin is highly active against most strains of staphylococci and other Gram-positive bacteria involved in shunt infections, although in centers where the drug is heavily used to treat other infections there may be a problem with resistant hospital-derived strains. However, it must never be used alone as this is followed by rapid development of resistance (79). Of the glycopeptides, most experience has been gained with vancomycin. Although this agent when given intravenously fails to give satisfactory CSF concentrations in the absence of inflammation, it has been given safely by the intraventricular route in relatively large doses with no ill effect (80,81). With very rare exceptions, staphylococci and most other Gram-positive bacteria associated with shunt infections are susceptible. Enterococci are not reliably susceptible to glycopeptides (82). Probably the first use of intraventricular vancomycin for a shunt infection was by Visconti and Peters (83), who successfully eradicated an infection due to CoNS with an intraventricular dose of 20 mg vancomycin daily and shunt removal. Since then there have been several accounts of its use in this way. However, the use of vancomycin alone is not to be recommended and the addition of oral or systemic rifampicin has been found to make a significant difference to the outcome. Ring et al. (71) treated a CoNS VP shunt infection by shunt removal, but the infection persisted during treatment with chloramphenicol and nafcillin, being resolved rapidly only after starting oral rifampicin and intravenous vancomycin. A similar case was reported by Gombert et al. (84). Similarly, Ryan et al. (80) treated a case of enterococcal meningitis with intravenous vancomycin and intraventricular gentamicin without success, due to very low CSF drug concentrations. After institution of intraventricular vancomycin, the CSF drug levels became satisfactory, but with no clinical improvement. When oral rifampicin was added, prompt recovery occurred.

Recommended Treatment

The lengthy course of intravenous antibiotics and the wide variety used, with implications for treatment failure or relapse and for secondary infection, has led to a review by the British Society for Antimicrobial Chemotherapy and the issue of treatment guidelines (85). The treatment recommended for staphylococcal shunt infection is as follows:

1. As soon as possible after diagnosis, the infected shunt should be removed and an EVD inserted.
2. Intraventricular vancomycin, 20 mg each day, should be administered via the EVD with the EVD then clamped for one hour, or alternatively via a separately placed reservoir. The dose is not determined by the age or weight of the patient, although in cases of small or slit ventricles, 10 mg/day can be substituted.
3. Intravenous rifampicin, 600 mg/day in two doses for adults and 15 mg/kg/day for children, should be administered. This can be changed to oral dosage after a few days. If the causative organism is resistant to rifampicin, other agents that give antimicrobial CSF concentrations in the absence of blood/CSF barrier inflammation, such as trimethoprim (not co-trimoxazole), can be substituted. Chloramphenicol, while penetrating well into the CSF, has poor antistaphylococcal cidal activity and cannot be recommended. Although fosfomycin has been used to treat staphylococcal meningitis, little is known of its use in shunt infections. In cases where the causative bacterium is resistant to other agents, intravenous vancomycin should be given in addition to that given intraventricularly.
4. CSF should be examined daily, using samples from the ventricular catheter rather than from the collection bag. Clinical and microbiological monitoring should show resolution of the infection by days 4–5, the final results being available by day 7 of treatment. If this is

the case, reshunting should be carried out at the earliest opportunity thereafter, with the last dose of intraventricular vancomycin being given during surgery. No postoperative antibiotic treatment is necessary, and under no circumstances should rifampicin alone be continued beyond the day of surgery.

CSF concentrations of vancomycin commonly exceed 100 mg/l but no central nervous system toxicity or other side effects have been recorded with concentrations of 200–300 mg/l. Because of this, monitoring of CSF vancomycin levels is usually considered to be unnecessary. The use of the aforementioned regimen has led to considerable reductions in hospital stay with greatly improved treatment success and with reduction in relapse rate and secondary EVD infections.

Concern about the possibility of resistance due to the presence of rifampicin alone in extradural compartments has led to the inclusion of other intravenous antibiotics such as flucloxacillin or, in the case of methicillin-resistance, vancomycin. Teicoplanin can be substituted on the grounds of its lower toxicity for intravenous use. Teicoplanin has been used intraventricularly in a few cases. Venditti et al. (86) treated two cases of methicillin-resistant *S. aureus* (MRSA) shunt infection with 20 mg and 40 mg daily intraventricularly, and Fernandez Guerrero et al. (87) used 10 mg daily in two cases due to methicillin-resistant *S. epidermidis* (MRSE) and one due to enterococci. In all four cases the shunt was removed. The CSF levels were greater than four to eight times the minimal inhibitory concentration (MIC), and the infections were rapidly eradicated. The two glycopeptides have been compared (88). The use of linezolid has been considered in infections due to glycopeptide-resistant cocci. The drug has been shown to give therapeutic CSF concentrations after 600 mg twice daily intravenously, when measured at between 6 and 12 days after start of treatment of meningitis due to MRSE or MRSA (89). It was assumed that the inflammatory response had subsided at this time. Linezolid has been shown to have good activity against teicoplanin-resistant CoNS (90). Although the recommended regimen includes shunt removal, and clinical evidence supports this, Brown and Jones (91) have reported success with CoNS but not *S. aureus* using intraventricular vancomycin and oral rifampicin without shunt removal in selected patients. In cases where further surgery is contra-indicated, this approach should be considered.

Treatment of Shunt Infection Caused by Gram-Negative Bacilli

Treatment should be similar to that for meningitis caused by these organisms but the shunt should be removed. Meningeal inflammation is usually sufficient to ensure therapeutic CSF concentrations of antimicrobials such as third-generation cephalosporins, carbapenems, and quinolones with intravenous administration. Duration of treatment will vary depending on clinical and microbiological response and will range from 10 to 20 days, but should be as short as possible to avoid secondary infection from external drainage.

Treatment of Shunt Infection Caused by Fungi

Shunt infections due to *Candida* or *Cryptococcus* should be treated by shunt removal and antifungal therapy such as fluconazole 6 mg/kg daily for 10–14 days (92). In some cases where intravenous administration of amphotericin does not give adequate CSF levels, intraventricular administration can be considered (46). However, it should be noted that this can cause serious side effects (93). Combination of amphotericin with flucytosine allows the use of lower doses of amphotericin (94).

Treatment of Community-Acquired Meningitis in Shunted Patients

Though the rule for successful treatment of shunt infection is shunt removal, community-acquired meningitis in shunted patients is an exception. In such cases the shunt should not be removed, as there appears to be no risk of its becoming colonized by the infecting bacteria, and shunted patients recover more quickly than those without shunts. Such infections should be treated in the same way as pneumococcal, meningococcal, or *Haemophilus* meningitis (1,95–99).

Infections Caused by Visceral Perforation

The lower catheter of a VP shunt sometimes perforates hollow viscera such as the large bowel, vagina, bladder, or scrotal sac. In such cases, the patient is often well with little or no clinical evidence of infection (47,48), though polymicrobial ventriculitis might be present. There is rarely evidence of peritonitis (49,50) and laparotomy is contraindicated, the perforation healing spontaneously. The shunt should be removed, with gentle traction on the lower catheter being all that is necessary to remove it. Broad-spectrum antimicrobials such as amoxicillin-clavulanate or a second-generation cephalosporin should be given along with metronidazole for 14 days or until the infection is eradicated. Reshunting, if necessary, may need to be by the VA route.

External Shunt Infections

As soon as external infection of the shunt is suspected, intravenous antimicrobials should be given. Cefuroxime is recommended for staphylococci and Gram-negative bacilli but, in the case of MRSA or MRSE, gentamicin and vancomycin or teicoplanin should be substituted. For resistant Gram-negative bacilli such as *Pseudomonas aeruginosa*, ceftazidime or a quinolone should be given. However, unless treatment is started early, the shunt is very unlikely to be salvaged. Signs of shunt obstruction or peritonitis, persistent fever, or continuing erythema or purulence around the shunt should prompt its immediate removal and continuance of antimicrobials for an additional 14 days before reshunting on the opposite side.

Prevention

General Measures

An appreciation of the etiology of shunt infections is essential to planned prevention. For practical purposes, all shunt infections are contracted at surgery to insert or revise them, and it is this event to which prevention strategies should be directed. One of the most powerful factors is the experience and expertise of the surgeon (100), but too often shunt surgery is delegated to juniors because of its apparent technical simplicity. As it is clear that most of the infecting organisms are derived from the patient's skin or mucous membranes (8,9,17), the lack of convincing reports of the benefit from measures such as ultraclean air or exhaust suits (7) is not unexpected. Review of agents for skin preparation prior to incision has shown that an alcoholic formulation is superior to an aqueous one, and that chlorhexidine is better than povidone iodine (1,16,17). However, it must be realized that the skin surface will remain free of viable bacteria for a limited time only (16,17). Extensive shaving of the scalp is unnecessary, and the value of any shaving is questionable (101,102). Shaving damages the skin and, if used, it must be carried out immediately before surgery rather than the previous day to avoid formation of microfoci of infection in the skin. In most cases, clipping of the scalp hair is sufficient. The hair should have been thoroughly shampooed and dried shortly before surgery, and should again be wetted with alcoholic chlorhexidine during skin preparation. Any alcoholic preparations must be allowed to dry completely before surgery commences, and any pooling of alcohol beneath the patient should be removed to avoid risk of burns when diathermy is used. Attempts have been made to reduce the infection rate using barriers of gauze soaked in an antibiotic or antiseptic (103,104) at the skin edges in the incision, but a proper trial has not been undertaken. Similarly, impervious adhesive plastic drapes have been used, but studies in other areas of surgery have either not shown a significant difference in wound contamination, or have shown an increase in contamination during shunt surgery (19,103,105).

Antimicrobial Prophylaxis

Many studies have been carried out to investigate the efficacy of prophylactic antimicrobials in shunt surgery. A variety of agents has been given intravenously preoperatively, with beta-lactams such as flucloxacillin, methicillin, oxacillin, or nafcillin being the most common. As stated previously, none of these agents gives antimicrobial concentrations in the CSF in the absence of meningeal inflammation, and are therefore unlikely to have any effect on the incidence of shunt infection, with the possible exception of external infection.

The same is true for aminoglycosides and glycopeptides (70). Tissue in the incision may show antimicrobial concentrations during surgery, but this is accompanied by an unchanged number of viable, susceptible bacteria, probably due to the extremely slow bactericidal action of antibiotics (106). Cotrimoxazole has been used (107) in a double-blind randomized controlled trial in the expectation that antimicrobial concentrations of trimethoprim would be attained, but there was no effect on infection rate. Interestingly, Blomstedt et al. (108) also used cotrimoxazole with a similar regimen and claimed a highly significant beneficial effect, but this could have been due to the very high rate (23%) in their control group compared to 6% in the prophylaxis group. In fact, only some of those studies involving very high infection rates have shown an effect of antimicrobial prophylaxis. A review of publications on antibiotic prophylaxis in shunt surgery has been carried out by Brown et al. (109), in which the validity of the published trials was assessed according to whether they were controlled, randomized, used historical controls, contained sufficient numbers of patients to overcome α and β errors, and other factors. Almost all the trials were flawed in their design so that the data could not be used. The most common flaws were the nature of the controls and the numbers of patients enrolled. If an infection rate of 5% to 7% in controls is expected from previous clinical audit, approximately 700 patients would be required to show a statistically significant result with satisfactory attention to α and β errors. It is now considered unlikely that a satisfactory, properly constructed trial of sufficient size will ever be undertaken successfully.

Three recent meta-analyses have been carried out in an attempt to resolve the issue. Reider et al. (110) analyzed five trials and did not detect a significant effect. Langley et al. (111) reviewed 37 studies from which they chose 12 that met their criteria for validity. In this group, only one trial claimed a significant benefit, but Langley et al. concluded, on the basis of their meta-analysis of the group, that antimicrobial prophylaxis was beneficial. Similarly, Haines and Walters (112) reviewed nine publications, eight of which appeared in Langley's study, and found a beneficial effect after meta-analysis. These three meta-analyses have been reviewed by Brown et al. (109). The findings of this review were that the meta-analyses themselves could be criticized for poorly discriminating inclusion criteria, some of the studies included not complying with the criteria laid down by the authors. The conclusion of statistically significant benefit on these grounds was therefore very weak. In addition, the protective effect of antimicrobial prophylaxis, where it reached statistical significance, was again limited to studies with control infection rates higher then 15%, different factors probably being involved. Internal and external infections were not usually distinguished. Also, many different antimicrobial agents and regimens were used such that the findings could not be used to guide the practitioner as to which to use, if any. Almost all reports forming the basis of assessments of the incidence of shunt infection are derived from studies where antimicrobial prophylaxis has been used, yet rates above 10% are not uncommon (113). The report of the British Society for Antimicrobial Chemotherapy (85) stated that there was no clearly proven benefit to be expected from the use of antimicrobial prophylaxis in shunt surgery. However, if surgeons felt that they should use prophylaxis, the report recommended that vancomycin 10 mg and gentamicin 3 mg be instilled into the ventricular system at operation. If external shunt infections are seen to be a particular local problem, a first- or second-generation cephalosporin such as cephradine or cefuroxime, or alternatively amoxicillin-clavulanate, should be given intravenously at induction of anesthesia.

Antimicrobial Prophylaxis in Dental and Other Procedures in Shunted Patients: Though a connection between dental procedures and shunt infection, particularly VA, has been assumed, no evidence exists to support this despite searches and surveys. All cases suspected to be due to bacteremia from dental procedures were shown to be unconnected (1). There is no evidence for the use of prophylactic antimicrobials in other procedures thought to constitute a risk to the shunt. Pittman et al. (114) reviewed 44 abdominal operations, 18 involving opening of the gastrointestinal tract, and there were no subsequent infections whether prophylactic antibiotics were used or not.

Shunt Soaking

The practice of soaking and flushing shunts with antibiotic solution is widespread, with gentamicin or a cephalosporin most popular. However, no trials have been carried out to investigate the efficacy. A recent study (115) of the time taken to kill bacteria by irrigation fluid containing either antibiotics or elemental iodine showed that antibiotics are very slow to kill bacteria, whereas 100% were killed by 40 ppm iodine in seconds. Further investigations showed that this concentration was not toxic to neural tissue in a rat study. No clinical data are yet available.

Antimicrobial Shunt Catheters

A variety of antimicrobial catheters is available for vascular access or for other sites such as the urinary tract. Most of these are coated either with a ligand or reservoir for antibiotics or with silver compounds and/or antiseptics. Few are applicable to central nervous system use. One which has been recommended for prevention of shunt infection is coated with hydrogel (116). The claims are that the hydrogel surface, being hydrophilic, reduces bacterial attachment to the catheter surface (and, by implication, reduces infection rate), and that if antibiotics are dissolved in the water used to soak the catheter and rehydrate the hydrogel before use, they are taken up and released after implantation, again reducing the infection rate. A laboratory study (116) showed that antibacterial activity on agar plates lasted for between 2 and

84 hours depending on the antibiotics used, but eventual attachment of bacteria to the catheters was not prevented. These results were obtained despite the authors' use of antibiotic concentrations typically 50,000 times higher than the MIC for the bacteria in question. An animal implantation study by the same authors (117) revealed a puzzling phenomenon of abscess formation around hydrogel-coated, but not plain, catheters in the presence of either live or dead *S. epidermidis*. Nevertheless, two clinical trials have been carried out. The first (118) did not show a statistically significant difference for gentamicin-soaked hydrogel catheters. The second (119) claimed a significant difference, again with gentamicin-soaked catheters, but used historical controls and stratified groups of small numbers of patients, and Type II (β) error cannot be ruled out. The question of whether the hydrogel catheters are coated on the inner surface, where the great majority of shunt infections begin, has been addressed using confocal microscopy of tetracycline-soaked catheters. At pH 4.0, this antibiotic fluoresces bright green in UV light. Fluorescence was confined to the outer surface (Roger Bayston, 2003) indicating no hydrogel on the inner surface. Anecdotal reports suggest that, in situations of high incidence of external shunt infection, the external hydrogel coating might be beneficial in reducing bacterial attachment.

In the early 1980s, we investigated processes by which antimicrobial agents could be impregnated into silicone catheters (120), and a range of agents was later tested for the ability to protect shunt catheters against bacterial challenge in a simulation model with flow conditions over several weeks (121). The two agents in combination that were clearly superior to any others were rifampicin and clindamycin, and extensive further testing of these agents was undertaken. The amount of antimicrobials in the catheters was relatively small (0.54%), but they appeared to be effective and to remain so over approximately 50 days in perfusion conditions. A similar process was used by Hampl et al. (122) to introduce rifampicin alone into shunt catheters, at a concentration of 9%. This led to crystal formation on the catheter surface which was said to be beneficial. We have shown that subtle changes in mechanical properties of silicone occur at rifampicin concentrations above 2% (123). The rifampicin plus clindamycin-impregnated catheters have been found to be unaffected by plasma protein conditioning film such as is found in neonates following periventricular hemorrhage or in adults with subarachnoid hemorrhage (124). These treated catheters have also been shown not to inhibit bacterial adherence but to kill all the adhered bacteria within 48–52 hours (125). In addition, all attempts to select resistant mutants have failed, probably due to the presence of two agents with different bacterial target sites. Shunt catheters impregnated in this way are now commercially available, and early clinical results are very encouraging, though formal clinical trial results are awaited.

Role of Staff Training and Experience in Prevention

The design and execution of many clinical trials in prevention of shunt infection are rendered ineffective by the failure to recruit the expected number of infections in the control group. The numbers, based on the pretrial infection rate, fall at commencement of the trial, often necessitating an extension to the trial period to achieve statistical power. This is known as the Hawthorn Effect (126). This phenomenon is due to a general increase in awareness of the problem and a corresponding heightening of enthusiasm and care taken by all personnel involved. This is perhaps the clearest indication that the most powerful preventive measure must be continuing education and training of all staff involved in shunting to ensure constant high standards. The tendency to delegate the relatively simple technique of shunt insertion or revision to less experienced surgeons should be resisted.

EXTERNAL VENTRICULAR DRAINAGE

Introduction

External Drainage Devices

External ventricular drainage is used as a temporary means of controlling CSF pressure, either following hemorrhage or trauma or in the course of shunt revision for infection. The drainage devices consist of a ventricular catheter resembling that of the CSF shunt, and a collecting system incorporating an antireflux component such as a drip chamber or a nonreturn valve, various injection ports and three-way taps, and a collection bag (Fig. 4). They are usually tunnelled under the scalp for several centimeters between the exit site and the burr hole.

Etiology and Pathogenesis of External Drainage Device Infections

Infection associated with external ventricular drainage can take the form of ventriculitis, exit-site infection, or tunnel infection, or a combination of these. The causative organisms are usually members of the skin flora, with *S. epidermidis* and *S. aureus* predominating. Bacteria can enter the EVD system on changing the collecting system or the bag, and this is also a potential source of both enteric and environmental Gram-negative bacilli. Infection becomes more likely the longer the EVD is in place, and after 8–10 days the incidence rises steeply. As patients become ambulant, the collecting system can become disconnected or the bag punctured or compressed. In the case of babies, contamination of the connection sites can occur from fecal soiling or from bathing. The paucity of published data on EVD infection probably reflects the view that EVD management is a nursing concern rather than a medical one, and nurses often receive little training in EVD management. The solution to this problem is obvious. Consequences of EVD infection include greatly increased resource expenditure with longer hospital stay, repeated surgery, delayed shunting, and sometimes death. Published studies are generally not illuminating. Mori and Raimondi (127)

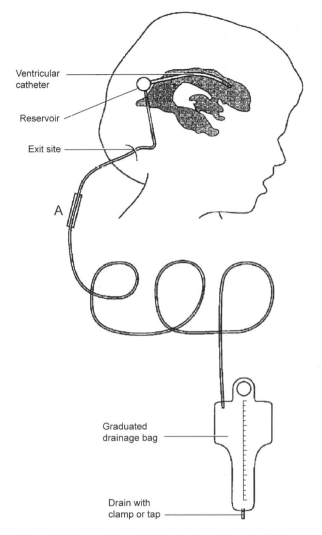

Figure 4 External ventricular drainage for raised intracranial pressure. (A) Either a drip chamber or a unidirectional valve to prevent reflux of fluid. Other designs may have an integral manometer for pressure measurement, three-way taps, injection ports, etc. The drainage bag is usually designed to be discarded when full, but some have a drain so that the bag can be emptied and reused without disconnection.

treated 23 cases of shunt infection with EVD for an average of three weeks, revising each electively after two weeks. Secondary infection, mainly due to Gram-negative bacilli, was encountered but the incidence was not stated. Santini et al. (128) treated 27 cases, eight with shunt infection, for an average of 13 days and reported secondary infection due to CoNS (two cases) and *P. aeruginosa.* Anwar (129) found two infections in 19 patients, and Leonhardt (130) and Chan et al. (131) found none in 13 cases and 34 cases, respectively. In a series of 37 preterm neonates reported by Berger et al. (132), in which the mean duration of EVD was 23 days, there were two cases of ventriculitis. Holloway et al. (133) reviewed the literature and reported infection rates of up to 40% but more commonly 10–17%. In a large series of 100 patients (134) treated for long periods (40 had EVD for 10–29 days), the infection rate was 2% but rose to 13% in those who had a CSF leak around the ventricular catheter. This can arise due to poor catheter placement or to inadequate CSF pressure control. It is clearly a significant risk factor for infection. One of the problems in comparing published accounts is that there is usually no distinction made between ventriculitis and tunnel or exit-site infection.

Clinical Features and Diagnosis

Pyrexia may be the first indication of EVD infection, especially in the case of ventriculitis. Exit-site infections or tunnel infections are indicated by erythema and exudate around the catheter. A boggy swelling around the tunnelled segment indicates a CSF leak around the outside of the catheter, which may not be infected but is likely to become so unless addressed urgently. Exit-site cultures can help to guide therapy. CSF samples for investigation should be aspirated from the reservoir (if present) or the ventricular catheter. Samples taken from the collection bag are unreliable (135).

Treatment

Except for trivial exit-site infection, there is little likelihood of salvaging an EVD catheter if infection occurs. The best chance is afforded by early, vigorous antibiotic treatment but the catheter almost always has to be removed. A replacement catheter may need to be retunnelled in another site. If ventriculitis is present, intraventricular treatment should also be given unless there is a vigorous inflammatory response. Initial treatment should consist of intravenous cefuroxime to cover most staphylococci and Gram-negative bacilli. This treatment may need adjustment when the causative organism has been identified and susceptibility tests completed. In the case of MRSA or MRSE, intravenous vancomycin or teicoplanin and oral (or intravenous) rifampicin should be given, and this supplemented with intraventricular vancomycin in the case of CoNS. The inflammatory response in the case of Gram-negative bacilli and *S. aureus* is usually sufficient to allow therapeutic drug concentrations in the CSF on intravenous administration. If revision surgery is undertaken for a CSF leak, this should be considered to be infected until culture results are available, and cefuroxime should be started preoperatively and continued until results are known.

Prevention

Prophylactic antimicrobials are contraindicated for EVD, even though patients undergoing EVD as part of treatment of a shunt infection will receive them as part of the treatment. Zingale et al. (136) found a 10% infection rate despite prophylactic antibiotics, and Alleyne et al. (137) found no difference in infection rate whether antimicrobial prophylaxis was used or not. They pointed out that antimicrobial prophylaxis was likely to select resistant strains which then present greater therapeutic problems. They also calculated that discontinuing prophylaxis would save their institution $80,000 each year. Elective changing of the EVD catheter has been considered, and though Mayhall et al. (138) found that the rate could be reduced by a change at five days, no benefit was found by Holloway et al. (133) when the catheter was changed at either five days or later. They recommended that EVD catheters should therefore not be changed electively to avoid infection. The British Society for Antimicrobial Chemotherapy Report (139) agrees with this recommendation, and also does not recommend routine prophylactic antibiotics for EVD.

The contribution of good care and management of the EVD system in order to prevent infection cannot be overemphasized. Nursing staff should be thoroughly trained in this aspect. In addition, the exit site should be kept clean and dry by means of a dry dressing or an occlusive, transparent adhesive one. If the latter is used, the site must be thoroughly cleaned with alcoholic chlorhexidine and allowed to dry for a few minutes before application of the dressing. Whichever dressing is used, the first one must be applied in the operating room. Any exudate from the exit site must be reported.

Antimicrobial EVD catheters similar to those used for CSF shunting are becoming available, and they might contribute significantly to prevention of infection.

VENTRICULAR ACCESS RESERVOIRS

Introduction

Ventricular Reservoirs

Frequent ventricular access may be required for sampling of CSF, for measuring CSF pressure, or for intraventricular administration of antibiotics or drugs to treat malignancy. The ventricular reservoir allows this percutaneously. The reservoir consists of a ventricular catheter, similar to that in a shunt, connected to a blind dome-shaped chamber whose roof is made of silicone elastomer. The base may be silicone or steel to prevent it from being pierced (Fig. 5). The chamber should be positioned extracranially under a scalp flap well away from the incision.

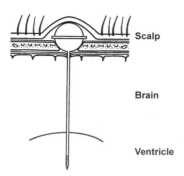
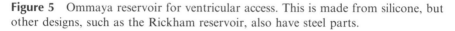

Scalp

Brain

Ventricle

Figure 5 Ommaya reservoir for ventricular access. This is made from silicone, but other designs, such as the Rickham reservoir, also have steel parts.

Etiology and Pathogenesis of Ventricular Reservoir Infections

The main causative bacteria are skin flora, with CoNS predominating. CSF leak around the reservoir is a risk factor for infection. Otherwise, repeated puncture of the reservoir, and overlying scalp, is the main risk, though if the scalp is properly prepared and fine needles are used, the risk is low. Nevertheless, Chamberlain and Dirr (140) treated patients with AIDS-related lymphoma by daily puncture for several months and found a 10%–15% infection rate.

Clinical Features

Apart from pyrexia and headache, erythema, and boggy swelling around the reservoir are indicators of infection.

Treatment

Treatment is relatively simple. Removal of the infected reservoir and insertion of a new one is advisable but some have succeeded without this (141). However, antibiotics must be administered intraventricularly via the reservoir. Sutherland et al. (142) were unsuccessful in an attempt to treat a patient with intravenous vancomycin for CoNS reservoir infection. The peak CSF vancomycin level was found to be subtherapeutic, but when the drug was given via the reservoir the infection was cleared. Lishner (143) also used intraventricular vancomycin successfully. It is therefore recommended that staphylococcal infections be treated with intraventricular vancomycin 10–20 mg daily for five days, preferably after changing the reservoir. It appears that the new reservoir can be inserted through the same burr hole after vancomycin treatment has begun without risk of reinfecting it. In the event of *P. aeruginosa* infection, the reservoir should be changed immediately, and high-dose intravenous ceftazidime given along with gentamicin 3–5 mg daily via the reservoir.

Prevention

As with EVD, prophylactic antimicrobials are not indicated, and prevention consists of care of the scalp over the reservoir and aseptic puncture technique.

INTRASPINAL DRUG DELIVERY DEVICES

Introduction

Intraspinal Drug Delivery Devices

The direct infusion of drugs into the spinal theca has been shown to give superior control of otherwise intractable pain and prolonged relaxation of spasticity, compared to intramuscular or intravenous injection. It is achieved by implantation of a delivery catheter into the theca and a reservoir incorporating a programmable infusion pump (Fig. 6) which is sited in the

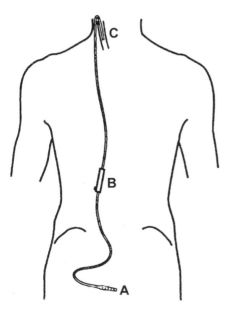

Figure 6 Peritoneovenous shunt for control of intractable ascites. (A) Peritoneal catheter with inlet holes; (B) unidirectional valve to prevent reflux; (C) distal catheter to jugular vein. Alternatively, the distal catheter may drain ascitic fluid to the portal vein. The shunt is made from silicone.

flank. The reservoir is charged subcutaneously. Infrequent change of the long-life batteries requires further surgery.

Etiology and Pathogenesis of Intraspinal Drug Delivery Device Infections

The sources of infection are contamination at the time of insertion, and of the reservoir when charging. Du Pen (144) reviewed the literature and reported an infection rate of up to 12%. Byers et al. (145) studied 81 catheter placements and found that, in seven infections (9%), the causative bacteria were again members of the skin flora. The main risk factor in their study was insertion time prolonged beyond 100 minutes. Six of the seven infections involved either the pocket or the tunnel with two showing meningeal involvement.

Clinical Features

Back pain, pyrexia, and erythema over the reservoir indicate infection.

Treatment

Intravenous flucloxacillin or vancomycin should be given for a staphylococcal pocket or tunnel infection, and if the infection fails to resolve or if meningitis develops, the system should be removed where possible. However, the device can be used to administer intrathecal vancomycin via the reservoir. In one case of infection by CoNS, Bennett et al. (146) charged the reservoir with 50 mg/l vancomycin and programmed the pump to deliver 5 mg daily intrathecally for 30 days. The addition of oral rifampicin, 600 mg twice daily, probably contributed significantly to the eradication of the infection without removal of the device. The CSF concentration of vancomycin was 54 mg/l but, as with CSF shunt infections, no toxicity resulted. Vancomycin also appeared to be chemically compatible with baclophen. Such considerations are important when considering intraspinal drug administration if arachnoiditis is to be avoided. The authors suggested that, in retrospect, a shorter course of treatment would have sufficed. In the series reported by Byers (145), three infections were cured by device removal and systemic antibiotics, but a further four were treated with antibiotics without surgery, and their symptoms were said to be "satisfactorily suppressed." This approach is recommended in terminally ill patients when there is no central nervous system (CNS) involvement.

Prevention

In view of the association of prolonged operating time with infection (145), prophylactic antibiotics can be expected to reduce the risk from this source. One dose of intravenous cefazolin or flucloxacillin immediately before surgery is recommended. However, routine prophylaxis during use of the system is not indicated. Meticulous skin preparation and aseptic technique when charging the reservoir is essential.

PERITONEOVENOUS SHUNTS FOR ASCITES

Introduction

Use of Ascites Shunts and Incidence of Infection

Devices resembling hydrocephalus shunts are available for the control of ascites in cirrhosis or malignant liver disease (Fig. 7). They drain ascitic fluid from the peritoneal cavity to the venous system via the jugular vein. Reflux of blood is prevented by a nonreturn valve. Patients with intractable ascites are in the late stages of liver failure and shunts are intended to remain in place for only one or two years. They are required to drain a large volume of fluid with a high protein content, and obstruction is a major problem. Infection can also occur, giving rise to peritonitis, colonization of the shunt, and bloodstream infection. *S. aureus* and enteric Gram-negative bacilli have been implicated in most cases, and while many infections appear to be introduced at insertion, some appear later. An important factor may be the grossly impaired immunity of the ascitic peritoneal cavity.

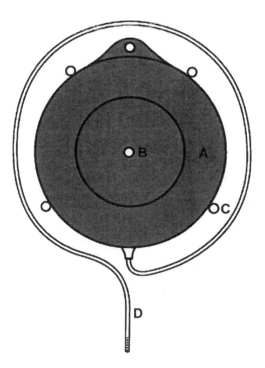

Figure 7 Totally implantable intraspinal drug delivery device. (A) Housing for reservoir, battery, and pump; (B) injection port for recharging reservoir; (C) loops for tissue fixation; (D) catheter to spinal theca.

Treatment of Infected Ascites Shunts

There are few published reports of infection in ascites shunts, but those that mention its management recommend shunt removal and intravenous antibiotics. The problem of the CNS compartment encountered with hydrocephalus shunts does not apply here, and the agents should be chosen on the basis of susceptibility test results, but gentamicin or cefuroxime should be given initially. The primary illness, the resulting impaired immunity, and the presence of bloodstream infection suggest that treatment should continue for at least three weeks.

Antimicrobial Prophylaxis

Although antimicrobial prophylaxis has been used at the time of insertion, the results have been disappointing. Smajda and Franco (147) used oral oxacillin, giving it for 10 days postoperatively, but 15 of 54 patients developed infection nevertheless. Hillaire et al. (148) reported similar results with ofloxacin and cefotetan. No clinical trial data are available to support any recommendations, but in view of the likely causative organisms, either gentamicin or cefuroxime should be given intravenously at induction of anesthesia, and not continued beyond 24 hours postoperatively.

SUMMARY AND CONCLUSION

In common with most implantable devices, those used in the CNS are prone to infection. In this instance almost all infecting bacteria are thought to originate on the patient's skin or mucous membranes. And the majority of infections are caused by staphylococci. Diagnosis, particularly of shunt infection, can be very difficult. The pharmacologically privileged nature of the CNS renders antimicrobial chemotherapy and prophylaxis problematic. While the mainstay of prevention is rigorous aseptic surgical technique, infection might be reduced still further by the use of new antimicrobial shunt catheters. Comprehensive clinical evidence of efficacy is awaited.

REFERENCES

1. Bayston R. Hydrocephalus Shunt Infections. London: Chapman and Hall, 1989.
2. Bayston R, Penny SR. Excessive production of mucoid substance by *Staphylococcus* SIIA: a possible factor in colonisation of Holter shunts. Dev Med Child Neurol 1972; 27(suppl 14):25–28.
3. Cochrane D, Kestle J, Steinbok P, Evans D, Heron N. Model for the cost analysis of shunted hydrocephalic children. Pediatr Neurosurg 1995; 23:14–19.
4. Drake J, Sainte-Rose C. The Shunt Book. Cambridge MA: Blackwell Science, 1995.

5. McClone DG, Czyzewski D, Raimondi AJ, Somers RC. Central nervous system infections as a limiting factor in the intelligence of children with meningomyelocele. Pediatrics 1982; 70:338–342.

6. Renier D, Sainte-Rose C, Pierre-Kahn A, Hirsch JF. Prenatal hydrocephalus: outcome and prognosis. Child's Nervous System 1988; 4:213–222.

7. Renier D, Lacombe J, Pierre-Khan A, Sainte-Rose C, Hirsch JF. Factors causing acute shunt infection. J Neurosurg 1984; 61:1072–1078.

8. Shapiro S, Boaz J, Kleiman M, Kalsbeck J, Mealey J. Origin of organisms infecting ventricular shunts. Neurosurgery 1988; 22:868–872.

9. Pople IK, Bayston R, Hayward RD. Infection of cerebrospinal fluid shunts in infants: a study of etiological factors. J Neurosurg 1992; 77:29–36.

10. George R, Leibrock L, Epstein M. Long-term analysis of cerebrospinal fluid shunt infections. J Neurosurg 1979; 51:804–811.

11. Ammirati M, Raimondi AJ. Cerebrospinal fluid shunt infections in children. A study of the relationship between the aetiology of hydrocephalus, age at time of shunt placement and infection rate. Child's Nervous System 1987; 3:106–109.

12. O'Kane MC, Richards H, Winfield P, Pickard JD. The United Kingdom Shunt registry. Europ J Pediatr Surg 1997; 7(suppl):56.

13. Walters BC, Hoffman HJ, Hendrick EB, Humphreys RP. Cerebrospinal fluid shunt infection. Influences on initial management and subsequent outcome. J Neurosurg 1984; 60:1014–1021.

14. Choux M, Genitori L, Lang D, Lena G. Shunt implantation: reducing the incidence of shunt infection. J Neurosurg 1992; 77:875–880.

15. Anderson FM. Ventriculo-auriculostomy in treatment of hydrocephalus. J Neurosurg 1959; 16:551–557.

16. Cohen SJ, Callaghan RP. Septicaemia due to colonisation of Spitz-Holter valves by Staphylococcus. Br Med J 1961; I:860–863.

17. Bayston R, Lari J. A study of the sources of infection in colonised shunts. Dev Med Child Neurol 1974; 16(suppl 32):16–22.

18. Raahave D. Bacterial density in operation wounds. Acta Chir Scand 1976; 140:585–593.

19. Raahave D. Effect of plastic skin and would drapes on the density of bacteria in operation wounds. Br J Surg 1976; 63:421–426.

20. Guevara JA, Zuccaro G, Trevisan A, Denoya CD. Bacterial adhesion to cerebrospinal fluid shunts. J Neurosurg 1987; 67:438–445.

21. Brydon HL, Kier G, Thompson EJ, Bayston R, Hayward RD, Harkness W. Protein adsorption to hydrocephalus shunt catheters. J Neurol Neurosurg Psychiatr 1998; 64:643–647.

22. Bayston R, Lambert E. Duration of protective activity of cerebrospinal fluid shunt catheters impregnated with antimicrobial agents to prevent bacterial catheter-related infection. J Neurosurg 1997; 87:247–251.

23. Brydon HL, Bayston R, Hayward R, Harkness W. Reduced bacterial adhesion to hydrocephalus shunts mediated by cerebrospinal fluid proteins. J Neurol Neurosurg Psychiatr 1996; 60:671–675.

24. Ljungh Å, Mortan AP, Wadström T. Interactions of bacterial adhesins with extracellular matrix and plasma proteins: pathogenic implications and therapeutic possibilities. FEMS Immunol Med Microbiol 1996; 16:117–126.

25. Gristina AG. Biomaterial-centred infection. Microbial adhesion versus tissue integration. Science 1987; 237:1588–1595.

26. Lundberg F, Schliamser S, Ljungh Å. Vitronectin may mediate staphylococcal adhesion to polymer surfaces in perfusing human cerebrospinal fluid. J Med Microbiol 1997; 46:285–296.

27. Lyte M, Neal C, Freestone P, Parkin J, Olson B, Bayston R, Williams PH. Catecholaminergic drug-induced *Staphylococcus epidermidis* biofilm formation in the presence of plasma. Lancet 2003; 361:130–135.

28. Kaplan K, Weinstein L. Diphtheroid infection of man. Ann Intern Med 1969; 70:919–929.

29. Bolton WK, Sande MA, Normansell DE, Sturgill BC, Westerbelt FB. Ventriculo-jugular shunt nephritis with *Corynebacterium bovis*. Successful therapy with antibiotics. Am J Med 1975; 59:417–423.

30. Moss SW, Gary NE, Eissinger RP. Nephritis associated with a diphtheroid-infected cerebrospinal fluid shunt. Am J Med 1977; 63:318–319.

31. O'Regan S, Makker SP. Shunt nephritis: demonstration of diphtheroid antigen in glomeruli. Am J Med Sci 1979; 278:161–165.

32. Hande KR, Witebski FG, Brown MS, Schulman CB, Anderson SE, Levine AS, Chabner BA. Sepsis with a new species of corynebacterium. Ann Intern Med 1976; 85:423–426.

33. Allen KD, Green HT. Infections due to "JK" coryneforms. J Infect 1986; 13:41–44.

34. Everett ED, Eickhoff TC, Simon RG. Cerebrospinal fluid shunt infections with anaerobic diphtheroids (propionibacterium species). J Neurosurg 1976; 44:580–584.

35. Beeler BA, Crowder JG, Smith JW, White A. *Propionibacterium acnes*: pathogen in central nervous system shunt infection. Report of three cases including immune complex glomerulonephritis. Am J Med 1976; 61:935–938.

36. Skinner PR, Taylor AJ, Coakham H. Propionibacteria as a cause of shunt and post neurosurgical infections. J Clin Pathol 1978; 31:1085–1089.

37. Brook I, Controni G, Rodriguez WJ, Martin WJ. Anaerobic bacteremia in children. Am J Dis Child 1980; 134:1052–1056.

38. Rekate HL, Ruch T, Nulsen FE. Diphtheroid infections of cerebrospinal fluid shunts. The changing pattern of shunt infection in Cleveland. J Neurosurg 1980; 52:553–556.

39. Lim BT, Avezaat CJ, Michel MF. Het voorkomen van propionibacterium acnes in bloed en liquor van neurochirurgische patienten. Ned Tjdschr Geneeskd 1980; 124:628–632.

40. Heck AF, Hameroff SB, Hornick RB. Chronic *Listeria monocytogenes* meningitis and normotensive hydrocephalus. Neurology 1971; 21:263–270.

41. Strife CF, McDonald BM, Ruley EJ, MacAdams AJ, West CD. Shunt nephritis: the nature of serum cryoglobulins and their relation to the complement profile. J Pediatr 1976; 88:403–413.

42. McLaurin RL. Infected cerebrospinal fluid shunts. Surg Neurol 1973; 1:191–195.

43. Caron C, Luneau C, Gervais MH, Plante GE, Sanchez G, Blain G. La glomerulonephrite de shunt: manifestations cliniques et histopathologiques. Can Med Assoc J 1979; 120:557–561.

44. Denoya CD, Trevisan AR, Zorzopulos J. Adherence of multiresistant strains of *Klebsiella pneumoniae* to cerebrospinal fluid shunts: correlation with plasmid content. J Med Microbiol 1986; 21:225–231.
45. Basset DC, Dickson JA, Hunt GH. Infection of Holter valve by Pseudomonas-contaminated chlorhexidine. Lancet 1973;i:1263–1264.
46. Sanchez-Portocarrero J, Martin-Rabadan P, Saldana CJ, Perez-Cecilia E. Candida cerebrospinal fluid shunt infection. Report of two new cases and review of the literature. Diagn Microbiol Infect Dis 1994; 20:33–40.
47. Brook I, Johnson N, Overturf G, Wilkins J. Mixed bacterial meningitis: a complication of ventriculo- and lumbo-peritoneal shunts. J Neurosurg 1977; 47:961–964.
48. Sami A, Ait Ben Ali S, Choukry M, Achouri M, Naja A, Ouboukhlik A, Elkamar A, Elazhari A, Boucetta M. Anal migration of ventriculoperitoneal shunt catheter. Apropos of 3 cases. Neuro-Chirurg 1995; 41:315–318.
49. Shinkawa H, Inoue T, Fujita T, Nojiri T, Furuya Y, Kuroda T, Naka S, Yasuhara H, Wada N. Unusual complication due to ventriculo-peritoneal shunt which peritoneal end perforated the rectum and protruded out of the anus: Report of a case. Jap J Gastroenterolog Surg 2001; 34:59–63.
50. Park C-K, Wang K-C, Seo Jeong Kee, Cho B-K. Transoral protrusion of a peritoneal catheter: A case report and literature review. Child's Nervous System 2000; 16:184–189.
51. Ingram CW, Haywood HB, Morris VM, Allen RL, Perfect JR. Cryptococcal ventricular-peritoneal shunt infection: clinical and epidemiological evaluation of two closely associated cases. Inf Control Hosp Epidemiol 1993; 14:719–722.
52. Tang IM. Ventriculoperitoneal shunt in cryptococcal meningitis with hydrocephalus. Surg Neurol 1990; 33:314–319.
53. Park MK, Hospenthal DR, Bennett JE. Treatment of hydrocephalus secondary to cryptococcal meningitis by use of shunting. Clin Infect Dis 1999; 28:629–633.
54. Upadhyaya P, Bhargava S, Sundaram KR, Mitra DK, George J, Singh DC. Hydrocephalus caused by tuberculous meningitis: clinical picture, CT findings and results of shunt surgery. Z Kinderchirurg 1983; 38(suppl II):76–80.
55. Lamprecht D, Schoeman J, Donald P, Hartzenberg H. Ventriculoperitoneal shunting in childhood tuberculous meningitis. Br J Neurosurg 2001; 15:119–125.
56. Bayston R, Swinden J. The aetiology and prevention of shunt nephritis. Zeit Kinderchirurg 1979; 28:377–384.
57. Stauffer UG. Shunt nephritis, a complication of ventriculo-atrial shunts. Dev Med Child Neuro 1970; 12(suppl 22):161–164.
58. Pinals RS, Tunnessen WW. Shunt arthritis. J Pediatr 1977; 91:681.
59. Nolan CM, Flanigan WJ, Rastogi SP, Brewer TE. Vancomycin penetration into CSF during treatment of patients receiving hemodialysis. South Med J 1980; 73:1333–1334.
60. Bayston R, Rodgers J. Role of serological tests in the diagnosis of immune complex disease in infection of ventriculoatrial shunts for hydrocephalus. Euro J Clin Microbiol Inf Dis 1994; 13:417–420.
61. Bayston R. Serological surveillance of children with CSF shunting devices. Dev Med Child Neurol 1975; 35(suppl 17):104–110.

62. Latchaw JP, Hahn JF. Intraperitoneal pseudocyst associated with ventriculoperitoneal shunt. Neurosurg 1981; 8:469–472.

63. Bayston R, Spitz L. Infective and cystic causes of obstruction of ventriculoperitoneal shunts for hydrocephalus. Zeit Kinderchirurg 1977; 22:419–424.

64. Castro-Gago M, Sanguinedo P, Garcia C, Pombo M, Ugarte J, Cabanas R, Pena J. Valor de la proteina C-reactiva (PCR) en el diagnostico de las complicaciones infecciosas de los "shunts" en nos ninos hidrocefalos. Ann Esp Pediatr 1982; 16:47–52.

65. Bayston R. Serum C-reactive protein test in diagnosis of septic complications of cerebrospinal fluid shunts for hydrocephalus. Arch Dis Child 1979; 54:545–547.

66. Bayston R, Leung TS, Wilkins BM, Hodges B. Bacteriological examination of removed cerebrospinal fluid shunts. J Clin Pathol 1983; 36:987–990.

67. Callaghan RP, Cohen SJ, Stewart GT. Septicaemia due to colonisation of Spitz-Holter valves by Staphylococcus. Br Med J 1961; 1:860–863.

68. Shurtleff DB, Foltz EL, Weeks RD, Loesser J. Therapy of *Staphylococcus epidermidis*: infections associated with cerebrospinal fluid shunts. Pediatr 1974; 53:52–62.

69. Spector R, Lorenzo AV. Inhibition of penicillin transport from the cerebrospinal fluid after intracisternal inoculation of bacteria. J Clin Invest 1974; 54:316–325.

70. Faillace WJ, Tan P. Serum and cerebrospinal fluid vancomycin and gentamicin concentrations during ventriculoperitoneal shunt surgery: An observational study. J Pharmacy Technol 2000; 16:155–160.

71. Ring JC, Cates KL, Bellani KK, Gaston TL, Sveum RJ, Marker SC. Rifampicin for CSF shunt infections caused by coagulase-negative staphylococci. J Pediatr 1979; 95:317–319.

72. Nau R, Prange HW, Menck S, Kolenda H, Visser K, Seydel JK. Penetration of rifampicin into the cerebrospinal fluid of adults with uninflamed meninges. 1992; 29:719–724.

73. Bayston R, Rickwood AMK. Factors involved in antibiotic treatment of cerebrospinal fluid shunt infections. Zeit Kinderchirurg 1981; 34:339–345.

74. Brown MRW, Collier PJ, Gilbert P. Influence of growth rate on susceptibility to antimicrobial agents: modification of cell envelope and batch and continuous culture studies. Antimicrob Ag Chemother 1990; 34:1623–1628.

75. Evans RC, Holmes CJ. Effect of vancomycin hydrochloride on *Staphylococcus epidermidis* biofilm associated with silicone elastomer. Antimicrob Ag Chemother 1987; 31:889–894.

76. James HE, Walsh JW, Wilson HD, Connor JD, Bean JR, Tibbs PA. Prospective randomised study of therapy in cerebrospinal fluid shunt infection. Neurosurg 1980; 7:459–463.

77. Chester DC, Penny SR, Emery JL. Fat-containing macrophages in the cerebrospinal fluid of children with hydrocephalus. Dev Med Child Neurol 1971; 13(suppl 25):33–38.

78. Grabb PA, Albright AL. Intraventricular vancomycin induced cerebrospinal fluid eosinophilia: report of two patients. Neurosurg 1992; 30:630–634.

79. Mandell GL, Moorman DR. Treatment of experimental staphylococcal

infections: effect of rifampicin alone and in combination on development of rifampicin resistance. Antimicrob Ag Chemother 1980; 17:658–662.

80. Ryan JL, Pachner A, Andriole VT, Root RK. Enterococcal meningitis: combined vancomycin and rifampicin therapy. Am J Med 1980; 68:449–451.

81. Young EJ, Ratner RE, Clarridge JE. Staphylococcal ventriculitis treated with vancomycin. South Med J 1981; 74:1014–1015.

82. Woodford N, Johnson AP, Morrison D, Speller DC. Current perspectives on glycopeptide resistance. Clin Microbiol Rev 1995; 8:585–615.

83. Visconti EB, Peters G. Vancomycin treatment of cerebrospinal fluid shunt infections. Report of two cases. J Neurosurg 1979; 51:245–246.

84. Gombert ME, Landesman SH, Corrado ML, Stein SC, Melvin ET, Cummings M. Vancomycin and rifampicin therapy for Staphylococcus epidermidis meningitis associated with CSF shunts. J Neurosurg 1981; 55:633–636.

85. Bayston R, de Louvois J, Brown EM, Hedges AJ, Johnston RA, Lees P. Treatment of infections associated with shunting for hydrocephalus. Working party on the use of antibiotics in neurosurgery of the British Society for Antimicrobial Chemotherapy. Br J Hosp Med 1995; 53:368–373.

86. Venditti M, Micozzi A, Serra P, Buniva G, Palma L, Martino P. Intraventricular administration of teicoplaninin shunt associated ventriculitis caused by methicillin resistant *Staphylococcus aureus*. J Antimicrob Chemother 1988; 21:513–515.

87. Fernandez Guerrero MLF, de Gorgolas M, Roblas RF, Campos JM. Treatment of cerebrospinal fluid shunt infections with teicoplanin. Eur J Clin Microbiol Inf Dis 1994; 13:1056–1058.

88. Murphy S, Pinney RJ. Teicoplanin or vancomycin in the treatment of gram-positive infections? J Clin Pharmacy and Therapeut 1995; 20:5–11.

89. Villani P, Regazzi MB, Marubbi F, Viale P, Pagani L, Cristini F, Cadeo B, Carosi G, Bergomi R. Cerebrospinal fluid linezolid concentrations in post-neurosurgical central nervous system infections. Antimicrob Ag Chemother 2002; 46:936–937.

90. Cercenado E, Garcia-Garrote F, Bouza E. In vitro activity of linezolid against multiply-resistant Gram positive clinical isolates. J Antimicrob Chemother 2001; 47:77–81.

91. Brown EM, Jones EM. Non-surgical management of CSF shunt infections. Eur J Pediatr Surg 1995; 5(suppl 1):26.

92. Cruciani M, Di Perri G, Mollesini M, Vento S, Concia E, Bassetti D. Use of fluconazole in the treatment of *Candida albicans* hydrocephalus shunt infection. Eur J Clin Microbiol Inf Dis 1992; 11:957.

93. Fisher JF, Dewald J. Parkinsonism associated with intraventricular amphotericin B. J Antimicrob Chemother 1983; 12:97–99.

94. Bennett JE, Dismukes WE, Duma RJ, Medoff G, Sande MA, Gallis H, Leonard J, Fields BT, Bradshaw M, Haywood II, McGee ZA, Cate TR, Cobbs CG, Warner JF, Alling DW. A comparison of amphotericin B alone and combined with flucytosine, in the treatment of cryptococcal meningitis. New Eng J Med 1979;301126–131.

95. Shurtleff DB, Foltz EL, Christie D. Ventriculoauriculostomy-associated infections: a 12 year study. J Neurosurg 1971; 35:686–694.

96. Rennels MB, Wald ER. Treatment of *Hemophilus influenzae* type b meningitis in children with cerebrospinal fluid shunts. J Pediatr 1980; 97:424–426.

97. Leggiadro RJ, Atluru VL, Katz SP. Meningococcal meningitis associated with cerebrospinal fluid shunts. Pediatr Inf Dis 1984; 3:489–490.

98. Stern S, Bayston R, Hayward R. *Hemophilus influenzae* meningitis in the presence of cerebrospinal fluid shunts. Child's Nerv Syst 1988; 4:164–165.

99. Patriarca PA, Lauer BA. Ventriculoperitoneal shunt-associated infection due to Hemophilus influenzae. Pediatr 1980; 65:1007–1009.

100. Borgbjerg BM, Gjerris F, Albeck MJ, Borgesen SE. Risk of infection after cerebrospinal fluid shunt: an analysis of 884 first-time shunts. Acta Neurochirurg 1995; 136:1–7.

101. Horgan MA, Piatt JH. Shaving of the scalp may increase the rate of infection in CSF shunt surgery. Pediatr Neurosurg 1997; 26:180–184.

102. Tang K, Yeh JS, Sgouros S. The influence of hair shave on the infection rate in neurosurgery. A prospective study. Pediatr Neurosurg 2001; 35:13–17.

103. Tabara Z, Forrest DM. Colonisation of CSF shunts: preventive measures. Zeit Kinderchirurg 1982; 37:156–158.

104. Fitzgerald R, Connelly B. An operative technique to reduce valve colonisation. Zeit Kinderchirurg 1984; 39(suppl II):107–109.

105. Jackson DW, Pollock AV, Tindall DS. The value of plastic adhesive drape in prevention of wound infection. A controlled trial. Br J Surg 1971; 58:340–342.

106. Bayston R. Antibiotic prophylaxis in shunt surgery. Dev Med Child Neurol 1975; 35(suppl 17):99–103.

107. Wang EEL, Prober CG, Hendrick EB, Hoffman HJ, Humphreys RP. Prophylactic sulphamethoxazole and trimethoprim in ventriculoperitoneal shunt surgery. A double blind, randomised, placebo-controlled trial. JAMA 1984; 251:1174–1177.

108. Blomstedt GC. Results of trimethoprim-sulphamethoxazole prophylaxis in ventriculostomy and shunting procedures. A double blind randomised trial. J Neurosurg 1985; 62:694–697.

109. Brown EM, de Louvois J, Bayston R, Hedges AJ, Johnston RA, Lees P. Antimicrobial prophylaxis in neurosurgery and after head injury. Lancet 1994; 344:1547–1551.

110. Reider MJ, Frewen TC, Del Maestro RF. The effect of cephalothin prophylaxis on postoperative ventriculoperitoneal shunt infections. Can Med Assoc J 1987; 136:935–938.

111. Langley JM, LeBlanc JC, Drake JM, Milner R. Efficacy of antimicrobial prophylaxis in cerebrospinal fluid shunt placement: a meta-analysis. Clin Inf Dis 1993; 17:98–103.

112. Haines SJ, Walters BC. Antibiotic prophylaxis for cerebrospinal fluid shunts: a meta-analysis. Neurosurg 1994; 34:87–92.

113. Sanchez-Carpintero R, Lopez de mesa R, Modesto C, Riol M, Sierrasesumaga L. Complications in the treatment of infantile hydrocephalus: retrospective study of cerebrospinal fluid derivations made at our center in the last fifteen years. Revista Espanola de Pediatria 1996; 52:327–330.

114. Pittman T, Williams D, Weber TR, Steinhardt G, Tracey T. The risk of abdominal operations in children with ventriculoperitoneal shunts. J Pediatr Surg 1992; 27:1051–1053.

115. Choi S, McComb JG, Levy ML, Gonzalez-Gomez I, Bayston R. Use of elemental iodine for shunt infection prophylaxis. J Neurosurg 2003; 52:908–913.
116. Boelens JJ, Tan W-F, Dankert J, Zaat SAJ. Antibacterial activity of antibiotic-soaked polyvinylpyrrolidone-grafted silicon elastomer hydrocephalus shunts. J Antimicrob Chemother 2000a; 45:221–224.
117. Boelens JJ, Zaat SAJ, Meeldijk J, Dankert J. Subcutaneous abscess formation around catheters induced by viable and nonviable *Staphylococcus epidermidis* as well as by small amounts of bacterial cell wall components. J Biomed Mater Res 2000b; 50:546–556.
118. Nomura S, Adachi H, Fujii M, Akimura T, Kakino S, Kubota H, Yamashita K, Ito H. Prevention and treatment of cerebrospinal fluid shunt-induced infections using silicone catheters with Bioglide modification. Curr Tr Hyd (Tokyo) 1999; 9:79–83.
119. Takahashi Y. Prevention of pediatric shunt infection-inhibitory effect on shunt infection by hydrogelprocessed shunt catheters. Curr Tr Hyd (Tokyo) 2001; 11:42–48.
120. Bayston R, Milner RDG. Antibacterial activity of silicone rubber used in hydrocephalus shunts, after impregnation with antimicrobial substances. J Clin Pathol 1981; 34:1057–1062.
121. Bayston R, Grove N, Seigel J, Lawellin D, Barsham S. Prevention of hydrocephalus shunt catheter colonization in vitro by impregnation with antimicrobials. J Neurol Neurosurg Psychiatr 1989; 52:605–609.
122. Hampl J, Schierholz J, Jansen B, Aschoff A. In vitro and in vivo efficacy of a rifampin-loaded silicone catheter for the prevention of CSF shunt infections. Acta Neurochir (Wien) 1995; 133:147–152.
123. Bayston R. Effect of antibiotic impregnation on the function of slit valves used to control hydrocephalus. Zeit Kinderchir 1980; 31:353–359.
124. Bayston R, Lambert E. Duration of activity of cerebrospinal fluid shunt cathetersimpregnated with antimicrobials toprevent bacterial catheter-related infection. J Neurosurg 1997; 87:247–251.
125. Bayston R, Ashraf W, Bhundia C. Mode of action of an antimicrobial shunt catheter. Eur J Pediatr Surg 2000; 12:S56.
126. Entwistle NJ, Nisbet JD. Educational Research in Action. London: University of London Press, 1972.
127. Mori K, Raimondi AJ. An analysis of external ventricular drainage as a treatment for infected shunts. Child's Brain 1975; 1:1975, 243–250.
128. Santini J-J, Billard C, Boissonnet H, Borderon JC. Surveillance bactériologique des dérivations ventriculaires externés chez l'enfant. Neurochururgie 1982; 28:379–382.
129. Anwar M, Doyle AJ, Kadam S, Hiatt M, Hegyi T. Management of posthemorrhagic hydrocephalus in the preterm infant. J Pediatr Surg 1986; 21:334–337.
130. Leonhardt A, Steiner H-H, Linderkamp O. Management of posthemorrhagic hydrocephalus with a subcutaneous ventricular catheter reservoir in preterm infants. Arch Dis Child 1989; 64:24–28.
131. Chan K-H, Mann KS. Prolonged therapeutic external ventricular drainage: a prospective study. Neurosurgary 1988; 23:436–438.
132. Berger A, Weninger M, Reinprecht A, Haschke N, Kolhauser C, Pollak A,

Steinbook P. Longterm experience with subcutaneously tunneled external ventricular drainage in preterm infants. Child's Nervous System 2000; 16:103–110.

133. Holloway KL, Barnes T, Choi S, Bullock R, Marshal LF, Eisenberg HM, Jane JA, Ward JD, Young HF, Marmarou A. Ventriculostomy infections: the effect of monitoring duration and catheter exchange in 584 patients. J Neurosurg 1996; 85:419–424.

134. Bogdahn U, Lau W, Hassel W, Gunreben G, Mertens HG, Brawanski A. Continuous pressure-controlled external ventricular drainage for treatment of acute hydrocephalus - Evaluation of risk factors. Neurosurgery 1992; 31:898–904.

135. Scarff TB, Nelson PB, Reigel DH. External drainage for ventricular infection following cerebrospinal fluid shunts. Child's Brain 1978; 4:129–136.

136. Zingale A, Ippolito S, Pappalardo P, Chibbaro S, Amoroso R, Humansky F, Di Rocco C, Brambilla G. Infections and re-infections in longterm external ventricular drainage: A variation upon a theme. J Neurol Sci 1999; 43:125–133.

137. Alleyne CH, Hassan M, Zabramski JM, Hall WA, Kelly DF, Macdonald RL, McComb JG, Milhorat TH. The efficacy and cost of prophylactic and periprocedural antibiotics in patients with external ventricular drains. 2000; 47:1124–1129.

138. Mayhall CG, Archer NH, Lamb VA, Spadora AC, Baggett JW, Ward JD, Narayan RK. Ventriculostomy-related infections. A prospective epidemiologic study. N Engl J Med 1984; 310:553–559.

139. Brown EM, de Louvois J, Bayston R, Lees PD, Pople IK. The management of neurosurgical patients with postoperative bacterial or aseptic meningitis or external ventricular drain-associated ventriculitis. Br J Neurosurg 2000; 14:7–12.

140. Chamberlain MC, Dirr L. Involved-filed radiotherapy and intra-Ommaya methotrexate/cytarabine in patients with AIDS-related lymphomatous meningitis. J Clin Oncol 1993; 11:1978–1984.

141. Hirsch BE, Amodio M, Einzig AI, Halevy R, Soeiro R. Instillation of vancomycin into a cerebrospinal fluid reservoir to clear infection. Pharmacokinetic considerations. J Infect Dis 1991; 163:197–200.

142. Sutherland GE, Palitang EG, Marr JJ, Lwedke SL. Sterilization of an Ommaya reservoir by instillation of vancomycin. Em J Med 1981; 71:1068–1070.

143. Lishner M, Scheinbaum R, Messner HA. Intrathecal vancomycin in the treatment of Ommaya reservoir infection by *Staphylococcus epidermidis*. Scand J Infect Dis 1991; 23:10–14.

144. Du Pen SL, Peterson DG, Williams A, Bogosian AJ. Infection during chronic epidural catheterization: diagnosis and treatment. Anesthesiol 1990; 73:905–909.

145. Byers K, Axelrod P, Michaerl S, Rosen S. Infections complicating tunneled intraspinal catheter systems used to treat chronic pain. Clin Infect Dis 1995; 21:403–408.

146. Bennett MI, Tai YMA, Symonds JM. Staphylococcal meningitis following Synchromed intrathecal pump implant: a case report. Pain 1994; 56:243–244.

147. Smajda C, Franco D. The leVeen shunt in the elective treatment of intractable ascites in cirrhosis. A prospective study on 140 patients. Ann Surg 1985; 210, 488–493.

148. Hillaire S, Labianca M, Borgonovo G, Smajda C, Grange D, Franco D. Peritoneovenous shunting of intractable ascites in patients with cirrhosis: improving results and predictive factors of failure. Surgery 1993; 113:373–379.

16

Infections Associated with Chronic Peritoneal Dialysis

Henri A. Verbrugh

Erasmus University Medical Center Rotterdam
Rotterdam, The Netherlands

INTRODUCTION

Chronic peritoneal dialysis (CPD) is increasingly used as the renal replacement therapy of choice in many countries. The number of patients on CPD was approximately 4000 in 1980 but reached 95,200 by the end of 1994 (1). The annual increase from 1991 to 1994 was 15%. The proportion of patients with end-stage renal disease treated by CPD (versus hemodialysis) varies considerably from country to country, being less than 10% in Italy, France, Germany, and Japan, and 50% or greater in the United Kingdom, New Zealand, and Mexico. These differences are thought to be largely due to national differences in the way renal replacement therapy is organized and reimbursed. The CPD technique per se is not questioned. In contrast, CPD has been validated in many studies, and, although there are limits in dialysis adequacy, CPD has several advantages over hemodialysis (2,3). Currently, two types of CPD are practiced: continuous ambulatory peritoneal dialysis (CAPD) and continuous cyclic peritoneal dialysis (CCPD). Continuous ambulatory peritoneal dialysis was first introduced in the late 1970s by Popovich et al. (4) and Oreopoulos et al. (5) as a machine-free regimen that entailed the continuous presence of dialysate in the peritoneal cavity. Approximately every 6 h, dialysate is exchanged for fresh PD fluid using only gravitational forces to drain and refill the abdominal cavity. CCPD was introduced in the early 1980s to take care of patients who were incapable of performing the exchanges manually or who were unwilling to interrupt their daily routines for dialysate exchanges (6). In CCPD, rapid nocturnal fluid exchanges are performed through a bedside cycling machine. Miniaturization technology has now allowed such machines to become easily portable, further improving patients' freedom to schedule their own activities. By the end of 1994, approximately 25% of all CPD in the United States was of the CCPD variety.

From the very beginning of peritoneal dialysis in the 1960s, the technique has been plagued by infectious complications—especially, high rates of acute bacterial peritonitis. The introduction by Tenckhoff and Schechter (7) of a tunnelled catheter segment with Dacron felt cuffs at either end of its track through the abdominal wall was the first major step forward in reducing the risk of infection (Fig. 1). With the popularization of CAPD in the 1980s, much attention has been given to further improve aseptic techniques, especially during the exchange procedure. Many devices have been proposed,

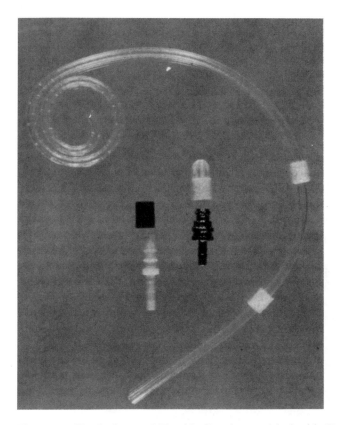

Figure 1 Classical curved Tenckhoff catheter with double Dacron felt cuffs.

including in-line bacterial filters, ultraviolet light-based germicidal boxes, and antiseptic-containing cuffs around the external connectors. Reductions in peritonitis rates have been consistently observed only in those centers that have switched to integrated "Y systems" that flush the potentially contaminated connector with sterile dialysate before fresh dialysate enters the peritoneum (8–10). Even so, peritonitis and infection at the exit site or in the tunnel track around the Tenckhoff catheter remain prevalent problems in most CPD programs around the world.

PATHOGENESIS OF CAPD PERITONITIS

Different routes of bacterial invasion into the peritoneal cavity exist in CAPD patients. The most common access for coagulase-negative staphylococci, *Staphylococcus aureus*, and other Gram-positive pathogens is via the Tenckhoff catheter. In contrast, enteric bacilli may reach the peritoneal cavity by direct transmigration (also known as translocation) from the gut across the intestinal wall (11–13). Intestinal pathologies including diverticulosis and ischemic or ulcerative bowel diseases may facilitate this mode of peritoneal contamination (14). A third route is hematogenous spread from a distant focus to the peritoneum; this route may be important in peritonitis due to streptococci, *Listeria*, and *Hemophilus* (15). Finally, infections ascending through the fallopian tubes may be the cause of peritonitis in women undergoing CAPD (15). Most episodes are due to organisms of the patient's own microflora. Thus, carriers of *S. aureus* are at a three- to fivefold increased risk of *S. aureus* exit-site infection when compared to noncarriers (as will be discussed later).

The sequence of events following peritoneal contamination in CAPD patients can be separated into three different scenarios.

1. Bacteria do not adhere to surfaces of the peritoneum or Tenckhoff catheter present in the abdominal cavity and are therefore likely to be flushed out again during subsequent fluid exchanges; no inflammation ensues. Thus, contamination does not always lead to clinical peritonitis (16,17).
2. Bacteria adhere to the surface of the plastic Tenckhoff catheter and form a biofilm on the foreign material. Biofilms per se do not necessarily induce inflammation that becomes clinically apparent. Biofilms are found on many, if not all, Tenckhoff catheters removed for various (infectious and noninfectious) reasons. In many cases, the presence of biofilm is not temporarily associated with the occurrence of clinical peritonitis (18–20). However, it has been proposed that biofilm-derived microorganisms may become the cause of peritonitis at some later stage, even though the forces that would drive such transition are presently unknown (21).

3. Bacteria adhere to the peritoneal membrane, either directly upon
   entry into the abdominal cavity or via an intermediate residence
   within the biofilm on the Tenckhoff catheter (as described in Point
   2). Bacterial adherence to the mesothelial cell monolayer of the
   peritoneal membrane is theoretically most probable, since these cells
   are the most prevalent type of cells present in the peritoneal cavity.
   In a relevant animal model, preferential adherence to the membrane
   has been demonstrated (22). It is presently thought that bacterial
   adherence to the membrane is the crucial first step in the pathogenesis of CAPD peritonitis (23). In contrast, the role of the free-
   floating leukocytes (macrophages, predominantly) in this phase is
   probably limited. It has been shown that at the prevailing densities
   of these cells in uninfected dialysate effluent ($<10^5$/ml), they are not
   likely to encounter invading bacteria (24). In addition, the levels of
   opsonins needed for efficient recognition of bacteria by leukocytes
   are so low that bacteria-leukocyte encounters may not be effective,
   i.e., result in bacterial engulfment by the leukocytes (25). Lack of
   leukocytes and opsonins is due to the repeated drainage and
   instillation of large volumes of dialysis fluid. In animal models such
   dilution has been shown to greatly diminish the phagocytic defense
   of the peritoneal cavity (26). At later stages of peritonitis, when
   massive numbers of leukocytes migrate into the cavity, these cells
   constitute the major host response to bacterial challenge.

The subsequent cascade of the inflammatory response following bacterial adherence to the peritoneal membrane is depicted in Fig. 2. Importantly,
mesothelial cells become directly activated by bacteria (27–29), or indirectly
via activated macrophages (30), to secrete chemotactic agents (IL-8 and
MCP-1) in a polarized fashion. These cytokines attract large numbers of
leukocytes into the peritoneal cavity (23). The peritoneal membrane may
further contribute to inflammation by generation of prostaglandins and other
cytokines (e.g., Il-6).

Migration of leukocytes from peritoneal capillaries across vascular
endothelium and peritoneal mesothelium is in itself a complex process
involving cell/cell interactions via specific ligands in the leukocyte membrane
(CR-3 and VLA-4) and receptors present on endothelial and mesothelial cells
(ICAM-1 and VCAM-1) (31). Leukocyte migration is accompanied by
exudation of serum proteins including opsonic molecules such as C3, IgG,
and fibronectin. In this manner, an intra-abdominal milieu is created that is
effectively antibacterial (24).

Recently, defensive-type antimicrobial peptides have been found in the
peritoneal cavity of CPD patients. Although their contribution to peritoneal
defenses is currently unknown, mesothelial cells produce beta-defensive
peptides in variable amounts that can be upregulated by cytokines and
growth factors (32). However, continued exchanges with fresh dialysis fluids

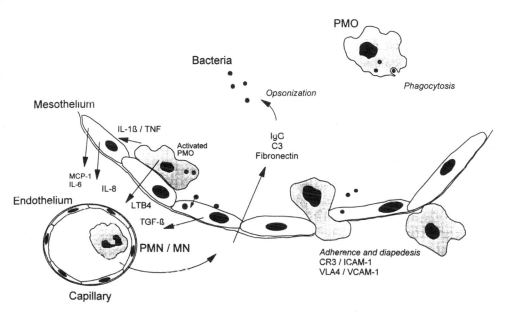

Figure 2 Schematic representation of the inflammatory response of the peritoneal membrane. Via activation of peritoneal macrophages, bacteria directly or indirectly stimulate mesothelial cells to excrete proinflammatory cytokines IL-6, IL-8, monocytic chemotactic protein-1 (MCP-1), and transforming growth factor β (TGF-β) that attract polymorphonuclear (PMN) and mononuclear (MN) leukocytes from nearby capillaries in the submesothelial loose connective tissue. Diapedesis of PMN and Mn require coordinated adhesion to mesothelial cells in which leukocyte adhesion molecules CR3 (on PMN) and VLA-4 (on MN) interact with ligands ICAM and VCAM on mesothelium. Exudation of opsonic proteins IgG, C3, and fibronectin also occurs.

that are intrinsically rather damaging for host defense cells and proteins (33–36) may partly neutralize the beneficial effect of the peritoneal inflammatory response. Thus, fresh fluids have recently been shown to induce mithochondrial DNA damage and heatshock protein synthesis in mesothelial cells, and to accelerate the rate of apoptosis among neutrophils exposed to the high glucose-containing fluids (37–39).

Once inside, bacteria may become sequestered at sites—e.g., within biofilm or within cells—where they cannot be attacked properly by the inflammatory cells (19,40). This feature may help explain the partial response to antibiotic therapies that do not specifically target such difficult-to-reach sites of microbial growth and survival (21). Patients who are further compromised—e.g., diabetics or others with immune function disorders affecting their phagocytes—are especially prone to experiencing recurrent infection (41–43). Also, higher rates of *S. epidermidis* peritonitis have been observed in patients whose dialysates fail to opsonize these coagulase-negative staphylococci (44).

EPIDEMIOLOGY AND ETIOLOGY

This chapter focuses on bacterial peritonitis and exit-site and tunnel infections around the permanent Tenckhoff catheter. This is not to say that CAPD patients may not also suffer from other types of infections related to the uremic state or to diseases underlying their renal insufficiency. However, the incidences of peritonitis and tunnel-track infections are such that they are largely responsible for the infectious morbidity seen among CPD patients. The incidence of bacterial peritonitis was high, approximately one episode per 2.5 patient-months CAPD, in the early years of CAPD. Infection rates were also high in the learning phases of most centers starting with this treatment modality in the early 1980s (rates of one episode per 3 to 6 months for European centers in 1985) (3,45). With more experience, and probably also due to changes in the vital statistics of the patients treated, most centers managed to achieve peritonitis rates of one episode per 6 to 12 patient-months prior to the introduction of the Y connector systems (referred to earlier). In that era the probability of remaining free from peritonitis after 12 months on CAPD was less than 50% (8–10). In centers using the Y sets, peritonitis rates now vary from one episode per 15 to 25 months, and perhaps up to one per 33 months in some centers (8–10,46–48).

The distribution of organisms causing acute peritonitis has previously been collated from the literature up to 1989 and published (49). Studies detailing the distribution of peritonitis-causing organisms published in 1991 to 1994 reveal a very similar pattern (Table 1). Thus, CAPD-causing organisms are predominantly divided among enteric bacilli and the *Acinetobacter*, *Pseudomonas*, and other glucose-nonfermenting species. Anaerobes are rarely isolated, and fungi, usually *Candida* spp., cause approximately 2% of peritonitis episodes in CAPD patients. However, even the most recently published studies do not all address the effect of the introduction of the Y systems on the species distribution in their respective centers. The few studies that have evaluated this specifically show that Y sets reduce the rate of infection due to coagulase-negative staphylococci but not those of the other species listed in Table 1 (46–48). Thus, the relative contribution to the total number of peritonitis episodes caused by Gram-negative bacilli and fungi in patients will most probably increase along with the introduction of Y sets.

The risk of peritonitis may also be influenced by ethnic factors and the premorbid state of the patients. Advanced age, diabetes mellitus, black race, and being HIV-positive have all been associated with higher incidences of CAPD-associated peritonitis (10,41,58). Also, *S. aureus* may cause more infections in children than *Pseudomonas*, and fungi may trouble HIV-positive patients on CAPD (41,49).

The risk of peritonitis is not equally distributed among all patients on CAPD. Patients who have had one episode of peritonitis have an increased risk of peritonitis recurring at a later date. In one national study in the United States, the peritonitis rate in the patients using Y sets was one episode per 20.6

Table 1 Species Distribution of Microbial Pathogens Causing Peritonitis in Patients Undergoing Chronic Peritoneal Dialysis

Microbial species	Mean (range) percentage of total isolates as published in the literature	
	1980s	1990s
Gram-positive bacteria	74 (41–87)	74 (46–84)
Coagulase-negative staphylococci	44 (16–58)	46 (19–56)
Staphylococcus aureus	14 (3–33)	14 (5–21)
Streptococcus, Enterococcus spp.	12 (1–16)	10 (1–20)
Corynebacterium spp.	3 (0–10)	3 (0–7)
Other[a]	1 (0–6)	1 (0–5)
Gram-negative bacilli	19 (1–36)	23 (14–36)
Enterobacteriaceae[b]	11 (0–17)	10 (7–25)
Glucose-nonfermenting[c]	8 (1–18)	13 (5–26)
Anaerobic bacteria	<1 (0–3)	<1 (0–1)
Fungi[d]	2 (0–9)	2 (0–9)
Miscellaneous[e]	2 (0–5)	1 (0–11)
Mixed species	2 (0–14)	<1 (0–5)

Note: Percentages for the 1980s are from Ref. 46 and are based on 1,569 episodes observed in adults. Data from the 1990s are pooled from Refs. 46 and 50–57 and are based on 1,661 episodes.
[a] *Bacillus* spp. predominantly.
[b] *Escherichia coli, Enterobacter, Klebsiella, Citrobacter,* and *Serratia* spp. primarily.
[c] *Acinetobacter* and *Pseudomonas* spp. predominantly.
[d] Predominantly *Candida* spp.
[e] Includes *Hemophilus, Neisseria, Pasteurella, Agrobacterium, Chlamydia,* and *Flavobacterium* spp., and mycobacteria and unidentified isolates.

patient-months for the first episode, but this increased to one per 8.2 patient-months for a subsequent episode (10). Vice versa, a small minority of patients will remain free of peritonitis for many years on CAPD.

Also, patients with a history of multiple episodes of peritonitis are prone to develop fungal or polymicrobial infection at a later stage of their CPD life (59,60). However, it remains difficult to predict from the onset of CPD which patient will develop peritonitis, and who will remain peritonitis-free. The exception is infection due to *S. aureus*. Patients who are nasal carriers of this species are at a three- to fourfold higher risk of developing CPD catheter-related *S. aureus* infections than those who do not carry *S. aureus* (as will be discussed later).

Infections of the exit site of the Tenckhoff catheter through the abdominal skin and, much less frequently, infection of the tunnel track through the abdominal wall are also observed regularly in CAPD patients. Today, incidence rates for exit-site infection equal those for peritonitis, usually one episode per 12 to 24 months on CAPD (41,48,55), but are

Table 2   Species Distribution of Microbial Pathogens Causing Exit-Site and
Tunnel-Track Infection in CAPD Patients

Microbial species	Mean (range) percentage of isolates
Staphylococcus aureus	42 (33–81)
Coagulase-negative staphylococci	28 (6–33)
Pseudomonas spp.	14 (6–21)
Enterobacteriaceae[a]	4 (3–8)
Others[b]	12 (0–16)

Note: Percentages computed from data pooled from Refs. 41, 45, 55, and 61 are based on
547 episodes observed in adults.
[a] *Escherichia coli, Proteus* spp., *Enterobacter* spp.
[b] *Corynebacterium, Enterococcus* spp., and fungi.

sometimes less frequent (61,62). These infections are commonly caused by
S. aureus, coagulase-negative staphylococci, and *Pseudomonas* spp.
(Table 2). Tunnel-track infections occur at approximately 20% the rate of
exit-site infections (45) and may be associated with concurrent exit-site
infection and subsequent peritonitis.

CLINICAL PRESENTATION AND COMPLICATIONS

The signs and symptoms of CAPD peritonitis are a cloudy dialysate effluent,
abdominal pain or tenderness, and fever. The earliest suggestive sign of
peritonitis is usually cloudy fluid. However, occasionally abdominal pain may
be the initial complaint, and in children an increased temperature may be the
earliest finding (Table 3).

Nausea, vomiting, and diarrhea may also be present, more often in
patients who have gastroenteritis due to the same organisms, e.g., *Campylobacter* (11) or *Aeromonas* (12). Cloudy dialysate alone may not be due to
infection and inflammation, unless cell count and differential count show the

Table 3   Clinical Presentation of CAPD Peritonitis

Signs and symptoms	Number (%) of episodes
Cloudy effluent	116 (99)
Abdominal pain	99 (85)
Fever	25 (21)
Nausea and vomiting	18 (15)
Diarrhea	11 (9)
Total episodes	117

Source: Ref. 49.

increased presence of polymorphonuclear neutrophils (PMN). Other causes of cloudy effluent include retrograde blood contamination during menstruation (63) and peritoneal fluid eosinophilia as an allergic manifestation to plasticizers or other foreign constituents in the dialysis fluid (64).

However, in bacterial or fungal peritonitis, the cell count uniformly reveals more than 100 cells/mm^3 effluent, with more than 50% of these cells being PMNs. Clearly, the clinical presentation is to a large extent determined by the pathogenic potential of the infecting species and by the virulence factors carried by the invading strain of a given species. Thus, wide variations in clinical presentations may be expected. In general, however, peritonitis caused by coagulase-negative staphylococci is clinically a mild disease. In contrast, infections due to *S. aureus*, hemolytic streptococci, and Gram-negative bacilli may be clinically severe and even fatal (15,65,66). However, mortality due to peritonitis in CAPD is low (2% to 3%) and may be due in part to secondary complications such as myocardial infarction and cachexia. The major complication of CAPD peritonitis and exit-site infection is technique failure. Technique failure entails the need to remove the Tenckhoff catheter and to transfer the patient to hemodialysis in order to control the infection, either in the acute phase or in case of repeatedly relapsing infection (1).

Exit-site infection is characterized by the presence of purulent drainage and erythema of the skin at the catheter–epidermal interface. Induration and tenderness along the tunnel track indicates tunnel infection, with or without discharge and positive culture. Sonography may help diagnose a tunnel-track infection. A positive culture from an exit site in the absence of signs of inflammation does not necessarily constitute or herald infection (62). Another important feature of CAPD-peritonitis is its tendency to relapse upon discontinuation of apparently successful therapy. Relapse rates are especially high following infections due to the *Staphylococcus*, *Pseudomonas*, and fungal species. Relapses and reinfection are also seen with exit-site and tunnel-track infections.

A separate entity, not of a directly infectious nature, is the so-called sclerosing peritonitis that may complicate CAPD. In sclerosing peritonitis, peritoneal thickening, laminar intestinal concrescence, and diffuse hemorrhage occur, often resulting in patient death from ileus. Intestinal obstruction and loss of ultrafiltration are also features of this dreaded complication. The etiology of sclerosing peritonitis remains uncertain, but recurrent episodes of bacterial or fungal peritonitis may well be a major risk factor (67). Fortunately, this complication is rare and, if it occurs, it is a late one.

DIAGNOSIS OF INFECTION

In patients with signs and symptoms, laboratory evaluation of effluent dialysate should include a total white cell count with differential, Gram stain, and culture. In patients who have only abdominal pain with or without fever but who have clear effluents containing less than 100 PMN/mm^3 the diagnosis of peritonitis is uncertain and immediate initiation of therapy is not necessary. In contrast, patients with cloudy fluid accompanied by abdominal pain or fever require prompt initiation of therapy, and diagnostic laboratory studies should be obtained expeditiously. A Gram stain is positive in up to 40% of episodes of peritonitis, and when positive, it is predictive of the type of organism in 85% of cases. Since fungi may grow slowly, a Gram stain is particularly useful in the early recognition of fungal peritonitis. Many techniques have been described for the isolation of pathogens from infected CAPD effluent (49). As in blood cultures, the sensitivity of the culture increases with the volume that is sampled. Generally, enrichment broths (e.g., blood-culturing systems) are reported to have superior sensitivity compared to direct plating of sediments. The yields of the direct plating methods are significantly increased if the cell sediment is first lysed (freeing cell-associated bacteria) through the action of detergents, sonication, or osmotic shock. More than 90% of the episodes of CAPD peritonitis are culture-positive. However, routine culture of clear dialysate from uninfected patients may also grow bacteria in up to 27% of the samples (17); such growth probably reflects the intermittant entry and outflow of low numbers of bacteria in and out of the peritoneal space (described earlier).

Purulent exudate from inflamed exit sites may be cultured by routine swabbing and forwarding to the medical microbiology laboratory utilizing standard transport media. Culturing of an erythematous exit site in the absence of a discharge does not provide clinically useful reports, and culture results usually demonstrate commensal skin flora. Gram stains should be routinely performed on all exudate material since this will reveal the presence or absence of leukocytes and the type(s) of organism(s) present.

If catheters are removed as a consequence of infection, culturing of several sections of the catheter (intraperitoneal, tunnel track, exit site) may be helpful in establishing the etiological role of the organisms attached. New molecular techniques including PCR-mediated DNA fingerprinting and pulsed-field gel electrophoresis of bacterial DNA will allow genotyping of virtually all pathogens causing infections in CAPD patients (68). Thus, sources of strains and routes of infections can be traced accurately.

TREATMENT

The majority of CAPD-related episodes of peritonitis are initially treated empirically, or on the basis of the result of a Gram stain. Many different antimicrobial agents and combinations thereof have been used to treat CAPD peritonitis (69). Both national and international working parties have set guidelines that are regularly updated (70,71). Based on published data on the types and resistance patterns of organisms isolated, the empirical regimen should include vancomycin (1 to 2 g every 7 days) and either an aminoglycoside (gentamicin, tobramycin, or netilmicin, 40 mg/day), or a third-generation cephalosporin with antipseudomonal activity (e.g., ceftazidime, 1 g/day). Vancomycin is needed since many staphylococci are methicillin-resistant. However, fear of emergence of vancomycin resistance among enterococci and staphylococci in many centers in the United States has led one consensus recommendation away from proposing this agent an empirical basis (71). Indeed, the first fully vancomycin-resistant *S. aureus* strain was recently isolated from a hemodialysis patient after receiving multiple courses of vancomycin for methicillin-resistant *S. aureus* infection (72).

All agents are preferentially given via the intraperitoneal route—amino-glycosides once daily, and the cephalosporin divided in equal doses/exchange. Once-daily cephalosporin may also be effective. Oral therapies with fluoro-quinolones are not recommended since their bioavailabilty may vary widely in these patients, and the low dialysate levels reached with these agents are associated with frequent relapses of peritonitis (73). A high rate of relapse (11/73; 15%) was also observed in one study when, through intraperitoneal dosing, mean dialysate levels of 10 mg/l ciprofloxacin were achieved; 10 of 11 relapsing organisms were Gram-positive organisms (74). Thus, fluoroquino-lone monotherapy may not suffice. However, a regimen that combines intraperitoneal fluoroquinolone with rifampin may well work (75). Failure may be due to inaccessibility of the organisms within intracellular sites or due to phenotypic antimicrobial resistance of sessile bacteria located within catheter-associated biofilm (referred to earlier). Also, peritoneal dialysis fluid may constitute a milieu in which bacteria display increased resistance to antibiotics (24,76). The carbapenem imipenem/cilastatin has also been used with some initial success, but high rates of gastrointestinal side effects were noted (50). Peritonitis due to yeasts may be amendable to medical treatment alone, although catheter removal is still recommended if the patient does not respond in 4 to 7 days. When culture results become available, the broad-spectrum empirical regimens should be streamlined. The optimal length of treatment is unknown but may be as short as 7 days, 10 to 14 days being considered sufficient by most centers.

In cases of failure to obtain resolution of signs and symptoms of infection or if the infection relapses repeatedly in the face of appropriate antimicrobial treatments, the patient needs to be reassessed carefully for the presence of occult pathologies within the abdomen or along the catheter and for the presence of unusual organisms. Patients with staphylococcal infections may have oral rifampicin added to their regimen since this agent is thought to kill biofilm-associated bacteria as well as staphylococci sequestered inside host cells (77). Fibrinolytic agents such as urokinase have also been used in this setting with some success (71,78); however, its exact mode of action remains unknown.

There are few data on the therapeutic efficacy of methods to cure exit-site infections. Combination therapy including rifampicin in the case of staphylococcal etiology or ciprofloxacin in the case of Gram-negative infection is recommended for 2 to 4 weeks. For pseudomonal or fungal exit-site infection associated with peritonitis, the treatment of choice is early catheter removal. Shaving off the Dacron cuff at the external exit site may, in some patients, result in cure (71). When needed, removal and replacement of the infected catheter in a single operative procedure is safe, as long as there are no signs of active intraperitoneal infection (79).

PREVENTION

Several strategies for the prevention of peritonitis and exit-site infections in CAPD patients are currently pursued. One strategy is to further increase the antimicrobial barriers for entry into the peritoneal cavity. Improvements in connector technology may still lower the rate of intraluminal contamination during the exchange procedures; in-line bacterial filters, if they can be made cost-effective, would also serve this goal. In addition, the choice of catheter design and the orientation of catheter placement in the patient may affect the likelihood of catheter contamination and the formation of progressive biofilm along its surfaces (71). Thus, catheters would ideally be made of a material that is fully biocompatible with the surrounding human tissues while also preventing the adherence of bacteria.

Of course, the catheter placement procedure should be performed under strict aseptic conditions, as is done for other types of implant surgery. Design and placement should avoid as much as possible the chance that catheters are subjected to trauma and repeated or continued mechanical stress.

The current state of the art is that double-cuffed Tenckhof catheters are better than single-cuffed ones (80), that delayed externalization of the catheter may be beneficial, and that a downward pointing exit site is less prone to infection compared to an upward pointing exit site (81). Also, antibiotic prophylaxis at the time of catheter infection may prevent infection (82). Catheters experimentally coated with antibacterial substances (silver sulphiadiazine plus chlorhexidine plus triclosan) may reduce that rate of infection, but a silver ring placed around the catheter at the level of the skin failed to prevent infection in a clinical trial (82,83). Postplacement prevention strategies should rely on thorough training (6–7 weeks) of patients new to CPD (84), and, perhaps, the daily application of antibacterials to the exit site. Ciprofloxacin solution and povidone-iodine ointment, applied daily, have both shown benefit, although daily spray with povidone-iodine dry powder did not (85–87).

Since the risk of *S. aureus* infections has now been firmly linked to the carrier-status of CPD patients, *S. aureus* infection may be open to further preventive measures. There are three types of *S. aureus* carriers. Persons may never carry *S. aureus* (noncarriers), carry *S. aureus* sometimes but not all the time (intermittent carriers), or are always positive for *S. aureus* when cultured (permanent carriers). To correctly distinguish among these three groups, multiple, serial cultures, preferably quantitative cultures, are needed (88,89). Generally, persistent carriers of *S. aureus* have higher numbers of staphylococci in their noses compared to intermittent carriers, and have the highest risk of *S. aureus* infections (85). However, in most studies on CPD patients, carriers have been defined as those that have at least one positive culture, thus lumping persistent and intermittent carriers together. Nevertheless, CPD patients defined as carriers in such manner have three- to fourfold higher rates of *S. aureus* exit-site infection and peritonitis (89). The sequence of events most probably is first colonization of the exit site with *S. aureus* from the nose of the patient prior to exit-site infection and peritonitis. Intervention strategies aimed at eliminating *S. aureus* from the nose or exit site of CPD patients have been successful in reducing the risk of *S. aureus* infection (90–94). Application of mupirocin ointment to the nose and to the exit site in proven carriers may be most effective since application of mupirocin to the nose alone may not eliminate *S. aureus* from exit sites. Alternative agents including oral rifampicin may also be effective but run more risk of side effects and the development of antibiotic resistance (95–97).

SUMMARY AND CONCLUSION

CPD has become the first choice of replacement therapy for most patients with end-stage renal failure, despite increased risks of catheter-related infection (exit-site, tunnel-track, or peritonitis). The high rates of infection observed in the early days of CPD have now come down due to better training programs, better connector technologies, and interventions aimed at eliminating *S. aureus* carriage. However, CPD carriers remain prone to developing biofilm-embedded microorganisms that cause infection at some stage of CPD-life, and such infections remain the major cause of CPD-technique failure. Strategies that further reduce the rate of biofilm formation, either through training patients or by use of biofilm-resistant catheters, are still needed. In our era of resistance, antibiotics, both systemic and topical, should be used prudently based on current information regarding the causative microbes and their resistance profiles. Thus, cyclic mupirocin ointment should be given prophylactically only to those CPD patients known to be (persistent) carriers of *S. aureus*.

REFERENCES

1. Nolph KD. Peritoneal dialysis registry update. Proceedings of the 15th Annual Conference on Peritoneal Dialysis, Baltimore, Feb. 12–14, 1995:179–182.
2. Serkes KD, Blagg ChR, Nolph KD, Vanesh EF, Shapiro F. Comparison of patient and technique survival in continuous ambulatory peritoneal dialysis (CAPD) and haemodialysis: A multi-center study. Perit Dial Int 1990; 10:15–19.

3. Gokal R, Jakubowski C, King J, Hunt L, Bogle S, Baillod R, Marse F, Ogg C, Wand M. Outcome in patients on continuous ambulatory peritoneal dialysis and haemodialysis: 4-year analysis of a prospective multicenter study. Lancet 1987; ii:1105–1109.

4. Popovich RP, Moncrief JW, Decherd JF, Bomar JB, Pyle W. The definition of a novel portable/wearable equilibrium peritoneal dialysis technique. Trans Am Soc Artif Intern Organs 1976; 5:64. Abstract.

5. Oreopoulos DG, Robson M, Izatt S, Clayton S, de Veber GA. A simple and safe technique for continuous ambulatory peritoneal dialysis. Trans Am Soc Artif Intern Organs 1978; 24:484–489.

6. Diaz-Buxo J, Walker P, Farmer C, Chandler J, Holt R. Continuous cyclic peritoneal dialysis: a preliminary report. Artif Organs 1981; 5:157–161.

7. Tenckhoff H, Schechter H. A bacteriologically safe peritoneal access device. Trans Am Soc Artif Intern Organs 1968; 14:181–187.

8. Fellin G, Gentile MG, Manna GM, Redaelli L, D'Amico G. Peritonitis prevention: a Y-connector and sodium hypochloride three years' experience. Report of the Italian CAPD study group. In: Khanna R, Nolph KD, Prowant B, Twardowski ZJ, Oreopoulo DG, eds. Advances in Continuous Peritoneal Dialysis. Toronto: Peritoneal Dialysis Bulletin, 1987:114–118.

9. Canadian CAPD Clinical Trials Group. Peritonitis in continuous ambulatory peritoneal dialysis. Randomized clinical trial comparing the Y connector disinfectant system to standard systems. Perit Dial Int 1989; 9:159–164.

10. Port FK, Held PJ, Nolph KD, Turenne MN, Wolfe RA. Risk of peritonitis and technique failure by CAPD connection technique: A national study. Kidney Int 1992; 42:867–974.

11. Wood CJ, Flemming V, Turnidge J, Thompson N, Atkins RC. *Campylobacter* peritonitis in continuous ambulatory peritoneal dialysis: report of eight cases and a review of the literature. Am J Kidney Dis 1992; 19:257–263.

12. Muñoz P, Fernández-Baca V, Peláez T, Sánchez R, Rodriquez-Créixems M, Bouza E. *Aeromonas* peritonitis. Clin Infect Dis 1994; 18:32–37.

13. Schweinburg FB, Seligman AM, Fine J. Transmural migration of intestinal bacteria. N Engl J Med 1950; 242:747–751.

14. Wu G, Khanna R, Vas S, Oreopoulos DG. Is extensive diverticulosis of the colon a contra-indication to CAPD? Perit Dial Bull 1983; 3:180–183.

15. Vas SI. Peritonitis. In: Nolph KD, ed. Peritoneal Dialysis. Dordrecht: Kluwer Academic, 1989:161–188.

16. Fijen JW, Struyk DG, Krediet RT, Boeschoten EW, de Vries JP, Arisz L. Dialysate leukocytosis in CAPD patients without clinical infection. Neth J Med 1988; 33:270–280.

17. Van Bronswijk G. Microbial invasion and peritoneal defence in CAPD patients. PhD thesis, Free University of Amsterdam, Amsterdam, Netherlands, 1988.

18. Marrie TJ, Bobel MA, Costerton JW. Examination of the morphology of bacteria adhering to peritoneal dialysis catheters by scanning and transmission election microscopy. J Clin Microbiol 1983; 18:1388–1398.

19. Holmes CJ. Catheter-associated biofilm. In: Coles GA, Davies M, Williams JD, eds. CAPD: Host Defence, Nutrition and UltrafiltrationContrib Nephrol 1990; 85:49–56.

20. Rodriquez-Carmona A, Fortán MP, Falcóa P, Lañedo FV. Prevalence of microbial colonization in removed peritoneal catheters: a prospective study. Adv Perit Dial 2000; 16:276–279.

21. Finkelstein ES, Jekel J, Troidle L, Gorbau-Brennan N, Finkelstein FO, Bia FJ. Patterns of infection in patients maintained on long-term peritoneal dialysis therapy with multiple episodes of peritonitis. Am J Kidney Dis 2002; 39:1318–1320.

22. Gallimore B, Gognon RF, Richards GK. Role of an intraperitoneal implant in the pathogenesis of experimental *Staphylococcus epidermidis* peritoneal infection in renal failure mice. Am J Nephrol 1988; 36:406–413.

23. Topley N, Williams JD. Role of the peritoneal membrane in the control of inflammation in the peritoneal cavity. Kidney Int 1994; 46(suppl 48):71–78.

24. Verbrugh HA, Keane WF, Conroy WE, Peterson PK. Bacterial growth and killing in chronic ambulatory peritoneal dialysis fluids. J Clin Microbiol 1984; 20:199–203.

25. Verbrugh HA, Keane WF, Hoidal JR, Freiberg MR, Elliott GR, Peterson PK. Peritoneal macrophages and opsonins: antibacterial defense in patients undergoing chronic peritoneal dialysis. J Infect Dis 1983; 147:1018–1029.

26. Dunn DL, Barke RA, Ahrenholtz DH, Humphrey EW, Simmons RL. The adjuvant effect of peritoneal fluid in experimental peritonitis. Mechanisms and clinical implications. Ann Surg 1984; 199:37–43.

27. Zeillemaker AM, Mul FPJ, Hoynck van Papendrecht AAGM, Diepersloot RJ. Polarized secretion of interleukin-8 by human mesothelial cells: a role in neutrophil migration. Immunol 1995; 84:227–232.

28. Kimaert P, De Wilde JP, Bournonville B, Husson C, Salmon L. Direct activation of human peritoneal mesothelial cells by heat-killed organisms. Ann Surg 1996; 224:749–754.

29. Mandl-Weber S, Haslinger B, Lederer SR, Sitter T. Heat-killed micro-organisms in induce PAI-1 expression in human peritoneal mesothelial cells: role of interleukin-1 alpha. Am J Kidney Dis 2000; 37:815–819.

30. Betjes MGH, Tuk CW, Struijk DG, Krediet RT, Arisz L, Beelem RH. Interleukin-8 production by human peritoneal mesothelial cells in response to tumor necrosis factor (interleukin-1, and medium conditioned by macrophages co-cultured with *Staphylococcus epidermidis*. J Infect Dis 1993; 168:1202–1210.

31. Jonjic N, Peri G, Bernasconi S, Jilek P, Anichini A, Romiani G, Montavani M. Expression of adhesion molecules and chemotactic cytokines in cultured human mesothelial cells. J Exp Med 1992; 176:1165–1174.

32. Zarriukalam KIT, Lezzvesley DI, Stanley JM, Atkins GJ, Faull RJ. Expression of defensin antimicrobial peptides in the peritoneal cavity of patients on peritoneal dialysis. Perit Dial Int 2001; 21:501–508.

33. Duwe AK, Vas SI, Weatherhead JW. Effects of the composition of peritoneal dialysis fluid on chemiluminescence, phagocytosis and bacterial activity in vitro. Infect Immun 1981; 33:130–135.

34. Van Bronswijk H, Verbrugh HA, Bos HJ, Heezius EC, De PL, Verhoef J. Cytotoxic effects of commercial continuous ambulatory peritoneal dialysis (CAPD) fluids and of bacterial exoproducts on human mesothelial cells in vitro. Perit Dial Int 1989; 9:197–202.

35. Keane WF, Comty CM, Verbrugh HA, Peterson PK. Opsonic deficiency of

peritoneal dialysis effluent in continuous ambulatory peritoneal dialysis. Kidney Int 1984; 25:539–543.

36. Holmes CJ. Biocompatibility of peritoneal dialysis solutions. Perit Dial Int 1993; 13:88–94.

37. Ishibashi Y, Sugimoto T, Ichikawa Y, Akatsuha A, Myata T, Naugak M, Tagawa H, Kurokawa K. Glucose dialysates induces mitochondrial DNA damage in peritoneal mesothelial cells. Perit Dial Int 2002; 22:11–21.

38. Arbeiter K, Bidmon B, Endemann M, Beuder TO, Eickelberg O, Ruffinpshofer D, Mueller T, Regele H, Herkner K, Aufrizht C. Peritoneal dialysis fluid composition determines heat shock protein expression patterns in human mesothelial cells. Kidney Int 2001; 60:1930–1937.

39. Catalan MP, Reyero A, Egido J, Ortiz A. Acceleration of neutrophil apoptosis by glucose-containing peritoneal dialysis solutions: role of caspases. J Am Soc Nephrol 2001; 12:2442–2449.

40. De Fijter CWH, Verbrugh HA, Heezius HCJM, van der Meulen J, De PL, Donkar AJ, Verhoef J. Effect of clindamycin on the intracellular bactericidal capacity of human peritoneal macrophages. J Antimicrob Chemother 1990; 26:525–532.

41. Tebben JA, Rigsby MO, Selwyn PA, Brennon N, Kliger A, Finkelstein FO. Outcome of HIV-infected patients on continuous ambulatory peritoneal dialysis patients. Am J Kidney Dis 1991; 18:674–677.

42. Khan GA, Bank N. An adult patient with hyperimmune globulinemia E (Job's) syndrome, end-stage renal disease and repeated episodes of peritonitis. Clin Nephrol 1994; 41:233–236.

43. Lewis SI, Young SA, Wood BJ, Morgan KS, Erickson DG, Holmes CJ. Relationships between frequent episodes of peritonitis and altered immune status. Am J Kidney Dis 1993; 22:456–461.

44. Holmes CJ. Peritoneal host defense mechanisms in peritoneal dialysis. Kidney Int 1994; 46(suppl 48):58–70.

45. Golper TA, Geerlings W, Selwood NH, Brunner FP, Wing AJ. Peritoneal dialysis results in the EDTA registry. In: Nolph KD, ed. Peritoneal Dialysis. Dordrecht: Kluwer Academic, 1989:414–428.

46. Domrongkitchaiporn S, Karim M, Watson L, Moriarty M. The influence of continuous ambulatory peritoneal dialysis connection technique on peritonitis rate and technique survival. Am J Kidney Dis 1994; 24:50–58.

47. Dryden MS, McCann M, Wing AJ, Phillips I. Controlled trial of a Y-set dialysis delivery system to prevent peritonitis in patients receiving continuous ambulatory peritoneal dialysis. J Hosp Infect 1992; 20:185–192.

48. Holley JL, Bernardini J, Piraino B. Infecting organisms in continuous ambulatory peritoneal dialysis patients on the Y-set. Am J Kidney Dis 1994; 23:569–573.

49. Verbrugh HA. Organisms causing peritonitis. In: Coles G, Davies M, Williams JD, eds. CAPD: Host Defence, Nutrition and Ultrafiltration. Contrib Nephrol 1990; 85:39–48.

50. Lui SF, Cheng AB, Leung CB, Wong KC, Li PKT, Lai KN. Imipenem/ cilastatin sodium in the treatment of continuous ambulatory peritoneal dialysis-associated peritonitis. Am J Nephrol 1994; 14:182–186.

51. Were AJ, Marsden A, Tooth A, Ramsden R, Mistry CD, Gokal R. Netilmicin

and Vancomycin in the treatment of peritonitis in CAPD patients. Clin Nephrol 1992; 37:209–213.

52. Dryden MS, Wing AJ, Phillips I. Low dose intraperitoneal ciprofloxacin for the treatment of peritonitis in patients receiving continuous ambulatory dialysis (CAPD). J Antimicrob Chemother 1991; 28:131–139.

53. Taylor PC. Routine laboratory diagnosis of continuous ambulatory peritoneal dialysis peritonitis using centrifugation/lysis and saponin-containing media. Eur J Clin Microbiol Infect Dis 1994; 13:249–252.

54. Ludlam HA. Infectious consequences of continuous ambulatory peritoneal dialysis. J Hosp Infect 1991; 18(suppl A):341–354.

55. Rotellar C, Black J, Winchester JF, Rakowski TA, Mosher WF, Mazzoui MJ, Amiranzari M, Garagwi Y, Alijani MR, Argy WP. Ten years' experience with continuous ambulatory peritoneal dialysis. Am J Kidney Dis 1991; 17:158–164.

56. Wilcox MH, Finch RG, Burden RP, Morgan AG. Peritonitis complicating continuous ambulatory peritoneal dialysis in Nottingham 1983–1988. J Med Microbiol 1991; 34:137–141.

57. Dryden M, Eykyn SJ. Short-course gentamicin in gram-negative CAPD peritonitis. Lancet 1993; 341:497.

58. Viglino G, Cancarini C, Catizone I., Cocchi R, De Vecchi A, Lupo A, Salomone M, Segoloui GP, Reuzetti GA. Ten years experience of CAPD in diabetics: comparison of results with non-diabetics. Nephrol Dial Transplant 1994; 9:1443–1448.

59. Goldie SJ, Hiernan-Troidle L, Torres C, Gorban-Brennas N, Dunne D, Kliger AS, Finkelstein FO. Fungal peritonitis in a large chronic peritoneal dialysis population: A report of 55 cases. Am J Kidney Dis 1996; 28:86–91.

60. Kim GC, Korbet SM. Polymicrobial peritonitis in continuous ambulatory peritoneal dialysis patients. Am J Kidney Dis 2000; 36:1000–1008.

61. Scalamogna A, Castelnouo C, de Vecchi A, Ponticelli C. Exit-site and tunnel infections in continuous ambulatory peritoneal dialysis. Kidney Int 1993; 44:191–198.

62. Luzar MA, Brown CB, Balf D, Hill L, Isaad B, Monnier B, Moulart J, Sabatier JC, Waugier JP, Peluso F. Exit-site care and exit-site infection in continuous ambulatory peritoneal dialysis (CAPD): results of a randomised multicenter trial. Periton Dial Int 1990; 10:25–29.

63. Steigbigel RT, Cross AS. Infections associated with haemodialysis and chronic peritoneal dialysis. In: Remington JS, Swartz MN, eds. Current Clinical Topics in Infectious Diseases. New York: McGraw-Hill, 1984:125–145.

64. Solary E, Cabanne JF, Tauter Y, Rifle G. Evidence for a role of plasticizers in 'Eosinophilic' peritonitis in continuous ambulatory peritoneal dialysis. Nephron 1986; 42:341–342.

65. Dratwa M, Glupczynski Y, Lameire N, Matthys D, Verschraegen G, Vaneechoutte M, Boelaert J, Schurpers M, Van Lauduyt H, Verheelen D. Treatment of gram-negative peritonitis with aztreonam in patients undergoing continuous ambulatory peritoneal dialysis. Rev Infect Dis 1991; 13(suppl):645–647.

66. Borra SI, Chandarana J, Kleinfeld M. Fatal peritonitis due to group B beta-hemolytic *Streptococcus* in a patient receiving chronic ambulatory peritoneal dialysis. Am J Kidney Dis 1992; 19:375–377.

67. Rubin J, Herrera GA, Collins D. An autopsy study of the peritoneal cavity from patients on continuous ambulatory peritoneal dialysis. Am J Kidney Dis 1991; 18:97–102.

68. Van Belkum A. DNA fingerprinting of medically important microorganisms by use of PCR. Clin Microbiology Rev 1994; 7:174–187.

69. Millikin SP, Matzke GR, Keane WF. Antimicrobial treatment of peritonitis associated with continuous ambulatory peritoneal dialysis. Perit Dial Int 1991; 11:252–260.

70. Murphy BF, Harris DCH, Disney A, Ibels LS, Saltissi D, Rigby R, Suranyi M, Collins J. Treatment of peritoneal dialysis related peritonitis—an Australian and New Zealand perspective. Aust NZ J nmed 1999; 29:552–555.

71. Keane WF, Bailie GR, Boeschoten E, Gokal R, Golper TA, Holmes CJ, Kawaguchi Y, Piraino B, Riella M, Vas S. Peritoneal dialysis-related peritonitis treatment recommendations: 2000 update. Perit Dial Int 2000; 20:396–411.

72. Rudrik JT, Brown W, Hafeez W, Lundstrom T, Flauapan E, Johnson R, Mitchell J, Chauf S. *Staphylococcus aureus* resistant to vancomycin—United Stated 2002. MMWR Morb Mortal Wkly Rep 2002: 51:565–567.

73. Bailie GR, Eisele G. Pharmacokinetic issues in the treatment of continuous ambulatory peritoneal dialysis-associated peritonitis. J Antimicrob Chemother 1995; 35:563–567.

74. Ludlam HA, Barton I, While L, McMullin C, King A. Phillips I Intraperitoneal ciprofloxacin for the treatment of peritonitis in patients receiving continuous ambulatory peritoneal dialysis (CAPD). J Antimicrob Chemother 1990; 25:843–851.

75. De Fijter CW, ter Wee PM, Oe LP, Verbrugh HA. Intraperitoneal ciprofloxacin and rifampicin versus cephradine as initial treatment of (C) APD-related peritonitis: A prospective, randomised, multicenter comparison (CIPPER trail). Perit Dial Int 2001; 21:480–486.

76. Wilcox MH, Geary I, Spencer RC. In-vitro-activity of imipenem, in comparison with cefuroxime and ciprofloxacin, against coagulase-negative staphylococci in broth and peritoneal dialysis fluid. J Antimicrob Chemother 1992; 29:49–55.

77. Zimmerman SW. Rifampin use in peritoneal dialysis. Perit Dial Int 1989; 9:241–243.

78. Innes A, Burden RP, Finch RG, Morgan AG. Treatment of resistant peritonitis in continuous ambulatory peritoneal dialysis with intraperitoneal urokinase: A double-blind clinical trial. Nephrol Dial Transplant 1994; 9:797–799.

79. Singhal MK, Vas SI, Oreopoulos D. Treatment of peritoneal dialysis catheter-related infections by simultaneous catheter removal and replacement. Is it safe? Perit Dial Int 1998; 18:565–567.

80. Prischl FC, Wallner M, Kalchmair It, Porac F, Kiamar R. Initial subutaneous embedding of the peritoneal dialysis catheter—a critical appraisal of this new implantation technique. Nephrol Dial Transplant 1997; 12:1661–1667.

81. Golpher TA, Brier ME, Buuke M, Schreiber MJ, Bartlett DK, Hewilton RW, Strife F, Hamburger RJ. Risk factors for peritonitis in long-term peritoneal dialysis: the network 9 peritonitis and catheter survival studies. Am J Kidney Dis 1996; 28:428–436.

82. Wikdahl AM, Engman U, Stegmayr BG, Sorenssen JG. One-dose cefuroxime

i.v. and i.p. reduces microbial growth in PD patients after catheter insertion. Nephrol Dial Transplants 1997; 12:157–160.

83. Kim CY, Kuman A, Sampath L, Sokol K, Modak S. Evaluation of an antimicrobial impregnated continuous ambulatory peritoneal dialyses catheter for infection control in rats. Am J Kidney Dis 2002; 39:165–173.

84. Pommer W, Brauner M, Westphale H-J, Brunkhorst R, Kramer R, Bundslu D, Hottken B, Sternhauer NB, Luttgen FM, Schillinger-Pokomy E, Schaefer F, Weude R, Offuer G, Netter S, Osten B, Zimmering M, Ehrich JH, Mausmanu U, Grosse-Siestrup C. Effect of a silver device in preventing catheter related infections in peritoneal dialysis patients: silver ring prophylaxis of the catheter exit study. Am J Kidney Dis 1998; 32:752–760.

85. Verrina E, Honda M, Warady R, Piraino B. Prevention of peritonitis in children on peritoneal dialysis. Perit Dial Int 2000; 20:625–630.

86. Waite NM, Webster N, Laurel M, Johnson M, Fong IWF. The efficacy of exit site povidone-iodine ointment in the prevention of early peritoneal dialysis-related infections. Am J Kidney Dis 1997; 29:763–768.

87. Montenegro J, Saracho R, Aquirre R, Martinez I, Iribar I, Ocharan J. Exit-site care with ciprofoxacin othologic solutions prevents polyurethane catheter infection in peritoneal dialysis patients. Petit Dial Int 2000; 20:209–214.

88. Wilson APR, Lewis C, O'Sullivan H, Shetty N, Neild GH, Mansell M. The use of Povidone-Iodine in exit site care for patients undergoing continuous peritoneal dialysis. J Hosp, Infect 1997; 35:287–293.

89. Nouwen JL, van Belkum A, Verbrugh HA. Determinants of *Staphylococcus aureus* nasal carriage. Neth J Med 2001; 59:126–133.

90. Kluytmans J, van Belkum A, Verbrugh HA. Nasal carriage of *Staphylococcus aureus*: epidemiology, underlying mechanisms, and associated risks. Clin Microbiol Rev 1997; 10:505–520.

91. Mupirocin Study Group. Nasal mupirocin prevents *Staphylococcus aureus* exit site infection during peritoneal dialysis. Am Soc Nephrol 1996; 7:240–248.

92. Thodis E, Passadakis P, Panagoutsos S, Bacharaki D, Euthimiadou A, Vargemezis V. The effectiveness of mupirocin preventing *Staphylococcus aureus* in catheter-related infections in peritoneal dialysis. Adv Periton Dial 2000; 16: 257–261.

93. Crabtree JH, Hadnott LL, Burchette RJ, Siddiqi RA. Outcome and clinical implications of surveillance program for *Staphylococcus aureus* nasal carriage in peritoneal dialysis patients. Adv Periton Dial 2000; 16:272–275.

94. Thodis E, Bhaskaran S, Pasadakis P, Bargman JM, Vas SI, Oreopoulos D. Decrease in *Staphylococcus aureus* exit-site infections and peritonitis in CAPD patients by local application of mupirocin ointment at the catheter exit site. Perit Dial Int 1998; 18:261–270.

95. Bernardini J, Nolph KD. A Randomised trial of *Staphylococcus aureus* prophylaxis in peritoneal dialysis patients: mupirocin calcium ointment 2% applied to the exit site versus cyclic oral rifampin. Am J Kidney Dis 1996; 27: 695–700.

96. Sanyal D, Williams AJ, Johnsons AP, Georgy RC. The emergence of vancomycin resistance in renal dialysis. J Hosp Infect 1993; 24:167–173.

97. Editorial. Prevention of peritonitis in CAPD. Lancet 1991; 337:22–23.

17

Infections Associated with Hemodialysis Vascular Accesses and with Catheters Used for Hemodialysis

Jerome I. Tokars and R. Monina Klevens

Division of Healthcare Quality Promotion
Centers for Disease Control and Prevention, National Center for Infectious Diseases
Atlanta, Georgia, U.S.A.

INTRODUCTION

Hemodialysis patients require a vascular-access site for blood removal and replacement after wastes have been removed. Modern types of vascular access include the native arteriovenous fistula (constructed of native vessels), arteriovenous graft (of synthetic materials), permanent (tunnelled, cuffed) catheters, temporary (nontunneled, noncuffed) catheters, and implanted port devices. In December 2001, the types of access used to treat hemodialysis patients in the United States were as follows: 44.4% of patients via an arteriovenous graft, 30.4% via an arteriovenous fistula, and 24.6% via a temporary or permanent central catheter (1).

Since the first dialysis was performed in 1943, impressive improvements have occurred in dialysis technology and in the care of persons with end-stage renal disease. At the same time, the number of dialysis patients and the percentage receiving in-center dialysis treatment have increased substantially (2). Furthermore, the frequency of comorbidity among new dialysis patients is higher than ever before (2).

Infections associated with vascular-access are among the most serious complications of chronic hemodialysis. Individuals on chronic hemodialysis are especially vulnerable to vascular-access infections because they are immunosuppressed and because of the frequent puncture of their vascular-access site. For these reasons, preventing infections from hemodialysis catheters and other accesses remains a challenge. In this chapter we describe these infections, highlighting the most recent literature on the subject, summarize effective prevention strategies, and provide resources for conducting surveillance and prevention (3).

PATHOGENESIS

The pathogenesis of infections associated with catheters among dialysis patients is similar to that among other patient groups. Briefly, resident skin flora can be introduced at the time of catheter insertion at the insertion/exit site. These organisms can colonize the catheter tip or contaminate the hub and enter the lumen of the catheter. In addition, extrinsically contaminated infusates can lead to catheter-associated infections (4). Once intraluminal, organisms can be embedded in a biofilm or disseminated over the catheter surface (5). Several factors are associated with the pathogenesis of infections associated with catheters.

Catheter Characteristics

The material the catheter is made of and the presence of irregularities on the surface can facilitate the adherence of microorganisms (4). In addition, the catheter material can promote the formation of thrombus and an environment for bacterial growth. Tunneled catheters have a cuff that prevents migration of organisms into the catheter tract by promoting the growth of a tissue seal (4,6).

Adherence Properties of the Organism

Both of the organisms most frequently isolated in hemodialysis-related bacteremia, coagulase-negative staphylococci and *Staphylococcus aureus*, adhere to catheters promoted by host proteins coating the catheter (4,7).

Duration of Placement

Recently inserted catheters are more likely to have been colonized on the external surface by skin flora. Longer-term catheters are more likely to have become contaminated from the catheter hub.

 The major cause of access failure in the case of fistula and grafts is thrombosis (8); stenosis predisposes to thrombosis in most cases. Stenosis develops from "intimal fibromuscular hyperplasia" and is distinct from other types of vascular injury due to the stress and vessel wall injury, among other factors, inherent in dialysis. Thrombi in grafts are associated with infection (9).

EPIDEMIOLOGY

Incidence

In several studies during 1997–2002, the incidence of hemodialysis access-associated bacteremia ranged from 0.31 to 1.2 infections per 1000 patient-days (Table 1) (10–16). The incidence of bacteremia among patients undergoing chronic hemodialysis in a large acute care facility was even higher (2.5 infections per 1000 patient-days) (17). A review of four recent studies used a consensus rate of 0.6 bacteremias per 1000 patient-days to estimate that 50,000 access-associated bacteremias occur per year in the United States (18). Wherever the issue was studied, the incidence of infection was highest with catheters and lowest with fistulas.

Because of the importance of bacterial infections in hemodialysis patients, the Centers for Disease Control and Prevention (CDC) initiated an ongoing surveillance project in 1999 (16). Hemodialysis centers treating outpatients are eligible to enroll. Only bacterial infections associated with hospital admission or receipt of intravenous antimicrobials were counted (i.e.,

Table 1 Measurement of Incidence of Vascular Access-Related Bacteremia per 1000 Patient-Days[a] among Patients in Hemodialysis

Author, year	Type of study	No. of centers	Vascular access type				
			All	Fistula	Graft	Tunneled catheter	Nontunneled catheter
Bonomo, 1997 (10)	Retrospective	1	—	0.82[b]		—	—
Hoen, 1998 (11)	Prospective	19	0.31	—	—	—	—
Taylor, 1998 (12)	Surveillance	1	1.20	—	—	—	—
D'Agata, 2000 (17)	Surveillance	1	2.5	—	—	—	—
Taylor, 2002 (13)	Surveillance	6	0.59	0.09	0.23	1.31	2.23
Dopirak, 2002 (14)	Surveillance	10	0.45	0.04[b]			1.14[c]
Stevenson, 2002 (15)	Surveillance	6	0.65	0.07	0.15	2.37	4.53
Tokars, 2002 (16)	Surveillance	109	0.59	0.08	0.18	1.61	2.91

[a] Where necessary, rates per 1000 sessions were converted to rates per 1000 patient-days by assuming 3 sessions per 7 days.
[b] For fistulas and grafts combined.
[c] For tunneled and nontunneled catheters combined.

infections treated with outpatient oral antimicrobials were excluded); therefore, this system likely detected only the more severe infections. During 1999–2001, 109 centers reported data. Rates of infection per 100 patient-months were 3.2 for all vascular-access infections (including access infections both with and without bacteremia), 1.8 for vascular access-associated bacteremias, 1.4 for local access infections, 1.3 for wound infections not related to the vascular access, 0.8 for pneumonias, and 0.3 for urinary tract infections. The rate of access-associated bacteremias per 100 patient-months varied by type of vascular access: 8.7 for noncuffed catheters, 4.8 for cuffed catheters, 0.5 for grafts, and 0.3 for fistulas (16). Note that, in this study, rates of infection were tabulated per 100 patient-months; these rates are approximately 3 times higher than rates per 1000 patient-days. A rate of 3.2 per 100 patient-months can be interpreted to mean that on average 3.2% of the patients have the infection each month, or that there are 0.38 infections per patient-year.

Risk Factors

Many risk factors have been assessed in epidemiologic studies.

Vascular-Access Type

The primary risk factor for access infection is access type. Risk is highest for catheters, intermediate for grafts, and lowest for native arteriovenous fistulas (11,16,19). Fistulas or grafts should be preferred to central venous catheters for permanent access in dialysis patients.

Location of the Access

Among patients with catheters, the subclavian site (rather than a jugular or a femoral site) is associated with lower infection (20) and colonization (21) rates in adult patients with a central venous catheter; however, neither of these studies involved hemodialysis patients. The Kidney Disease Outcomes Quality Initiative (KDOQI) guidelines recommend the right internal jugular vein for insertion of tunneled cuffed venous dialysis catheters; noncuffed catheters can be inserted in the femoral, internal jugular, or subclavian sites (22). Among patients with fistulas or grafts, location in the lower extremities has been associated with a higher risk of infections (10).

Characteristics of the Patient

Older age, uninsured, or having Medicaid insurance were associated with a higher risk of bacteremia (19).

Comorbidities

The following have been associated with a higher rate of vascular-access infection: a history of hospitalization, human immunodeficiency virus (HIV) infection (23), and previous history of bacteremia (11,19,23).

Serum Albumin

Low serum albumin is associated with increased risk of bacteremia (19,23).

Immunosupressive Therapy

In one study, current immunosuppressive therapy was associated with a threefold increase in risk of bacteremia (11).

Reuse of Dialyzers

In a large cohort study, 57% of 4005 patients on hemodialysis were treated with reused dialyzers; these patients had a risk ratio of bacteremia of 1.28 over the 7-year follow-up period compared to patients not treated with reused membranes (19). (Note: here and throughout this document we have replaced the term septicemia with bacteremia, although septicemia was originally used by many authors, and the significance of the terms can be somewhat different).

Dialysis Adequacy

The effectiveness, or adequacy, of dialysis treatment has been evaluated as a risk factor for bacteremia. Adequacy can be measured using the urea reduction ratio [100 × (the predialysis urea level − the postdialysis level/ predialysis level)] or the Kt/V (the dialyzer clearance × the duration of the dialysis session/the estimated volume of water in the patient's body). Higher levels of the urea reduction ratio may be associated with a lower risk of bacteremia (23); however, this finding is not consistent across studies (11). Kt/V was not a significant risk factor for bacteremia in one study (11) but has been associated with risk of death due to infection in dialysis patients (19).

Hematocrit

Lower hematocrit values have been associated with an increased risk of bacteremia (11), although not consistently (19,23).

Mortality

U. S. hemodialysis patients have a mortality rate of approximately 23% per year (234.6 per 1000 patient-years at risk). Infections are the second most common cause of death, accounting for 14% of deaths (2). Bacterial sepsis (11.1% of all deaths) is the most common infectious cause of mortality. Prevalent mortality rates for U.S. dialysis patients have fallen 10% since 1980; however, rates have fallen 22 and 15% for patients with <2 and 2–5 years on dialysis, respectively (2).

ETIOLOGY/MICROBIOLOGY

The majority of bacteremias associated with hemodialysis catheters are due to *S. aureus* and coagulase-negative staphylococci. Data from the Dialysis

Table 2 Microorganisms Isolated from Blood Cultures from Access-Related Bacteremias Reported to the Dialysis Surveillance Network, Oct. 1999–May 2001

Microorganism	Catheter-related bacteremia[a] [n (%)]	Fistula or graft access-related bacteremia[b] [n (%)]
Staphylococcus aureus	399 (32.1)	123 (53.0)
Coagulase-negative staphylococci	401 (32.3)	47 (20.3)
Other Gram-positive organisms		
Enterococcus spp.	125 (10.1)	11 (4.7)
Streptococcus spp.	30 (2.4)	15 (6.5)
Gram-negative rods	229 (18.4)	23 (9.9)
Other (including fungi)	59 (4.7)	13 (5.6)

[a] Total no. of cases = 1243.
[b] Total no. of cases = 232.

Surveillance Network (DSN) reported through May 2001 (16) indicate that the organisms most frequently isolated from blood cultures associated with catheter access-related bacteremias, in descending order of frequency, were coagulase-negative staphylococci (32%), *S. aureus* (32%), Gram-negative bacilli (18%), and nonstaphylococcal Gram-positive cocci, including enterococci (12%) (Table 2). The proportion of infections caused by *S. aureus* was higher among patients with fistulas or grafts (53%).

Antimicrobial pressure from therapy for hemodialysis-associated bacteremias is one of the factors increasing the prevalence of antimicrobial resistance. In the United States, five of the first six patients with vancomycin-intermediate *S. aureus* had received dialysis (24), and the first patient reported to be infected with vancomycin-resistant *S. aureus* was a hemodialysis patient (25). During 1995–2001, in a national survey of dialysis centers that receive reimbursement from the Centers for Medicare and Medicaid Services, the percentage of centers surveyed reporting that they had treated one or more patients with methicillin- or oxacillin-resistant *S. aureus* (MRSA or ORSA) increased from 40% to 72% (1). The percentage of centers reporting one or more patients with colonization or infection with vancomycin-resistant enterococci increased from 12 to 43% in the same period (1).

DIAGNOSIS

Diagnosis of vascular-access infection at the exit site can be based on the observation of tenderness, erythema, edema, exudate, or site induration along the subcutaneous tract of a tunnelled catheter (4). Purulent drainage from the exit site should be cultured. Fistulas and grafts presented with signs of local access infection including pus, redness, or swelling of the access site without signs of bacteremia in 54.6% and 61.0%, respectively, of infections at the vascular site reported to the DSN through 2001 (16). Local signs of vascular access infection are erythema, warmth, induration, swelling, tenderness, breakdown of skin, loculated fluid, and purulent exudates (10,26,27).

Catheter-related bloodstream infection should be suspected when a patient with signs of sepsis (fever, chills, or hypotension) has an intravascular catheter and positive cultures. Blood cultures should be obtained before antimicrobial treatment. It is preferable to draw all blood cultures from a peripheral vein rather than through a catheter, since contamination of the specimen is less likely. However, avoidance of peripheral venipuncture in hemodialysis patients may be desirable in cases when venous sites are limited or there is a need to preserve future arteriovenous access sites (28).

Although it is best to obtain a blood culture before initiating intravenous antimicrobial therapy, in practice, this does not always occur. In the DSN database, 60% of intravenous antimicrobial starts were preceded by a blood culture (16).

CATHETER MATERIAL/SPECIAL TYPES OF CATHETERS

Hemodialysis catheters differ from most other catheter types in that blood is pumped through them under relatively high pressure. This puts stress on the catheters and exposes them to the risk of mechanical failure and leakage. Several materials have been used over time for dialysis (29), including polyethylene, Teflon, silicone, polyurethane, and polyurethane with polycarbonate copolymers. Different materials have been used to achieve the physical properties necessary in the dialysis procedure; these properties can be difficult to balance and include wall thickness, flexibility, rigidity, resistance to crimping or kinking, moldability under heat or stress, capacity to bond to other materials, ability to conform to body shape, and resistance to dissolution by disinfectants. Adherence of microorganisms to the catheter and thrombogenicity of catheter materials are critical issues in the pathogenesis of infection. In the United States, most central venous catheters for dialysis are made of polyurethane or silicone, with polyurethane predominating. Teflon (29) and polyethylene (4) are not currently used in catheters for dialysis in the United States, since polyethylene catheters are less resistant to the adherence of microorganisms.

Grafts are made of polytetrafluoroethylene, a synthetic material that allows flexibility in insertion sites and high patency rates and that can be used promptly after surgery; however, they are also susceptible to thrombosis and access failure (8).

Alcohol disinfectants, including isopropyl alcohol and ointments containing polyethylene glycol, have been reported to degrade polyurethane catheters (29). Iodine weakens silicone catheters, but less so when formulated as part of a povidone-iodine solution. Manufacturers' guidelines should always be followed when choosing a disinfectant for a specific hemodialysis catheter type (4).

MANAGEMENT/THERAPY

For more comprehensive discussions of treatment of catheter- and access-associated infections, see guidelines produced by the Infectious Diseases Society of America, the American College of Critical Care Medicine, and the Society for Healthcare Epidemiology of America (IDSA/ACCCM/ SHEA) (6), the National Kidney Foundation (NKF) (22), and a recent summary (28). Guidelines prepared by the Healthcare Infection Control Practices Advisory Committee of the CDC (HICPAC/CDC) (4) for the prevention of infectious complications associated with the use of intravascular catheters are useful because they emphasize the removal of catheters that are no longer necessary.

Fistula- and Graft- Related Infections

Empiric therapy for infected fistulas or grafts should consist of antimicrobials with coverage against Gram-negative and Gram-positive organisms, including *Enterococcus* species (22). Either vancomycin or a beta-lactam and an aminoglycoside would be acceptable, depending on local susceptibility patterns. Arteriovenous grafts that are more than superficially infected should be surgically removed; newly placed grafts (i.e., <1 month old) should be removed regardless of the extent of infection (22).

Catheter-Related Infections

Recommendations for the management and treatment of catheter-related infections in hemodialysis patients specify the following issues:

1. Exit-site infections are typically associated with erythema, crusting, and exudate without systemic symptoms or positive blood cultures. When there is no evidence of a tunnel infection, exit-site infections in patients with cuffed, tunneled catheters generally can be treated with topical antibiotic ointments without catheter removal or systemic antibiotics (22). However, this recommendation does not apply for exit-site infections in noncuffed catheters (28).
2. Tunnel infections are manifested by tenderness, erythema, and/or induration. The IDSA/ACCCM/SHEA guidelines recommend that tunnel infections be treated with catheter removal as well as appropriate antibiotics (6). Tunnel infections are often accompanied by bacteremia that requires treatment as outlined subsequently.
3. Initial empiric antimicrobial therapy should be directed against both Gram-positive and Gram-negative organisms, with subse-

quent therapy based on blood culture results. Vancomycin and an aminoglycoside (i.e., gentamicin) or antipseudomonal cephalosporin are commonly used initially. A beta-lactam, such as cefazolin, with or without an aminoglycoside, may be reasonable initial therapy if the risk of infection with *S. aureus* resistant to oxacillin (MRSA or ORSA) is low (28). If blood cultures identify a beta-lactam-susceptible organism, vancomycin, if administered initially for empiric therapy, should be discontinued, and cefazolin or another alternate agent should be used.

4. Management of bacteremia related to indwelling double-cuffed hemodialysis catheters has been addressed in several recent reports and the NKF K/DOQI clinical practice guidelines (22), but remains controversial. Attempts at salvaging tunneled, cuffed hemodialysis catheters in patients with catheter-related bacteremia with antimicrobial agents alone without catheter removal are usually unsuccessful (30,31). CDC/HICPAC guidelines recommend that central venous catheters (including hemodialysis catheters) be replaced and not exchanged over a guidewire if there is suspicion that a bacteremia is catheter-related except as salvage therapy in selected hemodialysis patients with limited venous access (4). Guidelines from the IDSA indicate that in the presence of *S. aureus* bacteremia, tunneled hemodialysis catheters should be removed with the duration of antimicrobial therapy guided by findings on transesophageal echocardiography (14 days if no evidence of vegetation; 4–6 weeks if vegetation is present) (6). These same guidelines suggest that catheter-related bacteremia caused by coagulase-negative staphylococci can be treated without catheter removal, but may require more prolonged antimicrobial therapy (6). A few reports indicate that catheter replacement over a guidewire within 48 hours of initiating antimicrobials, followed by a period of appropriate antimicrobial therapy, can be successful in carefully selected patients who are not critically ill (31–35). Catheters should be removed promptly, rather than exchanged over a guidewire, if there is evidence of catheter tunnel or exit-site infection in clinically unstable patients with features of sepsis, and in patients who remain febrile or symptomatic for more than 36 hours after initiation of antimicrobial therapy or who have persistently positive blood cultures despite antimicrobial therapy (22). Periodic blood cultures should be obtained after completion of therapy to confirm eradication of the infection. Antimicrobial treatment for hemodialysis catheter-related bacteremias for at least three weeks is recommended (22), although the optimal duration of therapy has not been systematically explored. Circumstances in which a longer or shorter duration of therapy might be appropriate or necessary remain to be defined.

5. Although vancomycin is acceptable prophylaxis for major surgical procedures involving implantation of prosthetic materials or devices at institutions that have a high rate of MRSA (ORSA) or methicillin-resistant *Staphylococcus epidermidis*, this does not include placement or revision of hemodialysis catheters, fistulas, or grafts.
6. Vancomycin is discouraged for routine prophylaxis of infections in patients on hemodialysis (36) and for treatment (chosen for dosing convenience) of infections caused by beta-lactam-susceptible Gram-positive microorganisms in patients with renal failure.
7. Instillation of antimicrobial agents into hemodialysis catheters (antibiotic lock) is not recommended as a routine preventive measure, but has been recommended when there is a history of multiple catheter-related bacteremias despite optimal aseptic technique (4) or when the catheter is retained during an episode of catheter-related bacteremia (6). Guidelines from IDSA describe in greater detail the role of antibiotic lock therapy in the management of catheter-related bloodstream infections, including patient selection and duration of therapy issues (6).

PREVENTION AND CONTROL

Despite higher rates of bacteremia in patients treated with hemodialysis catheters than those treated with fistulas or grafts, the percentage of U.S. hemodialysis patients treated with catheters has increased substantially, from 13% to 25% during 1995 to 2001 (1). The most basic strategy to prevent catheter-related bacteremias among hemodialysis patients is to minimize the use of catheters; efforts to reduce the use of catheters for permanent vascular access should be a part of every prevention program (4,15,20).

Catheters are used for different reasons. In a survey of chronic hemodialysis centers, the reasons reported for using catheters for vascular access in 2001 were as follows: 40% of catheters were used as an access of last resort (i.e., no sites remained for creation of a fistula or graft), 28% were for established patients with a failed access awaiting a new implanted access, 25% were for new patients awaiting an implanted access, and 6% were for other reasons, including patient preference (1).

Here, we discuss and provide resources for three aspects of a prevention program: surveillance, prevention of infections, and prevention of antimicrobial resistance.

Surveillance for Infections

Although information from the literature is invaluable in preventing infections, local data provide the information needed to quickly identify problems and target control measures. A record keeping system, such as a log book or

electronic file, should be developed and maintained centrally (37). Information that should be collected at the individual patient level for aggregate
analyses includes episodes of bacteremia or loss of the vascular access due to
infection (including date of onset, site of infection, genus and species of the
infecting organism, and selected antimicrobial susceptibility results). A staff
person should be designated to periodically review episodes of bacteremia or
vascular-access infections and test results; a protocol should be specified for
actions required when findings from this review indicate action is needed.

For comparisons of data on infections or complications across outpatient facilities, it is necessary to adjust the number of events for the number of
days at risk or the number of dialysis sessions. Several recent articles outline
methods and definitions for surveillance for hemodialysis access infections
(13,15,16). The CDC sponsors a system available to all centers caring for
hemodialysis outpatients (see http://www.cdc.gov/ncidod/hip/default.htm);
forms are available as a resource, and dialysis centers can voluntarily
participate.

Preventing Infections

Recommendations for preventing vascular-access infections have been developed by NKF (22) and CDC/HICPAC (4) and represent the critical first
step in the CDC Campaign to Prevent Antimicrobial Resistance (3). Selected
recommendations for preventing hemodialysis catheter-associated infection
include the following: not routinely replacing the catheter; using sterile
technique (cap, mask, sterile gown, large sterile drapes, and gloves) during
catheter insertion; limiting use of noncuffed catheters to 3–4 weeks; using the
catheter solely for hemodialysis unless there is no alternative; restricting
catheter manipulation and dressing changes to trained personnel; replacing
the catheter-site dressing at each dialysis treatment or if damp, loose, or
soiled; disinfecting skin before catheter insertion and dressing changes (a 2%
chlorhexidine-based preparation is preferred); and ensuring that catheter-site
care is compatible with the catheter material (28).

The European Renal Association recommends the following measures
to reduce the susceptibility of hemodialysis patients to infection: ensure
optimal adequacy of hemodialysis, prevent or treat malnutrition, maintain
optimum hemoglobin concentration, avoid iron overload, and use a dialysis
membrane with the lowest degree of complement and leukocyte activation
(38). Vaccination might also be added to the list of measures to reduce
susceptibility to infections, e.g., a recent study describes successful limited
immunization of hemodialysis patients with a *S. aureus* vaccine (39).

In hemodialysis patients, the IDSA/ACCCM/SHEA guidelines recommend treatment with nasal mupirocin in documented *S. aureus* carriers who
have had a catheter-related bacteremia with *S. aureus* and continue to need
the hemodialysis catheter (6). Otherwise, the routine use of nasal mupirocin in

Table 3 Twelve Steps to Prevent Antimicrobial Resistance among Dialysis Patients

---

Prevent Infection
Step 1. Vaccinate Staff and Patients
- Get influenza vaccine
- Give influenza and pneumococcal vaccine to patients in addition to routine vaccines (e.g., hepatitis B)

Step 2. Get the Catheters Out
Hemodialysis
- Use catheters only when essential
- Maximize use of fistulas/grafts
- Remove catheters when they are no longer essential
Peritoneal Dialysis
- Remove/replace infected catheters

Step 3. Optimize Access Care
- Follow established KDOQI and CDC guidelines for access care
- Use proper insertion and catheter-care protocols
- Remove access device when infected
- Use the correct catheter

Diagnose and Treat Infection Effectively
Step 4. Target the Pathogen
- Obtain appropriate cultures
- Target empiric therapy to likely pathogens
- Target definitive therapy to known pathogens
- Optimize timing, regimen, dose, route, and duration

Step 5. Access the Experts
- Consult the appropriate expert for complicated infections

Use Antimicrobials Wisely
Step 6. Use Local Data
- Know your local antibiogram
- Get previous microbiology results when patients transfer to your facility

Step 7. Know When to Say "No" to Vanco
- Follow CDC guidelines for vancomycin use
- Consider 1st generation cephalosporins instead of vancomycin

Step 8. Treat Infection, Not Contamination or Colonization
- Use proper antisepsis for drawing blood cultures
- Get one peripheral vein blood culture, if possible
- Avoid culturing vascular catheter tips
- Treat bacteremia, not the catheter tip

Step 9. Stop Antimicrobial Treatment
- When infection is treated
- When infection is not diagnosed

Prevent Transmission
Step 10. Follow Infection Control Precautions
- Use standard infection control precautions for dialysis centers
- Consult local infection control experts

Table 3 Continued

Step 11. Practice Hand Hygiene
- Wash your hands or use an alcohol-based handrub
- Set an example

Step 12. Partner With Your Patients
- Educate on access care and infection control measures
- Re-educate regularly

patients with hemodialysis catheters is not recommended by either CDC or the NKF (4,22).

The KDOQI guideline recommends either povidone-iodine or mupirocin ointment at the exit site of the hemodialysis catheter, unless there is an interaction with the material of the catheter (22). Mupirocin should be avoided with polyurethane catheters because of potential material degradation (34,35). The HICPAC/CDC guideline recommends only povidone/iodine ointment (4). The practice of antibiotic lock is not routinely recommended for prevention of infections (4). However, an antibiotic lock may be used when there is a history of multiple catheter-related bacteremias despite optimal aseptic technique (4).

Preventing Antimicrobial Resistance

The CDC has developed the Campaign to Prevent Antimicrobial Resistance (3). For each of several subspecialties, including nephrology, a manuscript and series of 12 action steps was developed (http://www.cdc.gov/drugresistance/healthcare/patients.htm#dialysis). The 12 steps are grouped into the following four strategies: prevent infection, diagnose and treat infections effectively, use antimicrobials wisely, and prevent transmission. The steps address aspects of protecting patients with appropriate vaccination, eliminating unnecessary risk of infection, diagnosis and effective treatment of infections, judicious use of antimicrobials, and prevention of secondary transmission of infections (Table 3). Resources are available for public use and can be downloaded from the web site.

SUMMARY AND CONCLUSION

Hemodialysis patients are at high risk for infection because they are immunocompromised and require a vascular-access site for removal and replacement of blood. The vascular access may consist of an implanted access (fistula or graft) or a catheter. Rates of infection are highest for catheters, and the percent of U.S. hemodialysis patients treated with catheters increased to approximately 25% in 2001. Because of frequent infections and need for antimicrobial therapy, resistance to antimicrobials (particularly vancomycin) is high in hemodialysis patients. The most important infection control strategy is to use an implanted access rather than a catheter. For patients with catheters, strict adherence to guidelines for insertion and care are essential to minimize the risk of infection.

REFERENCES

1. Tokars JI, Finelli L, Alter MJ, Arduino MJ. National surveillance of dialysis-associated diseases in the United States, 2001. Report accessed from http://www.cdc.gov/ncidod/hip/SURVEILL/SURVEILL.HTM
2. U.S. Renal Data System, USRDS 2003 Annual Data Report: Atlas of End-Stage Renal Disease in the United States, National Institutes of Health, National Institute of Diabetes and Digestive and Kidney Diseases, Bethesda, MD, 2003.
3. Centers for Disease Control and Prevention. Campaign to Prevent Antimicrobial Resistance in Healthcare Settings. http://www.cdc.gov/drugresistance/healthcare/default.htm. Accessed on December 9, 2003.
4. Centers for Disease Control and Prevention. Guidelines for the prevention of intravascular catheter-related infections. MMWR 2002; 51(No.RR-10):1–29.
5. Raad I. Intravascular-catheter-related infections. Lancet 1998; 351:893–898.
6. Mermel LA, Farr BM, Sherertz RJ, Raad II, O'Grady N, Harris JS, Craven DE. Guidelines for the management of intravascular catheter-related infections. Clin Infect Dis 2001; 32(9):1249–1272.
7. Alter MJ, Tokars JI, Arduino MJ, Favero MS. Nosocomial Infections Associated with Hemodialysis. In: Mayhall CG, ed. Hospital Epidemiology and Infection Control. 3rd Ed. Philadelphia, PA: Lippincott Williams and Wilkins, 2004:1139–1160.
8. Joseph S, Adler S. Vascular access problems in dialysis patients. Pathogenesis and strategies for management. Heart Disease 2001; 3:242–247.
9. Ayus JC, Sheikh-Hamad D. Silent infection in clotted hemodialysis access grafts. J Am Soc Nephrol 1998; 9:1314–1317.
10. Bonomo RA, Rice D, Whalen C, Linn D, Eckstein E, Shlaes DM. Risk factors associated with permanent access-site infections in chronic hemodialysis patients. Infect Control Hosp Epidemiol 1997; 18:757–761.
11. Hoen B, Paul-Dauphin A, Hestin D, Kessler M. EPIBACDIAL: a multicenter prospective study of risk factors for bacteremia in chronic hemodialysis patients. J Am Soc Nephrol 1998; 9:869–876.
12. Taylor GD, McKenzie M, Buchanan-Chell M, Caballo L, Chui L, Kowalweska-Grochowska K. Central venous catheters as a source of hemodialysis-related bacteremia. Infect Control Hosp Epidemiol 1998; 19:643–646.
13. Taylor G, Gravel D, Johnston L, Embil J, Holton D, Paton S. Prospective surveillance for primary bloodstream infections occurring in Canadian hemodialysis units. Infect Control Hosp Epidemiol 2002; 23:716–720.
14. Dopirak M, Hill C, Oleksiw M, Dumigan D, Arvai J, English E, Carusillo E, Malo-Schlegel S, Richo J, Traficanti K, Welch B, Cooper B. Surveillance of the

hemodialysis-associated primary bloodstream infections: the experience of ten hospital based centers. Infect Control Hosp Epidemiol 2002; 23:721–724.

15. Stevenson KB, Hannah E, Lowder CA, Adcox MJ, Davidson RL, Mallea MC, Narasimhan N, Wagnild JP. Epidemiology of hemodialysis vascular-access infections from longitudinal infection surveillance data: predicting the impact of NKF-DOQI clinical practice guidelines for vascular access. Am J Kidney Dis 2002; 39:549–555.

16. Tokars JI, Miller ER, Stein G. New national surveillance system for hemodialysis-associated infections: initial results. Am J Infect Control 2002; 30:288–295.

17. D'Agata EMC, Mount DB, Thayer V, Schaffner W. Hospital-acquired infections among chronic hemodialysis patients. Am J Kidney Dis 2000; 35: 1083–1088.

18. Tokars JI. Bloodstream infections in hemodialysis patients: getting some deserved attention. Infect Control Hosp Epidemiol 2002; 23:713–715.

19. Powe NR, Jaar B, Furth SL, Hermann J, Briggs W. Septicemia in dialysis patients: incidence, risk factors, and prognosis. Kidney Int 1999; 55:1081–1090.

20. Merrer J, De Jonghe B, Golliot F, Lefrant JY, Raffy B, Barre E, Rigaud JP, Casciani D, Misset B, Bosquet C, Outin H, Brun-Buisson C, Nitenberg G, French Catheter Study Group in Intensive Care. Complications of femoral and subclavian venous catheterization in critically ill patients: a randomized controlled trial. JAMA 2001; 286:700–707.

21. Goetz A, Wagener MM, Miller JM, Muder RR. Risk of infection due to central venous catheters: effect of site of placement and catheter type. Infect Control Hosp Epidemiol 1998; 19:842–845.

22. National Kidney Foundation. KDOQI clinical practice guideline for vascular access, 2000. Am J Kidney Dis 2001; 37(suppl 1):S137–S181.

23. Tokars JI, Light P, Anderson J, Miller ER, Parrish J, Armistead N, Jarvis WR, Gehr T. A prospective study of vascular-access infections at seven outpatient hemodialysis centers. Am J Kidney Dis 2001; 37:1232–1240.

24. Fridkin SK. Vancomycin-intermediate and -resistant *Staphylococcus aureus*: what the infectious disease specialist needs to know. Clin Infect Dis 2001; 32:108–115.

25. Centers for Disease Control and Prevention. *Staphylococcus aureus* resistant to vancomycin: United States, 2002. MMWR 2002; 51:565–567.

26. Kaplowitz LG, Comstock JA, Landwehr DM, Dalton HP, Mayhall CG. A prospective study of infections in hemodialysis patients: patient hygiene and other risk factors for infection. Infect Control Hosp Epidemiol 1988; 9:534–541.

27. Padberg FT Jr, Lee BC, Curl GR. Hemoaccess site infection. Surg Gynecol Obstet 1992; 174:103–108.

28. Berns JS, Tokars JI. Preventing bacterial infections and antimicrobial resistance in dialysis patients. Am J Kidney Dis 2002; 40:886–898.

29. Ash SR. The evolution and function of central venous catheters for dialysis. Seminars in Dialysis 2001; 14:416–424.

30. Marr KA, Sexton DJ, Conlon PJ, Corey GR, Schwab SJ, Kirkland KB. Catheter-related bacteremia and outcome of attempted catheter salvage in patients undergoing hemodialysis. Ann Intern Med 1997; 127:275–280.

31. Saad TF. Bacteremia associated with tunneled, cuffed hemodialysis catheters. Am J Kidney Dis 1999; 34:1114–1124.
32. Beathard GA. Management of bacteremia associated with tunneled-cuffed hemodialysis catheters. J Am Soc Nephrol 1999; 10:1045–1049.
33. Shaffer D. Catheter-related sepsis complicating long-term, tunneled central venous dialysis catheters: management by guidewire exchange. Am J Kidney Dis 1995; 25:593–596.
34. Robinson D, Suhocki P, Schwab SJ. Treatment of infected tunneled venous access hemodialysis catheters with guidewire exchange. Kidney Int 1998; 53:1792–1794.
35. Tanriover B, Carlton D, Saddekni S, Hamrick K, Oser R, Westfall AO, Allon M. Bacteremia associated with tunneled dialysis catheters: comparison of two treatment strategies. Kidney Int 2000; 57:2151–2155.
36. Hospital Infection Control Practices Advisory Committee (HICPAC). Recommendations for preventing the spread of vancomycin resistance. Infect Control Hosp Epidemiol 1995; 16:105–113.
37. Centers for Disease Control and Prevention. Recommendations for preventing transmission of infections among chronic hemodialysis patients. MMWR 2001; 50(No.RR-5):1–43.
38. European Best Practice Guidelines Expert Group on Hemodialysis, European Renal Association. Section VI. Haemodialysis-associated infection. Nephrol Dial Transplant 2002; 17(S7):72–87.
39. Shinefield H, Black S, Fattom A, Horwith G, Rasgon S, Ordonez J, Yeoh H, Law D, Robbins JB, Schneerson R, Muenz L, Naso R. Use of a *Staphylococcus aureus* conjugate vaccine in patients receiving hemodialysis. N Engl J Med 2002; 346:491–496.

18

Catheter-Related Infections in Pediatric Patients

André Fleer, Tannette G. Krediet, Leo J. Gerards, and Tom F.W. Wolfs
Wilhelmina Children's Hospital, University Medical Center Utrecht
Utrecht, The Netherlands

John J. Roord
Department of Pediatrics, Free University Medical Center
Amsterdam, The Netherlands

INTRODUCTION

Central venous catheters (CVCs) have become a major asset in the treatment of infants and children with various forms of malignancy, nutritional disorders, and chronic debilitating diseases. Infection remains one of the most frequent and troublesome complications of CVCs in all categories of pediatric patients. In a large survey of nosocomial infections (NIs) in 4684 pediatric patients, it was found that the highest NI rate occurred in the neonatal intensive care unit (NICU) (14%), followed by neurosurgery (12%), hematology/oncology (12%), neonatal surgery (9%), and the pediatric intensive care unit (ICU) (6%) (1). Both this last study and the National Nosocomial Infections Surveillance (NNIS) study in the United States (2–4) revealed that NIs in pediatric patients, particularly in the ICU and among neonatal and hematology/oncology patients, are primarily bloodstream infections which are intravascular device-related.

For this reason this chapter will be mainly confined to the epidemiology, microbiology, clinical aspects, and issues of management of CVC-related infections (CRI) in those categories of pediatric patients in which they are most prominent, particularly premature newborns and children with cancer, and to their predominant pathogen: coagulase-negative staphylococci (CONS). A considerable experience has been gathered over the past 20 years with respect to CRIs in infancy and childhood. The data published up to 1988 were superbly reviewed by Decker and Edwards (5). That review was used as starting point for the chapter on Catheter-Related Infections in Children in the first edition of this book; in the present review we have extended and updated this information.

Since bacterial factors and pathogenetic mechanisms involved in these infections are dealt with in the various other chapters of this book, they will be discussed here only as far as they are relevant and specific for the pediatric situation.

PATHOGENESIS

As pointed out in the introduction, intravascular device-related infections in infants and children are most commonly encountered in the NICU and in hematology/oncology patients. A number of pathogenetic factors have been identified, particularly for the premature newborn, which may partially explain this enhanced susceptibility. The propensity for CONS bacteremia to occur in the most premature infants is probably explained by the decline in host defenses, particularly opsonic defense, to CONS with increasing prematurity (6,7). Opsonic defense to CONS in premature infants proved to be exclusively dependent on complement activation (6), which is deficient itself in the premature infant (6,8–10). Moreover, CONS strains from neonatal bacteremia may vary in their opsonic requirements (11–13). Particularly, some strongly hydrophobic CONS strains proved to be almost opsonization-resistant in neonatal serum (11). Based on these findings, it is not surprising that some of these CONS strains cannot be cleared by premature newborns from their bloodstream. In addition, we found transplacental IgG to be opsonically deficient for CONS, which adds to the neonate's host defense defects against these bacteria.

Another factor of potential pathogenetic importance is the ability of CONS strains to survive and persist in the NICU environment. Persistence of CONS strains in the NICU has been well documented in a number of studies (14–19). The capacity to develop antibiotic resistance appears to be one of the driving forces behind persistence of such strains (18–20). There are undoubtedly additional factors that determine persistence of CONS strains in the NICU, but very little definite information exists on the identity of such factors. The ease with which strains colonize both personnel and patients, enabling them to be transmitted within the unit, may be such a factor and another driving force behind persistence of certain CONS strains.

We indeed obtained evidence for this notion in a study using molecular typing methods that showed that neonatal CONS septicemia is most frequently caused by certain strains that are not only antibiotic-resistant, but also predominate in the unit and are widely distributed among both neonates and personnel (20). Apparently, these particular molecular types harbor characteristics that promote colonization. At the molecular level, these colonization factors are probably adhesins expressed at the surface of the staphylococcal cell wall, like the biomaterial adhesins of CONS (21), with which they possibly share expression on fimbriae-like surface appendages (22). It is an attractive hypothesis that these adhesins of CONS are a family of "multipurpose" adhesive molecules that may mediate adherence to skin and mucosal surfaces as well as to biomaterials. Strains possessing this kind of adhesins are clearly at a considerable advantage over other strains, provided that, in addition, they are also capable of quickly adapting and becoming resistant to antibiotics used in these units. It is evident that such CONS strains are not only supremely equipped for survival and persistence in the NICU, but also in other departments where biomaterials and antibiotics are widely used.

EPIDEMIOLOGY

Neonatal Intensive Care

Incidence

Nosocomial infections are an important cause of morbidity in NICUs and are primarily device-related, i.e., CVC-related. The incidence, expressed in different ways in various studies, varies from 5 to 32% in hospitalized infants and from 5 to 20 infections/1000 catheter-days, respectively (4,23–28). These variations can probably be explained by differences in the intensity of care, gestational age, and birthweight, duration of hospital stay between study populations, and possibly also differences in the definitions used in the studies. However, recent multicenter studies among NICUs in the United States have confirmed a considerable center-to-center variability in incidence of late-onset sepsis (25,26,28).

Risk Factors

Birthweight and gestational age were the risk factors with the strongest relationship with late-onset sepsis in all four recent surveys from the United States (25–28). A similar relation was found in an earlier multicenter study by Gaynes et al., in which it was found that infants of <1500-g birthweight were three times more likely to acquire a CVC-related bacteremia than infants of >1500 g (median infection rates of 14.6 and 5.1 bacteremias per 1000 catheter-days, respectively, $P = 0.0001$) (4). This highly significant inverse relation of infection rate with birthweight and gestational age was confirmed in more recent surveys (25,26,28).

Other factors, such as crowding, may also greatly influence the incidence rate of NIs in the NICU, as was demonstrated in the classic study of

Goldmann et al. (24), in which a fivefold decrease in NI rate was found after the NICU was moved to a new, more spacious facility.

In addition, changes in the mode of care, particularly increased instrumentation, have undoubtedly influenced the evolution in the pattern of NIs in the NICU, as we have observed in an epidemiological study over the last decade (1990–2000) in our own unit. An increasing incidence of nosocomial sepsis in general was noted in this last decade, from 5% in 1990 to 16% in 2000, and an emergence of nosocomial CONS sepsis in particular; these phenomena were parallelled by an increasing use of indwelling intravascular catheters, artificial ventilation and total parenteral nutrition (TPN) (Krediet et al., 2002, unpublished data). The data suggest that increased instrumentation, particularly IV access through CVCs and the administration of TPN, may be in part responsible for the current trends in NIs in the NICU, especially for the emergence of certain nosocomial pathogens, notably CONS, during the past decades. This trend of increased instrumentation, i.e., intravascular access and TPN use, and its association with nosocomial septicemia in the NICU has been noted in various surveys as well as in a number of studies from single centers (25,28–31).

The proportion of NIs that are CVC-related is evidently dependent on the extent to which CVCs are used in a particular NICU. As mentioned earlier, this rate is very high in the intensive care nursery of today. As a result, CVC-related bacteremia presently exists as one of the most important NIs in NICUs, with rates of 10 to 15%. This was exemplified in a nationwide survey conducted in the Netherlands on complications of parenteral nutrition in neonates involving seven NICUs, in which it was found that CVC-related sepsis was the most frequent complication, occurring in 11.7% of infants (32).

The results of the NNIS study (4) clearly showed that the use of devices characterized the NICU in terms of invasive practices as well as the average severity of illness of the infants. In addition, the NNIS study convincingly demonstrated that the utilization of devices was an important risk factor for the occurrence of NIs. Thus, the incidence of nosocomial bacteremia was found to be related mainly to the use of central catheters. These findings were corroborated in four more recent NICU surveys (25–28).

However, it should be emphasized that other modes of care of hospitalized premature newborns may independently influence NI rates. For example, lipid parenteral nutrition not only may promote CVC-related sepsis by specific agents such as the yeast *Malassezia furfur* (33,34), but also appears to be an independent risk factor for CONS bacteremia (29,30) and candidemia (35–37). In addition, Shah et al. (38) found that CVC use was an independent risk factor for Gram-negative bacteremia in the NICU.

It can be concluded that, although the complexity of modern neonatal care makes it difficult to disentangle the various possible risk factors for nosocomial septicemia, the aid of statistical methods including logistic regression analysis has permitted identification of the most important ones.

The aforementioned studies have clearly documented that prematurity, low birthweight, CVC use, and the administration of TPN, particularly lipids, are the predominant risk factors.

Molecular Epidemiology

Until recently, molecular epidemiologic studies were difficult to realize because reliable molecular typing methods of causative agents were unavailable. However, modern molecular typing methods have, in the meantime, revolutionized epidemiologic studies of microbial infections and have, in fact evolved into essential tools for such studies (39). By using various methods, notably RAPD (randomly amplified polymorphic DNA), ribotyping and PFGE (pulsed-field gel electrophoresis), a number of features of the epidemiologic behavior of CONS strains in the hospital environment and in the NICU, in particular, has been clarified. For example, Bingen et al. (40) demonstrated that RAPD provided differentiation of CONS blood isolates from a pediatric hospital, revealing cross-infection in one ward but not in another. By molecular typing of CONS bloodstream isolates collected over periods of up to 10 years in a neonatal unit, Huebner et al. (14) and Lyytikäinen et al. (15) showed that certain CONS types can become endemic over longer periods of time and can repeatedly cause bloodstream infections in neonates, and that cross-infection is probably common. A number of studies have confirmed these observations (16–19). Moreover, the studies of Burnie et al. (17) and Vermont et al. (18) demonstrated that different units could harbor different predominant epidemic clones, even within one hospital. In addition, two recent studies (17,20) have documented colonization of personnel of the unit with the predominant types causing bloodstream infections, indicating a role of staff members in cross-infection with these predominant clones. Together these data suggest that each unit selects and generates its own predominant CONS clones, which may persist for long periods of time in the unit and can become a source of bloodstream infection if sufficiently susceptible hosts are present.

Another interesting application of molecular typing was reported by Hammerberg et al. (41). They provided evidence that CONS blood isolates from neonates are only rarely found (in only 7% of cases) on the skin venipuncture site after skin cleansing by iodine and alcohol. Accordingly, the authors conclude that in the vast majority of cases, neonatal CONS blood isolates represent true bacteremia rather than contamination.

It is evident that nucleic acid-based methods have quickly become the gold standard of typing of CONS isolates, as is true for other microbes, and are therefore essential and indispensable tools for epidemiologic studies.

Morbidity and Mortality

Mortality directly attributable to CVC-related septicemia tends to be low, i.e., only a few percent or even zero in most studies. It should be realized, however, that the overwhelming majority of these infections are due to CONS and it is generally observed that CVC-related CONS infections tend to have a low mortality (25,28). Despite this, it should be mentioned that the NICU surveys of Stoll and Fanaroff still found that infants with CVC-related sepsis were more likely to die during hospitalization (25,27,28). Although it was difficult to directly relate death to infection because of associated morbidity, infants with Gram-negative sepsis were at the greatest risk to die (25,28). This is another important point emphasized by these surveys, that the death rate of the more rare causes of CVC-related septicemia is considerably higher than for CONS infections, e.g., for *Staphylococcus aureus* it is 18% and for Gram-negative bacilli it is 40 to 60%. Despite its low overall mortality, late-onset CVC-related septicemia is still a significant problem in NICUs, because associated morbidity is extensive. In addition, there is prolongation of hospital stay, and considerably increased cost and resource use (25,27,28,42,43).

In summary, it is evident from a large number of studies during the past 20 years that CVC-related bacteremia is an important NI in the NICU and that CONS dominate as causative agents (4,24–28,44–46). Mortality is low, but morbidity is extensive and associated costs are considerable; therefore, CVC-related CONS septicemia has evolved into a major problem in neonatal intensive care.

Hematology/Oncology

Epidemiology

Infection is one of the major complications of the use of long-term right atrial catheters of the Hickman–Broviac type in children with cancer (47–59). The incidence varies widely, from 0.15 to 6.8 episodes per 1000 catheter-days (Table 1). Catheter-related bacteremia, the most serious infectious complication of CVCs, occurs with a frequency of 0.52 to 6.8/1000 catheter-days (Table 1). As with CRI in neonates, the wide variation in incidence rates is probably explained by differences in patient populations and in the definition of CRI.

Risk Factors

Risk factors for the occurrence of CRI in pediatric oncology patients have been assessed in a number of studies, particularly the role of variables such as neutropenia, chemotherapy, and age. Hartman and Shochat (50) found that neutropenia was associated with 70% of CRI, but also that 75% of all other infections occurred during neutropenia. Thus, in this study, neutropenia per se did not appear to increase the risk of CRI. However, insertion of a CVC during a neutropenic episode was associated with a more than twofold increased risk of bacteremia. In contrast, a large European Organisation for Research and Treatment of Cancer (EORTC) survey by Viscoli et al. (51) revealed that neutropenia did not impose an increased risk for CRI. This finding was confirmed in at least four other studies (56,58,60,61).

Table 1 Incidence of Central Venous Catheter-Related Infections in Neutropenic Children[a]

	Incidence (rate/1000 catheter-days)	
Study	Local infection	Bacteremia
Darbyshire et al. (77)	—[b]	6.8
Johnson et al. (78)	2.8	1.4
Hartman and Shochat (80)	2.5	2.1
Viscoli et al. (81)	0.16	0.52
Van Hoff et al. (82)	0.54	2.3
Rizzari et al. (83)	0.15	4.4
Uderzo et al. (84)	2.5	0.58
Rikkonen et al. (85)	0.22	0.75
Das et al. (56)	—	1.7
Elishoov et al. (59)	2.6	5.3
Ertem et al. (57)	0.6	4.9
Stamou et al. (58)	1.4	0.75

[a] Data compiled from twelve studies, 1985–1999 (Refs. 56–59, 77, 78, and 80–85).
[b] — = not stated.

Contrary to these latter findings, Hiemenz et al. (49) reported that from their experience with CVCs at the National Cancer Institute in Bethesda, Maryland, neutropenic patients had a fourfold increased risk of developing bacteremia if they had a CVC in place. Rizzari et al. also noted an increased risk of CRI during neutropenia (53), and similar observations were obtained by Elishoov et al. (59) in a recent prospective study in bone marrow transplant patients. Thus, the question whether neutropenia poses a risk factor for CRI in children with cancer appears to be unresolved. The only valid conclusion seems to be that placement of a catheter increases the risk of infection in both neutropenic and nonneutropenic oncological patients. Whether bone marrow transplantation (BMT) poses an independent risk for CRIs is another unresolved issue, although in a recent review of CRIs in BMT recipients, the authors concluded that in non-BMT patients with malignant disease rates of CRI were indeed lower (59). However, in the strict sense, these populations are not comparable, because the decision to perform a BMT in a cancer patient places the patient, by definition, in another category. Therefore, calculation of an independent risk associated with BMT will be difficult, if not impossible.

With respect to patient age in relation to the risk of CVC infection, Johnson et al. (48) clearly found an increased risk for Broviac catheter infections in younger children. Toddlers (1 through 4 years of age) had a rate of 3.9 infections per 1000 catheter-days compared to rates of 2.7/1000 catheter-days for school children and 0.5/1000 catheter-days for adolescents. Similar observations were made by Mulloy et al. (62), who found that children

<2 years of age were 2.6 times more likely to experience sepsis associated with tunneled CVCs than older children.

The type of device also influences the rate of infection. A study from the Memorial Sloan-Kettering Cancer Center (63) reported that the rate of CRI in 1431 cancer patients was tenfold lower in those with implanted ports (0.21/1000 catheter-days) than in those with Hickman-type silastic tunneled CVCs (2.77/1000 days). Similar findings were obtained by Rikkonen et al. (55), who observed that Hickman–Broviac type catheters carried a higher risk for bacteremia (0.75/1000 catheter-days) than implanted ports (0.14/1000 days). Moreover, these authors noted that CVCs in place for >300 days tended to be safer in this regard than those of shorter duration, although the difference was not statistically significant. It should be noted that patients with long infection-free intervals had leukocyte counts >1000/µl at the time of insertion of the CVC; thus, it is likely that their better host defenses contributed to the prevention of CRI, although the precise role of neutrophils in the pathogenesis of foreign body-related infections is still uncertain (64). However, it has also been observed in several studies that there is a subpopulation of patients that never develops an infection (47,48,55,56,59). Therefore, there may be a subpopulation of cancer patients that as a result of as yet unknown characteristics is less likely to develop a CRI a priori, apart from higher leukocyte counts at the time of insertion of a CVC. There are recent data indicating an association between infection risk in hemato-oncological patients and gene polymorphisms in determinants of innate immunity, specifically mannose-binding lectin (64a,64b). Further analysis of these determinants may yield valuable information for the management and control of CRI, not only in this particular group of patients, but presumably also for other categories. A possible explanation for the phenomenon that CVCs with long infection-free intervals are safer is offered by the experimental studies by Sherertz et al. (65,66). These studies demonstrated both in a mouse and in a rabbit model of subcutaneous catheter infection that catheters residing in the animal for 2 to 4 days before inoculation with microorganisms had up to 40% lower infection rate than catheters challenged immediately after insertion. Presumably, if one allows an inflammatory reaction to be formed around the catheter, the likelihood of a subsequent CVC infection is less.

Molecular Epidemiology

Molecular epidemiologic studies have revealed that, similar to the situation in the NICU, there are persistent CONS clones in hematology units carried by personnel and capable of causing bloodstream infections in susceptible patients (17,67).

Morbidity and Mortality

Mortality attributable to CRI is low, varying from 0 to 6% in the studies cited (47–59), and even if death ensues it is often difficult to specifically relate it to CVC infection. In this respect, the causative agent appears more important, i.e., death from CRI is more likely to occur with agents such as Gram-negative bacilli, particularly *Pseudomonas aeruginosa*, *S. aureus* and *Candida* spp., than with CONS (59).

Other Categories

Cystic Fibrosis

Other patient categories in which long-term cannulae are used are cystic fibrosis (CF) patients and patients on long-term home parenteral nutrition (HPN). There is relatively little information on risk factors and infection rates in these pediatric populations. Recently, the ten-year experience with regard to CRI in CF patients from a single center was reported (68). This study found only nine infections during a total of 75,660 catheter-days, for a rate of only 0.12 CVC infections per 1000 catheter-days.

Long-Term Parenteral Nutrition

A French study of CRI in children on HPN (69) noted an interesting dichotomy in the patient group: those with relatively few infections and a group with more frequent infections. The group with relatively few infections was characterized by a longer duration of HPN and a longer delay between start of HPN and the first CRI episode. These findings suggest that as yet unknown patient characteristics determine a priori the likelihood of CRI in patients on long-term HPN.

MICROBIOLOGY

In all categories of pediatric patients, CONS feature as the foremost agents of CRI. The CONS have "invaded" and perhaps even surprised the medical world during the last decades as versatile pathogens in patients fitted with intravascular or prosthetic devices. A number of reviews have highlighted virtually all aspects of CONS (70–75), among these two excellent reviews dealing with their exceptional significance as the foremost agents of CRI in the premature neonate (74,75). Also, in pediatric hematology/oncology patients, CONS dominate as causative agents of CRIs. In the present section we will discuss the microbiology of CRI in these two pediatric risk categories separately.

Neonatal Intensive Care

Coagulase-Negative Staphylococci

The CONS cause 50 to 80% of nosocomial septicemias in the NICU, according to reviews covering the last 15 to 20 years (25–28). These septicemias emerged in the 1980s when a number of NICUs noted an increase in bloodstream infections due to CONS (24,30,44–46,76). It soon became evident that this phenomenon could no longer be regarded as contamination of blood culture bottles due to improper aseptic techniques. These latter studies clearly documented CONS bacteremia in the premature neonate as a separate disease entity which is almost exclusively intravascular device-related. In fact, catheter-related sepsis in prematures has become almost synonymous with CONS bacteremia.

A number of features of CONS make this species particularly well equipped for causing infection with CVCs and other prosthetic devices. These properties have been highlighted in the preceding chapters on pathogenesis and will not be reiterated here, as these bacterial factors are likely to play a similar role in the pathogenesis of catheter-related infection in adults and children. However, the finding that slime production may characterize invasive CONS isolates and thus represent a risk factor for CONS bacteremia in infants colonized with such strains (77,78) could not be verified in our study (79).

With the emergence of CONS as important pathogens in certain hosts, typing became particularly important and in 1988 an evaluation of CONS typing methods was presented in a review on the clinical significance of CONS by Pfaller and Herwaldt (72). This review was updated in 1994 by Kloos and Bannerman (80).

Phenotyping of CONS strains from neonatal bacteremia cases associated with CVCs by biochemical profile-based methods such as API Staph-Ident has revealed that the majority of isolates belong to *S. epidermidis* (75% or more), the remainder to *S. haemolyticus*, *S. hominis*, and *S. warneri* (76–78). However, a clear disadvantage of phenotype-based methods is their lack of discriminatory power in epidemiologic studies (72, 80). For the latter purpose, molecular typing methods are much better suited and in the meantime have proven to be an invaluable tool for epidemiologic typing of CONS isolates, as already discussed in the section on Epidemiology.

Staphylococcus aureus

Staphylococcus aureus, Gram-negative enteric bacilli, and *Candida* spp. feature as causative agents of CVC-related sepsis next to CONS, however, with considerably lower incidence rates, varying from around 3 to 10% (25, 26, 28). According to two large recent surveys, *S. aureus* ranks second or third among nosocomial pathogens in pediatrics (1,81), and its position as a nosocomial pathogen in the NICU is the same; in two large, recent NICU surveys it ranked second or third (25,26,28). Moreover, in a report from a single Swedish neonatal center, it even surpassed CONS as the most important nosocomial blood isolate (82).

Gram-Negative Bacilli

CVC-related infections due to Gram-negative enteric bacilli occur with rates up to 10% in the NICU and have been reported in association with contaminated TPN infusion fluids (83). Contamination with *Klebsiella* and *Enterobacter* was traced to repeated entry of lipid emulsion bottles which had been extrinsically contaminated by hands of personnel. The importance of a CVC as a risk factor also for Gram-negative nosocomial bacteremias was highlighted in a retrospective study by Shah et al. that found a substantially increased incidence of Gram-negative rod septicemia in the NICU during recent years (1995–1997 compared to 1988–1994), from 10.2 to 25.5 episodes/1000 NICU admissions, respectively (38). Risk factors associated with Gram-negative rod septicemia were maternal intrapartum antibiotics and the presence of a CVC.

All surveys note that CVC-related bloodstream infection due to *P. aeruginosa* is rare (around 2%), but runs a devastating course with a high mortality (60 to 100%) (25,26,28,84).

Candida

The incidence of CVC-related fungemia in the NICU, with *Candida* spp. as the predominant agent, ranges from 7 to 12% in most surveys, making it the second or third most frequent nosocomial bloodstream infection in the NICU (25, 26, 28, 84). A recent prospective multicenter NICU study from the United States clearly identified the presence of a central catheter as a highly significant risk factor for neonatal candidemia (37).

A CRI due to the lipophilic yeast *M. furfur* has been observed in neonates and older infants receiving IV lipid emulsions (33,34,85).

Hematology/Oncology

In most studies, Gram-positive organisms constitute the majority of bloodstream isolates of CVC-related bacteremias in hematology/oncology patients, accounting for up to 78% of isolates (Table 2). In the previously cited studies (47–59), CONS rank first among the Gram-positive agents, comprising 13 to

Table 2 Causative Agents of Central Venous Catheter-Related Infection in Neutropenic Children: Predominance of Gram-Positive Organisms[a]

Study	Gram-positive (%)	CONS[b](%)
Darbyshire et al. (77)	67	51
Johnson et al. (78)	46	13.5
Hartman and Shochat (80)	46	19
Viscoli et al. (81)	78	30
Van Hoff et al. (82)	59	30
Rizzari et al. (83)	56	43
Uderzo et al. (84)	75	50
Rikkonen et al. (85)	55	25
Das et al. (56)	66	51
Elishoov et al. (59)	41	17
Ertem et al. (57)	48	25
Stamou et al. (58)	90	60

[a] Data compiled from twelve studies, 1985–1999 (Refs. 56–59, 77, 78, and 80–85).
[b] CONS = Coagulase-negative staphylococci.

60% of all agents, but 30 to almost 80% of gram-positive isolates (Table 2). Other causative agents include *S. aureus*, viridans streptococci, enterococci, a variety of Gram-negative bacilli, with *Escherichia coli, Klebsiella, Entero- bacter*, and *P. aeruginosa* as predominant isolates, and fungi and yeasts, primarily *Candida* spp. More rare pathogens include *Bacillus* spp. (86) and *Mycobacterium chelonae/fortuitum* (87). Apart from the fact that these infections occurred in immunocompromised patients (mostly children treated for leukemia and lymphoma) and in the obvious presence of a Hickman catheter, there were no predisposing factors to distinguish these cases.

CLINICAL MANIFESTATIONS

Neonatal Intensive Care

The clinical picture of CVC-related CONS bacteremia in the premature neonate has been described in some detail in a number of studies (27,30, 44–46,76). All studies mentioned the relatively indolent clinical presentation of CONS bacteremia. A summary of clinical manifestations and laboratory values most frequently found to be abnormal is presented in Table 3. It should be realized that most of these signs and symptoms are rather nonspecific. These infections tend to occur during the second and third week of hospital- ization, primarily in low-birthweight, severely ill, premature infants with a CVC in situ (umbilical or inserted through a peripheral vein), often being on TPN and treated with broad-spectrum antibiotics. It should be mentioned that the data in all these studies were examined retrospectively; therefore, conclusions are inevitably biased.

Table 3 Signs and Symptoms and Laboratory Abnormalities in Infants with Coagulase- Negative Staphylococcal Bacteremia

Signs and symptoms
Recurrent bradycardia
Recurrent apneic attacks
Pallor and/or cyanosis
Fever or temperature instability
Increased oxygen requirement
Lethargy
Feeding intolerance
Laboratory abnormalities
Leukocytosis
Increased immature:total neutrophil ratio (I:T)
Decreased platelet count
C-reactive protein increased

For this reason a more detailed analysis of clinical risk factors and manifestations was attempted in a few prospective studies. The essential findings of a prospective clinical study by Schmidt et al. (88) were that infants with CONS bacteremia had temperature elevation, an increased oxygen requirement, lethargy, and feeding intolerance significantly more often than noninfected matched controls. The most frequently found laboratory abnormalities were an increased leukocyte count, particularly an increased immature:total neutrophil (I:T) ratio; a decreased platelet count; and an elevated C-reactive protein (CRP). In addition, Schmidt et al. identified an elevated CRP as the best discriminating laboratory variable.

However, in a prospective study of the value of I:T ratio and CRP as diagnostic tools in early- and late-onset neonatal sepsis, including CONS bacteremia, we could not confirm these results. We found the positive predictive value of both I:T ratio and CRP to be too low to be of any diagnostic value in both early-onset (41 and 36%, respectively) and late-onset neonatal sepsis (68 and 63%, respectively) (89). The negative predictive value of these parameters was found to be higher (90 to 98%); therefore they seem to be more suitable in excluding infection in the neonate.

The clinical picture of CVC-related *S. aureus* bloodstream infections in the NICU is, in our experience, usually similar to that of CONS infections, and only a minority may present with a more severe clinical syndrome. A similar experience was noted in a Swedish study (82), and although in this study it was not clearly stated whether *S. aureus* infections were CVC-related or not, it was thought that the increased rate of staphylococcal nosocomial septicemias (both *S. aureus* and CONS) was due to an increased use of invasive procedures. In one of the surveys from the United States, it was found that *S. aureus* infections were more commonly linked to surgery (26). Two of the other surveys from the United States (25,28) found a higher mortality rate for nosocomial sepsis due to *S. aureus* than for CONS sepsis (18 vs. 10% and 17 vs. 9%, respectively), but both rates were considerably lower than those for sepsis due to Gram-negative bacilli (around 40%) and to *Candida* spp. (around 30%). These latter data indicate that CVC-related septicemia due to Gram-negative rods and candidemia may run a more severe course in the neonate than CONS infections. This is particularly true for Gram-negative sepsis associated with contaminated infusion fluids.

In a study on an outbreak caused by lipid emulsions contaminated with *Klebsiella* and *Enterobacter*, there was substantial morbidity and mortality: five of 20 infants developed a severe, life-threatening illness, and two of these five died (83). This report underscores the need for rigorous hygienic measures when administering TPN to small infants, particularly hand hygiene during preparation of TPN fluids.

Candidemia is a much feared infection in the neonate, because of the mortality rate of up to 50% reported in earlier studies (90,91). However, the prognosis of CVC-related candidemia may be less terrifying. Two recent studies, both reporting on long-term experience, found mortality rates directly attributable to CVC-related *Candida* infection of 20 and 12%, respectively (35,36), which corresponds to the generally relatively mild clinical picture of CVC-related candidemia. Clinical findings are usually not helpful in distinguishing CVC-related candidemia in the neonate from other causes of CRI, with temperature instability, respiratory deterioration, and attacks of apnea and bradycardia predominating, i.e., much like the indolent picture of CONS sepsis (27,35,36,92). Apart from the relatively benign clinical presentation, another reason for the significantly better prognosis when compared to the older reports may be an earlier awareness of candidemia in neonates with a CVC, and thus less reluctance to discard *Candida* as a contaminant. This increased vigilance when *Candida* is isolated from cultures may be clinically important, considering the nonspecific clinical findings. Colonization with *Candida* may direct attention to this agent as a possible cause, as in a recent multicenter study from NICUs in the United States, colonization was found to be a risk factor for nosocomial candidemia in univariate analysis (37). Early diagnosis and, as a result, prompt and aggressive treatment, i.e., removal of catheters and antifungal therapy, may be instrumental in improving outcome of neonatal candidemia. Even in the earlier reports it was noted, despite a mortality rate of 50%, that rapid initiation of treatment resulted in a much better outcome than when there was a delay in diagnosis and initiation of therapy. In fact, these earlier studies reported that as much as 20 to 30% of cases of neonatal systemic candidiasis may go undiagnosed during life and are only documented at autopsy, and therefore, supposedly, inadequately treated or not treated at all.

Most CRIs with the lipophilic yeast *M. furfur* are usually clinically not very severe. Most patients develop a mild-to-moderate infection with apneic and bradycardic attacks, low-grade fever, and respiratory symptoms.

Hematology/Oncology

A CRI in the child with cancer usually manifests itself as a febrile episode. Fever is a common event in neutropenic patients, often alerting the physician to an impending infection in a vulnerable patient. In the absence of signs of any other site of infection, notably lungs, urinary tract, or gastrointestinal tract, an indwelling CVC is often suspected to be the source of infection, especially if the exit site and/or the tunnel tract of the CVC are inflamed. In addition, fever is often included in the definition of CRI, and therefore necessarily present in most patients with such an infection. Local signs, e.g., at the exit site or along the tunnel tract, are present only in a minority of patients with CRIs. Only one study reports an incidence of 50% (58); others find local signs in 20 to 40% of cases of CVC-related sepsis, or even much less. Thus, absence of local signs certainly does not exclude a CRI.

DIAGNOSIS

Diagnostic guidelines have been published by the Centers for Disease Control and Prevention (CDC) (93) and more recently by the Infectious Diseases Society of America (IDSA) (94). For a detailed discussion the reader is referred to these guidelines and to the Chapter on Diagnosis of Catheter-Related Infections. It is commonly recommended that two blood cultures be obtained, one from the CVC and one from a peripheral vein. Both cultures should yield the same organism, and an effort should be made to implicate the CVC as a source of infection, either by quantification of CVC and peripheral blood culture (cfu/ml blood) or by the recently introduced and more economical differential time-to-positivity method (95,96). These procedures are especially recommended when skin commensals such as CONS are implicated as causative agents of CVC-related bacteremia.Thus, in neutropenic children the same diagnostic approach as in adults can be used. However, in small premature infants, it is not always possible to meet these requirements because of the small blood volume, problems with access to a peripheral vein, etc. This has resulted in a continuous debate as to whether CONS isolated from the blood of neonates with signs of sepsis represent true bacteremia or contamination. Various studies have attempted to resolve this issue, by quantification of blood cultures (97,98), by evaluating time to positivity (98,99), or by comparing blood and skin isolates by molecular typing (41). The results of the latter study of Hammerberg et al., already referred to in the section on Epidemiology, provided evidence that CONS blood isolates from neonates are only rarely found on the infant's skin, and therefore the authors concluded that in the vast majority of cases, neonatal CONS blood isolates represent true bacteremia rather than contamination. Although we concur with this latter conclusion, it will probably be impossible to resolve this issue of true bacteremia versus contamination satisfactorily for neonatal CONS blood isolates. For this reason we propose a more realistic approach by adapting the aforementioned guidelines for the premature neonate: A CVC-related septicemia is defined as a positive culture from both a CVC and a peripheral blood sample (if possible), yielding growth of the same organism within 24 to 48 h in a patient with signs of sepsis, as specified in the section on Clinical Manifestations. The reason that we recommend using the 24- to 48-h interval for time-to-blood culture positivity is because this was found to be a sensitive indicator for detecting neonatal CVC-related septicemia (98,99).

MANAGEMENT

Recently, the IDSA published guidelines for the management of intravascular catheter-related infections, including a chapter on treatment of CRI in pediatric patients (94). It is specifically stated in this paper that "data to support most of the recommendations in these guidelines have been garnered from small clinical trials in which patients were not randomized, therapy was not blinded, and data analysis was limited. In fact, to date, there have been no published reports of randomized, double-blind, clinical trials with regard to the clinical diagnosis or management of iv-catheter-related infections." This is perhaps even more true for the pediatric situation. Although a number of recent studies have provided important information with respect to the management of catheter-related infections in neonates, particularly whether or not a catheter should be removed, all studies were retrospective and, no matter how important, their conclusions should be viewed with caution.

Neonatal Intensive Care

Coagulase-Negative Staphylococci

The CONS are well-known for their propensity to develop resistance to antibiotics (72,80). Indeed, most NICUs report widespread resistance of CONS isolates to penicillin, methicillin, oxacillin, cephalosporins, and gentamicin (74,75). Despite this widespread, high degree of resistance, vancomycin resistance among CONS is still rare, and this is why this antibiotic is often recommended as the drug of choice for treating CONS infections in the NICU. The high degree of beta-lactam resistance undoubtedly correlates with the high *mecA* carriage of CONS blood isolates from the NICU, as we (100) and others (19,101,102) have detected, although the precise relation between *mecA* carriage, penicillin-binding protein (PBP) 2′ expression, and beta-lactam susceptibility in CONS is still not determined. Vancomycin resistance of CONS appears to be confined to some strains of *S. haemolyticus* (72,80). It should be mentioned, however, that already in 1991 Herwaldt et al. (103) succeeded in generating vancomycin-resistant strains of both *S. haemolyticus* and *S. epidermidis* by serial passage in broth as well as on agar plates containing vancomycin. Decreased susceptibility to the other registered glycopeptide compound, teicoplanin, is more widespread than to vancomycin among CONS isolates, notably in *S. epidermidis* and *S. haemolyticus* (80). Glycopeptide resistance may be an emerging phenomenon in both CONS and *S. aureus* (104,105), and in 2002 the first fully vancomycin-resistant *S. aureus* (VRSA) clinical isolate was reported (106). This VRSA isolate contained the *vanA* resistance gene from enterococci, suggesting gene transfer between the two species, which is a rather worrisome phenomenon. In view of these alarming developments, it may be prudent and worthwhile to reconsider the recommendation to treat with vancomycin. Both we (100) and others (107) have documented that either cephalothin or ampicillin-sulbactam is effective in the treatment of CONS septicemia in the premature neonate. This is possibly explained by the more effective binding to PBP 2′ of first-generation cephalosporins and ampicillin, compared to methicillin/oxacillin (108,109). Another explanation may be suppression or lack of expression of methicillin resistance in vivo as a result of phase variation (110), despite widespread carriage of *mecA* by CONS clinical isolates. This latter notion is supported by a recent paper by Karlowicz et al., documenting in a retrospective analysis that a switch from vancomycin to oxacillin had no adverse effect on the outcome of CONS sepsis in the NICU (111).

Although catheter removal is often advocated, in our experience and that of others, this is not necessary with CONS bacteremia (74–76,100,112), since most infections quickly respond to appropriate antibiotic therapy without removal of the catheter. In each case it may be worthwhile to carefully consider whether a CVC is needed any longer, since early removal will improve response to therapy (110). A course of seven days of antibiotic therapy is considered adequate in most cases, although formal proof to substantiate this notion is lacking. If infection persists despite adequate antibiotic treatment, the existence of focal infection, particularly endocarditis, should be considered (113). This is a potentially dangerous condition usually associated with an umbilical catheter in the right atrium. It is probably one of the few types of CONS bacteremia in the newborn necessitating prompt removal of the catheter in addition to antibiotic therapy. The other type requiring removal of the catheter is persistent CONS bacteremia lasting >4 days without any focus other than the CVC, as was demonstrated by Karlowicz et al. in a retrospectively analyzed cohort study (112). However, in a small open study of 10 neonates, the addition of rifampin to vancomycin also proved to be effective in clearing persistent CONS bacteremia in 90% of infants within 48 h, without removal of the catheter (114).

Staphylococcus aureus

Management of *S. aureus* CVC-related sepsis in a manner similar to that for CONS infections, i.e., antibiotic therapy without removal of the catheter, is a hazardous approach. We therefore recommend following an approach similar to that used for adults, in which catheter removal is required to prevent relapse and sepsis-related death (115). Thus, in the (premature) neonate with *S. aureus* CRI, it is prudent to also remove the catheter, which is particularly true in case of a CRI due to methicillin-resistant *S. aureus* (MRSA), as will be pointed out later. Antibiotic treatment should be continued for at least 10 days even in uncomplicated cases (115).

Some cases of *S. aureus* CVC-related sepsis in the neonate may follow a protracted course with severe complications, particularly a destructive arthritis of the hip. Removal of the catheter and a prolonged (6- to 8-week) course of intravenous antibiotics are required to combat such complicated infections.

The regimen of antibiotic therapy, i.e., whether or not vancomycin should be the agent of choice, depends on the local susceptibility data. In the

Scandinavian countries and in the Netherlands, most *S. aureus* are still oxacillin-sensitive, although MRSA may prevail in other countries (116). Epidemics with MRSA in NICUs have occurred in various countries, if only sporadically (117–124). A nationwide survey of the prevalence of MRSA (both colonization and infection) in children's hospitals in the United States revealed that the presence of a pediatric ICU or NICU was not a risk factor for MRSA (125). Apparently, in pediatric hospitals in the United States, MRSA occurs just as likely in the ICU as in other departments. As with methicillin-susceptible *S. aureus*, MRSA infection in the neonate may disseminate, particularly to the bone (126). The latter report also found that an intravascular device was the most frequent port of entry of disseminated MRSA infection. Prompt treatment with vancomycin resulted in a good short-term response (95% cure rate) with minimal toxicity and no significant loss of function of the affected limb.

Gram-Negative Bacilli

Apart from sporadic reports, there is little information on the course and management of CVC-related Gram-negative bacteremia in neonates and infants. For example, there are no controlled studies about the need for catheter removal. However, in view of findings in older children and adults (59, 115), it seems advisable to do so. Findings from a recent retrospective cohort study corroborated this notion (127).

Yeasts

Removal of the catheter is considered to be essential for optimal management of CRIs due to yeasts; whether antifungal agents are needed depends on the isolate. Patients with a CRI due to lipophilic yeast *M. furfur* promptly recover upon removal of the catheter. Antifungal therapy without removal of the catheter appears to be more problematic (85). Therefore, prompt removal of the catheter is recommended as the treatment of choice for CVC-related *M. furfur* fungemia in infants.

Antifungal treatment and removal of the catheter is considered to be absolutely required for adequate management of CVC-related candidemia in the premature neonate. As already mentioned, with prompt and adequate treatment, the mortality rate of CVC-related candidemia is probably 10 to 20%. Even in earlier reports (90,91) it was noted that, despite an overall mortality rate of 50%, rapid initiation of treatment with amphotericin B and 5-flucytosine resulted in a much better outcome than when there was a delay in diagnosis and initiation of therapy. More recent studies (35,36,128,129) demonstrate that treatment with amphotericin B with or without 5-flucytosine and with concurrent removal of the catheter is efficacious in 80 to 90% of cases. In all reports it is emphasized that removal of the catheter is absolutely required to ensure effective management of neonatal CVC-related candidemia, a recommendation strongly supported by a recent paper (130). This retrospective study found that failure to remove the CVC within three days after diagnosis of candidemia resulted in a significantly increased mortality (39% vs. zero in neonates with removal of the CVC within three days). On the other hand, a recent evidence-based review failed to find objective data to substantiate this consensus recommendation (131).

Of the newer antimycotic agents, fluconazole and itraconazole, the former has been evaluated in the treatment of neonatal candidiasis with promising results (132,133). Fluconazole has attractive pharmacokinetic properties in the neonate (134) and proven efficacy in *Candida* infections in older children. One of the aforementioned studies showed fluconazole to be equally as effective as amphotericin B in the treatment of neonatal fungal septicemia (132). Because of its more convenient use and much lower toxicity than amphotericin B, it appears, therefore, the agent of choice for treating invasive neonatal *Candida* infections including CVC-related candidemia. Finally, two new antifugal agents, voriconazole and the echinocandin caspofungin, are promising new drugs for the treatment of mycoses, including *Candida* and *Aspergillus* infections, but data on safety and clinical efficacy in infants and children are not yet available.

Hematology/Oncology

Although removal of a foreign device is still the most effective way of treating a device-related infection, this is no longer considered to be necessary in the management of CRIs in children with cancer, particularly in the case of infection with CONS. Numerous studies have clearly demonstrated that antibiotic treatment without removal of the catheter is highly successful in CVC-related CONS bacteremia in children with cancer, resulting in eradication rates of more than 90% (Table 4). Treatment is usually started empirically with parenteral antibiotics and continued for 10 to 14 days, depending on the patient's response. However, as mentioned earlier, optimal duration of therapy has not been determined (94). Apart from clinical signs, laboratory parameters such as CRP may be useful in determining the duration of therapy. Continuation of treatment beyond two weeks may be indicated when there is a slow but definite response or when fever and neutropenia persist (55). It should be remembered that CVCs are often a real "lifeline" in these pediatric cancer patients, and sacrificing a CVC may be a much less attractive option than extending the antibiotic treatment course. The optimal choice of empirical antibiotic therapy should be guided by the predominant isolates in a particular setting. As pointed out in the preceding section, these are usually CONS, many of which are oxacillin- (methicillin-) resistant. Therefore, vancomycin is considered to be the antibiotic of choice for empiric treatment of CRIs in neutropenic children. This choice is further supported by the excellent results that have been obtained with this drug in the treatment of CVC-related

Table 4 Central Venous Catheter-Related Infection in Neutropenic Children: Response to Antibiotic Therapy Without Catheter Removal[a]

| Study | Cure (%) | |
	Local infection	Bacteremia
Darbyshire et al. (77)	—[b]	38 (mult. isolates)
		88 (single isolates)
		72 (total)
Johnson et al. (78)	71	83
Hartman and Shochat (80)	—	93
Viscoli et al. (81)	0 (tunnel)	71
Van Hoff et al. (82)	14	68
Rizzari et al. (83)	0 (tunnel)	90
Uderzo et al. (84)		72[c]
Rikkonen et al. (85)	—	78
Das et al. (56)		71[d]
Ertem et al.(57)	100 (exit site)	79
	0 (tunnel)	
Stamou et al. (58)	82	63

[a] Data compiled from eleven studies, 1985–1999 (Refs. 56–59, 77, 78, and 80–85).
[b] — = not stated.
[c] Response not specified separately for local and bacteremic infection.
[d] Only septicemia cases included in study.

bacteremias. Trials comparing the efficacy of vancomycin to other potentially active drugs are lacking, however, in pediatric cancer patients.

When Gram-negative bacilli are suspected, treatment should include an antipseudomonal beta-lactam agent such as ceftazidime or piperacillin. However, current data indicate that Gram-negative CVC-related bacteremias, especially when due to *Pseudomonas*, are less succesfully treated with antibiotics alone—i.e., without removal of the catheter (135). Similar considerations apply to CVC-related bacteremia due to more unusual pathogens, notably *Bacillus* spp. (86), *M. chelonae* and *M. fortuitum* (87), and CVC-related candidemia (128–130). In these cases, catheter removal appears necessary to succesfully treat CVC-related bloodstream infections. If *S. aureus* has been identified as the causative pathogen, one should be more cautious about leaving the CVC in place, although definite data are unavailable (94,115). In relation to this consensus recommendation, it is interesting to note that in a recent study Rubin et al. (136) documented that, in pediatric hematology–oncology patients, implanted port-associated staphylococcal bacteremias, including a small number of *S. aureus* bacteremias, could be cured safely by antibiotics alone, without removal of the port. Nevertheless, removal of a catheter or port must be the primary option with *S. aureus* device-related bacteremia.

In the recent U.S. guidelines (94), the antibiotic-lock technique is discussed as an alternative or additional treatment method to salvage difficult-to-replace tunneled CVCs. Initial uncontrolled studies in children have yielded favorable results (137,138), but prospective, randomized trials are needed to ascertain whether antibiotic-lock technique is a valuable adjunct or alternative to systemic treatment.

Finally, catheter removal seems to be the only effective treatment in 70 to 75% of tunnel infections. However, exit-site infections rarely necessitate catheter removal and can be treated by antibiotics alone in up to 80% of cases (48,135), with the exception of exit-site and tunnel infections due to *M. chelonae* and *M. fortuitum*, which require surgical excision of the exit site or tunnel tract and surrounding tissues in addition to removal of the catheter (87).

PREVENTION

Recently, revised guidelines for the prevention of catheter-related infections were issued, developed by a working group from the Society of Critical Care Medicine in collaboration with many other professional organizations, among these the IDSA and the CDC (139). In this document, recommendations for the placement and care of intravascular catheters in adults and children are specified, with indications of the strength of the recommendations. Important issues that cannot be overemphasized are the education of personnel, the value of specialized "IV teams," and proper hygiene during insertion and maintenance of catheters. This not only is true for NIs due to Gram-negative bacilli, but also has become a key issue in prevention of CONS infections, since molecular epidemiologic studies have revealed that medical personnel play an important role in the persistence and spread of isolates capable of causing NIs. Therefore, comments in the present section will be restricted to specific issues in infants and children. For more complete and detailed information, the reader is referred to the aforementioned document.

Neonatal Intensive Care

Because of the extensive morbidity and considerable associated costs, measures to prevent CVC-related bacteremia are obviously important and urgently needed, as emphasized in large NICU surveys on nosocomial, late-onset bacteremia in the premature neonate (25–28). In the present section on neonatal intensive care, we will focus on umbilical catheters, catheter care, and prophylaxis with antibiotics and antibodies.

Umbilical Catheters

There are few data on the prevalence of infection of umbilical catheters (summarized in Ref. 139), but these data indicate that umbilical catheter-related bacteremia occurs in 5% (umbilical artery catheters) and 3 to 8% (umbilical vein catheters) of cases. These rates are lower than for CVC-related bacteremia rates in the NICU in general, which vary from 11 to 32% (25,28). This seems to indicate that umbilical catheters are less prone to bacteremia than nonumbilical catheters, which is in agreement with our own observation that umbilical catheter-related bacteremia is relatively rare. However, this relatively low rate of bacteremia is more likely due to the common policy of removing umbilical catheters within the first week of life. Therefore, we concur with the recommendation to restrict the use of umbilical catheters as much as possible and to remove them preferably within five days (umbilical artery) to two weeks (umbilical vein) (139), although in our own institution umbilical catheters are by protocol removed within one week.

Catheter Care

There is very little evidence-based information on catheter care in neonates. One randomized, controlled trial in neonates evaluating the efficacy of a chlorhexidine-impregnated sponge for the prevention of catheter tip colonization and CVC-related bacteremia concluded that the sponge was more efficacious than alcohol disinfectant in preventing catheter tip colonization, but CVC bacteremia rates did not differ between the two groups (140).

Antibiotic Prophylaxis

There have been two reports of prospective randomized trials of long-term vancomycin prophylaxis in premature neonates that were accompanied by a critical commentary (141–143). Although the trials were successful in preventing CONS bacteremia in this patient group, both in the reports and in the editorial comment, concern was expressed that widespread implementation of this kind of prophylaxis might induce development of vancomycin resistance among CONS and *S. aureus* (106). However, vancomycin resistance among CONS was detected in neither of the two studies. Despite this lack of resistance development, we concur with the recommendation that this approach should not be followed on a large scale until better data on the emergence of vancomycin-resistant staphylococci are available (144). In addition, such a policy of prudent vancomycin use is in agreement with recommendations to prevent the spread of vancomycin resistance among enterococci and staphylococci issued by the CDC (145). Therefore, alternative strategies should be explored before embarking on large-scale vancomycin prophylaxis.

Prophylaxis with Antibodies

An alternative approach to prevent CONS bacteremia in the premature newborn may be to boost antibacterial defenses. Considering the deficient host defenses against CONS found in this population, particularly the low level of antibacterial IgG, which may, in addition, be opsonically deficient (6), prophylaxis with intravenous immunoglobulin (IVIG) is an apparently logical approach. Hill summarized in a recent review (146) the data of 10 studies of IVIG prophylaxis in the neonatal ICU. He concluded that "prophylactic administration of IVIG to human neonates may never be shown to alter the overall instance of nosocomial infections, especially if catheter- and procedure-related infections are included." A short while after publication of this review, the results of a large multicenter trial on prophylaxis of nosocomial infections in the NICU were reported, essentially confirming the conclusions of Hill (147). Hill added that this lack of efficacy of IVIG is probably explained by the fact that antibody alone may not play a major role against infections associated with indwelling devices. This notion is, however, not supported by our experimental findings in a study of the opsonic requirements of surface-adherent CONS which showed that IgG sufficed as an opsonin for efficient uptake by neutrophils (12). Moreover, lack of efficacy of IVIG against CONS bacteremia might be explained by variations in the opsonic titer to CONS between IVIG lots, as was demonstrated by Fischer et al. in an animal model (148). Those IVIG lots with high opsonic activity promoted bacterial clearance and enhanced survival in this suckling rat model. It is feasible, therefore, that specific (monoclonal) antibodies with a high and broad-spectrum activity to CONS might provide a valuable contribution in the prevention of CVC-related CONS bacteremia in the future. Data on the safety and pharmacokinetics of a candidate monoclonal antibody directed to CONS in neonates were recently presented (149), and efficacy studies are planned for the near future.

Antimicrobial-Coated Catheters

There have been successful trials with antibiotic- and disinfectant-coated catheters in adults (150,151), but data for infants and children are not yet available.

Hematology/Oncology

Infection is a significant cause of morbidity and mortality in children with cancer and, because a CVC is an important risk factor in this regard, prevention is, as in neonatology, a major goal. As already mentioned in the neonatal section, an approach successfully used in adults, i.e., antibiotic- or disinfectant-coated catheters, has not yet resulted in studies in infants and children. As a consequence, data in children are still lacking, but they are eagerly awaited (152). In addition, data are awaited on the development of resistance to the antimicrobial agents used for coating.

Second, apart from the type of material of the device, the way in which the device is inserted may influence infection rates. As mentioned in the preceding section, totally implanted devices, i.e., without skin exit site, such as Port-a-Caths, may have lower infection rates than Hickman–Broviac type CVCs (55,63). Overall, tunneled catheters are less prone to catheter infection than nontunneled CVCs.

Third, prevention may be accomplished by administration of antibiotics during CVC placement, by antibiotic flushing, or by long-term administration of vancomycin. Although the latter regimen proved to be effective in preventing CVC-related CONS bacteremia in newborns (141,142), the results in pediatric cancer patients both with short-term prophylaxis protocols and with antibiotic flushing were not as unequivocal as the long-term administration of vancomycin in the neonate (153–156). Thus, antibiotic prophylaxis during catheter insertion or antibiotic flushing cannot be recommended at present in pediatric oncology patients.

Two studies, one of which was performed in children (137,138), reported that the antibiotic-lock technique was effective in treating this type of CVC-related sepsis. A recent prospective trial showed that the antibiotic-lock technique was also effective in preventing CVC-related bacteremia, thus supporting the results of the earlier, uncontrolled studies (157). Although obviously successful, we do not advocate this approach on a regular basis in all patients with long-term venous access, for objections similar to those mentioned for long-term vancomycin prophylaxis in neonates in the preceding section, i.e., the potential threat for emergence and dissemination of vancomycin resistance or resistance to other antibiotics prophylactically used.

CONCLUSIONS

Central venous catheters are an integral part of modern medicine, especially in the care of ICU and oncological patients. This is true for both children and adults, although incidence rates of catheter-related infection in infants and children tend to be higher than in adults. In pediatrics, the highest incidence of CRI is observed in hospitalized premature newborns and neutropenic children. Coagulase-negative staphylococci are the predominant pathogens in both patient groups. Considering the fact that CVCs are invaluable tools in the treatment of many patient categories, the main thrust of future studies should be to minimize the rate of infection. Although vancomycin prophylaxis seemed to be effective in both neonates and neutropenic children, the general consensus is that it should not be considered as a general measure to prevent CRI. The threat of vancomycin resistance among CONS is sufficiently frightening to preclude this solution. Prophylaxis with IVIG in the premature neonate does not seem to be effective.

There are now ample data to conclude that CRI due to CONS can be treated by antibiotics alone, with a few exceptions. Treatment of a CRI due to *S. aureus*, Gram-negative bacteria, *Bacillus* species, *M. fortuitum*, *M. chelonae*, *Candida* spp., and *M. furfur* requires removal of the catheter.

There is a continuous emergence of "new" pathogens associated with CRI (158,159), which is especially true for the immunocompromised host, that confronts the physician constantly with new treatment problems. These uncertainties and problems in management strongly emphasize the need for effective prevention, which has become an issue of major importance. A new approach for further improvements in hygienic care of catheters is the development of anti-infective biomaterials, which in a number of trials have proven their efficacy. There continue to be interesting developments in this field, pioneered by Jansen et al. (158) and Sherertz et al. (65,66). These and other issues on prevention will be discussed in more detail in the chapter on prevention and control of catheter-related infections.

REFERENCES

1. Ford-Jones EL, Mindorff CM, Langley JM, Allen U, Navas L, Milner R, Gold R. Epidemiologic study of 4684 hospital-acquired infections in pediatric patients. Pediatr Infect Dis J 1989; 8:669–675.
2. Gaynes RP, Banerjee S, Emori G, Culver DH, Martone WJ, Emori TG, Horan TC, Edwards JR, Jarvis WR, Tolson JS, Henderson TS, Hughes JM. The national nosocomial infections surveillance system: plans for the 1990s and beyond. Am J Med 1991; 91(suppl 3B):116S–120S.
3. Jarvis WR, Edwards JR, Culver DH, Hughes JM, Horan TC, Emori TG, Banerjee S, Tolson J, Henderson T, Gaynes RP, Martone WJ. Nosocomial infection rates in adult and pediatric intensive care units in the United States. Am J Med 1991; 91(suppl 3B):185S–191S.
4. Gaynes RP, Martone WJ, Culver DH, Emori TG, Horan TC, Edwards JR, Jarvis WR, Tolson JS, Henderson TS. Comparison of rates of nosocomial infections in neonatal intensive care units in the United States. Am J Med 1991; 91(suppl 3B):192S–196S.
5. Decker MD, Edwards KM. Central venous catheter infections. Pediatr Clin North Am 1988; 35:579–612.
6. Fleer A, Gerards LJ, Aerts P, Westerdaal NA, Senders RC, Van Dijk H, Verhoef J. Opsonic defense to *Staphylococcus epidermidis* in the premature neonate. J Infect Dis 1985; 152:930–937.
7. Cates KL, Goetz C, Rosenberg N, Pantschenko A, Rowe JC, Ballow M. Longitudinal development of specific and functional antibody in very low birthweight premature infants. Pediatr Res 1988; 23:14–22.
8. Shaio MF, Yang KD, Bohnsack JF, Hill HR. Effect of immune globulin intravenous on opsonization of bacteria by classic and alternative complement pathways in premature serum. Pediatr Res 1989; 25:634–640.
9. Notarangelo LD, Chirico G, Chiara A, Colombo A, Rondini G, Plebani A, Martini A, Ugazio AG. Activity of classical and alternative pathways of complement in preterm and small for gestational age infants. Pediatr Res 1984; 18:281–285.
10. Geelen SPM, Fleer A, Bezemer AC, Gerards LJ, Rijkers GT, Verhoef J. Deficiencies in opsonic defense to pneumococci in the human newborn despite adequate levels of complement and specific IgG antibodies. Pediatr Res 1990; 27:514–518.
11. Fleer A, Gerards LJ, Pascual A, et al. Coagulase-negative staphylococcal

septicemia in premature neonates. Epidemiological features and the role of host defence and bacterial factors. In: Pulverer G, Quie PG, Peters G, eds. The Pathogenicity and Clinical Significance of Coagulase-Negative Staphylococci. Stuttgart: Gustav Fischer Verlag, 1987:215–223.

12. Pascual A, Fleer A, Westerdaal NAC, Berghuis M, Verhoef J. Surface hydrophobicity and opsonic requirements of coagulase-negative staphylococci in suspension and adhering to a polymer substratum. Eur J Clin Microbiol Infect Dis 1988; 7:161–166.

13. Van Bronswijk H, Verbrugh HA, Heezius CJM, Renders NH, Fleer A, der Meulen J, Oe PL, Verhoef J. Heterogeneity in opsonic requirements of *Staphylococcus epidermidis*: relative importance of surface hydrophobicity, capsules and slime. Immunology 1989; 67:81–86.

14. Huebner J, Pier GB, Maslow JN, Muller E, Shiro H, Parent M, Kropec A, Arbeit RD, Goldmann DA. Endemic nosocomial transmission of *Staphylococcus epidermidis* bacteremia isolates in a neonatal intensive care unit over 10 years. J Infect Dis 1994; 169:526–531.

15. Lyytikäinen O, Saxén H, Ryhänen R, Vaara M, Vuopio-Varkila J. Persistence of a multiresistant clone of *Staphylococcus epidermidis* in a neonatal intensive-care unit for a four-year period. Clin Infect Dis 1995; 20:24–29.

16. Neumeister B, Kastner S, Conrad S, Klotz G, Bartmann P. Characterization of coagulase-negative staphylococci causing nosocomial infections in preterm infants. Eur J Clin Microbiol Infect Dis 1995; 14:856–863.

17. Burnie JP, Naderi-Nasab M, Loudon KW, Matthews RC. An epidemiological study of blood culture isolates of coagulase-negative staphylococci demonstrating hospital-acquired infection. J Clin Microbiol 1997; 35:1746–1750.

18. Vermont CL, Hartwig NG, Fleer A, de Man P, Verbrugh H, Van den Anker J, de Groot R, Van Belkum A. Persistence of clones of coagulase-negative staphylococci among premature neonates in neonatal intensive care units: two-center study of bacterial genotyping and patient risk factors. J Clin Microbiol 1998; 36:2485–2490.

19. Villari P, Sarnataro C, Iacuzio L. Molecular epidemiology of *Staphylococcus epidermidis* in a neonatal intensive care unit over a three year period. J Clin Microbiol 2000; 38:1740–1746.

20. Krediet TG, Jones ME, Janssen K, Gerards LJ, Fleer A. Prevalence of molecular types and *mecA* gene carriage of coagulase-negative staphylococci in a neonatal intensive care unit: relation to nosocomial septicemia. J Clin Microbiol 2001; 39:3376–3378.

21. Timmerman CP, Fleer A, Besnier JM, De Graaf L, Cremers F, Verhoef J. Characterization of a proteinaceous adhesin of *Staphylococcus epidermidis* which mediates attachment to polystyrene. Infect Immun 1991; 59:4187–4192.

22. Veenstra GJC, Cremers FFM, Van Dijk H, Fleer A. Ultrastructural organization and regulation of a biomaterial adhesin of *Staphylococcus epidermidis*. J Bacteriol 1996; 178:537–541.

23. Hemming VG, Overall JC, Britt MR. Nosocomial infections in a newborn intensive care unit. Results of forty-one months of surveillance. N Engl J Med 1976; 294:1310–1316.

24. Goldmann DA, Durbin WA Jr, Freeman J. Nosocomial infections in a neonatal intensive care unit. J Infect Dis 1981; 144:449–459.

25. Stoll BJ, Gordon T, Korones SB, Shankaran S, Tyson JE, Bauer CR, Fanaroff AA, Lemons JA, Donovan EF, Oh W, Stevenson DK, Ehrenkranz RA, Papile LA, Verter J, Wright LL. Late-onset sepsis in very low birthweight neonates: a report from the National Institute of Child Health and Human Development Neonatal research network. J Pediatr 1996; 129:63–71.

26. Gaynes RP, Edwards JR, Jarvis WR, Culver DH, Tolson JS, Martone WJ. Nosocomial infections among neonates in high-risk nurseries in the United States. Pediatrics 1996; 98:357–361.

27. Fanaroff AA, Korones SB, Wright LL, Verter J, Poland RL, Bauer CR, Tyson JE, Philips JB III, Edwards W, Lucey JF, Catz CS, Shankaran S, Oh W. Incidence, presenting features, risk factors and significance of late onset septicemia in very low birthweight infants. Pediatr Infect Dis J 1998; 17:593–598.

28. Stoll BJ, Hansen N, Fanaroff AA, Wright LL, Carlo WA, Ehrenkranz RA, Lemons JA, Donovan EF, Stark AR, Tyson JE, Oh W, Bauer CR, Korones SB, Shankaran S, Laptook AR, Stevenson DK, Papile LA, Poole WK. Late-onset sepsis in very low birthweight neonates: the experience of the NICHD neonatal research network. Pediatrics 2002; 110:285–291.

29. Freeman J, Goldmann DA, Smith NE, Sidebottom DG, Epstein MF, Platt R. Association of intravenous lipid emulsion and coagulase-negative staphylococcal bacteremia in neonatal intensive care units. N Engl J Med 1990; 323:301–308.

30. Munson DP, Thompson TR, Johnson DE, Rhame FS, Van Drunen N, Ferrieri P. Coagulase-negative staphylococcal septicemia: experience in a newborn intensive care unit. J Pediatr 1982; 101:602–605.

31. Mahieu LM, De Muynck AO, Ieven MM, De Dooy JJ, Goosens HJ, Van Reempts PJ. Risk factors for central vascular catheter-associated bloodstream infections among patients in a neonatal intensive care unit. J Hosp Infect 2001; 48:108–116.

32. Liem KD, Van Lingen RA, Krediet TG. Complications of central venous catheters in neonates: a multicenter study. Abstracts of the 17th Annual Meeting of the Dutch Society for Pediatrics, Veldhoven, Netherlands, Netherlands, November 1–3, 1995. Abstract 156.

33. Powell DA, Aungst J, Snedden S, Hansen N, Brady M. Broviac catheter-related *Malassezia furfur* sepsis in five infants receiving intravenous fat emulsions. J Pediatr 1984; 105:987–990.

34. Azimi PH, Levernier K, Lefrak LM, Petru AM, Barrett T, Schenck H, Sandhu AS, Duritz G, Valesco M. *Malassezia furfur*: a cause of occlusion of percutaneous central venous catheters in infants in the intensive care nursery. Pediatr Infect Dis J 1988; 7:100–103.

35. Weese-Mayer DE, Wheeler Fondriest D, Brouillette RT, Shulman ST. Risk factors associated with candidemia in the neonatal intensive care unit: a case control study. Pediatr Infect Dis J 1987; 6:190–196.

36. Leibovitz E, Iuster-Reicher A, Amitai M, Mogilner B. Systemic candidal infections associated with use of peripheral venous catheters in neonates: a 9-year experience. Clin Infect Dis 1992; 14:485–491.

37. Saiman L, Ludington E, Pfaller M, Rangel-Frausto S, Wiblin RT, Dawson J, Blumberg HM, Patterson JE, Rinaldi M, Edwards JE, Wenzel RP, Jarvis W.

Risk factors for candidemia in neonatal intensive care unit patients. Pediatr Infect Dis J 2000; 19:319–324.

38. Shah SS, Ehrenkranz RA, Gallagher PG. Increasing incidence of Gram-negative rod bacteremia in a newborn intensive care unit. Pediatr Infect Dis J 1999; 18:591–595.

39. Van Belkum A. DNA fingerprinting of medically important microorganisms by use of PCR. Clin Microbiol Rev 1994; 7:174–184.

40. Bingen E, Barc M-C, Brahimi N, Vilmer E, Beaufils F. Randomly amplified polymorphic DNA analysis provides rapid differentiation of methicillin-resistant coagulase-negative *Staphylococcus* bacteremia isolates in pediatric hospital. J Clin Microbiol 1995; 33:1657–1659.

41. Hammerberg O, Bialkowska-Hobrzanska H, Gregson D, Potters H, Gopaul D, Reid D. Comparison of blood cultures with corresponding venipuncture site cultures of specimens from hospitalized premature neonates. J Pediatr 1992; 120:120–124.

42. Freeman JG, Epstein MF, Smith NE, Platt R, Sidebottom DG, Goldman DA. Extra hospital stay and antibiotic usage with nosocomial coagulase-negative staphylococcal bacteremia in two neonatal intensive care unit populations. Am J Dis Child 1990; 144:324–329.

43. Gray JE, Richardson DK, McCormick MC, Goldman DA. Coagulase-negative staphylococcal bacteremia among very low birthweight infants: relation to admission illness severity, resource use and outcome. Pediatrics 1995; 95:225–230.

44. Battisti O, Mitchison R, Davies P. Changing blood culture isolates in a referral neonatal intensive care unit. Arch Dis Child 1983; 56:775–778.

45. Baumgart S, Hall SE, Campos JM, Polin RA. Sepsis with coagulase-negative staphylococci in critically ill newborns. Am J Dis Child 1983; 137:461–463.

46. LaGamma EF, Drusin LM, Mackles AW, Machalek S, Auld PA. Neonatal infections. An important determinant of late NICU mortality in infants less than 1,000 g at birth. Am J Dis Chil 1983; 137:838–841.

47. Darbyshire PJ, Weightman NC, Speller DCE. Problems associated with indwelling central venous catheters. Arch Dis Child 1985; 60:129–134.

48. Johnson PR, Decker MD, Edwards KM, Schaffner W, Wright PF. Frequency of Broviac catheter infections in pediatric oncology patients. J Infect Dis 1986; 154:570–578.

49. Hiemenz J, Skelton J, Pizzo PA. Perspective on the management of catheter-related infections in cancer patients. Pediatr Infect Dis 1986; 5:6–11.

50. Hartman GE, Shochat SJ. Management of septic complications associated with Silastic® catheters in childhood malignancy. Pediatr Infect Dis J 1987; 6:1042–1047.

51. Viscoli C, Garaventa A, Boni L, Melodia A, Dini G, Cuneo R, Rizzo A, Moroni C, Rogers D, De Bernardi B. Role of Broviac catheters in infections in children with cancer. Pediatr Infect Dis J 1988; 7:556–560.

52. VanHoff J, Berg AT, Seashore JH. The effect of right atrial catheters on infectious complications of chemotherapy in children. J Clin Oncol 1990; 8:1255–1262.

53. Rizzari C, Palamone G, Corbetta A, Uderzo C, Vigano EF, Codecasa G.

Central venous catheter-related infections in pediatric hemotology-oncology patients: role of home and hospital management. Pediatr Hematol Oncol 1992; 6:115–123.

54. Uderzo C, D'Angelo P, Rizzari C, Vigano EF, Rovelli A, Gornati G, Codecasa G, Locasciulli A, Masera G. Central venous catheter-related complications after bone marrow transplantation in children with hematological malignancies. Bone Marrow Transpl 1992; 9:113–117.

55. Rikkonen P, Saarinen UM, Lähteenoja K-M, Jalanko H. Management of indwelling central venous catheters in pediatric cancer patients with fever and neutropenia. Scand J Infect Dis 1993; 25:357–364.

56. Das I, Philpott C, George RH. Central venous catheter-related septicaemia in paediatric cancer patients. J Hosp Infect 1997; 36:67–76.

57. Ertem M, Yavuz G, Aysev D, Unal E, Gozdasoglu S, Tacyildiz N, Cavdar A, Clin S. Right atrial catheter-related complications in pediatric oncology patients: the situation in a developing country. Pediatr Hematol Oncol 1999; 16:299–309.

58. Stamou SC, Maltezou HC, Pourtsidis A, Psaltopoulou T, Skondras C, Aivazoglou T. Hickman–Broviac catheter-related infections in children with malignancies. Mt Sinai J Med 1999; 66:320–326.

59. Elishoov H, Or R, Strauss N, Engelhard D. Nosocomial colonization, septicemia, and Hickman–Broviac catheter-related infections in bone marrow transplant recipients. Medicine 1998; 77:83–101.

60. Gorelick MH, Owen WC, Seibel NL, Reaman GH. Lack of association between neutropenia and the incidence of bacteremia associated with indwelling central venous catheters in febrile pediatric cancer patients. Pediatr Infect Dis J 1991; 10:506–510.

61. Gray JW, Pedler SJ, Craft AW, Kernahan J, Windebank KP, Pearson AD. Changing causes of septicemia in paediatric oncology patients: effect of imipenem use. Eur J Pediatr 1994; 153:84–89.

62. Mulloy RH, Jadaji T, Russell ML. Tunneled central venous catheter sepsis: risk factors in a pediatric hospital. J Parenter Enter Nutr 1991; 15:460–463.

63. Groeger JS, Lucas AB, Thaler HT. Infectious morbidity associated with long-term use of venous access devices in patients with cancer. Ann Intern Med 1993; 119:1168–1174.

64. Zimmerli W, Lew PD, Waldvogel FA. Pathogenesis of foreign body infection: evidence for a local granulocyte defect. J Clin Invest 1984; 73:1191–1200.

64a. Peterslund NA, Koch C, Jensenius JC, Thiel S. Association between deficiency of mannose-binding lectin and severe infections after chemotherapy. Lancet 2001; 358:637–638.

64b. Mullighan CG, Heatley S, Doherty K, Szabo F, Grigg A, Hughes TP, Schwarer AP, Szer J, Tait BD, Bik To L, Bardy PG. Mannose-binding lectin polymorphisms are associated with major infection following allogeneic hemopoietic stem cell transplantation. Blood 2002; 99:3524–3529.

65. Sherertz RJ, Forman DM, Solomon DD. Efficacy of dicloxacillin-coated polyurethane catheters in preventing subcutaneous *Staphylococcus aureus* infection in mice. Antimirob Agents Chemother 1989; 33:1174–1178.

66. Sherertz RJ, Carruth WA, Hampton AA, Byron MP, Solomon DD. Efficacy

of antibiotic-coated catheters in preventing subcutaneous *Staphylococcus aureus* infection in rabbits. J Infect Dis 1993; 167:98–106.

67. Nouwen JL, Van Belkum A, De Marie S, Sluijs J, Wielenga JJ, Kluytmans JA, Verbrugh HA. Clonal expansion of *Staphylococcus epidermidis* strains causing Hickman catheter-related infections in a hemato-oncologic department. J Clin Microbiol 1998; 36:2696–2702.

68. Aitken ML, Tonelli MR. Complications of indwelling catheters in cystic fibrosis. Chest 2000; 118:1598–1602.

69. Colomb V, Fabeiro M, Goulet O, Merckx J, Ricour C. Central venous catheter-related infections in children on long-term home parenteral nutrition; incidence and risk factors. Clin Nutr 2000; 19:355–359.

70. Lowy FD, Hammer SM. *Staphylococcus epidermidis* infections. Ann Intern Med 1983; 99:834–839.

71. Christensen GD. The confusing and tenacious coagulase-negative staphylococci. Adv Intern Med 1987; 32:177–192.

72. Pfaller MA, Herwaldt LA. Laboratory, clinical and epidemiological aspects of coagulase-negative staphylococci. Clin Microbiol Rev 1988; 1:281–299.

73. Patrick CC. Coagulase-negative staphylococci: pathogens with increasing clinical significance. J Pediatr 1990; 116:497–507.

74. Hall SL. Coagulase-negative staphylococcal infections in neonates. Pediatr Infect Dis J 1991; 10:57–67.

75. St. Geme JW, Harris MC. Coagulase-negative staphylococcal infection in the neonate. Clin Perinatol 1991; 18:281–302.

76. Fleer A, Senders RC, Visser MR, Bijlmer RP, Gerards LJ, Kraaijeveld CA, Verhoef J. Septicemia due to coagulase-negative staphylococci in a neonatal intensive care unit: clinical and bacteriological features and contaminated parenteral fluids as a source of sepsis. Pediatr Infect Dis 1983; 2:426–431.

77. Hall RT, Hall SL, Barnes WG, Izuegbu J, Rogolsky M, Zorbas I. Characteristics of coagulase-negative staphylococci from infants with bacteremia. Pediatr Infect Dis J 1987; 6:377–383.

78. Hall SL, Hall RT, Barnes WG, Riddell S. Colonization with slime-positive coagulase-negative staphylococci as a risk factor for invasive coagulase-negative staphylococcal infections in neonates. J Perinatol 1988; 8:215–221.

79. Fleer A, Verhoef J. New aspects of staphylococcal infections: emergence of coagulase-negative staphylococci as pathogens. Antonie van Leeuwenhoek 1984; 50:729–744.

80. Kloos WE, Bannerman RL. Update on clinical significance of coagulase-negative staphylococci. Clin Microbiol Rev 1994; 7:117–140.

81. Milliken J, Tait GA, Ford-Jones EL, Mindorff CM, Gold R, Mullins G. Nosocomial infections in a pediatric intensive care unit. Crit Care Med 1988; 16:233–237.

82. Källman J, Kihlström E, Sjöberg L, Schollin J. Increase of staphylococci in neonatal septicemia: a fourteen-year study. Acta Paediatr 1997; 86:533–538.

83. Jarvis WR, Highsmith AK, Allen J, Halley RW. Polymicrobial bacteremia associated with lipid emulsion in a neonatal intensive care unit. Pediatr Infect Dis 1983; 2:203–208.

84. Cordero L, Sananes M, Ayers LW. Bloodstream infections in a neonatal

intensive-care unit: 12 years' experience with an antibiotic control program. Infect Control Hosp Epidemiol 1999; 20:242–246.

85. Powell DA, Marcon MJ. Failure to eradicate *Malassezia furfur* Broviac catheter infection with antifungal therapy. Pediatr Infect Dis J 1987; 6:579–580.

86. Saleh RA, Schorin MA. *Bacillus* sp. sepsis associated with Hickman catheters in patients with neoplastic disease. Pediatr Infect Dis J 1987; 6:851–856.

87. Flynn PM, vanHooser B, Gigliotti F. Atypical mycobacterial infections of Hickman catheter exit sites. Pediatr Infect Dis J 1988; 7:510–513.

88. Schmidt BK, Kirpalani HM, Corey M, Low DE, Philip AG, Ford-Jones EL. Coagulase-negative staphylococci as true pathogens in newborn infants: a cohort study. Pediatr Infect Dis J 1987; 6:1026–1031.

89. Krediet TG, Gerards LJ, Fleer A, Van Stekelenburg G. The predictive value of CRP and I/T ratio in neonatal infection. J Perinat Med 1992; 20:479–485.

90. Johnson DE, Thompson TR, Green TP, Ferrieri P. Systemic candidiasis in very low-birthweight infants (1,500 grams). Pediatrics 1984; 73:138–143.

91. Faix RG. Systemic *Candida* infections in infants in intensive care nurseries: high incidence of central nervous system involvement. J Pediatr 1984; 105:616–622.

92. Fairchild KD, Tomkoria S, Sharp E, Mena FV. Neonatal *Candida glabrata* sepsis: clinical and laboratory features compared with other *Candida* species. Pediatr Infect Dis J 2002; 21:39–43.

93. Pearson ML, Hierholzer WJ, Garner JS, et al. Guideline for the prevention of intravascular device-related infections. Am J Infect Control 1996; 24:262–293.

94. Mermel LA, Farr BM, Sherertz RJ, Raad II, O'Grady N, Harris JS, Craven DE. Guidelines for the management of intravascular catheter-related infections. J Infect Dis 2001; 32:1249–1272.

95. Blot F, Schmidt E, Nitenberg G, Tancrede C, Leclercq B, Laplanche A, Andremont A. Earlier positivity of central-venous- versus peripheral-blood cultures is highly predictive of catheter-related sepsis. J Clin Microbiol 1998; 36:105–109.

96. Blot F, Nitenberg G, Chachaty E, Raynard B, Germann N, Antoun S, Laplanche A, Brun-Buisson C, Tancrede C. Diagnosis of catheter-related bacteraemia: a prospective comparison of the time to positivity of hub–blood versus peripheral-blood cultures. Lancet 1999; 354:1071–1077.

97. St Geme JW, Bell LM, Baumgart S, D'Angio CT, Harris MC. Distinguishing sepsis from blood culture contamination in young infants with blood cultures growing coagulase-negative staphylococci. Pediatrics 1990; 86:157–162.

98. Phillips SE, Bradley JS. Bacteremia detected by lysis direct plating in a neonatal intensive care unit. J Clin Microbiol 1990; 28:1–4.

99. Jawaheer G, Neal TJ, Shaw NJ. Blood culture volume and detection of coagulase-negative staphylococcal septicaemia in neonates. Arch Dis Child 1997; 76:F57–F58.

100. Krediet TG, Jones ME, Gerards LJ, Fleer A. Clinical outcome of cephalothin versus vancomycin therapy in the treatment of coagulase-negative staphylococcal septicemia in neonates: relation to methicillin resistance and *mecA* gene carriage of blood isolates. Pediatrics 1999; 103:1–5. http://www.pediatrics.org/cgi/content/full/103/3/e29.

101. Nesin M, Projan S, Kreiswirth B, Bolt Y, Novick RP. Molecular epidemiology of *Staphylococcus epidermidis* blood isolates from neonatal intensive care unit patients. J Hosp Infect 1995; 31:111–121.

102. De Giusti M, Pacifico L, Tufti D, Panero A, Boccia A, Chiesa C. Phenotypic detection of nosocomial *mecA*-positive coagulase-negative staphylococci from neonates. J Antimicrob Chemother 1999; 44:351–358.

103. Herwald L, Boyken L, Pfaller M. In vitro selection of resistance to vancomycin in bloodstream isolates of *Staphylococcus haemolyticus* and *Staphylococcus epidermidis*. Eur J Clin Microbiol Infect Dis 1991; 10:1007–1012.

104. Hiramatsu K, Hanaki H, Ino T, Yabuta K, Oguri T, Tenover FC. Methicillin-resistant *Staphylococcus aureus* clinical strain with reduced vancomycin susceptibility. J Antimicr Chemother 1997; 40:135–136.

105. Hiramatsu K, Hanaki H. Glycopeptide resistance in staphylococci. Curr Opin Infect Dis 1998; 11:653–658.

106. CDC. *Staphylococcus aureus* resistant to vancomycin—United States, 2002. MMWR 2002; 51:565–567.

107. Wang SM, Liu CC, Tseng HW, Yang YJ, Lin CH, Huang AH, Wu YH. *Staphylococcus capitis* bacteremia of very low birthweight premature infants at neonatal intensive care units: clinical significance and antimicrobial susceptibility. J Microbiol Immunol Infect 1999; 32:26–32.

108. Chambers HF, Sachdeva M. Binding of β-lactam antibiotics to penicillin-binding proteins in methicillin-resistant staphylococci. J Infect Dis 1990; 161:1170–1176.

109. Chambers HF, Sachdeva M, Kennedy S. Binding affinity for penicillin-binding protein 2a correlates with in vivo activity of β-lactam antibiotics against methicillin-resistant *Staphylococcus aureus*. J Infect Dis 1990; 162:705–710.

110. Mempel M, Feucht H, Ziebuhr W, Endres M, Laufs R, Gruter L. Lack of *mecA* transcription in slime-negative phase variants of methicillin-resistant *Staphylococcus epidermidis*. Antimicrob Agents Chemother 1994; 38:1251–1255.

111. Karlowicz MG, Buescher ES, Surka AE. Fulminant late-onset sepsis in a neonatal intensive-care unit, 1988-1997, and the impact of avoiding empiric vancomycin therapy. Pediatrics 2000; 106:1387–1390.

112. Karlowicz MG, Furigay PJ, Croitoru DP, Buescher ES. Central venous catheter removal versus in situ treatment in neonates with coagulase-negative staphylococcal bacteremia. Pediatr Infect Dis J 2002; 21:22–27.

113. Noel GJ, O'Loughlin JE, Edelson PJ. Neonatal *Staphylococcus epidermidis* right-sided endocarditis: description of five catheterized infants. Pediatrics 1988; 82:234–239.

114. Tan TQ, Mason EO, Ching-Nan O, Kaplan SL. Use of intravenous rifampin in neonates with persistent staphylococcal bacteremia. Antimicrob Ag Chemother 1993; 37:2401–2406.

115. Raad II, Bodey GP. Infectious complications of indwelling vascular catheters. Clin Infect Dis 1992; 15:197–210.

116. Voss A, Milatovic D, Wallrauch-Schwarz C, Rosdahl VT, Braveny I.

Methicillin-resistant *Staphylococcus aureus* in Europe. Eur J Clin Microb Infect Dis 1994; 13:50–55.

117. Graham DR, Correa-Villasenor A, Anderson RL, Vollman JH, Baine WB. Epidemic neonatal gentamicin–methicillin-resistant *Staphylococcus aureus* infection associated with nonspecific topical use of gentamicin. J Pediatr 1980; 97:972–987.

118. Dunkle LM, Naqvi SH, MacCallum R, Lofgren JP. Eradication of epidemic neonatal methicillin–gentamicin-resistant *Staphylococcus aureus* in an intensive care nursery. Am J Med 1981; 70:455–458.

119. Armington LA, Mooney BR. Early recognition and control of methicillin-resistant *Staphylococcus aureus* in a newborn ICU. Am J Infect Control 1986; 14:84.

120. Mulhern B, Griffin E. An epidemic of gentamicin/cloxacillin resistant staphylococcal infection in a neonatal unit. Irish Med J 1987; 74:228–229.

121. Price EH, Brain A, Dickson JAS. An outbreak of infection with a gentamicin and methicillin-resistant *Staphylococcus aureus* in a neonatal unit. J Hosp Infect 1980; 1:221–228.

122. Trallero EP, Arenzana JG, Castaneda AA, Grisolia LP. Unusual multi-resistant *Staphylococcus aureus* in a newborn nursery. Am J Dis Child 1981; 135:689–692.

123. Gilbert GL, Asche V, Hewstone AS, Mathiesen JL. Methicillin-resistant *Staphylococcus aureus* in neonatal nurseries. Med J Aust 1982; 1:455–459.

124. Reboli AC, John JF, Levkoff AH. Epidemic methicillin–gentamicin-resistant *Staphylococcus aureus* in a neonatal intensive care unit. Am J Dis Child 1989; 143:34–39.

125. Jarvis WR, Thornsberry C, Boyce J, Hughes JM. Methicillin-resistant *Staphylococcus aureus* at children's hospitals in the United States. Pediatr Infect Dis 1985; 4:651–655.

126. Ish-Horowicz MR, McIntyre P, Nade S. Bone and joint infections caused by multiply resistant *Staphylococcus aureus* in a neonatal intensive care unit. Pediatr Infect Dis J 1992; 11:82–87.

127. Nazemi KJ, Buescher ES, Kelly RE, Karlowicz MG. Central venous catheter removal versus in situ treatment in neonates with Enterobacteriaceae bacteremia. Pediatrics 2003; 111:e269–e274. URL: http://www.pediatrics. org/cgi/content/full/111/3/e269.

128. Eppes SC, Troutman JL, Gutman LT. Outcome of treatment of candidemia in children whose central catheters were removed or retained. Pediatr Infect Dis J 1989; 8:99–104.

129. Dato VM, Dajani AS. Candidemia in children with central venous catheters: role of catheter removal and amphotericin B therapy. Pediatr Infect Dis J 1990; 9:309–314.

130. Karlowicz MG, Hashimoto LN, Kelly RE, Buescher ES. Should central venous catheters be removed as soon as candidemia is detected in neonates? Pediatrics 2000; 106:1–5. http://www.pediatrics.org/cgi/content/full/106/5/e63.

131. Nucci M, Anaissie E. Should vascular catheters be removed from all patients with candidemia? An evidence-based review. Clin Infect Dis 2002; 34:591–599.

132. Driessen M, Ellis JB, Cooper PA, Wainer S, Muwazi F, Hahn D, Gous H, De

Villiers FP. Fluconazol vs. amphotericin B for the treatment of neonatal fungal septicemia: a prospective randomized trial. Pediatr Infect Dis J 1996; 15:1107–1112.

133. Wainer S, Cooper PA, Gouws H, Akierman A. Prospective study of fluconazol therapy in systemic neonatal fungal infection. Pediatr Infect Dis J 1997; 16:763–767.

134. Van De Anker JN, Van Popele NML, Sauer PJJ. Antifungal agents in neonatal systemic candidiasis. Antimicrob Agents Chemother 1995; 39:1391–1397.

135. Benezra D, Kiehn TE, Gold JW, Brown AE, Turnbull AD, Armstrong D. Prospective study of infections in indwelling central venous catheters using quantitative blood cultures. Am J Med 1988; 85:495–498.

136. Rubin LG, Shih S, Shende A, Karayalcin G, Lanzkowsky P. Cure of implantable venous port-associated bloodstream infections in pediatric hematology–oncology patients without catheter removal. Clin Infect Dis 1999; 29:102–105.

137. Messing B, Peitra-Cohen S, Debure A, Beliah M, Bernier JJ. Antibiotic-lock technique: a new approach to optimal therapy for catheter-related sepsis in home-parenteral nutrition patients. J Parenter Enter Nutr 1988; 12:185–189.

138. Johnson DC, Johnson FL, Goldman S. Preliminary results treating persistent central venous catheter infections with the antibiotic-lock technique in pediatric patients. Pediatr Infect Dis J 1994; 13:930–931.

139. O'Grady NP, Alexander M, Dellinger EP, Gerberding JL, Heard SO, Maki DG, Masur H, McCormick RD, Mermel LA, Pearson ML, Raad II, Randolph A, Weinstein RA. Guidelines for the prevention of intravascular catheter-related infections. Pediatrics 2002; 110(5). URL: http://www.pediatrics.org/cgi/content/full/110/5/e51.

140. Garland JS, Alex CP, Mueller CD, Otten D, Shivpuri C, Harris MC, Naples M, Pellegrini J, Buck RK, McAuliffe TL, Goldmann DA, Maki DG. A randomized trial comparing povidone-iodine to a chlorhexidine gluconate-impregnated dressing for prevention of central venous catheter infections in neonates. Pediatrics 2001; 107:1431–1436.

141. Kacica MA, Horgan MJ, Ochoa L, Sandler R, Lepow ML, Venezia RA. Prevention of gram-positive sepsis in neonates weighing less than 1500 grams. J Pediatr 1994;125:253–258.

142. Spafford PS, Sinkin RA, Cox C, Reubens L, Powell KR. Prevention of central venous catheter-related coagulase-negative staphylococcal sepsis in neonates. J Pediatr 1994; 125:259–263.

143. Barefield ES, Philips JB. Vancomycin prophylaxis for coagulase-negative staphylococcal bacteremia. J Pediatr 1994; 125:230–232.

144. Krediet TG, Fleer A. Should we use vancomycin as prophylaxis to prevent neonatal nosocomial coagulase-negative staphylococcal septicemia? Pediatr Infect Dis J 1998; 17:763–764.

145. CDC. Recommendations for preventing the spread of vancomycin resistance. Infect Contr Hosp Epidemiol 1995; 16:105–113.

146. Hill HR. Intravenous immunoglobulin use in the neonate: role in prophylaxis and therapy of infection. Pediatr Infect Dis J 1993; 12:549–559.

147. Fanaroff AA, Korones SB, Wright LL, Wright EC, Poland RL, Bauer CB,

Tyson JE, Philips JB III, Edwards W, Lucey JF, Shankaran S, Oh W. A controlled trial of intravenous immunoglobulin to reduce nosocomial infection in very-low-birthweight infants. New Engl J Med 1994; 330:1107–1113.

148. Fischer GW, Cieslak TJ, Wilson SR, Weisman LE, Hemming VG. Opsonic antibodies to *Staphylococcus epidermidis*: In vitro and in vivo studies using human intravenous immune globulin. J Infect Dis 1994; 169:324–329.

149. Weisman LE, Mandy GT, Garcia-Prats JA, et al. Safety and pharmacokinetics of a human chimeric anti-staphylococcal monoclonal antibody for prevention of coagulase-negative staphylococcal infection in very low birth-weight infants: preliminary report [abstr]. Pediatr Res 2003; 53:315A.

150. Raad I, Darouiche R, Dupuis J, Abi-Said D, Gabrielli A, Hachem R, Wall M, Harris R, Jones J, Buzaid A, Robertson C, Shenaq S, Curling P, Burke T, Ericsson C. Central venous catheters coated with minocycline and rifampin for the prevention of catheter-related colonization and bloodstream infections: a randomized, double-blind trial. Ann Intern Med 1997; 127:267–274.

151. Maki DG, Stolz SM, Wheeler S, Mermel LA. Prevention of central venous catheter-related bloodstream infection by use of an antiseptic-impregnated catheter: a randomized, controlled trial. Ann Intern Med 1997; 127:257–266.

152. Schutze GE. Antimicrobial-impregnated central venous catheters. Pediatr Infect Dis J 2002; 21:63–64.

153. Schwartz C, Henrickson KJ, Roghmann K, Powell K. Prevention of bacteremia attributed to luminal colonization of tunneled central venous catheters with vancomycin-susceptible organisms. J Clin Oncol 1990; 8:1591–1597.

154. Rackoff WR, Weiman M, Jakobowski D, Hirschl R, Stallings V, Bilodeau J, Danz P, Bell L, Lange B. A randomized, controlled trial of the efficacy of a heparin and vancomycin solution in preventing central venous catheter infections in children. J Pediatr 1995; 127:147–151.

155. Henrickson KJ, Axtell RA, Hoover SM, Kuhn SM, Pritchett J, Kehl SC, Klein JP. Prevention of CVC-related infections and thrombotic events in immunocompromised children by the use of vancomycin/ciprofloxacin/heparin flush solutions in a randomized, multicenter, double-blind trial. J Clin Oncol 2000; 18:1269–1278.

156. Dawson S, Fitzgerald P, Langer JC, Walton M, Winthrop A, Lau G, Wiernikowski J, Barr RD. A protocol for the prevention of infection in children with tunneled right atrial catheters. Oncol Rep 2000; 7:1239–1242.

157. Carratala J, Niubo J, Fernandez-Sevilla A, Juve E, Castellsague X, Berlanga J, Linares J, Gudiol F. Randomized, double-blind trial of an antibiotic-lock technique for prevention of Gram-positive central venous catheter-related infection in neutropenic patients with cancer. Antimicrob Agents Chemother 1999; 43:2200–2204.

158. Jansen B. Vascular catheter-related infection: aetiology and prevention. Curr Opin Infect Dis 1993; 6:526–531.

159. Goldmann DA, Pier GB. Pathogenesis of infections related to intravascular catheterization. Clin Microbiol Rev 1993; 6:176–192.

19

Infections Associated with Urinary Catheters

Carol E. Chenoweth

Division of Infectious Diseases
University of Michigan
Ann Arbor, Michigan, U.S.A.

Sanjay Saint

Division of General Medicine
Ann Arbor VA Medical Center and
University of Michigan Health System
Ann Arbor, Michigan, U.S.A.

INTRODUCTION

Urinary tract infection (UTI) is the most frequently reported nosocomial infection, accounting for up to 40% of infections. The vast majority of these infections are associated with urinary catheters. Urinary catheters are widely used in health care today, especially in the intensive care unit (ICU) setting, in long-term care facilities, and in patients with spinal cord injury. Indwelling urinary catheters are similar to other catheters, such as intravascular catheters, in that they disrupt the normal host immune mechanisms and allow for the formation of biofilm. Urinary catheters, however, are unique in the frequency of bacterial colonization, the etiologic organisms, and the types of components that make up their biofilm. These factors have important implications for treatment and prevention of UTI in the catheterized patient.

551

PATHOGENESIS

The normal urinary tract has a number of defense mechanisms that prevent attachment of potential pathogens to the uroepithelium (1–6). These mechanisms include length of the urethra, micturation, and urine flow, which effectively clears bacteria from the bladder. Urine osmolality, pH, and organic acids inhibit growth of most microorganisms. Antibacterial properties of urinary tract mucosa and urinary inhibitors of bacterial adhesion (i.e., Tamm-Horsfall proteins and bladder mucopolysaccharides) prevent attachment of pathogens (3,5,6). The use of a urinary catheter can interfere with these normal defenses, allowing colonization and attachment of microorganisms (1,2,4–6).

Most catheter-associated UTIs are caused by organisms entering the bladder through an ascending route. Rarely, hematogenously spread organisms, such as *Staphylococcus aureus*, may cause upper tract infection (7,8). Organisms ascend into the bladder in one of two ways. First, organisms may enter through an extraluminal route via direct inoculation early or through migration in the mucous film surrounding the external aspect of the catheter. Organisms entering through this route are primarily endogenous organisms, originating from the rectum and colonizing the patient's perineum (4,9–11). This is the route that most organisms enter the bladder; approximately 70% of episodes of bacteriuria in women involved the extraluminal route (9). The second mechanism of entry into the bladder is via intraluminal reflux or migration. This occurs when organisms gain access to the internal lumen of the catheter through failure of a closed drainage system or contamination of the collection bag (4,11,12). Most of these organisms are from exogenous sources and often are the result of cross-transmission of organisms introduced via the hands of health care personnel (5,11,12).

In a recent prospective study designed to determine the probable route that microorganisms used to gain access to the catheterized bladder, Tambyah and colleagues performed serial paired quantitative cultures of the specimen port and the collection bag. The probable mechanism of infection could be determined for 173 catheter-related UTIs. Of these, 115 (66%) were acquired through extraluminal migration of organisms ascending from the perineum in the mucous along the external surface of the catheter. A smaller proportion of infections (34%) were acquired from intraluminal contamination of the collection system (11).

While most UTIs with Enterobacteriaceae are thought to be from an endogenous source, recent epidemiologic studies suggest that clonal spread of a virulent, antibiotic-resistant strain may have occurred in the community setting (13). Virulence factors associated with *Escherichia coli* in patients with acute, uncomplicated, community-acquired UTI have not been associated with catheter-related UTI (1,13,14). However, microorganisms causing nosocomial UTI are easily transmitted from one patient to another in an institution. About 15% of episodes of nosocomial bacteriuria occur in clusters, and they often involve highly antibiotic-resistant organisms (4,12,15–18). Most hospital-based outbreak investigations indicate that lack of proper hand-washing by health care personnel is largely responsible for the transmission of these organisms (19). Despite these occasional epidemics, however, most cases of nosocomial UTI reflect endemic acquisition.

Once inserted, urinary catheters readily acquire biofilms on their inner and outer surfaces (12,20–23). Adhesion of microorganisms to catheter materials is dependent on the hydrophobicity of organisms and catheter surface; catheters with both hydrophobic and hydrophilic regions allow for colonization with the widest variety of organisms (21). Once microorganisms attach and multiply, the resultant sheet of organisms secretes an extracellular matrix of bacterial glycocalyces, embedding the microorganisms (4,5,21,22). Organisms in the biofilm grow slower than planktonic bacteria which grow within the urine itself, probably because of limited nutrients or oxygen (21,23). Even so, microorganisms located within the biofilm may ascend the inner surface of the catheter in 1 to 3 days (21,22). This rate may be affected by the presence of swarming organisms, such as *Proteus mirabilis* (24).

Urinary catheter biofilms are unique in that some organisms in the biofilm, such as *Proteus* spp., *Pseudomonas aeruginosa*, *Klebsiella pneumoniae*, and *Providencia* spp., have the ability to hydrolyze urea in the urine to free ammonia. This increases the local pH and allows precipitation of minerals such as hydroxyapetite or struvite (25). These minerals may then deposit in the catheter biofilm causing mineral encrustations (21,22,26). Encrustations are seen typically on the inner surface of the catheter and can build to completely block catheter flow (21,22,25).

The presence of urinary catheter biofilms has important implications for prevention and treatment of catheter-related UTIs. Since the glycocalyx matrix may inhibit activity of antimicrobials, the question of whether long-term urinary catheters should be replaced during treatment of bacteriuria has been raised. From a prevention standpoint, the need to develop catheters with materials that prevent microorganism attachment and biofilm ascent is paramount. Until such catheters are widely used, it is probably prudent to replace catheters in patients suspected of having symptomatic catheter-related urinary tract infection.

EPIDEMIOLOGY

Prevalence of Urinary Catheters

Up to 25% of patients have a urinary catheter placed at some time during their hospital stay (27,28). In one hospital, prevalence surveys performed between 1985 and 1999 revealed a significantly increased utilization of urinary catheters from 9% to 16% (29). The use of urinary catheters is highest in the ICU setting. Data from the National Nosocomial Infection Surveillance (NNIS) System between January 1992 and April 2000 reveal urinary catheter utilization in participating ICUs ranging from 0.32 to 0.88 urinary catheter-days/patient-days. Utilization was highest in cardiothoracic, trauma, and surgical ICUs, 0.88, 0.87, and 0.85 catheter-days/patient-days, respectively, and lowest in pediatric ICUs, 0.32 catheter-days/patient-days (30,31). Urinary catheter use approaches 100% in patients with the highest acuity in surgical ICUs (32). The duration of catheterization varies with hospital ward and patient population, but the mean and median durations in acute care hospitals are 2 and 4 days, respectively. Catheters are removed within 7 days in 70% of patients (33).

Several studies highlight the fact that urinary catheters are overutilized, and documentation surrounding catheterization is poor (27,34–39). In recent prospective studies of catheterized patients, the decision for catheterization was judged to be inappropriate 21 to 50% of the time (27,34,36,38,39). Furthermore, a written order or procedure note is often not documented in the medical record (36,37). In one study at three institutions, 28% of health care providers were unaware that their patient had an indwelling urinary catheter. The level of unawareness increased with the level of training; 21% of medical students, 22% of interns, 28% of residents, and 38% of attending physicians were unaware of catheters in their patients (27). Unawareness was correlated with inappropriate catheter use (27).

Incidence of Catheter-Related Urinary Tract Infection

Historically, UTIs have accounted for up to 40% of nosocomial infections (28,40), but account for a smaller proportion of nosocomial infections occurring in the ICU setting. Specfically, UTIs account for 15 to 21% of nosocomial infections in pediatric ICU patients, 23% of nosocomial infections in adult ICU patients in the United States, and 18% of ICU infections in the European EPIC study (31,41–43). Urinary catheters account for the vast majority of nosocomial UTI; up to 97% of UTIs in ICUs are associated with urinary catheters (43,44).

The overall incidence of bacteriuria in patients with an indwelling urinary catheter in place for 2 to 10 days is 26%, with an average daily risk of 3–10% per day (45–49). At this rate, after a month, nearly all catheterized patients will be bacteriuric, making this the dividing line between short- and long-term catheterization (6,50).

Rates of catheter-related UTIs reported through the NNIS System between January 1995 and April 2000 ranged from 3.1 infections/1000 catheter-days in cardiothoracic ICUs to 10.2 infections/1000 catheter-days in burn ICUs (30). Even within the ICU setting, some patient populations have a higher rate of infection; adult patients on extracorporeal membrane oxygenation had a much higher rate of UTI than other surgical ICU patients

(13.8 infections/1000 catheter-days vs. 5.6 infections/1000 catheter-days) (32). The rate of UTI in pediatric ICUs was 5.9 infections/1000 catheter-days, lower than the rate seen in an equivalent adult medical–surgical ICU population of 9.5 infections/1000 catheter-days (31,43). Nosocomial UTI is an infrequent complication in neonatal ICUs (51,52).

Risk Factors for Bacteriuria

In several prospective studies, risk factors for catheter-related bacteriuria have been evaluated. The most important and consistent risk factor for bacteriuria is the duration of catheterization [odds ratio (OR) = 2.3–22.4, depending on duration] (53–58). Females have a substantially higher risk of bacteriuria than males [relative risk (RR) = 1.7–3.7] (53,55,56,58,59). Since systemic antibiotics have a protective effect on bacteriuria, the lack of systemic antimicrobials significantly increases the risk of bacteriuria (RR = 2.0–3.9) (53–56,58,59). Catheter care violations have also been associated with increased risk of bacteriuria (12,53,55). Other risk factors identified in one or more studies include: rapidly fatal underlying illness (RR = 2.5) (53); age > 50 years (RR = 2) (53,56); nonsurgical disease (RR = 2.2) (53); hospitalization on an orthopedic (RR = 51) or urology service (RR = 4) (57); catheter insertion after the sixth day of hospitalization (RR = 8.6) (57); catheter inserted outside the operating room (RR = 5.3) (55); diabetes mellitus (OR = 2.3) (55); and serum creatinine greater than 2 mg/dL at the time of catheterization (OR = 2.1) (55). Heavy periurethral colonization with bacteria has also been associated with increased risk of bacteriuria (60). A summary of significant risk factors for catheter-related bacteriuria is shown in Table 1.

Table 1 Risk Factors Associated with Development of Catheter-Associated Bacteriuria

Risk factor	References
Increasing duration of catheterization	54–58
Not receiving systemic antibiotic therapy	53–59
Female sex	53, 55, 56, 58, 59
Diabetes mellitus	55
Older age	53, 56
Rapidly fatal underlying illness	53
Nonsurgical disease	53
Faulty aseptic management of the indwelling catheter	53
Bacterial colonization of drainage bag	55
Azotemia (serum creatinine concentration greater than 2.0 mg/dL)	55, 59
Catheter not connected to a urine meter	55
Periurethral colonization with uropathogens	60

Risk Factors for Bacteremia

Risk factors for UTI-related bacteremia are less clearly defined than for catheter-related bacteriuria. Because fewer than 4% of patients with catheter-related bacteriuria develop catheter-related bacteremia (61–63), detecting independent risk factors for bacteremia is difficult. Nevertheless, attempts have been made to identify risk factors for bacteremia. During a 23-month prospective study by Krieger et al., 1233 patients with nosocomial UTI were identified. Nosocomial bloodstream infections from a urinary tract origin were found in 32 patients (2.6%). Univariate analysis identified risk factors for secondary nosocomial bloodstream infections as UTI due to *Serratia marcescens*, compared with other organisms (RR = 3.5), and male sex (RR = 2.0) (62). No other factors (e.g., age, race, underlying disease, hospital service) were found to significantly predispose a bacteriuric patient to bacteremia (62). Of note is the perplexing finding that women are at greater risk for bacteriuria while men are at greater risk for bacteremia from a urinary source.

Attributable Morbidity, Mortality, Cost of Catheter-Related UTI

The estimated excess duration of hospitalization due to nosocomial UTI is 1 to 4 days, with an estimated average cost of infection between $558 and $676 (64,65). In a retrospective study of adult acute care hospitals in the United States, Haley and colleagues estimated that nosocomial UTI occurred at a rate of 2.39 per 100 admissions, prolonged hospitalization of 1 day, and cost $593 (40,66). In another study, nosocomial UTI resulted in an average increase in length of stay of 2.4 days, and an associated cost of $558 (67). More recent data suggest that each episode of bacteriuria is expected to cost an additional $676, and urinary catheter-related bacteremia increases costs by as much as $2836 per episode (65).

In prospective studies of patients with catheter-related nosocomial UTI, a mortality rate of 14–19% was found in infected patients. Infected patients were nearly three times more likely to die during hospitalization than patients without such an infection, even after a multivariate analysis excluded 20 other variables (68,69). The attributable case-fatality rate from UTI-related nosocomial bacteremia is approximately 12.7% (61), with severely ill patients at highest risk. The presence of a urinary catheter was independently associated with an increased risk of death in an elderly population residing in nursing homes (70).

Special Issues

Spinal Cord Injury

Due to disturbances in the urinary system that commonly affect individuals with spinal cord injury, urinary catheterization of some type is frequently used in this population. Until the mid-1970s, renal failure and UTI were the most frequent causes of death among those with injured spinal cords (71–73). Given the high prevalence of urinary catheterization, it is not surprising that UTI remains the most frequent medical complication during acute rehabilitation following spinal cord injury (74); 22% of patients with acute spinal cord injury have clinical UTI within a period of 50 days (71,75). Recently, Shekelle and colleagues reviewed risk factors for UTI in adults with spinal cord dysfunction (76). Their main finding was that persons using intermittent catheterization had fewer infections than individuals using indwelling catheterization (76).

Urinary tract infection remains the fifth most common primary or secondary cause of death in individuals with spinal cord dysfunction, and individuals with spinal cord injury are 82 times more likely to die of septicemia compared with the general population (72). In addition, bacteriuria due to the long-term use of urinary collection devices remains an important source of antimicrobial resistance; 33% of Gram-negative urinary isolates from persons with spinal cord injury had resistance to two or more classes of drugs (77).

Long-Term Care Facilities

Urinary incontinence affects 20–30% of older adults living in the community, and is one of the leading factors in the decision to place family members in a long-term care facility (78). This condition is more frequent in those living in long-term care facilities, where 35–50% of residents are incontinent of urine (79–81). The daily prevalence of urethral catheter use by 4259 aged residents of 53 long-term care facilities in Maryland was 7.5% (79). This number has been used to estimate that 99,000 patients in long-term care facilities nationally have indwelling urethral catheters (79). In a review of the Maryland patients (82), 10% of women and 15% of men used a urine collection device of some kind. Among bedfast patients, 47% of the women and 58% of the men used such devices. Among women using a urinary collection system, 93% were using urethral catheters. Among men using some kind of device, 43% used urethral catheters, 39% used condom catheters, and 15% used suprapubic catheters (82).

UTI is the most common infection seen in long-term care facilities, with prevalence rates of 15–50% (83–85). The incidence of bacteriuria is 3–10% per day, which is similar to the rate seen in short-term catheterization (50). UTI is the most common source of bacteremia in long-term care, accounting for up to 55% of cases (86, 87). The presence of a urethral catheter increases the risk of bacteremia 60-fold (86). It is estimated that the urinary tract is the source of two-thirds of febrile episodes seen in residents of long-term care facilities (88). Residents of nursing homes that receive long-term indwelling catheterization are three times more likely to die within a year compared to similar patients without catheters (70).

MICROBIOLOGY

The microbial etiology of catheter-related UTI has changed over the past few decades, and varies between ward types (Table 2) (31,43,89,90). The most common pathogens associated with hospital-wide catheter-related UTI are the Enterobacteriaceae, including *E. coli, Klebsiella* spp., and *Enterobacter* spp. Other significant pathogens, which are more common in the ICU setting, include *P. aeruginosa*, enterococci, and *Candida* spp. European hospitals report a similar spectrum of bacteria associated with nosocomial UTI, except for *Pseudomonas* spp. which were isolated in only 7% of urine cultures (91). The prevalence of enterocococci as a cause of nosocomial UTI increased between 1975 and 1984 (92). Enterococci have remained a significant pathogen, especially with the emergence and spread of vancomycin-resistant enterococci (43,93–95). In one rehabilitation facility, enterococcal species accounted for 35% of urinary tract isolates (93). During DNA analysis, no single clone of enterococcus was identified, suggesting that in this setting, enterococci in the urine are primarily acquired from endogenous sources (93). This supports previous studies suggesting that enterococcal UTIs were endogenous infections from the patient's fecal flora (10).

Candida spp. are another emerging urinary pathogen, especially in the ICU where 25% of UTIs are associated with *Candida* spp. (31,43,96). Risk factors for candiduria include prolonged catheterization and use of broad-spectrum antimicrobials (97,98). Most *Candida* UTIs are asymptomatic, but fungus balls of the bladder or kidney, renal abscesses, or disseminated candidiasis may occasionally occur (99,100). Candidemia occurs most frequently in the setting of urinary tract abnormalities or procedures (99).

Coagulase-positive staphylococci (CPS) are an infrequent cause of catheter-related UTI (8,31,43). Coagulase-positive staphylococci are frequently found in the urine in association with CPS bacteremia or endocar-

Table 2 Percentage of Major Pathogens Associated with Catheter-Related Urinary Tract Infections Reported Through National Nosocomial Surveillance System

Microorganism	Hospital-wide 10/1986–12/1990	All ICUs 1/1992–5/1999	Medical–surgical ICUs 1992–1998	Pediatric ICUs 1992–1997
Escherichia coli, %	26.0	17.5	18.5	19.0
Candida spp., %	9.0	15.8	24.8	21.1
Enterococci, %	16.0	13.8	14.3	10.0
Pseudomonas aeruginosa, %	12.0	11.0	10.3	13.1
Klebsiella pneumoniae, %	6.4	6.2	5.2	7.3
Enterobacter spp., %	—	5.1	4.0	10.3

Source: Refs. 43, 89, 90, and 90a.

ditis; 27% of CPS bacteremia was associated with bacteriuria (8,31,43). Coagulase-negative staphylococci are rarely associated with urinary catheter infections (101). Anaerobic bacteria have been isolated in polymicrobial infections in urine from patients with long-term catheters, but are not found through routine urine cultures (102).

While 80% of infections associated with short-term indwelling urinary catheters are due to single organisms, infections in long-term catheters are frequently polymicrobial (4,5,50). UTI in long-term catheters are associated with two or more organisms in 77–95% of cases, and 10% have more than five species of organisms present (6,50). Certain strains of organisms, such as *Providencia stuartii, Pseudomonas* spp., enterococci, or *Proteus* spp. persist in the urinary tract for 4–10 weeks once present, while other organisms appear to spontaneously cycle in and out (4,50).

CLINICAL MANIFESTATIONS AND COMPLICATIONS

Catheter-associated UTIs may present in a spectrum from completely asymptomatic bacteriuria to overwhelming urosepsis associated with death (35,49,63,88). Symptoms of UTI include local symptoms of lower abdominal pain or discomfort or flank pain, or systemic symptoms such as nausea, vomiting, or fever (65). Only 10–32% of catheterized patients with bacteriuria develop symptoms referable to the urinary tract (35,49,63,65). In a recent study of 235 cases of nosocomial catheter-related bacteriuria, approximately 90% of infections were asymptomatic (63). There were no significant differences between patients with and without infection with respect to fever, dysuria, urgency, flank pain, or leukocytosis. Patients with bacteriuria who die may have autopsy findings of acute pyelonephritis, renal calculi, or perinephric abscesses (6,61,88,103).

Bacteremia is an important complication of catheter-related UTI. The urinary tract is the source of infection in 11 to 40% of nosocomial bacteremia (104–106). However, in prospective studies of nosocomial bacteriuria, secondary bacteremia occurs only infrequently; 0.4–3.9% of patients with nosocomial UTI have associated bacteremia (49,61–63,68). Bacteremia is less likely to occur with asymptomatic bacteriuria and is more likely to be associated with major underlying disease and comorbidities (63). Transient bacteremia may also occur following routine replacement of long-term urinary catheters. One study found that out of 120 catheter changes, five patients (4.2%) developed bacteremia (107).

Long-term catheterization may be associated with other complications, including catheter obstruction, urinary tract stones, and chronic renal inflammation (6,108). Encrustations on the surface of indwelling catheters may act as a nidus for formation of renal calculi (25,108,109). Occasionally, knots may complicate suprapubic or urethral catheters (110,111). Purple urine bag syndrome is an uncommon complication of chronically catheterized patients, which is due to an altered metabolism of tryptophan in the presence of *P. stuartii*, *K. pneumoniae*, or *Enterobacter agglomerans* (112). Finally, an under-appreciated complication of urinary catheterization is physical restraint of the patient, with substantial limitation of ability to function freely and with dignity (113).

DIAGNOSIS OF CATHETER-RELATED URINARY TRACT INFECTION

The definition of catheter-related UTI used in published reports varies, and the terms bacteriuria and UTI are often used interchangeably. The distinction between bacteriuria and the clinically more relevant symptomatic UTI is an important one. In most patients with asymptomatic catheter-related bacteriuria, the risk of bacteremia is low and treatment with antimicrobials is unnecessary (61–63,68). Most studies of catheter-related UTI use bacteriuria as the primary outcome. The term bacteriuria or candiduria implies the presence of a significant number of microorganisms in quantitative urine cultures (46,63). Once low levels of candiduria or bacteriuria are identified in a catheterized urine specimen, growth usually progresses within 72 h to concentrations of greater than 10^5 cfu/mL, unless antibiotic therapy is given (46). Therefore, growth of $\geq 10^2$ cfu/mL of a predominant pathogen from a catheterized urine specimen, collected aseptically from a sampling port, is a standard definition for catheter-related UTI (12,19).

The Centers for Disease Control and Prevention (CDC) have developed surveillance definitions for identifying hospital-acquired UTIs (114). The definitions differentiate between symptomatic (presence of fever, urgency, frequency, dysuria, or suprapubic tenderness) and asymptomatic infection, but do not allow for classification of asymptomatic bacteriuria with less than 10^5 cfu/mL. The definitions do allow for consistent application of definitions, allowing for interhospital comparison of infection rates (Table 2) (30,31,43).

While pyuria is considered an important indicator of UTI in the noncatheterized patient, pyuria is less strongly correlated with UTI in the catheterized patient (115,116). Musher and colleagues found that pyuria was nearly always present with bacteriuria in catheterized men, but pyuria was also present in 30% of catheterized patients without bacteriuria (115). In a recent prospective study of 761 catheterized patients, pyuria was most strongly associated with infection caused by Gram-negative bacilli, whereas infections caused by coagulase-negative staphylococci, enterococci, or yeast produced much less pyuria (116). Urinary white blood count >5/high-power field had a specificity of 90% for predicting infections with $>10^5$ cfu/mL, but had a sensitivity of less than 37% (116).

The urinary dipstick test for pyuria or nitrite has been used to screen for asymptomatic catheter-related UTI in an ICU (117). In 144 patients, the incidence of asymptomatic infection was 31.3%. The sensitivity of the test was 87%, with a specificity of 61% for predicting bacteriuria in the asymptomatic patient. More studies are necessary to determine if evaluating urine for the presence of white blood cells using dipstick tests are useful for predicting bacteriuria in catheterized patients (118). Culturing the tip of a removed urinary catheter has been shown to have no benefit in diagnosing infection (119).

In patients with long-term indwelling urinary catheters, neither urinalysis nor urine cultures are reliable tests for diagnosing symptomatic UTI (120). Bacteriuria in this setting is chronic and universal, and cultures obtained from the catheter may not reflect bladder cultures (6,50,121). Fever and chills may be the only symptoms of catheter-related UTI (71,88,103). UTI in patients with spinal cord lesions may be particularly difficult to diagnose because the ability to sense localizing symptoms is lacking (122).

Symptoms of UTI in this population may include fever, chills, diaphoresis, abdominal discomfort, costovertebral angle tenderness, or increased muscle spasticity (71). Nevertheless, a consensus panel of rehabilitation medicine experts suggested the following criteria for diagnosing bacteriuria from long-term catheterized patients: $\geq 10^2$ cfu/mL from patients undergoing intermittent catheterization; any detectable growth from those with an indwelling catheter; and $\geq 10^4$ cfu/mL from a clean-voided specimen from a man using a condom catheter (123).

SPECIAL TYPES OF URINARY CATHETERS

Indwelling Urinary Catheters

In the 1920s, Foley introduced the indwelling catheter which could be held in place by an intravesicular balloon (5). Routine indwelling urinary catheters are made of latex or silicone; some have a hydrogel or teflon coating (24,124). A variety of temperature-sensing urinary catheters are available for use in the operating room or intensive care setting (125).

Anti-Infective Coated Catheters

Several novel urinary catheters with anti-infective properties to reduce adherence of bacteria to the catheter have been developed and studied. Silver, a highly effective antibacterial substance, is a commonly used anti-infective on silicone urinary catheters. Reported results in eight randomized controlled trials evaluating silver-coated catheters were mixed (56,59,126–131). A recent meta-analysis, however, suggested that silver alloy catheters may be beneficial in preventing UTI whereas silver oxide catheters are not (132). Since publication of the meta-analysis, the results of additional studies have indicated somewhat mixed results with silver alloy urinary catheter use (133–137). A lecithin/silver-coated catheter is in development (138).

Catheters impregnated with antimicrobial agents other than silver have also been evaluated (139,140). A randomized study of catheters coated with minocycline and rifampin found that patients using the antimicrobial catheters had significantly lower rates of Gram-positive bacteriuria than the control group that used standard catheters (7.1% vs. 38.2%; $P < 0.001$), but similar rates of Gram-negative bacteriuria (46.4% vs. 47.1%) and candiduria (3.6% vs. 2.9%) (140). A study of catheters impregnated with nitrofurazone also showed a significant reduction in bacteriuria (12). A new gentamicin-releasing catheter was effective in preventing catheter-related UTI in animals (141). However, the theoretical risk of developing resistance to these antimicrobial agents, which are occasionally used systemically, may limit the use of urinary catheters coated with these substances.

External (Condom) Catheters

External urine collection systems for men are applied to the outside of the penis and empty through a collection tube into a drainage bag. Although devices have been developed for women (142), these systems are almost exclusively used with men. External urine collection systems may be associated with a lower risk of bacteriuria than indwelling catheters. One prospective study found that the risk of developing bacteriuria in men wearing a condom catheter was approximately 12% per month (143). However, in men who frequently manipulated their catheters, the rate was substantially higher (143). In cohort studies in a Veterans Affairs (VA) nursing home, the incidence of symptomatic UTI was about 2.5 times greater in men with a chronic indwelling catheter compared to those wearing a condom catheter (144,145). On the other hand, a cross-sectional study in Denmark found the risk of UTI in hospitalized patients was higher in patients wearing condom catheters than in those using indwelling catheters (146). Randomized trials comparing these devices need to be performed before any definitive statements are made about the relative efficacy of these urinary collection devices. Until such trials are reported, condom catheters should be considered in men who are unlikely to manipulate their catheters frequently (147).

Suprapubic Catheters

Suprapubic catheters are inserted through the lower abdominal wall, which is less heavily colonized with bacteria than the perineum, directly into the bladder. These devices have been compared to indwelling urethral catheters in a number of studies with varying results (148–156). Some trials indicate that patients with suprapubic catheters have a lower risk of UTI (148,149,155,156). Patient satisfaction has also been rated higher with this type of catheter than with urethral catheters (148,152,156). In several studies, however, mechanical complications, including failed introduction, catheter dislodgment, or leakage of urine after suprapubic catheter removal, were more frequent in those patients with suprapubic catheters (148,150,155). For men who require long-term catheterization, suprapubic catheterization may reduce the risk of local genitourinary complications such as meatal erosion, prostatitis, and epididymitis.

Intermittent Catheterization

Another strategy used for urinary collection is intermittent catheterization, i.e., inserting and removing a sterile or clean urinary catheter several times daily (157,158). Intermittent catheterization is an especially common method of urinary collection in persons with spinal cord injury (123,159,160), and may reduce the risk of bacteriuria compared with an indwelling catheter (74). Because the incidence of bacteriuria is about 1 3% per insertion, however, most patients likely become bacteriuric within a few weeks (6). Intermittent catheterization may be associated with a lower risk of local and systemic complications of bacteriuria compared with indwelling catheterization (76,161). Terpenning and colleagues evaluated 35 elderly patients receiving intermittent urethral catheterization in a VA hospital (161). Thirty-one of the 35 patients developed bacteriuria; the mean time from catheter initiation to bacteriuria was about six days. Only four patients (11%) developed symptomatic UTI (161). A prelubricated nonhydrophilic catheter may be associated with less symptomatic and asymptomatic bacteriuria (162).

Several studies have shown that long-term use of intermittent catheterization is associated with substantial improvement in urinary continence, risk of UTI, renal function, and the emotional status of the patient (163–165). Thus, intermittent catheterization seems to be a reasonable alternative for long-term catheterization and is currently the preferable form of urinary collection in persons with spinal cord dysfunction (76,160). Drawbacks of intermittent catheterization in hospitalized and nursing home patients, however, include the increased amount of nursing time required and the reliance on a very cooperative patient (166).

Patient Satisfaction with Types of Catheters

Few studies have looked carefully at patient preferences regarding urinary catheterization. In a survey of elderly men on medical wards at a VA medical center, patients were more likely to respond that a condom catheter was comfortable (86%), compared to those patients with an indwelling urethral catheter (58%, $P = 0.04$) (167). Patients also felt that condom catheters were less likely to be painful or restrictive of activities of daily living (24% vs. 61%, $P = 0.008$) (167). Another survey of patients and family of residents in long-term care revealed that 85% preferred diapers and 77% preferred prompted voiding to indwelling urinary catheterization (168).

MANAGEMENT OF INFECTIONS ASSOCIATED WITH URINARY CATHETERS

The treatment of asymptomatic bacteriuria in the catheterized patient is controversial. One study suggested that treatment of catheterized women with a short course of trimethoprim–sulfamethoxazole (TMP/SMX) was beneficial (169). However, the risk of complications from asymtomatic bacteriuria is low, treatment does not prevent bacteriuria from recurring, and treatment may select for resistant bacteria (62,63,88). Thus, most authorities would recommend against treating asymtomatic infection, unless the patient has an abnormal urinary tract or will undergo genitourinary tract manipulation or instrumentation (5,6,73,170).

Catheterized patients who develop symptoms of UTI or bacteremia should be treated with antibiotics (Table 3). Blood and urine cultures taken prior to instituting antibiotics may help with the selection of antimicrobials. Empirical antimicrobials should be selected based on knowledge of organisms, previous resistance patterns from the patient, and resistance patterns in the medical unit or geographic area. Once culture and susceptibilities are available, antibiotics should then be directed toward the specific pathogen with the narrowest spectrum antibiotic possible (5,73,170). Parenteral antibiotics are recommended if bacteremia is present or suspected (5). Oral ciprofloxacin is as effective as the intravenous formulation for the treatment of complicated UTI (171). While there are no adequate clinical studies to guide the length of therapy for catheter-related UTI, treatment for 7 to 14 days appears to be adequate (5,170).

Candiduria presents a treatment dilemma. While it is clear that symptomatic candiduria requires treatment, it is controversial whether asymptomatic candiduria requires treatment (5,96,172). Frequently, candiduria resolves without treatment if the catheter can be removed (5,172). In a recent randomized double-blind study of a 14–day treatment of asymptomatic or minimally symptomatic candiduria with fluconazole vs. placebo, there was overall 50% clearance of candiduria in the fluconazole-treated group compared to 29% clearance in the untreated group ($P < 0.001$). Of the 64 catheterized patients who completed 14 days of therapy, short-term eradication occurred in 33 (52%). Since long-term eradication of *Candida* was not

Table 3   Options for Empirical Treatment of Infections Associated with Urinary Catheters

	Route	Antimicrobials	Duration
Mild-to-moderate infection	Oral	Ciprofloxacin Trimethoprim/sulfamethoxazole	7–14 d
Severe illness, possible bacteremia	Intravenous	Piperacillin/tazobactam Ticarcillin/clavulanic acid Ampicillin plus gentamicin Imipenem or meropenem Ciprofloxacin	14–21 d[a]

[a]May switch to oral therapy after 2–3 days if patient becomes afebrile.
Source: Refs. 5, 31, 43, 71, 170, and 171.

achieved, the clinical benefit of this practice remains questionable (96). Candiduria in a patient with local or constitutional symptoms or in a patient with diabetes, immunosuppression, or urologic abnormality deserves a more aggressive approach. These patients likely require evaluation for disseminated candidiasis and may require systemic antifungal therapy (172,173).

Biofilms that develop on long-term indwelling urinary catheters make treatment difficult when the catheter remains in place. Antibiotics are unable to penetrate the biofilm to eradicate microorganisms, and normal immune defenses are ineffective within the biofilm (21–23). A recent prospective randomized controlled trial compared patients with symptomatic UTI who received indwelling catheter replacement prior to initiation of antibiotic therapy with patients who had no catheter replacement (174). Bacteriuria was significantly decreased in the patients who received a new catheter three days after initiation of therapy and seven days and 28 days after discontinuing therapy (174). In addition, patients who had their catheters exchanged became afebrile sooner, had improved clinical status at 72 h, and had a lower rate of symptomatic clinical relapse 28 days after therapy (174). This study supports the recommendation of most authorities to replace a catheter that had been in place for more than a week when a patient is treated for symptomatic UTI (5,6,170).

PREVENTION AND CONTROL

Two decades ago, the CDC developed guidelines for the prevention of nosocomial UTI, which emphasize the use of aseptic technique and closed urinary drainage (175). Great Britain has recently updated guidelines for insertion and maintenance of urinary catheters in the acute-care setting (176). Despite existence and knowledge of these guidelines, adherence to guidelines varies between institutions. At one institution, errors in compliance with guidelines were found in 11% of catheter-days and overall in 29% of catheterized patients (177). Surveillance and feedback of nosocomial UTI rates to staff may be an effective way to improve compliance with recommendations and decrease UTI rates (178–180). Several measures for the prevention of catheter-related UTI are discussed later.

Avoidance of Use of Indwelling Catheters

Since as many as 80% of nosocomial UTIs and 97% of UTIs in ICUs are associated with a urinary catheter, the best strategy for prevention is avoidance of urinary catheterization (4,6,43,62,147,181). Unfortunately, unjustified and excessively prolonged catheter use is common (27,35,39). Nevertheless, urinary catheters are important for patients requiring drainage of anatomic or physiologic outlet obstruction, patients undergoing surgery of the genitourinary tract, patients requiring accurate urinary output measurements, and patients with sacral or perineal wounds (39,147,175,182). Table 4 summarizes these and other indications for an indwelling urinary catheter.

If temporary or long-term urinary collection is required, options other than indwelling catheterization should be considered (catheter types were discussed earlier). In oliguric patients, ultrasound may be used for measuring urine output (183). Intermittent catheterization may reduce the risk of bacteriuria in patients with neurogenic bladder or spinal cord injuries (157–159,161,164). Clinicians may consider a suprapubic catheter in patients without contraindications (e.g., bleeding diatheses, previous lower abdominal surgery, morbid obesity, or prior radiation to the lower abdomen) who require long-term indwelling catheterization (148,149,155,156). Finally, external or condom catheters are a reasonable alternative to indwelling catheters in men requiring long-term catheterization who are unlikely to frequently manipulate their condom catheters (143,144,184). For men with prostatic enlargement causing bladder outlet obstruction, many observational studies describe an intraprostatic spiral or intraurethral stent that allows bladder emptying without the need for bladder catheterization (185–190). These devices may be considered in men with a contraindication to prostatic surgery who have urinary retention despite pharmacological treatment.

Use of Aseptic Insertion and Catheter Care Techniques

Proper aseptic technique, including aseptic insertion and maintenance of the catheter and drainage bag, remains essential in preventing catheter-related UTI (12,19,53,175,176). Although use of antiseptic cleansing at urinary catheter insertion has been widely recommended, this practice has not been well studied. A recent randomized trial of water or 0.1% chlorhexidine cleansing of the periurethral area prior to catheter insertion revealed no difference in occurrence of bacteriuria (191). Similarly, rigorous routine

Table 4 Appropriate Indications for Short-Term Indwelling Urinary Catheter Use

---

Monitoring of urine output required:
- Frequent or urgent monitoring is needed, as for critically ill patients.
- Patient is unable or unwilling to collect urine.

Urinary incontinence (without obstruction):
- Patient with an open sacral or perineal wound.
- At patient request.

Bladder outlet obstruction:
- Temporary relief of anatomical or functional obstruction.
- Longer term drainage if surgical correction is not indicated.

Prolonged surgical procedures with general or spinal anesthesia.

Source: Refs. 39, 147, 175, and 182.

meatal cleaning of catheterized patients has shown no benefit (192,193). The collection bag should always remain below the level of the bladder to prevent reflux of urine into the bladder. Use of gloves and proper hand-washing during insertion and manipulation of catheters is essential to prevent exogenous acquisition of hospital pathogens (15–17,194,195).

Use of Closed Drainage Systems

The most important advance in the prevention of urinary catheter-related infection was the introduction, approximately three decades ago, of the closed catheter drainage system (45,196–198). Effective maintenance of a closed drainage system includes the use of sealed urinary catheter junctions (68,69,199,200). A recent evaluation of two closed drainage systems compared a complex system (including a preattached catheter, antireflux valve, drip chamber, and povidone-iodine-releasing cartridge) with a two-chamber system. The authors found no difference in the rate of bacteriuria between the two systems (201). Nevertheless, improper catheter care and breaches of the closed system remain an important factor in the development of bacteriuria in clinical settings (53,177).

Other Catheter Care Practices

Recent efforts to prevent bacteriuria have also included irrigating the bladder, instilling antibacterial solutions in the urinary collecting bag, and prescribing short-term prophylactic antibiotics. Antibacterial agents, including povidone-iodine, chlorhexidine, neomycin, or polymixin, have been instilled either continuously or intermittently as bladder irrigation. Although this practice had some benefit in preventing UTI when an open drainage system was used, little overall effect has been seen in studies using closed systems (202–206). Because this practice allows for flow of organisms colonizing the catheter into the bladder, and in view of the potential for local toxicity and the complexity of this method, antibacterial irrigation cannot currently be recommended.

Several studies have evaluated the effect of adding various antibacterial agents (e.g., chlorhexidine, hydrogen peroxide, povidone-iodine) to the urinary catheter drainage bag. While several reports suggested that this intervention may prevent catheter-related UTI (207–210), some were flawed by using a before/after design (208,210), or by using other interventions in addition to the antibacterial agents (207,208). Other better-designed randomized trials have shown no benefit from the addition of antibacterials (211–213). Importantly, adding solutions to the drainage bag requires breaking the closed drainage system, and the bulk of evidence does not favor this approach.

A variety of other interventions to prevent catheter-related UTI have also been evaluated and have not clearly shown benefit. These include using meatal lubricants and creams (both antibacterial and nonantibacterial) (214–218), or urinary catheters that have been coated with antibiotics (214,219), heparin (220), or polymer (221). In addition, drinking cranberry juice did not prevent biofilm production in catheterized patients, and therefore is unlikely to prevent UTI (222).

Use of Anti-Infective Urinary Catheters

Several studies support the use of anti-infective urinary catheters as adjunct to the aforementioned proven methods of prevention in patients at high risk for catheter-related UTI (132,135–137,223). The cost of a silver-coated urinary catheter tray is significantly more than a standard, noncoated urinary catheter tray. A recent analysis of the clinical and economic consequences of urinary catheters indicates that silver alloy catheters may provide both clinical and economic benefits in patient populations receiving indwelling catheterization for 2 to 10 days, including the critically ill (65,224). Silver alloy urinary catheters appear to be a promising method of reducing bacteriuria in the catheterized patient. The effect silver alloy urinary catheters will have on the more important clinical outcomes of urinary catheter-related bacteremia and mortality is not clear from current studies.

Use of Systemic Antimicrobials

Receiving systemic antibiotic therapy has been shown in a number of studies to lower the risk for developing a catheter-related UTI (53–55,57). Several investigators have studied this intervention in a variety of settings. Comparing results of these studies is difficult due to variable inclusion criteria, differences in definitions of UTI, timing and duration of antibiotic therapy agents used, outcomes measured, and the retrospective nature of some of the studies. In general, systemic antibiotic therapy tends to be most useful in patients requiring urinary catheterization for durations between 3 and 14 days (225–230). Those catheterized for shorter durations are not at high risk for UTI, and those with longer durations develop bacteriuria regardless of antibiotic therapy. Prophylaxis with TMP/SMX has been shown to be beneficial for the prevention of UTI after renal transplantation (231,232). The available data from randomized controlled trials published in the past two decades suggest that antibiotic prophylaxis is justifiable for men undergoing transurethral resection of the prostate, especially in those with an indwelling catheter or preoperative bacteriuria (233). Most experts do not recommend routine use of prophylactic antibiotics for catheterized patients because of their cost, potential adverse effects, and potential for selection of antibiotic-resistant organisms (4,5,198,234). Several studies demonstrated that antibiotic prophylaxis increased the rate of isolation of resistant organisms in catheterized patients (50,225,226,228).

Use of Methenamine Hippurate

Methenamine, available as a salt of mandelate or hippurate, has been used for preventing catheter-associated UTI for over 30 years (147). Its antibacterial activity is thought to be related to its breakdown products, hippuric acid and formaldehyde, which acidify the urine. In small nonrandomized studies, oral methenamine hippurate therapy (2–6 g daily) has been found to reduce the incidence of bacteriuria (235,236), symptomatic UTI (237), and pyuria (238). It has also been associated with fewer courses of antibiotic therapy for symptomatic UTI and mechanical catheter complications (239). Other studies, however, have not found any benefit of methenamine in suppressing catheter-associated bacteriuria (240). While methenamine hippurate is not currently recommended, randomized controlled trials evaluating this intervention should be considered (147).

SUMMARY AND CONCLUSIONS

Urinary catheter-related infections are a common hospital infection, especially in the ICU setting. In addition, they are associated with significant cost and morbidity. The available data suggest that urinary catheter-associated bacteriuria may be preventable for the short-term (i.e., less than a few weeks), but at best is only postponed if the device is needed for a longer period. Proven interventions for the prevention of catheter-associated UTI include avoidance and curtailing use of catheters whenever possible. Measures should be taken to insert a catheter aseptically, use a closed drainage system, and properly maintain the catheter during use. Use of alternative drainage systems, including suprapubic catheters or condom catheters, may be desirable in selected patient populations. An anti-infective catheter should be considered in those patients at high risk for complications of catheter-associated bacteriuria. More well-designed clinical trials are necessary to further define methods of decreasing this serious catheter-related complication.

REFERENCES

1. Amundsen SK, Wang CC, Schwan WR, Duncan JL, Schaeffer AJ. Role of *Escherichia coli* adhesins in urethral colonization of catheterized patients. J Urol 1988; 140:651–655.
2. Daifuku R, Stamm WE. Bacterial adherence to bladder uroepithelial cells in catheter-associated urinary tract infection. N Engl J Med 1986; 314:1208–1213.
3. Sobel JD. Pathogenesis of urinary tract infection. Role of host defenses. Infect Dis Clin North Am 1997; 11(3):531–549.
4. Stamm WE. Catheter-associated urinary tract infections: epidemiology, pathogenesis, and prevention. Am J Med 1991; 91(3B):65S–71S.

5. Warren JW. Catheter-associated urinary tract infections. Int J Antimicrob Agents 2001; 17:299–303.
6. Warren JW. Catheter-associated urinary tract infections. Infect Dis Clin North Am 1997; 11(3):609–622.
7. Lee BK, Crossley K, Gerding DN. The association between *Staphylococcus aureus* bacteremia and bacteriuria. Am J Med 1978; 65:303–306.
8. Demuth PJ, Gerding DN, Crossley K. *Staphylococcus aureus* bacteriuria. Arch Intern Med 1979; 139:78–80.
9. Daifuku R, Stamm WE. Association of rectal and urethral colonization with urinary tract infection in patients with indwelling catheters. JAMA 1984; 252(15):2028–2030.
10. Gross PA, Messinger Harkavy L, Barden GE, Flower MF. The epidemiology of nosocomial enterococcal urinary tract infection. Am J Med Sci 1976; 272(1):75–81.
11. Tambyah PA, Halvorson KT, Maki DG. A prospective study of pathogenesis of catheter-associated urinary tract infections. Mayo Clin Proc 1999; 74(2):131–136.
12. Maki DG, Tambyah PA. Engineering out the risk of infection with urinary catheters. Emerging Infect Dis 2001; 7(2):1–6.
13. Manges AR, Johnson JR, Foxman B, O'Bryan TT, Fullerton KE, Riley LW. Widespread distribution of urinary tract infections caused by a multidrug-resistant *Escherichia coli* clonal group. N Engl J Med 2001; 345(14):1007–1013.
14. Ikaheimo R, Siitonen A, Karkkainen U, Makela PH. Virulence characteristics of *Escherichia coli* in nosocomial urinary tract infection. Clin Infect Dis 1993; 16:785–791.
15. Schaberg DR, Weinstein RA, Stamm WE. Epidemics of nosocomial urinary tract infection caused by multiply resistant gram-negative bacilli: epidemiology and control. J Infect Dis 1976; 133(3):363–366.
16. Schaberg DR, Haley RW, Highsmith AK, Anderson RL, McGowan JE Jr, Nosocomial bacteriuria: a prospective study of case clustering and antimicrobial resistance. Ann Intern Med 1980; 93(3):420–424.
17. Sotto A, deBoever CM, Fabbro-Peray P, Gouby A, Sirot D, Jourdan J. Risk factors for antibiotic-resistant *Escherichia coli* isolated from hospitalized patients with urinary tract infections: a prospective study. J Clin Microbiol 2001; 39(2):438–444.
18. Whiteley GR, Penner JL, Stewart IO, Stokan PC, Hinton NA. Nosocomial urinary tract infections caused by two O-serotypes of *Providencia stuartii* in one hospital. J Clin Microbiol 1977; 6(6):551–554.
19. Stamm WE. Urinary tract infections. In: Bennett JV, Brachman PS, eds. Hospital Infections. 4th ed. Philadephia: Lippincott-Raven, 1998.
20. Dunne WM Jr. Bacterial adhesion: seen any good biofilms lately? Clin Microbiol Rev 2002; 15(2):155–166.
21. Donlan RM, Costerton JW. Biofilms: survival mechanisms of clinically relevant microorganisms. Clin Microbiol Rev 2002; 15(2):167–193.
22. Donlan RM. Biofilms and device-associated infections. Emerging Infect Dis 2001; 7(2):1–4.

23. Donlan RM. Biofilm formation: a clinically relevant microbiological process. Clin Infect Dis 2001; 33:1387–1392.
24. Sabbuba N, Hughes G, Stickler DJ. The migration of *Proteus mirabilis* and other urinary tract pathogens over Foley catheters. BJU International 2002; 89:55–60.
25. Stickler DJ, King JB, Winters C, Morris SL. Blockage of urethral catheters by bacterial biofilms. J Infect 1993; 27(2):133–135.
26. Choong S, Wood S, Fry C, Whitfield H. Catheter associated urinary tract infection and encrustation. Int J Antimicrob Agents 2001; 17:305–310.
27. Saint S, Wiese J, Amory JK, Bernstein ML, Patel UD, Zemencuk JK, Bernstein SJ, Lipsky BA, Hofer TP. Are physicians aware of which of their patients have indwelling urinary catheters? Am J Med 2000; 109:476–480.
28. Haley RW, Hooton TM, Culver DH, Stanley RC, Emori TG, Hardison CD, Quade D, Shachtman RH, Schaberg DR, Shah BV, Schatz GD. Nosocomial infections in US hospitals, 1975–1976: estimated frequency by selected characteristics of patients. Am J Med 1981; 70(4):947–959.
29. Weinstein JW, Mazon D, Pantelick E, Reagan-Cirincione P, Dembry LM, Hierholzer WJ Jr. A decade of prevalence surveys in a tertiary-care center: trends in nosocomial infection rates, device utilization, and patient acuity. Infect Control Hosp Epidemiol 1999; 20(8):543–548.
30. Anonymous. National Nosocomial Infections Surveillance (NNIS) System Report, Data Summary from January 1992 April 2000, Issued June 2000. Am J Infect Control 2000; 28:429–448.
31. Richards MJ, Edwards JR, Culver DH, Gaynes RP, System N. Nosocomial infections in pediatric intensive care units in the United States. Pediatrics 1999; 103(4):1–7.
32. Burket JS, Bartlett RH, Vander Hyde K, Chenoweth CE. Nosocomial infections in adult patients undergoing extracorporeal membrane oxygenation. Clin Infect Dis 1999; 28:828–833.
33. Scheckler WE. Nosocomial infections in a community hospital. Arch Intern Med 1978; 138:1792–1794.
34. Munasinghe RL, Yazdani H, Siddique M, Hafeez W. Appropriateness of use of indwelling urinary catheters in patients admitted to the medical service. Infect Control Hosp Epidemiol 2001; 22:647–649.
35. Hartstein AI, Garber SB, Ward TT, Jones SR, Morthland VH. Nosocomial urinary tract infection: a prospective evaluation of 108 catheterized patients. Infect Control 1981; 2(5):380–386.
36. Gardam MA, Amihod B, Orenstein P, Consolacion N, Miller MA. Overutilization of indwelling urinary catheters and the development of nosocomial urinary tract infections. Clinical Performance and Quality Health Care 1998; 6:99–102.
37. Conybeare A, Pathak S, Imam I. The quality of hospital records of urethral catheterisation. Ann R Coll Surg Engl 2002; 84:109–110.
38. Bouza E, Rodriguez-Bouza H, Munoz P, Bernaldo de Quiros JCL, Rodriguez-Creixems M, Fernandez-Baca V. Evaluation of indwelling bladder catheterization in a general hospital. Infect Dis Clin Pract 1994; 3:358–362.

39. Jain P, Parada JP, David A, Smith LG. Overuse of the indwelling urinary tract catheter in hospitalized medical patients. Arch Intern Med 1995; 155(13): 1425–1429.

40. Haley RW, Culver DH, White JW, Morgan WM, Emori TG. The nationwide nosocomial infection rate. A new need for vital statistics. Am J Epidemiol 1985; 121(2):159–167.

41. Singh-Naz N, Sprague BM, Patel KM, Pollack MM. Risk factors for nosocomial infection in critically ill children: a prospective cohort study. Crit Care Med 1996; 24(5):875–878.

42. Vincent JL, Bihari DJ, Suter PM, Bruining HA, White J, Nicolas Chanoin MH, Wolff M, Spencer RC, Hemmer M. The prevalence of nosocomial infection in intensive care units in Europe. Results of the European Prevalence of Infection in Intensive Care (EPIC) Study. EPIC International Advisory Committee [see comments]. JAMA 1995; 274(8):639–644.

43. Richards MJ, Edwards JR, Culver DH, Gaynes RP. Nosocomial infections in combined medical–surgical intensive care units in the United States. Infect Control Hosp Epidemiol 2000; 21(8):510–515.

44. Krieger JN, Kaiser DL, Wenzel RP. Nosocomial urinary tract infections: secular trends, treatment and economics in a university hospital. J Urol 1983; 130(1):102–106.

45. Kunin CM, McCormack RC. Prevention of catheter-induced urinary-tract infections by sterile closed drainage. N Engl J Med 1966; 274(21):1155–1161.

46. Stark RP, Maki DG. Bacteriuria in the catheterized patient. What quantitative level of bacteriuria is relevant? N Engl J Med 1984; 311(9):560–564.

47. Saint S, Veentra DL, Lipsky BA. The clinical and economic consequences of nosocomial central venous catheter-related infection: are antimicrobial catheters useful? Infect Control Hosp Epidemiol 2000; 21:375–380.

48. Haley RW, Schaberg DR, Crossley KB, Von Allmen SD, McGowan JE Jr, Extra charges and prolongation of stay attributable to nosocomial infections: a prospective interhospital comparison. Am J Med 1981; 70(1):51–58.

49. Garibaldi RA, Mooney BR, Epstein BJ, Britt MR. An evaluation of daily bacteriologic monitoring to identify preventable episodes of catheter-associated urinary tract infection. Infect Control 1982; 3(6):466–470.

50. Warren JW, Tenney JH, Hoopes JM, Muncie HL, Anthony WC. A prospective microbiologic study of bacteriuria in patients with chronic indwelling urethral catheters. J Infect Dis 1982; 146(6):719–723.

51. Gaynes RP, Edwards JR, Jarvis WR, Culver DH, Tolson JS, Martone WJ. Nosocomial infections among neonates in high-risk nurseries in the United States. Pediatrics 1996; 98(3):357–361.

52. Langley JM, Hanakowski M, LeBlanc JC. Unique epidemiology of nosocomial urinary tract infection in children. Am J Infect Control 2001; 29:94–98.

53. Garibaldi RA, Burke JP, Dickman ML, Smith CB. Factors predisposing to bacteriuria during indwelling urethral catheterization. N Engl J Med 1974; 291(5):215–219.

54. Hustinx WN, Mintjes de Groot AJ, Verkooyen RP, Verbrugh HA. Impact of concurrent antimicrobial therapy on catheter-associated urinary tract infection. J Hosp Infect 1991; 18(1):45–56.

55. Platt R, Polk BF, Murdock B, Rosner B. Risk factors for nosocomial urinary tract infection. Am J Epidemiol 1986; 124(6):977–985.

56. Riley DK, Classen DC, Stevens LE, Burke JP. A large randomized clinical trial of a silver-impregnated urinary catheter: lack of efficacy and staphylococcal superinfection. Am J Med 1995; 98(4):349–356.

57. Shapiro M, Simchen E, Izraeli S, Sacks TG. A multivariate analysis of risk factors for acquiring bacteriuria in patients with indwelling urinary catheters for longer than 24 hours. Infect Control 1984; 5(11):525–532.

58. Tissot E, Limat S, Cornette C, Capellier G. Risk factors for catheter-associated bacteriuria in a medical intensive care unit. Eur J Clin Microbiol Infect Dis 2001; 20:260–262.

59. Johnson JR, Roberts PL, Olsen RJ, Moyer KA, Stamm WE. Prevention of catheter-associated urinary tract infection with a silver oxide-coated urinary catheter: clinical and microbiologic correlates. J Infect Dis 1990; 162(5):1145–1150.

60. Garibaldi RA, Burke JP, Britt MR, Miller MA, Smith CB. Meatal colonization and catheter-associated bacteriuria. N Engl J Med 1980; 303(6):316–318.

61. Bryan CS, Reynolds KL. Hospital-acquired bacteremic urinary tract infection: epidemiology and outcome. J Urol 1984; 132(3):494–498.

62. Krieger JN, Kaiser DL, Wenzel RP. Urinary tract etiology of bloodstream infections in hospitalized patients. J Infect Dis 1983; 148(1):57–62.

63. Tambyah PA, Maki DG. Catheter-associated urinary tract infection is rarely symptomatic: a prospective study of 1,497 catheterized patients. Arch Intern Med 2000; 160(5):678–682.

64. Jarvis WR. Selected aspects of the socioeconomic impact of nosocomial infections: morbidity, mortality, cost, and preventions. Infect Control Hosp Epidemiol 1996; 17(8):552–557.

65. Saint S. Clinical and economic consequences of nosocomial catheter-related bacteriuria. Am J Infect Control 2000; 28(1):68–75.

66. Haley RW, White JW, Culver DH, Hughes JM. The financial incentive for hospitals to prevent nosocomial infections under the prospective payment system. An empirical determination from a nationally representative sample. JAMA 1987; 257(12):1611–1614.

67. Givens CD, Wenzel RP. Catheter-associated urinary tract infections in surgical patients: a controlled study on the excess morbidity and costs. J Urol 1980; 124(5):646–648.

68. Platt R, Polk BF, Murdock B, Rosner B. Mortality associated with nosocomial urinary-tract infection. N Engl J Med 1982; 307(11):637–642.

69. Platt R, Polk BF, Murdock B, Rosner B. Reduction of mortality associated with nosocomial urinary tract infection. Lancet 1983; 1(8330):893–897.

70. Kunin CM, Douthitt S, Dancing J, Anderson J, Moeschberger M. The association between the use of urinary catheters and morbidity and mortality among elderly patients in nursing homes. Am J Epidemiol 1992; 135(3):291–301.

71. Biering-Sorensen F, Bagi P, Hoiby N. Urinary tract infections in patients with spinal cord lesions: treatment and prevention. Drugs 2001; 61(9):1275–1287.

72. DeVivo MJ, Black KJ, Stover SL. Causes of death during the first 12 years after spinal cord injury. Arch Phys Med Rehabil 1993; 74(3):248–254.

73. Siroky MB. Pathogenesis of bacteriuria and infection in the spinal cord injured patient. Am J Med 2002; 113(1A):67S–79S.

74. Cardenas DD, Hooton TM. Urinary tract infection in persons with spinal cord injury. Arch Phys Med Rehabil 1995; 76(3):272–280.

75. Maynard FM, Diokno AC. Urinary infection and complications during clean intermittent catheterization following spinal cord injury. J Urol 1984; 132:943–946.

76. Shekelle PG, Morton SC, Clark KA, Pathak M, Vickrey BG. Systematic review of risk factors for urinary tract infection in adults with spinal cord dysfunction. J Spinal Cord Med 1999; 22(4):258–272.

77. Waites KB, Chen Y, DeVivo MJ, Canupp KC, Moser SA. Antimicrobial resistance in gram-negative bacteria isolated from the urinary tract in community-residing persons with spinal cord injury. Arch Phys Med Rehabil 2000; 81(6):764–769.

78. Langa KM, Fultz N, Saint S, Kabeto MU, Herzog A. Informal caregiving time and costs for urinary incontinence among elderly individuals in the United States. J Am Geriat Soc 2002; 50:733–737.

79. Warren JW, Steinberg L, Hebel JR, Tenney JH. The prevalence of urethral catheterization in Maryland nursing homes. Arch Intern Med 1989; 149(7):1535–1537.

80. Ouslander JG, Palmer MH, Rovner BW, German PS. Urinary incontinence in nursing homes: incidence, remission and associated factors. J Am Geriatr Soc 1993; 41(10):1083–1089.

81. Ouslander JG, Schnelle JF. Incontinence in the nursing home. Ann Intern Med 1995; 122(6):438–449.

82. Hebel JR, Warren JW. The use of urethral, condom, and suprapubic catheters in aged nursing home patients. J Am Geriatr Soc 1990; 38(7):777–784.

83. Nicolle LE. Urinary tract infections in long-term care facilities. Infect Control Hosp Epidemiol 1993; 14:220–225.

84. Nicolle LE, Garibaldi RA. Infection control in long-term-care facilities. Infect Control Hosp Epidemiol 1995; 16:348–353.

85. Nicolle LE. Urinary tract infection in long-term-care facility residents. Clin Infect Dis 2000; 31:757–761.

86. Rudman D, Hontanosas A, Cohen Z, Mattson DE. Clinical correlates of bacteremia in a Veterans Administration extended care facility. J Am Geriatr Soc 1988; 36(8):726–732.

87. Muder RR, Brennen C, Wagener MM, Goetz AM. Bacteremia in a long-term-care facility: a five-year prospective study of 163 consecutive episodes. Clin Infect Dis 1992; 14:647–654.

88. Warren JW, Damron D, Tenney JH, Hoopes JM, Deforge B, Muncie HL Jr, Fever, bacteremia, and death as complications of bacteriuria in women with long-term urethral catheters. J Infect Dis 1987; 155(6):1151–1158.

89. Jarvis WR, Martone WJ. Predominant pathogens in hospital infections. J Antimicrob Chemother 1992; 29(suppl A):19–24.

90. Anonymous. National Nosocomial Infections Surveillance (NNIS) System

Report, Data Summary from January 1990-May 1999, Issued June 1999. Am J Infect Control 1999; 27:520–532.

90a. Richards MJ, Edwards JR, Culver DH, Gaynes RP. Nosocomial infections in medical intensive care units in the United States. National Nosocomial Infections Surveillance System [see comments]. Crit Care Med 1999; 27(5):887–892.

91. Bouza E, San Juan R, Munoz P, Voss A, Kluytmans J. A European perspective on nosociomial urinary tract infections. I. Report on the microbiology workload, etiology and antimicrobial susceptibility (ESGNI-003 study). Clin Microbiol Infect 2001; 7:523–531.

92. Morrison AJ, Wenzel RP. Nosocomial urinary tract infections due to enterococcus. Arch Intern Med 1986; 146:1549–1551.

93. Lloyd S, Zervos M, Mahayni R, Lundstrom T. Risk factors for enterococcal urinary tract infection and colonization in a rehabilitation facility. Am J Infect Control 1998; 26:35–39.

94. Cetinkaya Y, Falk P, Mayhall CG. Vancomycin-resistant enterococci. Clin Microbiol Rev 2000; 13(4):686–707.

95. Murray BE. Vancomycin-resistant enterococcal infections. N Engl J Med 2000; 342(10):710–721.

96. Sobel JD, Kauffman CA, McKinsey D, Zervos M, Vazquez JA, Karchmer AW, Lee J, Thomas C, Panzer H, Dismukes WE, Group NMS. Candiduria: a randomized, double-blind study of treatment with fluconazole and placebo. Clin Infect Dis 2000; 30:19–24.

97. Wise GJ, Silver DA. Fungal infections of the genitourinary system. J Urol 1993; 149:1377–1388.

98. Hamory BH, Wenzel RP. Hospital-associated candiduria: predisposing factors and review of the literature. J Urol 1978; 120:444–448.

99. Ang BSP, Telenti A, King B, Steckelberg JM, Wilson WR. Candidemia from a urinary tract source: Microbiological aspects and clinical significance. Clin Infect Dis 1993; 17:662–666.

100. Wainstein MA, Graham RC Jr, Resnick MI. Predisposing factors of systemic fungal infections of the genitourinary tract. J Urol 1995; 154:160–163.

101. Huebner J, Goldmann DA. Coagulase-negative staphylococci: role as pathogens. Annu Rev Med 1999; 50:223–236.

102. Alling B, Brandberg A, Seeberg S, Svanborg A. Aerobic and anaerobic microbial flora in the urinary tract of geriatric patients during long-term care. J Infect Dis 1973; 127(1):34–39.

103. Warren JW, Muncie HL Jr, Hebel JR, Hall Craggs M. Long-term urethral catheterization increases risk of chronic pyelonephritis and renal inflammation [see comments]. J Am Geriatr Soc 1994; 42(12):1286–1290.

104. Kreger BE, Craven DE, McCabe WR. Gram-negative bacteremia. IV. Re-evaluation of clinical features and treatment in 612 patients. Am J Med 1980; 68(3):344–355.

105. Lark RL, Chenoweth CE, Saint S, Zemencuk JK, Lipsky BA, Plorde JJ. Four year prospective evaluation of nosocomial bacteremia: epidemiology, microbiology, and patient outcome. Diagn Microbiol Infect Dis 2000; 38:131–140.

106. Weinstein MP, Towns ML, Quartey SM, Mirrett S, Reimer LG, Parmigiani G, Reller LB. The clinical significance of positive blood cultures in the 1990s: a prospective comprehensive evaluation of the microbiology, epidemiology, and outcome of bacteremia and fungemia in adults. Clin Infect Dis 1997; 24(4):584–602.

107. Bregenzer T, Frei R, Widmer AF, Seiler W, Probst W, Mattarelli G, Zimmerli W. Low risk of bacteremia during catheter replacement in patients with long-term urinary catheters. Arch Intern Med 1997; 157:521–525.

108. Grases F, Sohnel O, Costa-Bauza A, Ramis M, Wang Z. Study on concretions developed around urinary catheters and mechanisms of renal calculi development. Nephron 2001; 88:320–328.

109. Stickler DJ, Zimakoff J. Complications of urinary tract infections associated with devices used for long-term bladder management. J Hosp Infect 1994; 28(3):177–194.

110. Polychronidis A, Kantartzi K, Touloupidis S, Nikolaidis I, Simopoulos C. A true knot in a suprapubic catheter around a urethral catheter: a rare complication. J Urol 2001; 165(6):2001.

111. Foster H, Ritchey M, Bloom D. Adventitious knots in urethral catheters: Report of 5 cases. J Urol 1992; 148(5):1496–1498.

112. de Bruyn G, Eckman CD, Atmar RL. Purple discoloration in a urinary catheter bag. Clin Infect Dis 2002; 34:210, 285–286.

113. Saint S, Lipsky BA, Goold SD. Indwelling urinary catheters: a one-point restraint? Ann Intern Med 2002; 137(2):125–127.

114. Garner JS, Jarvis WR, Emori TG, Horan TC, Hughes JM. CDC definitions for nosocomial infections, 1988 [Published erratum appears in Am J Infect Control Aug;(4):177]. Am J Infect Control 1988; 16(3):128–140.

115. Musher DM, Thorsteinsson SB, Airola VM II. Quantitative urinalysis: diagnosing urinary tract infection in men. JAMA 1976; 236:2069–2072.

116. Tambyah PA, Maki DG. The relationship between pyuria and infection in patients with indwelling urinary catheters: a prospective study of 761 patients. Arch Intern Med 2000; 160:673–677.

117. Tissot E, Woronoff-Lemsi M-C, Cornette C, Plesiat P, Jacquet M, Capellier G. Cost-effectiveness of urinary dipsticks to screen asymptomatic catheter-associated urinary infections in an intensive care unit. Intensive Care Med 2001; 27(12):1842–1847.

118. Anonymous. Leukocyte esterase tests detect pyuria, not bacteriuria. Ann Intern Med 1993; 118(3):230–231.

119. Gross PA, Messinger Harkavy L, Barden GE, Kerstein M. Positive Foley catheter tip cultures—fact or fancy? JAMA 1974; 228:72–73.

120. Steward DK, Wood GL, Cohen RL, Smith JW, Mackowiak PA. Failure of the urinalysis and quantitative urine culture in diagnosing symptomatic urinary tract infections in patients with long-term urinary catheters. Am J Infect Control 1985; 13:154–160.

121. Bergqvist D, Bronnestam R, Hedelin H, Stahl A. The relevance of urinary sampling methods in patients with indwelling Foley catheters. Br. J Urol. 1980; 52:92–95.

122. Fisk DT, Saint S, Tierney LM. Clinical problem solving: "Back to the basics". N Engl J Med 1999; 341:747–750.

123. Anonymous. The prevention and management of urinary tract infections among people with spinal cord injuries. National Institute on Disability and Rehabilitation Research Consensus Statement. January 27–29, 1992. J Am Paraplegia Soc 1992; 15(3):194–204.

124. Bruce AW, Plumpton KJ, Willett WS, Chadwick P. Urethral response to latex and Silastic catheters. Can Med Assoc J 1976; 115(11):1099–1100.

125. Fallis WM. Monitoring urinary bladder temperature in the intensive care unit: State of the science. Am J Crit Care 2001; 10:38–47.

126. Schaeffer AJ, Story KO, Johnson SM. Effect of silver oxide/trichloroisocyanuric acid antimicrobial urinary drainage system on catheter-associated bacteriuria. J Urol 1988; 139(1):69–73.

127. Lundeberg T. Prevention of catheter-associated urinary-tract infections by use of silver-impregnated catheters [letter]. Lancet 1986; 2(8514):1031.

128. Liedberg H, Lundeberg T, Ekman P. Refinements in the coating of urethral catheters reduces the incidence of catheter-associated bacteriuria. An experimental and clinical study. Eur Urol 1990; 17(3):236–240.

129. Liedberg H, Lundeberg T. Silver alloy coated catheters reduce catheter-associated bacteriuria. Br J Urol 1990; 65(4):379–381.

130. Liedberg H, Lundeberg T. Prospective study of incidence of urinary tract infection in patients catheterized with bard hydrogel and silver-coated catheters or bard hydrogel-coated catheters [abstr]. J Urol 1993; 149 (4): 405A.

131. Takeuchi H, Hida S, Yoshida O, Ueda T. Clinical study on efficacy of a Foley catheter coated with silver-protein in prevention of urinary tract infections. Hinyokika Kiyo 1993; 39(3):293–298.

132. Saint S, Elmore JG, Sullivan SD, Emerson SS, Koepsell TD. The efficacy of silver alloy-coated urinary catheters in preventing urinary tract infection: A meta-analysis. Am J Med 1998; 105:236–241.

133. Verleyen P, De Ridder D, Van Poppel H, Baert L. Clinical application of the Bardex IC Foley catheter. Eur Urol 1999; 36(3):240–246.

134. Thibon P, Le Coutour X, Leroyer R, Fabry J. Randomized multi-centre trial of the effects of a catheter coated with hydrogel and silver salts on the incidence of hospital-acquired urinary tract infections. J Hosp Infect 2000; 45(2):117–124.

135. Newton T, Still JM, Law E. A comparison of the effect of early insertion of standard latex and silver-impregnated latex foley catheters on urinary tract infections in burn patients. Infect Control Hosp Epidemiol 2002; 23:217–218.

136. Karchmer TB, Giannetta ET, Muto CA, Strain BA, Farr BM. A randomized crossover study of silver-coated urinary catheters in hospitalized patients. Arch Intern Med 2000; 160(21):3294–3298.

137. Bologna RA, Tu LM, Polansky M, Fraimow HD, Gordon DA, Whitmore KE. Hydrogel/silver ion-coated urinary catheter reduces nosocomial urinary tract infection rates in intensive care unit patients: A multicenter study. Urology 1999; 54(6):982–987.

138. Kumon H, Hashimoto H, Nishimura M, Monden K, Ono N. Catheter-associated urinary tract infections: Impact of catheter materials on their management. Int J Antimicrob Agents 2001; 17:311–316.

139. Darouiche RO, Safar H, Raad II. In vitro efficacy of antimicrobial-coated bladder catheters in inhibiting bacterial migration along catheter surface. J Infect Dis 1997; 176:1109–1112.

140. Darouiche RO, Smith JA Jr, Hanna H, Dhabuwala CB, Steiner MS, Babaian RJ, Boone TB, Scardino PT, Thornby JI, Raad II. Efficacy of antimicrobial-impregnated bladder catheters in reducing catheter-associated bacteriuria: a prospective, randomized, multicenter clinical trial. Urology 1999; 54(6):976–981.

141. Cho Y-H, Lee S-J, Lee JY, Kim SW, Kwon IC, Chung SY, Yoon MS. Prophylactic efficacy of a new gentamicin-releasing urethral catheter in short-term catheterized rabbits. BJU International 2001; 87:104–109.

142. Johnson DE, Muncie HL, O'Reilly JL, Warren JW. An external urine collection device for incontinent women. Evaluation of long-term use. J Am Geriatr Soc 1990; 38(9):1016–1022.

143. Hirsh DD, Fainstein V, Musher DM. Do condom catheter collecting systems cause urinary tract infection? JAMA 1979; 242(4):340–341.

144. Ouslander JG, Greengold B, Chen S. External catheter use and urinary tract infections among incontinent male nursing home patients. J Am Geriatr Soc 1987; 35(12):1063–1070.

145. Ouslander JG, Greengold B, Chen S. Complications of chronic indwelling urinary catheters among male nursing home patients: a prospective study. J Urol 1987; 138(5):1191–1195.

146. Zimakoff J, Stickler DJ, Pontoppidan B, Larsen SO. Bladder management and urinary tract infections in Danish hospitals, nursing homes, and home care: a national prevalence study. Infect Control Hosp Epidemiol 1996; 17:215–221.

147. Saint S, Lipsky BA. Preventing catheter-related bacteriuria: Can we? Should we? How? Arch Intern Med 1999; 159:800–808.

148. Shapiro J, Hoffmann J, Jersky J. A comparison of suprapubic and transurethral drainage for postoperative urinary retention in general surgical patients. Acta Chir Scand 1982; 148(4):323–327.

149. Sethia KK, Selkon JB, Berry AR, Turner CM, Kettlewell MG, Gough MH. Prospective randomized controlled trial of urethral versus suprapubic catheterization. Br J Surg 1987; 74(7):624–625.

150. Schiotz HA, Malme PA, Tanbo TG. Urinary tract infections and asymptomatic bacteriuria after vaginal plastic surgery. A comparison of suprapubic and transurethral catheters. Acta Obstet Gynecol Scand 1989; 68(5):453–455.

151. Ratnaval CD, Renwick P, Farouk R, Monson JR, Lee PW. Suprapubic versus transurethral catheterisation of males undergoing pelvic colorectal surgery. Int J Colorectal Dis 1996; 11(4):177–179.

152. O'Kelly TJ, Mathew A, Ross S, Munro A. Optimum method for urinary drainage in major abdominal surgery: a prospective randomized trial of suprapubic versus urethral catheterization. Br J Surg 1995; 82(10):1367–1368.

153. Perrin LC, Penfold C, McLeish A. A prospective randomized controlled trial comparing suprapubic with urethral catheterization in rectal surgery. Aust N Z J Surg 1997; 67(8):554–556.

154. Ichsan J, Hunt DR. Suprapubic catheters: a comparison of suprapubic versus urethral catheters in the treatment of acute urinary retention. Aust N Z J Surg 1987; 57(1):33–36.

155. Horgan AF, Prasad B, Waldron DJ, O'Sullivan DC. Acute urinary retention. Comparison of suprapubic and urethral catheterisation. Br J Urol 1992; 70(2):149–151.

156. Andersen JT, Heisterberg L, Hebjorn S, Petersen K, Stampe Sorensen S, Fischer Rasmussen W, Molsted Pedersen L, Nielsen NC. Suprapubic versus transurethral bladder drainage after colposuspension/vaginal repair. Acta Obstet Gynecol Scand 1985; 64(2):139–143.

157. Lapides J, Diokno AC, Silber SJ, Lowe BS. Clean, intermittent self-catheterization in the treatment of urinary tract disease. J Urol 1972; 107(3): 458–461.

158. Lapides J, Diokno AC, Lowe BS, Kalish MD. Followup on unsterile intermittent self-catheterization. J Urol 1974; 111(2):184–187.

159. Kuhn W, Rist M, Zaech GA. Intermittent urethral self-catheterisation: long term results (bacteriological evolution, continence, acceptance, complications). Paraplegia 1991; 29(4):222–232.

160. Jamil F. Towards a catheter free status in neurogenic bladder dysfunction: A review of bladder management options in spinal cord injury (SCI). Spinal Cord 2001; 39:355–361.

161. Terpenning MS, Allada R, Kauffman CA. Intermittent urethral catheterization in the elderly. J Am Geriatr Soc 1989; 37(5):411–416.

162. Giannantoni A, Di Stasi SM, Scivoletto G, Virgili G, Dolci S, Porena M. Intermittent catheterization with a prelubricated catheter in spinal cord injured patients: A prospective randomized crossover study. J Urol 2001; 166(1):130–133.

163. Lapides J, Diokno AC, Gould FR, Lowe BS. Further observations on self-catheterization. J Urol 1976; 116(2):169–171.

164. Diokno AC, Sonda LP, Hollander JB, Lapides J. Fate of patients started on clean intermittent self-catheterization therapy 10 years ago. J Urol 1983; 129(6):1120–1122.

165. Pearman JW. Urological follow-up of 99 spinal cord injured patients initially managed by intermittent catheterisation. Br J Urol 1976; 48(5):297–310.

166. Kunin CM. Urinary Tract Infections: Detection, Prevention, and Management. 5th ed. Baltimore: Williams and Wilkins, 1997:419.

167. Saint S, Lipsky BA, Baker PD, McDonald LL, Ossenkop K. Urinary catheters: What type do men and their nurses prefer? J Am Geriatr Soc 1999; 47(12):1453–1457.

168. Johnson TM, Ouslander JG, Uman GC, Schnelle JF. Urinary incontinence treatment preferences in long-term care. J Am Geriatr Soc 2001; 49(6):710–718.

169. Harding GKM, Nicolle LE, Ronald AR, Preiksaitis JK, Forward KR, Low DE, Cheang M. How long should catheter-acquired urinary tract infection in women be treated? Ann Intern Med 1991; 114:713–719.

170. Stamm WE, Hooton TM. Management of urinary tract infections in adults. N Engl J Med 1993; 329(18):1328–1334.

171. Mombelli G, Pezzoli R, Pinoja-Lutz G, Monotti R, Marone C, Franciolli M. Oral vs. intravenous ciprofloxacin in the initial empirical management of severe pyelonephritis or complicated urinary tract infections. Arch Intern Med 1999; 159:53–58.

172. Fisher JF, Newman CL, Sobel JD. Yeast in the urine: Solutions for a budding problem. Clin Infect Dis 1995; 20:183–189.

173. Rex JH, Walsh TJ, Sobel JD, Filler SG, Pappas PG, Dismukes WE, Edwards JE. Practice guidelines for the treatment of candidiasis. Clin Infect Dis 2000; 30:662–678.

174. Raz R, Schiller D, Nicolle LE. Chronic indwelling catheter replacement before antimicrobial therapy for symptomatic urinary tract infection. J Urol 2000; 164(4):1254–1258.

175. Wong ES. Guideline for prevention of catheter-associated urinary tract infections. Am J Infect Control 1983; 11(1):28–36.

176. Anonymous. Guidelines for preventing infections associated with the insertion and maintenance of short-term indwelling urethral catheters in acute care. J Hosp Infect 2001; 47(suppl):S39–S46.

177. Burke JP, Larsen RA, Stevens LE. Nosocomial bacteriuria: Estimating the potential for prevention by closed sterile urinary drainage. Infect Control 1986; 7(suppl 2):96–99.

178. Haley RW, Morgan WM, Culver DH, White JW, Emori TG, Mosser J, Hughes JM. Update from the SENIC project. Hospital infection control: recent progress and opportunities under prospective payment. Am J Infect Control 1985; 13(3):97–108.

179. Haley RW, Quade D, Freeman HE, Bennett JV. The SENIC Project. Study on the efficacy of nosocomial infection control (SENIC Project). Summary of study design. Am J Epidemiol 1980; 111(5):472–485.

180. Goetz AM, Kedzuf S, Wagener M, Muder RR. Feedback to nursing staff as an intervention to reduce catheter-associated urinary tract infections. Am J Infect Control 1999; 27(5):402–404.

181. Aylett V, Lynch O. Catheterisation in elderly women is no "easy" option. Br Med J 2001; 322(7292):997.

182. Kunin CM. Can we build a better urinary catheter? [editorial]. N Engl J Med 1988; 319(6):365–366.

183. Kunin CM. Nosocomial urinary tract infections and the indwelling catheter: What is new and what is true? Chest 2001; 120(1):10–12.

184. Ouslander JG, Fowler E. Management of urinary incontinence in Veterans Administration nursing homes. J Am Geriatr Soc 1985; 33(1):33–40.

185. Nissenkorn I. The intraurethral catheter—three years of experience. Eur Urol 1993; 24(1):27–30.

186. Nissenkorn I. A simple nonmetal stent for treatment of urethral strictures: a preliminary report. J Urol 1995; 154(3):1117–1118.

187. Nissenkorn I, Slutzker D. The intraurethral catheter: long-term follow-up in patients with urinary retention due to infravesical obstruction. Br J Urol 1991; 68(3):277–279.

188. Nissenkorn I, Richter S, Slutzker D. A simple, self-retaining intraurethral catheter for treatment of prostatic obstruction. Eur Urol 1990; 18(4):286–289.

189. Nielsen KK, Klarskov P, Nordling J, Andersen JT, Holm HH. The intraprostatic spiral. New treatment for urinary retention. Br J Urol 1990; 65(5):500–503.

190. Slutzker D, Richter S, Lang R, Nissenkorn I. The use of a prostatic stent in high risk patients over 80 years old with benign prostatic hyperplasia and chronic retention. J Am Geriatr Soc 1994; 42(9):1004–1005.

191. Webster J, Hood RH, Burridge CA, Doidge ML, Phillips KM, George N. Water or antiseptic for periurethral cleaning before urinary catheterization: A randomized controlled trial. Am J Infect Control 2001; 29:389–394.

192. Burke JP, Jacobson JA, Garibaldi RA, Conti MT, Alling DW. Evaluation of daily meatal care with poly-antibiotic ointment in prevention of urinary catheter-associated bacteriuria. J Urol 1983; 129(2):331–334.

193. Burke JP, Garibaldi RA, Britt MR, Jacobson JA, Conti M, Alling DW. Prevention of catheter-associated urinary tract infections. Efficacy of daily meatal care regimens. Am J Med 1981; 70(3):655–658.

194. Pittet D. Improving adherence to hand hygiene practice: A multidisciplinary approach. Emerging Infect Dis 2001; 7(2):234–240.

195. Larson EL. APIC guideline for hand washing and hand antisepsis in health-care settings. Am J Infect Control 1995; 23:251–269.

196. Wolff G, Gradel E, Buchman B. Indwelling catheter and risk of urinary infection: a clinical investigation with a new closed-drainage system. Urol Res 1976; 4(1):15–18.

197. Thornton GF, Andriole VT. Bacteriuria during indwelling catheter drainage. II Effect of a closed sterile drainage system. JAMA 1970; 214(2):339–342.

198. Meares EM. Current patterns in nosocomial urinary tract infections. Urology 1991; 37(suppl 3):9–12.

199. Huth TS, Burke JP, Larsen RA, Classen DC, Stevens LE. Clinical trial of junction seals for the prevention of urinary catheter-associated bacteriuria. Arch Intern Med 1992; 152(4):807–812.

200. Finkelberg Z, Kunin CM. Clinical evaluation of closed urinary drainage systems. JAMA 1969; 207(9):1657–1662.

201. Leone M, Garnier F, Dubuc M, Bimar MC, Martin C. Prevention of nocosomial urinary tract infection in ICU patients: Comparison of effectiveness of two urinary drainage systems. Chest 2001; 120(1):220–224.

202. Warren JW, Platt R, Thomas RJ, Rosner B, Kass EH. Antibiotic irrigation and catheter-associated urinary-tract infections. N Engl J Med 1978; 299(11):570–573.

203. Kirk D, Dunn M, Bullock DW, Mitchell JP, Hobbs SJ. Hibitane bladder irrigation in the prevention of catheter-associated urinary infection. Br J Urol 1979; 51(6):528–531.

204. Gelman ML. Antibiotic irrigation and catheter-associated urinary tract infections [editorial]. Nephron 1980; 25(5):259.

205. Dudley MN, Barriere SL. Antimicrobial irrigations in the prevention and treatment of catheter-related urinary tract infections. Am J Hosp Pharm 1981; 38(1):59–65.

206. Bastable JR, Peel RN, Birch DM, Richards B. Continuous irrigation of the

bladder after prostatectomy: its effect on post-prostatectomy infection. Br J Urol 1977; 49(7):689–693.

207. al Juburi AZ, Cicmanec J. New apparatus to reduce urinary drainage associated with urinary tract infections. Urology 1989; 33(2):97–101.

208. Anonymous. Evaluation of aseptic techniques and chlorhexidine on the rate of catheter-associated urinary-tract infection. Southampton Infection Control Team. Lancet 1982; 1(8263):89–91.

209. Maizels M, Schaeffer AJ. Decreased incidence of bacteriuria associated with periodic instillations of hydrogen peroxide into the urethral catheter drainage bag. J Urol 1980; 123(6):841–845.

210. Sujka SK, Petrelli NJ, Herrera L. Incidence of urinary tract infections in patients requiring long-term catheterization after abdominoperineal resection for rectal carcinoma: does Betadine in the Foley drainage bag make a difference? Eur J Surg Oncol 1987; 13(4):341–343.

211. Sweet DE, Goodpasture HC, Holl K, Smart S, Alexander H, Hedari A. Evaluation of H2O2 prophylaxis of bacteriuria in patients with long-term indwelling Foley catheters: a randomized controlled study. Infect Control 1985; 6(7):263–266.

212. Thompson RL, Haley CE, Searcy MA, Guenthner SM, Kaiser DL, Groschel DH, Gillenwater JY, Wenzel RP. Catheter-associated bacteriuria. Failure to reduce attack rates using periodic instillations of a disinfectant into urinary drainage systems. JAMA 1984; 251(6):747–751.

213. Gillespie WA, Simpson RA, Jones JE, Nashef L, Teasdale C, Speller DC. Does the addition of disinfectant to urine drainage bags prevent infection in catheterised patients? Lancet 1983; 1(8332):1037–1039.

214. Butler HK, Kunin CM. Evaluation of polymyxin catheter lubricant and impregnated catheters. J Urol 1968; 100(4):560–566.

215. Cohen A. A microbiological comparison of a povidone-iodine lubricating gel and a control as catheter lubricants. J Hosp Infect 1985; 6:55–161.

216. Huth TS, Burke JP, Larsen RA, Classen DC, Stevens LE. Randomized trial of meatal care with silver sulfadiazine cream for the prevention of catheter-associated bacteriuria. J Infect Dis 1992; 165(1):14–18.

217. Kunin CM, Finkelberg Z. Evaluation of an intraurethral lubricating catheter in prevention of catheter-induced urinary tract infections. J Urol 1971; 106(6):928–930.

218. Weinberg SR, Sanford RS, Myman L, Bertoni G, Tanenbaum B. Evaluation of a catheter-care ointment. J Urol 1972; 108(1):89–90.

219. Cheng HJ. Manufacture and clinical employment of an antibiotic silicon-rubber catheter. Eur Urol 1988; 14(1):72–74.

220. Ruggieri MR, Hanno PM, Levin RM. Reduction of bacterial adherence to catheter surface with heparin. J Urol 1987; 138(2):423–426.

221. Monson T, Kunin CM. Evaluation of a polymer-coated indwelling catheter in prevention of infection. J Urol 1974; 111(2):220–222.

222. Morris NS, Stickler DJ. Does drinking cranberry juice produce urine inhibitory to the development of crystalline, catheter-blocking *Proteus mirabilis* biofilms? BJU International 2001; 88:192–197.

223. Plowman R, Graves N, Esquivel J, Roberts JA. An economic model to assess

the cost and benefits of the routine use of silver alloy coated urinary catheters to reduce the risk of urinary tract infections in catheterized patients. J Hosp Infect 2001; 48(1):33–42.

224. Saint S, Savel RH, Matthay MA. Enhancing the safety of critically ill patients by reducing urinary and central venous catheter-related infections. Am J Respir Crit Care Med 2002; 165(11):1475–1479.

225. van der Wall E, Verkooyen RP, Mintjes de Groot J, Oostinga J, van Dijk A, Hustinx WN, Verbrugh HA. Prophylactic ciprofloxacin for catheter-associated urinary-tract infection [see comments]. Lancet 1992; 339(8799):946–951.

226. Verbrugh HA, Mintjes de Groot AJ, Andriesse R, Hamersma K, van Dijk A. Postoperative prophylaxis with norfloxacin in patients requiring bladder catheters. Eur J Clin Microbiol Infect Dis 1988; 7(4):490–494.

227. Vollaard EJ, Clasener HA, Zambon JV, Joosten HJ, van Griethuysen AJ. Prevention of catheter-associated gram-negative bacilluria with norfloxacin by selective decontamination of the bowel and high urinary concentration. J Antimicrob Chemother 1989; 23(6):915–922.

228. Mountokalakis T, Skounakis M, Tselentis J. Short-term versus prolonged systemic antibiotic prophylaxis in patients treated with indwelling catheters. J Urol 1985; 134(3):506–508.

229. Little PJ, Pearson S, Peddie BA, Greenslade NF, Utley WL. Amoxicillin in the prevention of catheter-induced urinary infection. J Infect Dis 1974; 129(suppl): S241–S242.

230. Britt MR, Garibaldi RA, Miller WA, Hebertson RM, Burke JP. Antimicrobial prophylaxis for catheter-associated bacteriuria. Antimicrob Agents Chemother 1977; 11(2):240–243.

231. Tolkoff Rubin NE, Cosimi AB, Russell PS, Rubin RH. A controlled study of trimethoprim–sulfamethoxazole prophylaxis of urinary tract infection in renal transplant recipients. Rev Infect Dis 1982; 4(2):614–618.

232. Fox BC, Sollinger HW, Belzer FO, Maki DG. A prospective, randomized, double-blind study of trimethoprim–sulfamethoxazole for prophylaxis of infection in renal transplantation: clinical efficacy, absorption of trimethoprim–sulfamethoxazole, effects on the microflora, and the cost-benefit of prophylaxis. Am J Med 1990; 89(3):255–274.

233. Amin M. Antibacterial prophylaxis in urology: a review. Am J Med 1992; 92(4A):114S–117S.

234. Platt R, Polk BF, Murdock B, Rosner B. Prevention of catheter-associated urinary tract infection: a cost-benefit analysis. Infect Control Hosp Epidemiol 1989; 10(2):60–64.

235. Norberg B, Norberg A, Parkhede U, Gippert H. Effect of short-term high-dose treatment with methenamine hippurate on urinary infection in geriatric patients with an indwelling catheter. IV Clinical evaluation. Eur J Clin Pharmacol 1979; 15(5):357–361.

236. Nilsson S. Long-term treatment with methenamine hippurate in recurrent urinary tract infection. Acta Med Scand 1975; 198(1-2):81–85.

237. Norrman K, Wibell L. Treatment with methenamine hippurate in the patient with a catheter. J Int Med Res 1976; 4(2):115–117.

238. Norberg A, Norberg B, Parkhede U, Gippert H, Ekman R. The effect of short-term high-dose treatment with methenamine hippurate of urinary infection in geriatric patients with indwelling catheters. II Evaluation by means of a quantified urine sediment. Ups J Med Sci 1979; 84(1):75–82.

239. Nyr'en P, Runeberg L, Kostiala AI, Renkonen OV, Roine R. Prophylactic methenamine hippurate or nitrofurantoin in patients with an indwelling urinary catheter. Ann Clin Res 1981; 13(1):16–21.

240. Vainrub B, Musher DM. Lack of effect of methenamine in suppression of, or prophylaxis against, chronic urinary infection. Antimicrob Agents Chemother 1977; 12(5):625–629.

Index

5-flucytosine, 532

Abdominal adhesions, secondary to shunt infections, 448
Abdominal surgery, as risk factor for fungal infections, 237
Abnormal skin, as risk factor for developing CRIs, 25
Abscess formation, in hydrogel-coated shunts, 461
Absolute time to positivity, 61
Accumulation, in pathogenesis of coagulase-negative staphylococci infection, 166, 171–174
Accumulation-associated protein (AAP), 167
Achromobacter spp., 266, 274
  Achromobacter piechaudii, 258, 264
  Achromobacter xylosoxidans, 258, 264
Acinetobacter spp., 196, 200, 203, 274
  Acinetobacter baumannii, catheter-related infections caused by, 210–211

[*Acinetobacter* spp.]
  catheter-related infections caused by, 210–212
  common in polymicrobial infections, 282
Acremonium, 256
Acridine-orange leucocyte cytospin test, 63–65, 68
  cost-effectiveness of, 68
  in diagnosis of pulmonary artery catheter-related infection, 392
  in diagnosis of PVC-related colonization/infection, 348
Actinomycetes, 256, 260, 272
Acute bacterial peritonitis, 480. *See also* Peritonitis
Adherence. *See also* Bacterial adherence; Fungal adherence:
  in pathogenesis of CRI, 92
Adhesive matrix molecules (MSCRAMM), 170
Administration sets:
  in prevention of PVC-related infection, 361–362
  recommendations for CRI prevention, 99–100